# PHARMACY STUDENT SURVIVAL GUIDE

## Third Edition

# PHARMACY STUDENT
## SURVIVAL GUIDE

Third Edition

**Ruth E. Nemire, BSPh, PharmD, EdD**
*Associate Executive Vice President*
*American Association of Colleges of Pharmacy*
*Alexandria, Virginia*

**Karen L. Kier, PhD, MSc, RPh, BCPS, BCACP**
*Professor of Clinical Pharmacy*
*Director of Assessment*
*Preventive Care Specialist, ONU Healthwise*
*Raabe College of Pharmacy*
*Ohio Northern University*
*Ada, Ohio*

**Michelle Assa-Eley, PhD, RPh**
*Princeton, New Jersey*

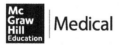

New York  Chicago  San Francisco  Athens  London  Madrid  Mexico City
Milan  New Delhi  Singapore  Sydney  Toronto

**Pharmacy Student Survival Guide, Third Edition**

1 2 3 4 5 6 7 8 9 0  DOC/DOC  18 17 16 15 14

ISBN 978-0-07-182847-5
MHID 0-07-182847-8

---

### Notice

Medicine is an ever-changing science. As new research and clinical experience broaden our knowledge, changes in treatment and drug therapy are required. The author and the publisher of this work have checked with sources believed to be reliable in their efforts to provide information that is complete and generally in accord with the standards accepted at the time of publication. However, in view of the possibility of human error or changes in medical sciences, neither the author nor the publisher nor any other party who has been involved in the preparation or publication of this work warrants that the information contained herein is in every respect accurate or complete, and they disclaim all responsibility for any errors or omissions or for the results obtained from use of the information contained in this work. Readers are encouraged to confirm the information contained herein with other sources. For example and in particular, readers are advised to check the product information sheet included in the package of each drug they plan to administer to be certain that the information contained in this work is accurate and that changes have not been made in the recommended dose or in the contraindications for administration. This recommendation is of particular importance in connection with new or infrequently used drugs.

---

This book was set in Minion Pro by MPS Limited.
The editors were Michael Weitz and Kim J. Davis.
The production supervisor was Catherine H. Saggese.
Project management was provided by Asheesh Ratra of MPS Limited.
RR Donnelley was the printer and binder.

This book is printed on acid-free paper.

**Library of Congress Cataloging-in-Publication Data**

Pharmacy student survival guide / [edited by] Ruth E. Nemire, Karen L. Kier, Michelle Assa-Eley. —Third edition.
   p. ; cm.
Includes bibliographical references and index.
ISBN 978-0-07-182847-5 (pbk. : alk. paper)—ISBN 0-07-182847-8 (pbk. : alk. paper)
I. Nemire, Ruth E., editor. II. Kier, Karen L., editor. III. Assa-Eley, Michelle, editor.
[DNLM: 1. Pharmacy. 2. Education, Pharmacy. 3. Pharmacy Administration. QV 704]
RS101
615'.4076—dc23
                    2014008003

*This book is dedicated to our teachers, mentors, friends, and colleagues in Colleges and Schools of Pharmacy across the United States and Canada. Your guidance, questions, and caring recognition are the foundations for the creation and development of this text. This book is meant to support the growth and development of student pharmacists across the globe who will impact pharmacy and the profession in ways we haven't yet realized, and your spirit goes with them.*

.

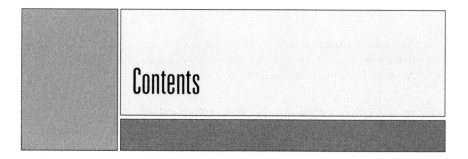

# Contents

## SECTION 1   Systems and Expectations

## 5 Rounding, Documentation, and Patient Education . . . . . . . 111

*Jacquelyn L. Bainbridge*

## 6 Monitoring Drug Therapy . . . . . . . . . . . . . . . . . . . . . . . . 128

*Chasity M. Shelton, Kelly C. Rogers*

## 7 Legal Implications for Pharmacy: Regulatory Agencies with Pharmacy Oversight, Legal Requirements for Filling a Prescription and Political Advocacy . . . . . . . . . . . . . . . . . 158

*Dean L. Arneson, Harold Bobrow, Loretta Brickman*

## SECTION 2  Patient Care Tool Box

## SECTION 3  Topics in Pharmacy Practice

## 17 Public Health  . . . . . . . . . . . . . . . . . . . . . . . . . . . . . . . . . . . 529
### Stuart Feldman, Ruth E. Nemire

## 18 Taking It to the Streets: Reducing Health Disparities through Domestic and Global Outreach to the Underserved  . . . . . . . . . . . . . . . . . . . . . . . . . . . . . . . . . . . 543
### Kelly L. Scolaro, Lisa Inge Stewart, Hazel H. Seaba

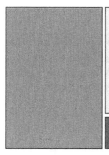

# Contributors

**Dean L. Arneson, PharmD, PhD**
Dean; Associate Professor of
  Pharmacy Administration
School of Pharmacy
Concordia University Wisconsin
Mequon, Wisconsin

**Michelle Assa-Eley, PhD, RPh**
Princeton, New Jersey

**Jacquelyn L. Bainbridge, PharmD**
Professor, Skags School of Pharmacy
  and Pharmaceutical Sciences
University of Colorado
Aurora, Colorado

**Cristina E. Bello-Quintero, MD,
PharmD**
Facilitator, Department of Continuing
  Education
College of Pharmacy
University of Florida
Gainesville, Florida

**Harold Bobrow, RPh**
Temple University School of
  Pharmacy
Philadelphia, Pennsylvania
Fairleigh Dickinson University School
  of Pharmacy
Madison, New Jersey
Rutgers University Ernest Mario
  School of Pharmacy
Piscataway, New Jersey

**Nancy Borja-Hart, PharmD, BCPS**
Assistant Director of Research
Medimix Specialty Pharmacy
Jacksonville, Florida

**Loretta Brickman, RPh**
Temple University School of
  Pharmacy
Philadelphia, Pennsylvania
Fairleigh Dickinson University School
  of Pharmacy
Madison, New Jersey
Rutgers University Ernest Mario
  School of Pharmacy
Piscataway, New Jersey

**Sherry Clayton, PharmD, BCPS**
Senior Drug Information Specialist
Wellpoint, Inc.
Mason, Ohio

**Nancy S. Collins, MD**
Epilepsy.com

**Sandra B. Earle, PharmD, BCPS**
Associate Professor, College of
  Pharmacy
University of Findlay
Findlay, Ohio

**A. Timothy Eley, RPh, PhD**
Bristol Myers Squibb
Princeton, New Jersey

**Stuart Feldman, PhD**
Professor Emeritus Pharmacy and
    Public Health
University of Georgia College of
    Public Health
Athens, Georgia

**Stephanie D. Garrett, PharmD,
    BCPS**
Network Clinical Pharmacy Specialist
    Internal Medicine,
Clinical Assistant Professor
Seton Healthcare Family
University of Texas at Austin College
    of Pharmacy
Austin, Texas

**Kevin R. Kearney, PhD**
Professor, Department of
    Pharmaceutical Sciences
Massachusetts College of Pharmacy
    and Health Sciences, School of
    Pharmacy-Worcester/Manchester
Worcester, Massachusetts

**Karen L. Kier, PhD, MSc, RPh,
BCPS, BCACP**
Professor of Clinical Pharmacy
Director of Assessment
Preventive Care Specialist, ONU
    Healthwise
Raabe College of Pharmacy
Ohio Northern University
Ada, Ohio

**Maria Maniscalco-Feichtl, PharmD**
Clinical Pharmacist, Team Lead
Pharmacotherapy Management Center
XLHealth, A UnitedHealthcare
    Company
Sunrise, Florida

**Karen Martin, PharmD, MBA, CGP**
Value Assessment Committee Director
Clinical Pharmacy Services, WellPoint,
    Inc.
Lebanon, Ohio

**Ruth E. Nemire, BSPh, PharmD,
EdD**
Associate Executive Vice President
American Association of Colleges of
    Pharmacy
Alexandria, Virginia

**Kelly C. Rogers, PharmD**
Professor, Clinical Pharmacy
University of Tennessee College of
    Pharmacy
Memphis, Tennessee

**Kelly L. Scolaro, PharmD**
Clinical Assistant Professor
UNC Eshelman School of Pharmacy
University of North Carolina-Chapel
    Hill
Chapel Hill, North Carolina

**Hazel H. Seaba, PharmMS**
Associate Dean and Professor
College of Pharmacy
The University of Iowa
Iowa City, Iowa

**Kathryn Shalek, PharmD**
Express Scripts
Mason, Ohio

**Chasity M. Shelton, PharmD, BCPS, BCNSP**
Assistant Professor, Department of
Clinical Pharmacy
The University of Tennessee Health
Science Center College of Pharmacy
Memphis, Tennessee

**Elizabeth Frenzel Shepherd, PharmD, MBA, BS Pharmacy, FASCP**
Assistant Dean Experiential Education
and Student Services
Assistant Professor Pharmacy Practice
College of Pharmacy
Nova Southeastern University
Fort Lauderdale, Florida

**Lisa Inge Stewart, PharmD, BCPS, BCACP, AAHIVE**
Medical Science Liaison - VIrology
(HIV/HCV) /Tuberculosis
Janssen Therapeutics

**Ceressa T. Ward, PharmD**
Clinical Coordinator, Critical Care
Medicine Clinical Pharmacy Specialist,
Metabolic Nutrition Support/
Cardiothoracic Surgery Critical
Care, Emory University Hospital
Midtown
Atlanta, Georgia

**Karen L. Whalen, PharmD, BCPS, CDE**
Assistant Dean for Clinical Education
Clinical Associate Professor
Department of Pharmacotherapy and
Translational Research
University of Florida College of
Pharmacy
Gainesville, Florida

**Antonia Zapantis, PharmD, MS, BCPS**
Director of Experiential Education
Associate Professor
Cleveland Clinic Florida
Nova Southeastern University College
of Pharmacy

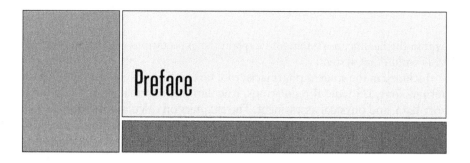

# Preface

Student pharmacists need a textbook to use for learning in general about etiquette, ethics, law, and other topics for practice courses. It should be a book that is the right size for quickly reading and referencing information when in a classroom or completing introductory and advanced practice courses. We feel this text will fulfill that need for students.

## TO THE STUDENT

This handbook is one of a few texts that you will use through your entire pharmacy school education. So take a pencil or pen and start scribbling notes in the margins, keep track of the "pearls" you learn in class here in a book where you can find them later. There is no one right way to use this handbook. The important thing is that it does not sit on your shelf as a required text, never to be opened. You bought the book; take the time to see what information is contained within. Think of it as your road map to practice courses; calculations, kinetics, drug information, medical terminology, and laboratory data book all in one.

## TO THE FACULTY/PRECEPTOR

Faculty/preceptors often find themselves looking for material that quickly acquaints students with a certain theory, process, or practice. We hope that this text meets those expectations. This text can be used both in the classroom to introduce ideas and during practice courses to help guide students in learning terminology, organizing case information, improving problem-solving skills, and rounding. The book is divided into three working sections: systems and expectations, patient care tool box, and topics in pharmacy practice.

In the systems and expectations section, the authors discuss topics for introductory and advanced pharmacy practice courses, etiquette, ethical issues, service-learning, communication skills, monitoring patients, and the function of a medical team. All chapters are written to help students become comfortable within the healthcare system and explain the expectations of student pharmacists within that system.

Included in the student pharmacist tool box section are chapters on medical terminology, US federal regulations, calculations, pharmacokinetics, laboratory data, and physical assessment. The chapters on calculations and pharmacokinetics may be used in a beginning classroom setting when students need to understand big concepts; it will supplement the regular textbook. Instructive chapters dealing with the technical and interpretive aspects of the practice of pharmacy, such as physical assessment, and laboratory testing are included in the tool box section and can be used by the student during their advanced practice courses to interpret patient findings. Students will be able to use this book early in their pharmacy school curriculum, keep note of their learning, and indicate "pearls" in the margins that they will use later to practice.

The last section of the book contains specific topics for pharmacy practice, including chapters addressing the practices of community and institutional pharmacy, the pharmacist as drug information specialist, managed care, public health, and global pharmacy. These chapters are included to round out the text so that it becomes the student practice guide from beginning to end. The final section touches on topics such as missions and the responsibility to advocate for the profession and advance the pharmacist's involvement in public health. All of the topics are meant to support the knowledge and professional growth of student pharmacists across a curriculum.

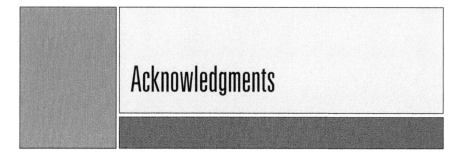

# Acknowledgments

When there is an accomplishment such as this book, do not presume that those listed as editors are the soul of the book. The authors are at the heart of each individual chapter. They take the seed of an idea and make it their own. The short amount of time, and amount of work required is not sufficiently awarded with thanks. To each of the authors and contributors to this book, you have our abiding gratitude. To those who contributed to the previous editions but could not participate in this book, your work laid the foundation for a much improved volume. Last but not least we would be remiss not to thank the people who helped shape ideas into an actual text. Laura Libretti had to collect, and e-mail, and collect information again and again from the authors; thanks for your part in making sure that every author and contributor receives recognition. Thanks to Kim Davis at McGraw-Hill Education (our project development editor yet again) because she is so easy to work with, and makes doing a text book fun. Without Kim the book would not be the excellent product that you are reading. The e-book is available because of Kim's extra efforts on our behalf. To other staff at McGraw-Hill Education who worked on the book but don't always get acknowledged, thanks; you know who you are. The last thanks, but not least at all, is for Michael Weitz who champions this book at every opportunity. We will always be grateful for your patience and understanding through a very trying year. This is our best book yet thanks to you. Our heartfelt thanks.

# 1

# Systems and Expectations

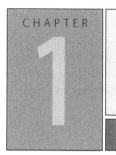

CHAPTER

# First Practice Course Expectations

*Elizabeth Frenzel Shepherd*

**Objectives: Upon completion of the chapter and exercises, the student pharmacist will be able to**

1. Define *profession* and *professional*.
2. Explain and portray a professional appearance and attitude.
3. Describe the ideal first day of practice experience and the responsibility of the student to make that happen.
4. Compose an appropriate cover letter to a preceptor.
5. Develop student curriculum vitae (CV).
6. Explain the expectations of introductory pharmacy practice experiences at your institution.

## INTRODUCTION

A group of learned individuals who agree to practice by a defined set of rules of conduct is loosely defined as a *profession*. The profession has an oversight board and the individuals are given autonomy to practice. A *professional* has the right academic qualifications, expert and specialized knowledge, and a standard of ethics. A profession has the power to exclude and control admission to the profession. Congratulations on your decision to become a part of the profession of pharmacy.

The specialized academic qualifications to become a pharmacist require both classroom and experiential education practice courses to complete the requirements for graduation. Experiential education courses range from 30% of the curricula in some schools to approximately 50% for others. While college curricula vary in length, in the United States they must all meet a certain set of defined standards for education of professionals. The Accreditation Council for Pharmacy Education (ACPE) provides the oversight and set guidelines for colleges to follow. In Canada, it is the Canadian Council for Accreditation of Pharmacy Programs that provide oversight and guidelines for the education of professional students.

This textbook is meant to support you through the development of the knowledge, skills, attitudes, and beliefs needed to practice pharmacy now and in the future. When you leave college, you will not stop learning; you will have the drive and desire to add continually to your body of knowledge. However, before you can get there, you have to start at the very beginning.

This book is a guide to help you integrate knowledge from the classroom, and practical examples, into your practice expertise. The first chapter introduces you to a broad set of goals and expectations for experiential courses in the first years of your pharmacy education that are required by ACPE. Schools not accredited by ACPE do not have these requirements. Becoming a professional should be one of your principal goals at this stage. Dress and attitude are primary objectives for developing professionalism. Dress and attitude are discussed in the first chapter as they are an important foundation for your success in pharmacy school classrooms and at practice sites. In this chapter, achievable goals are restricted to actions in and out of the classroom and the basics of what you should expect to achieve on your introductory pharmacy practice experiences. The goals listed in this chapter ought to support those specific objectives required by the institution you attend. If you are an advanced student, then later chapters of this book provide you with information and expectations for further growth and development in advanced practice courses.

*Never underestimate the value of the first impression!*

A checklist to prepare you for your first day of a practice experience course is provided in Table 1.1. If the directions in this table are different than those provided by your school faculty, then you should always follow the guidelines as required at the institution you attend.

---

### TABLE 1.1. PREPARATION CHECKLIST

- Mail preceptor your curriculum vitae and cover letter.
- Phone preceptor 10 days before beginning the experience. (Remember to ask about parking, directions to site, required documents, and readings before beginning experience.)
- If preceptor is unavailable, speak to designee.
- Review goals and objectives in your School or College's Introductory Professional Experience Manual.
- Confirm transportation to the site and/or drive by site before beginning the experience.
- Prepare list of student goals for the course.
- Make copies of immunization records and have them available.
- Complete additional site-required paperwork.
- Review wardrobe for enough professional attire and comfortable shoes.
- Put a smile on your face and get a good night's sleep.

## PROFESSIONAL ATTRIBUTES

### Appearance

Let's begin with appearance. "Dress for success" is a common cliché, but there is a lot of power in that statement. Now that you are in a professional school, appearance counts. Professional attire is important. Neatness and cleanliness are priorities. An ironed lab jacket should be worn over your clothes as directed by your faculty. The lab jacket should have your college of pharmacy school insignia in the chest area or upper arm area or elsewhere if required by your school. Always wear an identification/intern badge with your name attached to your lab coat. For men, a shirt and tie are appropriate with dress or casual pants. Shoes should be comfortable and look clean and polished. Remember to wear socks. For women, slacks, skirts, and dresses are all appropriate. Skirts and dresses should be of an appropriate length for comfort and not be too tight or too distracting for others. Shoes should be comfortable for wearing and walking all day long. Jewelry should not be excessive. Earrings should not hang down to your shoulders as it may be a hazard if they get caught and pulled. Do not wear a multitude of bracelets on one wrist as they too can be caught and cause damage to self or others. Long hair should be tied back or put into a stylish updo. Would you be embarrassed if a patient returned a prescription because hair was in the vial with the medicine? Introductory practice experiences facilitate meeting other health-care professionals, and help you to begin making professional contacts. The right appearance will help you create a professional image and you will make an appropriate first impression.

### Attitude

The next step in creating an appropriate image is presentation of the right attitude. You worked hard completing prerequisite courses and maintaining a high grade point average in order to achieve matriculation to a professional program. Be positive. Let everyone know you are glad to be in a pharmacy school. Wear a genuine smile. Be energetic and eager. Your preceptors will notice your positive attitude. Be honest and flexible. Pharmacists are regularly considered by the public to be highly ethical and trusted professionals.[1,2] Your preceptor and patients will notice your positive attitude. A smile is contagious.

Let's talk about how to handle yourself when small problems happen outside or even inside the pharmacy. Consider what your attitude may be on a day you do not feel well, or have a test in the afternoon, or received a traffic citation on the way to your practice site because you overslept. The patient and other health-care providers still need to have your full attention, and professional attitude. If you are going to be late, or absent, call the preceptor as soon as you know you will be unable to reach your practice site on time. Continuing to use the traffic citation as an example, in this case you may need to explain that you will be late because you received a speeding ticket. Do not over exaggerate and never lie. Leave your personal issues at the door of the pharmacy. Keep in mind that your preceptor was a pharmacy student and juggled tests, work, school, and home life all at the same time, and do not take advantage of them because they do remember what it is like, and want to be kind to you. Pharmacists often have to work when they are not feeling well. Discuss with your preceptor the appropriateness of going to the site if you are ill. Sometimes the preceptor may prefer you stay home as opposed to spreading disease among the staff. If you have an exam on a day when you are to be at a practice site, this is not an excuse for a less than positive attitude or lack of attendance. Remember that these opportunities to learn from the preceptor are not infinite. Maintaining a positive work ethic and professional attitude will also improve your learning.

## Timeliness

Before the first day, you should map your transportation route and the amount of time needed to arrive at your assigned practice site. If you are going to be driving to your site, you should do a preliminary drive to the site to see how long the commute is from your home. If you do this on the weekend, when traffic is light, remember to add additional travel time. If you are commuting by train or bus, make sure you have a schedule and know when and where you may have to transfer. Five minutes before you are scheduled to start at your site is sufficient time to arrive. Do not arrive too early and no more than 15 minutes before you are scheduled. Even though you are eager and want to put your best foot forward, your very early arrival will be distracting to your preceptor.

Notify your preceptor as soon as possible if you will be tardy or absent. Time off for holidays should be discussed with your preceptor at the beginning of the experience. Not all pharmacies will close for holidays, and you may be expected to be at your site on a holiday, especially if your preceptor is working.

## CURRICULUM VITAE AND COVER LETTER

Technology provides many alternatives for contacting a preceptor prior to the first day of your experiential education course. Whatever manner you are to use, it is always important to facilitate preparation for your arrival. You should be sure the preceptor receives an introductory letter (Fig. 1.1) and curriculum vitae (CV) about 5 to 10 days before you are scheduled to begin the experience. In the letter introduce yourself, include the start and stop dates of the experience, your address, e-mail address, telephone number, and when you will be contacting him or her in person. Make sure you know the appropriate title for your preceptor and how he or she should be addressed, Doctor, Mister, or Ms. Include in the introductory letter that you are looking forward to meeting them and learning with them during the course. You may be directed to provide this information

**Figure 1.1.** Cover letter.

Your Address

Date

Preceptor Name

Preceptor Title

Name of Institution

Address of Institution

Dear Dr. Smith,

This letter is to introduce myself. My name is Student Pharmacist. I am a student at Smart College of Pharmacy. I will be at your site from 00/00/00 through 00/00/00 for an early experience rotation. My phone number is 123-4567. I will be calling you Monday morning of next week to receive directions to your facility, where and what time I should meet you, and which readings or other preparatory work I can do before I begin the rotation. I am looking forward to meeting you and learning from your experience.

Sincerely,

Smart Pharmacy Student

by e-mail, or give access to your preceptor to your portfolio, instead of a cover letter. Follow the guidelines in your school student manual. A formal letter of introduction will always be in style, and set the stage for a professional and open learning experience.

Your CV should include your name, address, phone number, e-mail address, previous college attendance, current college attendance, professional experience, work experience, and any awards and honors you have received during your college years. If you read, write, or speak any languages other than English, include this in your CV. High school honors and awards should not be included. The phrase "references on request" should also be omitted because the college is your reference. Your professional experience should include any positions you have held in the field of pharmacy and any pharmacy certifications. Describe what you have done in pharmacy using action verbs. Examples of action terms are filled prescriptions, communicated with health-care professionals, and managed inventory. You may have counted capsules and tablets, spoken to nurses, and put away the stock, but on your CV you should use professional terms to describe your activities. In addition, include your specific job title for all jobs (technician, data entry clerk). If you worked as a professional other than a pharmacist, for example, a teacher or an engineer, you may include this as other professional experience. Be sure to include the dates of attendance at all colleges, any degrees you have earned, and the dates on which they were conferred. As you progress through practice experiences, include them on your CV. Put your most recent experience first, the rest in reverse chronological order. Remember that professional experience is gained while you are a student pharmacist. Even though practice experiences are part of your academic requirements, they still are part of your professional experience. Figure 1.2 illustrates a sample CV.

There are numerous primary and secondary sources and templates for writing a resume or CV. Your college library should have these, both in hard copy and online. *Drug Topics*, a pharmacy professional publication, gives graduating students tips on resume writing and interviewing skills in their March/April publication every year.

Make sure that you review and know the paperwork procedures and requirements for each of your scheduled sites, and send all required information with your cover letter, or earlier, if required. Your college may require you to keep this information as part of a portfolio or other program. Ensure that this documentation is appropriate with the preceptor. Some introductory experience sites may require special applications. Many sites will require copies of your immunization records and negative urine drug screens. Some sites may accept as proof a signature from your faculty that these forms are on file at the college. Other sites may require that you bring copies of these records on your first day of the practice experience course. Some sites may require that students have background checks, beyond what has been required by the college, and require

**Figure 1.2.** Student curriculum vitae.

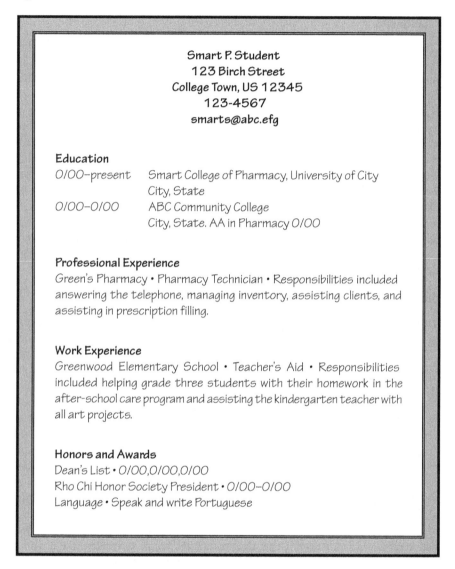

Smart P. Student
123 Birch Street
College Town, US 12345
123-4567
smarts@abc.efg

**Education**

O/OO–present    Smart College of Pharmacy, University of City
                City, State
O/OO–O/OO       ABC Community College
                City, State. AA in Pharmacy O/OO

**Professional Experience**

Green's Pharmacy • Pharmacy Technician • Responsibilities included answering the telephone, managing inventory, assisting clients, and assisting in prescription filling.

**Work Experience**

Greenwood Elementary School • Teacher's Aid • Responsibilities included helping grade three students with their homework in the after-school care program and assisting the kindergarten teacher with all art projects.

**Honors and Awards**

Dean's List • O/OO,O/OO,O/OO
Rho Chi Honor Society President • O/OO–O/OO
Language • Speak and write Portuguese

students to submit their social security numbers. Some introductory experience sites, especially schools and school programs, may require fingerprinting and photo identification badges. Be prepared by carrying two forms of identification with you to sites, and a copy of immunizations, and your intern certificate just in case.

## THE PRACTICE SITE

### Expectations

On the first day at the pharmacy, what can you expect? It really depends on what type of practice setting you are scheduled to attend. You are likely to be at an institution/hospital or a community pharmacy. Other possible places for experiential education courses include nursing home pharmacies, prisons, methadone facilities, or home health-care agencies. All of these facilities require the services of a pharmacist. Whatever your assignment for the first course, you should expect to be busy learning to become a pharmacist. From the moment you enter the pharmacy there will be phones ringing and people talking. The staff in the pharmacy or facility will be in constant motion, and you will be wondering where you should sit or stand. By your second week at the practice site you ought to be in motion too. Do not be disappointed or frustrated after the first day or even the second or third. You may feel that you are in the way, and in some manner, you will be. However, you will not be in the way for very long. It takes time to accommodate to the environment and to new responsibilities. It is your responsibility, not your preceptor's, to accommodate to the culture and activities in the pharmacy.

### Orientation

The best first day you can have during an experiential education course is to be early to the site. The preceptor gives you a tour of the facility and pharmacy, and provides a full-day orientation. This orientation will cover preceptor expectations, objectives for the experience, assignments, and outcomes expected. You ought to be introduced to all staff members. Preceptors should inform the student of the role of each staff member. It is essential that you understand individual roles, so you know who to ask what questions, as you progress through the course. You should share with the preceptor what you expect to get out of the experience, your concerns, and your desired goals. The objectives of the experience ought to be discussed at length. You will want to develop a plan with the preceptor to meet the objectives and establish due dates and guidelines for turning in assignments. Most preceptors will provide you with grading forms and a calendar of assignment due dates and meetings. These grading forms may also be found in your school manual with instructions from the faculty. This is the ideal situation and truly the best way to begin a practice experience. It may not always happen this way, and you must remember that you are in an experiential learning situation and that flexibility and adaptability are important attributes.

### Pharmacy Technicians

Pharmacy technicians are essential for the daily activities and success of a pharmacy. Technicians are in the pharmacy to assist the pharmacist. In some states, technicians are required to register with the State Board of Pharmacy and be certified as a Pharmacist Technician. In most states, the technicians are not yet required to have a license and will be closely controlled by the supervisor. Some pharmacy technicians are certified, but others are not. Most states allow the pharmacist to work with two technicians at a time, check state or national laws to make sure you know the required ratio. Technicians do not have the same responsibilities as pharmacy interns. Pharmacy interns must follow pharmacist laws and practice as a pharmacist and may complete every step in the dispensing and counseling process as long as the pharmacist supervises. Technicians cannot practice as a pharmacist in the United States and all their work must be checked by a pharmacist. You may find that the job responsibilities are very much the same. You will discover yourself doing what you think is a technician's work, or work that you feel is not your job as an intern. All effort in the pharmacy is the responsibility of the pharmacist and pharmacy intern. Because of this, all tasks are yours to make sure they are completed accurately and efficiently. You cannot supervise or manage a pharmacy if you do not know how the work is done or what the tasks are. Your positive working relationship with the technicians will improve your learning opportunities. Good technicians keep the workflow smooth and steady. As a student and pharmacist, you will come to depend on good technician support.

## Confidentiality and Success

### Goals

You discuss with your preceptor your goals for the experience, and you get started. How do you have a successful experience? There are a few things to keep in mind at all times. Remember your professional behavior and conduct while on practice experiences. You will have access to patients' medical records, charts, and data. Keep all information you know and have access to in the strictest confidence. Do not discuss patient information outside the pharmacy. If you must use patient information for a presentation or a school project, remember to use initials and not full names. Also, keep confidential all fee systems and professional policies that you may encounter. It is a good rule to keep all information to yourself and discuss it only in a pharmacy; elevators and hallways do not lend themselves to confidentiality.

Always be courteous and respectful of your preceptor. If you believe you witnessed your preceptor giving out incorrect information or practicing in the gray area of the law, do not confront him or her in front of others. Wait until you can discuss the matter in private. You may not be correct in your interpretation of the circumstance and might embarrass yourself or your preceptor. If you believe your preceptor is violating any pharmacy laws and cannot discuss the issue with him or her, seek advice of a faculty member at your college. The experiential director is probably the best person to share this information with because he or she is in a position to take action.

### Professional Decisions

Never dispense prescriptions before being double checked by your preceptor or another pharmacist. You do have liability as a pharmacy intern if you make a mistake in filling a prescription. Do not make professional decisions without first discussing them with your preceptor. Your answer may be incorrect or may violate policies of the institution. Always let your preceptor know of any information you will be giving to patients or health-care professionals.

*Communication*

Do not let the above cautionary statements keep you from initiating communication with other health-care professionals. You will be expected, as a student pharmacist, to call physicians and nurses on the phone. Always identify yourself as a student pharmacist and be courteous and professional on the telephone. Use common sense when interacting with patients and other health-care professionals. Always state why you are calling and remember to include the patient's name. Most of the time a nurse will be clarifying components of prescriptions written by physicians. Make sure the nurse understands what you need. If the strength of a medication is missing from a prescription, inform the nurse of the available strengths. Remember that it is possible that the physician does not know. When the nurse clarifies the prescription with the physician, she will give him the strength options. If you do not supply the information, it is possible the physician will indicate a strength he believes is available when it is not, and you will be starting the telephone process of seeking the medication strength all over again.

*Law*

You should be aware of the laws governing the practice of pharmacy and begin to incorporate them into your knowledge base immediately (Chap. 7 of this book discusses basic US federal regulations). You should have a copy of all the state and federal laws that apply to the practice of pharmacy. Read the laws. If you are unsure of procedures in the pharmacy, look up the law first before going to your preceptor. Your preceptor will be able to clarify any points that are unclear to you and explain the gray areas of the law. Some laws apply only to hospital pharmacies and not to community pharmacies. The opposite is also true. Your preceptor is the best person to clarify any questions you may have.

*Work Schedule*

Stick with the work schedule that you and your preceptor agree to, or if your college determines your schedule, adhere to the predetermined hours. Remember it will be necessary to devote time beyond the hours at the site, at home, and in the library, to meet the learning goals of your practice experiences. You ought to plan to spend additional time at your site to take advantage of unique experiences.

## PRACTICE EXPERIENCE COURSES

What are the goals of introductory pharmacy practice experiences? The main goal of the introductory experiences is to apply ideas learned in the classroom to practical experiences and integrate the information in order to improve understanding of concepts. Introductory experiences are designed to assist you in developing the practical aspects of the profession. You ought to develop advanced communication skills with patients and with other health-care professionals while on the introductory experiences.

Most colleges of pharmacy provide students with objectives and outcomes for the introductory pharmacy practice experiences. Faculty at colleges and universities and the ACPE Board want students to be immersed in hospital and community practices as introductory pharmacy practice experiences. You ought to want to build skills that will be effective for completing advanced practice experiences. Some college curricula may require that students be assigned to public health activities, community service activities, nursing homes, and home health-care agencies as early experience courses. Others emphasize continuity of patient care, and students are assigned to monitor one patient for an entire year or across years.

Introductory pharmacy practice experiences lead to building skills necessary for completing advanced pharmacy practice experiences. These advanced practice experiences enable you to apply your knowledge and skills learned in class to a clinical practice. During advanced pharmacy practice experiences, you become a part of the health-care team (Chaps. 5 and 6) and this is the only time you will be able to practice the position of pharmacist. Time passes quickly and you will be licensed before you are ready if you do not spend time practicing while in school. While completing advanced practice experiences you will learn to treat patients with disease and develop endpoints of therapy. Students enrolled in advanced pharmacy practice experience courses are directed to learn advanced practical applications of knowledge while progressively informing their clinical judgment.

## INTRODUCTORY PRACTICE COURSES

General goals for community, and hospital experiences in addition to service to the community, are discussed below and offer foundational objectives for beginning your student pharmacist career. Chapters 3, 14, and 15 provide in-depth information on community service, practice in the community pharmacy, and institutional settings. In addition, your own college of school will have a practice manual, goals, and objectives that will need to be met.

### Community Service Course

What can you expect if you are assigned to a community service course? You will have your own personal goals that you desire to achieve, in addition to those required by the school. You may be asked to spend time reflecting on your experiences to determine if you achieved your goals. Barbara Jacoby defines service learning as "a form of experiential education in which students engage in activities that address human and community needs together with structured opportunities intentionally designed to promote student learning and development. Reflection and reciprocity

---

**TABLE 1.2.** COMMUNITY SERVICE OBJECTIVES

........................................................................................................................................

- Display attitudes, habits, and values appropriate to a pharmacist.
- Promote awareness of health and prevention of disease.
- Articulate personal values and ethical principles.
- Display an understanding of unmet community needs and be able to provide examples in the community.
- Discuss issues of diversity.
- Choose appropriate levels of communication.
- Understand a health-care professional's role in the community.
- Work as a group leader and a team member.

---

are key concepts of service learning."[3] You may be asked to work on a project that will contribute in some way to the benefit of the community. Examples of projects in which you may participate include food and clothing drives, after-school care programs, and providing health care to underserved populations. Generally, these experiences help students improve listening, and observation skills with real people who may be your patients. You may well expand your knowledge of community and develop a professional demeanor. Learning through service will help you meet community needs while developing critical thinking and group problem-solving skills (Table 1.2).

## Institution Experience

What can you expect if you are assigned to an introductory hospital, or institution course? As a student pharmacist, you will be assigned to all areas of the pharmacy. You will be working with pharmacists, administrative personnel, and technicians. You may spend hours learning about a different aspect of pharmacy or other areas of an institution each time you are at your site. Learning how to fill a prescription in an institution pharmacy and interacting with other health-care professionals are the two major objectives of this course. You will want to participate in various aspects of institutional practice, including dispensing and management. Introductory courses in a hospital promote exposure and participation in drug distribution and enhance your awareness of the many aspects of practice. Experiences gained ought to include the role and responsibilities of a professionally oriented institutional pharmacist; the importance of effective communication with other health-care providers; the importance of monitoring drug utilization; organizational requirements necessary to achieve efficient operations; and the application of local, state, and federal regulations governing the prescription-dispensing process. Introductory pharmacy practice experience courses in a hospital setting also enable a student to develop the role and respect the responsibilities of the pharmacist in the health-care delivery system.

---

**TABLE 1.3.** INSTITUTIONAL PRACTICE OBJECTIVES
..................................................................................................................................

- Explain the process of receiving, interpreting, clarifying, and verifying medication orders for accuracy and completeness.
- Select the appropriate drug product to be used in filling medication orders.
- Package and label medication in compliance with hospital pharmacy policy and local and federal pharmacy laws.
- Describe the process for drug control, storage, and security functions in drug distribution.
- Describe the process for recording the medication order following established pharmacy policies and procedures.
- Participate in the drug distribution process for timely delivery of ordered medications, including STAT orders, to the appropriate location.
- Communicate effectively with other members of the health-care team including nurses, technicians, and other staff members.
- Observe aseptic technique in the IV room and recognize its importance.
- Discuss management issues as they pertain to inventory, formularies, budgets, regulation of narcotics, and quality assurance.

---

You ought to practice applying information learned in pharmacodynamics, pharmacy law, and basic sciences during this course. New and advanced technologies are being integrated into the practice of pharmacy in institutions, including Pyxis and computer medication administration records, direct-order entry. These technologies will change the practice, allowing the pharmacist to be more actively involved in patient care than in the past. Expect to incorporate advanced technologies into your practice at each new opportunity (Table 1.3).

## Community Experience

What can you expect if you are assigned to an introductory community course? As a student pharmacist assigned to an introductory community experience, you will learn aspects of managing and the operations of a community pharmacy. Every detail of filling a prescription will be reviewed and practiced regularly, including the ordering of prescription and nonprescription medications supplied from the pharmacy. Some of the activities you will be exposed to include inventory management, patient counseling, third-party plans, and state and federal pharmacy laws. An introductory course in a community pharmacy promotes competency in drug distribution and enhances awareness of many aspects of community pharmacy practice. You will be exposed to the role and responsibilities of the pharmacist; the importance of effective communication between pharmacists, patients, and other health-care providers; and the application of local, state, and federal regulations governing the

---

**TABLE 1.4.** COMMUNITY PRACTICE OBJECTIVES

- Receive, interpret, check, and verify prescriptions for accuracy and completeness.
- Select the most appropriate drug product to be used in filling a prescription, taking into account factors that will enhance patient care.
- Interact with health insurance companies to provide the patient with the most effective and lowest-cost medication.
- Describe the legal constraints governing the dispensing process.
- Package and label the prescription in compliance with local, state, and federal laws.
- Dispense the prescription to the patient in a professional manner that complies with all legal requirements.
- Maintain the confidentiality of patient information, especially during data collection, patient interviews, prescription clarification, and patient counseling.
- Participate in interactions with patients to obtain information relevant to filling the prescription.
- Participate in interactions with patients to create and/or expand the patient profile.
- Participate in interactions with other health-care providers with regard to the provision of patient care.

---

prescription-filling process and patient counseling. During the course, you ought to want to enhance patient care and contribute to the practice. The objectives of an introductory community experience are to facilitate the application of skills, concepts, and knowledge acquired in the classroom. Activities completed while on a community experience will be selection of drug products; prescription dispensing; interactions with patients; and interactions with nurses, physicians, and other health-care professionals (Table 1.4).

## CONCLUSION

After reading this chapter, you may have a better understanding of the professional role you play as a student pharmacist. There are vital attributes that you ought to want to master early in your career, such as appearance, attitude, and timeliness. It is important to write an appropriate cover letter, and develop a CV as directed by college faculty. Make sure that your preceptor has access to these documents if you are not sending them by mail. Setting goals for yourself before beginning your experiences and letting your preceptor know what they are is a way to gain the most knowledge. Learn the culture of a site and adapt to it early so that you are comfortable in your environment. The definitions, goals, expectations, and ideals discussed here are foundational requirements that may help you achieve your desired level of learning and comfort.

The information in this chapter is meant to support goals and objectives set forth by your own college of pharmacy. In all cases, follow the directions of your own faculty; and where this book disagrees, it is because the practice of pharmacy is not perfect, and many ways of doing things may be correct. That is why they call it practice.

## APPLICATION EXERCISES

1. What is considered professional dress for male and female pharmacists?
2. What is a professional attitude?
3. What can a student expect on the first day of practice experience in a pharmacy?
4. What goals will a pharmacy student have completed at the end of his or her introductory pharmacy practice experiences?
5. How do hospital and community practice experiences differ in expectations?

## REFERENCES

1. Facts about pharmacists—brief summary about pharmacists. USPharmD +. Available at http://www.uspharmd.com/student/Facts_about_Pharmacist.html. Accessed March, 2014.
2. Jones JM. Lobbyists Debut at Bottom of Honesty and Ethics List. Gallop Poll December 10, 2007. Available at http://www.gallup.com/poll/103123/Lobbyists-Debut-Bottom-Honesty-Ethics-List.aspx. Accessed March, 2014.
3. Jacoby B, ed. *Service Learning in Higher Education: Concepts and Practices*. San Francisco, CA: Jossey-Bass; 1996:5.

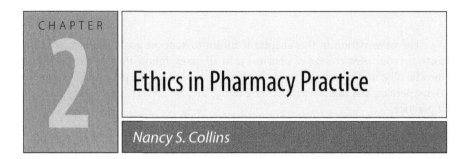

# Ethics in Pharmacy Practice

*Nancy S. Collins*

**Objectives: Upon completion of the chapter and exercises, the student pharmacist will be able to**

1. Identify and explain why the core of clinical ethics is the doctor/clinician-patient relationship, what responsibilities and potential abuses are inherent in that relationship, and why there need to be guidelines for clinicians.
2. Recognize what behavior is ethically their duty to provide to the patient and what is ethically unacceptable behavior.
3. Use the Jonsen and Siegler four topics box system of clinical ethics—(1) medical indications, (2) patient preferences, (3) quality of life, and (4) contextual features—when approaching cases of ethical decision making.
4. Reference and incorporate the four Georgetown bioethics principles of autonomy, beneficence, nonmaleficence, and justice into decision-making processes.
5. Follow codified ethical practices such as those published by the American College of Physicians.
6. Appreciate that ethical duties also extend to the family, to your profession, to society, and to patient research.

---

### Patient Encounter

### ETHICS

A 26-year-old African American Gold Medal Olympic bicyclist was struck by a car, flung 30 ft into the air, and fell into an embankment. He was training for his second Olympic trial and was well known in the community as being devoted to his sport. He was unconscious at the scene. After stabilization in the hospital, it was determined that his spinal cord was completely severed below T10. He sustained a serious head injury, but it was anticipated that he would probably be able to talk and communicate his wishes over time. However, a long

---

*(continued on next page)*

rehabilitation period was anticipated for the head injury with uncertain degree of return to full preaccident mental abilities, and the paraplegia was permanent. During his recovery period, he needed surrogates (proxies) to make decisions for him because of his temporary lack of decision-making capacity. The patient had several medical complications including pneumonia and urosepsis. After several weeks, several family members, including his wife, who was the main surrogate decision maker, voiced their concern that the patient, given his athletic prowess, would "never want to be a cripple" and suggested that, because of the patient's poor quality of life, antibiotics be withheld and the patient be allowed to "die with dignity." Both the patient and his wife were avid athletes, and the subject of paraplegia had never been discussed. Because of his love of the sport and their lifestyle of athleticism, she was sure he would not want to be a "cripple." You, as the pharmacist, are approached by the family to cease administration of antibiotics.

### DISCUSSION—A CASE INVOLVING QUALITY OF LIFE

It is difficult to know what a patient's preferences are when he cannot speak for himself. Quality-of-life assessment is often made by a third party making pronouncements about someone else's quality of life. It is important to note that there is significant bias introduced here.

Studies consistently show that physicians (not to mention family members) consistently rate the quality of life of their patients lower than the patients do themselves. Rehabilitation literature abounds that documents that although the initial grief and shock of disability are profound, paraplegics, even quadriplegic patients, gradually learn to find life worthwhile and cope with the disabilities and find pleasures in life.

This case is based largely on a case from Jonsen et al.[1]

## INTRODUCTION

This chapter is addressed to clinicians; a clinician is a professional involved in clinical care of patients. This includes physicians, nurses, physical therapists, occupational therapists, and others. Ethical decision making is involved in every patient case.

The chapter is set up in five sections:

1. Codes of ethics for the physician and pharmacist.
2. Two philosophical theories are often referred to in biomedical ethics: utilitarianism and deontology.
3. History of (a) how biomedical ethics evolved and the fundamental principles of biomedical ethics, (b) how clinical ethics evolved, and (c) clinical applications of those principles (clinical ethics) with case examples—these clinical applications are described in Jonsen and Siegler's four topics of clinical ethics: (1) medical indications, (2) patient preferences, (3) quality of life, and (4) contextual features.
4. Codes of conduct in the professions and, specifically, clinical ethics.
5. Conclusion: The doctor/clinician-patient relationship is the core of clinical ethics.

## THE CODES OF PROFESSIONAL ETHICS IN MEDICINE AND PHARMACY

When we choose a career in a health profession, there comes with it the power to restore health or, at the very least, lessen the suffering of the patient. In this very special relationship, the patient must assume the patient's role, that of asking for help from the clinician, and the clinician must assume the clinician's role, that of trying to restore health or at least lessen the suffering of the patient. These roles will always put the patient in the less powerful position and the clinician in the more powerful one. It is important that the clinician understands and accepts the responsibilities and potential abuses of the power in that relationship. Through the centuries it was recognized that because of this power differential, there needed to be guidelines for clinicians so that once a patient entrusted his or her health to the clinician's care, the clinician could recognize what behavior was ethically his or her duty to provide to the patient and what was ethically unacceptable behavior.

It has been recognized since the days of Hippocrates that physicians needed a shared understanding of the goals of medicine, their role in the practice of medicine, and what behavior was appropriate and what behavior was not appropriate toward patients. Written documentation of professing the ethical principles involved in patient care dates back to the Hippocratic Oath (Fig. 2.1) taken by physicians. The doctor-patient relationship is used in this chapter as the classic model of the clinician-patient relationship. The principles are the same for all clinicians.

The Hippocratic Oath is a physician's obligation to safeguard the life and welfare of the patient. The moral centerpiece of the Hippocratic Oath is that "the physician will use judgment to help the sick according to his ability and judgment, but never with the view to injury and wrongdoing." In book I on "Epidemics" attributed to Hippocrates, it is also said that "Physicians must

**Figure 2.1.** Hippocratic Oath as interpreted by Steven Miles.[2] (This version is closely based on the translation of von Staden H. *J Hist Med Allied Sci.* 1996;51:406 and the analysis of its cultural meaning in Miles SH. The Hippocratic Oath and the Ethics of Medicine, Oxford University Press, 2006.)

> I swear by Apollo the Physician and by Asclepius, Hygia, and Panacea, and by all the deities, making this testimony before them that I will keep this oath to the best of my power and judgement. I will regard those who taught me this art and science as equal to my patients. I will share with my teachers according to their necessities. I will impart the art, science, lectures, and all the rest of learning to those students who have sworn to live up to this profession. I will use treatments for the benefit of the ill according to my ability and judgement and from what is to their harm or injustice I will keep them. I will not give a poison to anyone if asked for it, nor will I suggest such a course. Likewise I will not give a woman a destructive pessary. In a pure and holy way, I will guard my life, my art, and my science. Into the households I enter, I will go to benefit the ill, while being far from all voluntary and destructive injustice, especially from sexual acts upon women's or men's bodies whether they be free or enslaved. Of whatever I see or hear in my personal or professional life that should not be aired, I will remain silent, holding such things to be unspeakable. If I observe this oath, and do not blur and evade it, may I enjoy the benefits of life and of this work and be held in good repute by all persons for all time. However, if I transgress and perjure myself, may the opposite befall me.

take a habit of two things—to help or at least to do no harm. The art of medicine has three factors, the disease, the patient, and the physician. The physician is the servant of the Art. The patient must cooperate with the physician in combating the disease."[2] Once the patient seeks the physician's help, the patient must ultimately trust that the Hippocratic physician will provide the best available treatment for the medical condition and end treatment if it turns out to be harmful.

The Oath of a Pharmacist (Table 2.1) and the Pharmacists Code of Ethics (Table 2.2) developed by the American Pharmacists Association give deference to the principles applied by Hippocrates, and delineate specific responsibilities to the profession and patient.[3,4]

---

**TABLE 2.1.  THE OATH OF A PHARMACIST[3]**

At this time, I vow to devote my professional life to the service of all humankind through the profession of pharmacy.

I will consider the welfare of humanity and relief of human suffering my primary concerns.

I will apply my knowledge, experience, and skills to the best of my ability to assure optimal drug therapy outcomes for the patients I serve.

I will keep abreast of developments and maintain professional competency in my profession of pharmacy.

I will maintain the highest principles of moral, ethical, and legal conduct.

I will embrace and advocate change in the profession of pharmacy that improves patient care.

I take these vows voluntarily with the full realization of the responsibility with which I am entrusted by the public.

---

## TWO PHILOSOPHICAL THEORIES ARE OFTEN REFERRED TO IN BIOMEDICAL AND CLINICAL ETHICS: UTILITARIANISM AND DEONTOLOGY

When you look through textbooks on ethics, you will see thousands of pages devoted to many philosophic theories. However, when these theories are applied to clinical practice, two are highly regarded as sound ethical principles.

Utilitarian philosophy is based on the belief that the morality of an act is based solely on the basis of its consequences. In the words of the most famous of the utilitarian philosophers, John Mill, "Actions are right in proportion as they tend to

---

**TABLE 2.2.  CODE OF ETHICS FOR PHARMACISTS[4]**

A *pharmacist* respects the covenantal relationship between the patient and pharmacist.

A *pharmacist* promotes the good of every patient in a caring, compassionate, and confidential manner.

A *pharmacist* respects the autonomy and dignity of each patient.

A *pharmacist* acts with honesty and integrity in professional relationships.

A *pharmacist* maintains professional competence.

A *pharmacist* respects the values and abilities of colleagues and other health professionals.

A *pharmacist* serves individual, community, and societal needs.

A *pharmacist* seeks justice in the distribution of health resources.

---

Adopted by the membership of the American Pharmacists Association October 27, 1994.

promote happiness, wrong as they tend to produce the reverse of happiness."[5] The degree of moral rightness of an act is directly proportional to its net utility, defined as the difference between its overall utility and disutility or, in medical terminology, its benefits and burdens.

Deontological philosophy is based on the belief that the morality of an act is based solely on the basis of the moral rightness of intentions, termed the *categorical imperative*. In this paradigm, the intentions and sense of duty behind a given act determine the degree of moral rightness of an act. Immanuel Kant is the most famous of the philosophers of deontologism.

## HISTORY OF (A) HOW BIOMEDICAL ETHICS EVOLVED AND THE FUNDAMENTAL PRINCIPLES OF BIOMEDICAL ETHICS, (B) HOW CLINICAL ETHICS EVOLVED, AND (C) CLINICAL APPLICATIONS OF THOSE PRINCIPLES (CLINICAL ETHICS) WITH CASE EXAMPLES

### (a) History of How Biomedical Ethics Evolved and the Fundamental Principles of Biomedical Ethics

*Nuremberg Code*[6]

After the Second World War, the Nuremberg trials revealed the terrible abuses, called "medical experimentation," perpetuated by Nazi doctors on concentration camp prisoners. The Nuremberg Code, 10 rules set down to protect human subjects in medical research in perpetuity, was formulated in August 1947 in Nuremberg, Germany by American judges sitting in judgment of 23 physicians and scientists accused of murder and torture in the conduct of medical experiments in the concentration camps. These rules were a merger of the physician-centered duties set down in the Hippocratic Oath and the patient/subject-centered assertion of patient/subject protections. Within the text of the Nuremberg Code was the assertion of the unequivocable, absolute protection of the rights of patients/subjects and of their autonomy. Those protections affirmed two important rights—that of informed consent and the right to withdraw from research.

Since that time, the informed consent requirement of the Code is now seen as an ethical necessity not only in research but also in the treatment.

*Famous Historical Examples of Ethical Dilemmas and Scandals in the 1960s: Recognition of Medical and Nonmedical Selection Bias while Attempting to Ethically Ration Hemodialysis; Exposure of the Flagrant but Unrecognized Racial Bias in the Tuskegee Syphilis Study; Beginnings of Debate over Definition of Death in Organ Transplantation and in Brain Death*

After the Nuremberg Code, more ethical dilemmas were recognized in the United States. In the early 1960s, with the advent of hemodialysis, there were many more candidates than hemodialysis machines. Determination of selection of patients for hemodialysis was ultimately recognized as an ethical dilemma—what medical and nonmedical criteria should be used to select suitable candidates?

Later, the research carried out over several decades (1932-1972) by the US Public Health Service in Tuskegee, Alabama, on hundreds of black men with known syphilis who were never offered penicillin in order that the progression of the disease could be studied was made known. This led to acknowledgment of physician bias, racial arrogance, and unethical treatment of racial minorities in the United States.[7]

In 1967, Dr. Christiaan Barnard transplanted a human heart from a dead (or dying) person into a patient with a terminal cardiac disease. This led to some wondering about the organ donor's state—was the source truly dead, and what were the wishes of the donor about donating his heart while living?

In the early 1960s ventilators had been invented, and patients with polio were being saved from certain death. However, other patients, including those in irreversible coma, were placed on ventilators as well. This led to a large number of cases where physicians were faced with the ethical dilemma of withdrawing ventilator support from patients who had functioning cardiorespiratory systems but who had had cessation of total brain functions. The standard definition of death was when a doctor determined that the heart and/or lungs ceased to function. However, these patients on ventilator support had functioning hearts and lungs, but brain function had ceased. Adding to this concern was the growing recognition that these patients' organs were of great value in transplantation. Therefore, in 1968, the Harvard Ad Hoc Committee on Brain Death was established and published its definition and recommendations for the diagnosis of brain death. Under these recommendations, patients who met the brain death criteria were considered medically unequivocally dead, and ventilator withdrawal was deemed medically and ethically appropriate. Also, organ removal for transplantation from these patients was deemed ethically appropriate (assuming consent from the family) because these patients were medically unequivocally dead.

*Famous Historical Examples of Ethical Dilemmas in the 1970s and 1980s: Ethical Dilemmas Arising from Famous Cases of Patients in Persistent Vegetative State (Recognition and Definition of Persistent Vegetative State; Who Can Make Decisions Regarding Administering and Withdrawing Hydration and Nutrition in These No Longer Autonomous Patients); Belmont Report's Critical Role in Codifying Protection of Human Subjects in Research and Stating the Three General Principles of Biomedical Ethics[6] (Respect for Persons, Beneficence, Justice) and Their Applications (Informed Consent, Assessment of Risks and Benefits, and Fair Selection of Subjects); the Four Principles of Biomedical Ethics[7]*

By the 1970s and 1980s, several court cases arose concerning patients (Quinlan, Cruzan, Brophy) in persistent vegetative state (a state in which the brain stem, which controls various vegetative functions such as wake/sleep cycles, breathing, and pupillary responses, is still functioning but the higher levels of cortical functioning such as meaningful interaction with the environment permanently cease to function), raising questions of the ethics surrounding the withdrawal of ventilator, hydration, and nutrition in nonautonomous (ie, without decision-making capacity) patients.

By 1974, the Congress established the National Commission for the Protection of Human Subjects of Biomedical and Behavioral Research to recommend policies that would guide researchers in the design of ethical research. That commission, which sat from 1974 to 1978, engaged the help of a wide variety of scholars from many disciplines and solicited public opinion on many issues. Out of this commission developed *The Belmont Report: Ethical Principles and Guidelines for the Protection of Human Subjects of Research* (April 18, 1979) published by the Department of Health, Education, and Welfare. *The Belmont Report* asserted three general principles of biomedical ethics[8]:

1. *Respect for persons*, which includes two moral requirements: (a) the requirement to acknowledge *autonomy* and (b) the requirement to protect those with diminished autonomy.
2. *Beneficence*, which is the obligation to secure the patient's well-being. Two general rules apply: (a) do no harm and (b) maximize possible benefits and minimize possible harms.
3. *Justice*, fairness in distribution; the importance of explaining in what respects people should be treated equally.[8]

Applications of the three general principles include[8] (1) informed consent, which includes three elements: (a) information, (b) comprehension, and (c) voluntariness; (2) assessment of risks and benefits, which include (a) the nature and scope of risk and benefits and (b) the systematic assessment of risks and benefits; and (3) selection of subjects, with fair procedures and outcomes in the selection of research subjects.[8]

*The Belmont Report* then led to the publishing of the landmark work of Beauchamp and Childress, *The Principles of Biomedical Ethics*.[9] This system is taught at the Kennedy Institute of Ethics at Georgetown University and is labeled the Principles of Biomedical Ethics. In this system there are four essential ethical principles[9]:

1. *Respect for Autonomy*: *Autonomy* is the moral right to choose and follow one's own plan of life and action. Respect for autonomy is the moral attitude that disposes one to refrain from interference with others' autonomous beliefs and actions in the pursuit of their goals.
2. *Nonmaleficence*: *Nonmaleficence* is the moral duty to do no harm.
3. *Beneficence*: *Beneficence* is the moral duty to assist persons in need.
4. *Justice*: *Justice* is the ethics of fair and equitable distribution of burdens and benefits within a community.[9]

These ethical principles of *beneficence*, *nonmaleficence*, *autonomy*, and *justice* as set forth by Beauchamp and Childress remain well established in the bioethics field. However, at the bedside or clinic, it was often difficult to see how these principles can be applied to medical decision making in individual cases. This led to the development of *clinical ethics* decision making as described in the next section.

## (b) History of How Clinical Ethics Evolved

The term "clinical ethics" was coined by Siegler in the 1970s.[10] Clinical ethics is an approach to assisting clinicians in identifying, analyzing, and resolving ethical issues in clinical medicine. Albert Jonsen, Mark Siegler, and William Winslade published their first of many classic editions of *Clinical Ethics* in 1982 in which they wrote:

> The practice of good clinical medicine requires some working knowledge about ethical issues such as informed consent, truth telling, confidentiality, end of life care, pain relief, and patient rights. Medicine, even at its most technical and scientific, is an encounter between human beings, and the physician's work of diagnosing disease, offering advice, and providing treatment is embedded in a moral context. Usually values such as mutual respect, honesty, trustworthiness, compassion, and a commitment to pursue shared goals make a clinical encounter between physician and patient morally unproblematic. Occasionally physicians and patients may disagree about values or face choices that challenge their values. It is then that ethical problems arise. Clinical ethics is both about the ethical features that are present in every clinical encounter and about the ethical problems that occasionally arise in those encounters.[1]

## (c) Clinical Applications of Biomedical Ethics Using the Siegler Method of Four Boxes

When you are seeing patients in the outpatient or inpatient setting and a dilemma arises as to how to best resolve an ethical question, I suggest you use the following "four box" system developed by Jonsen et al[1] (Fig. 2.2). It was developed because clinicians have long found it difficult to see how ethical principles of autonomy, beneficence, nonmaleficence, and justice, as valued as they are, can be brought back down to practical application at the bedside or clinic setting. In their book, *Clinical Ethics,* Jonsen et al pooled their extensive experiences and incorporated all the important bioethical principles into a "hands on" practical approach to solving ethical dilemmas in clinical practice. In the Jonsen et al's clinical ethics approach,[1] each clinical case, when seen as an ethical problem, should be analyzed by using four topics (Fig. 2.2).

1. *Medical indications*: Medical indications refer to the relation between the pathophysiology presented by the patient and the diagnostic and therapeutic interventions that are "indicated," that is, appropriate to evaluate and treat the problem. The ethical discussion will not only review the medical acts but also focus on the purposes and goals of any indicated interventions.
2. *Patient preferences*: The preferences of the patient are based on the patient's own values and personal assessment of benefits and burdens. This is the clinical application of autonomy. The systematic review of this topic requires further questions including decision-making capacity, informed consent, the authority to decide on behalf of the patient (surrogate decision maker), the legal and ethical limits of that authority, and so on.

**Figure 2.2.** The "four box" method for ethical decision making.[1] (From Jonsen A, Siegler M, Winslade W. *Clinical Ethics: A Practical Approach to Ethical Decisions in Clinical Medicine.* 6th ed. New York: McGraw-Hill; 2006.)

| ■ MEDICAL INDICATIONS | ■ PATIENT PREFERENCES |
|---|---|
| The Principles of Beneficence and Nonmaleficence<br><br>1. What is the patient's medical problem? history? diagnosis? prognosis?<br>2. Is the problem acute? chronic? critical? emergent? reversible?<br>3. What are the goals of treatment?<br>4. What are the probabilities of success?<br>5. What are the plans in case of therapeutic failure?<br>6. In sum, how can this patient be benefited by medical and nursing care, and how can harm be avoided? | The Principle of Respect for Autonomy<br><br>1. Is the patient mentally capable and legally competent? Is there evidence of incapacity?<br>2. If competent, what is the patient stating about preferences for treatment?<br>3. Has the patient been informed of benefits and risks, understood this information, and given consent?<br>4. If incapacitated, who is the appropriate surrogate? Is the surrogate using appropriate standards for decision making?<br>5. Has the patient expressed prior preferences, eg, Advance Directives?<br>6. Is the patient unwilling or unable to cooperate with medical treatment? If so, why?<br>7. In sum, is the patient's right to choose being respected to the extent possible in ethics and law? |
| ■ QUALITY OF LIFE | ■ CONTEXTUAL FEATURES |
| The Principles of Beneficence and Nonmaleficence and Respect for Autonomy<br><br>1. What are the prospects, with or without treatment, for a return to normal life?<br>2. What physical, mental, and social deficits is the patient likely to experience if treatment succeeds?<br>3. Are there biases that might prejudice the provider's evaluation of the patient's quality of life?<br>4. Is the patient's present or future condition such that his or her continued life might be judged undesirable?<br>5. Is there any plan and rationale to forgo treatment?<br>6. Are there plans for comfort and palliative care? | The Principles of Loyalty and Fairness<br><br>1. Are there family issues that might influence treatment decisions?<br>2. Are there provider (physicians and nurses) issues that might influence treatment decisions?<br>3. Are there financial and economic factors?<br>4. Are there religious or cultural factors?<br>5. Are there limits on confidentiality?<br>6. Are there problems of allocation of resources?<br>7. How does the law affect treatment decisions?<br>8. Is clinical research or teaching involved?<br>9. Is there any conflict of interest on the part of the providers or the institution? |

3. **Quality of life:** This is less worked out in the literature of medical ethics but is important in all medical situations. Any injury or illness threatens patients with actual or potential reduced quality of life. The clinician has a duty to restore, maintain, or improve quality of life. However, it is usually a third party such as the clinician or family members rather than the patient who is involved in quality-of-life decisions. Because the patients themselves may not be able to assert their own preferences, and it is third parties rather than the patient who are trying to judge the patient's quality of life, these decisions are perilous and must be recognized as such because these decisions open the door for bias and prejudice. Nevertheless, quality-of-life issues must be confronted in the context of analysis of clinical ethical problems.

4. **Contextual features:** The doctor-patient relationship, defined by the patient's asking for help and the physician's fiduciary duty to help, is at the core of clinical ethics. But every medical case is embedded in a larger context of persons; religious beliefs; institutions; and financial, legal, and social arrangements. These contextual features are important in understanding and resolving clinical problems.[1]

Each topic organizes the varying facts of the case and identifies the moral principles appropriate to the case. These topics help clinicians understand where the moral principles meet the circumstances of the clinical case.[1]

Notice in the "four box" system above, medical indications and patient preferences are above the quality of life and contextual features. This is intentional. Although in any clinical situation all four aspects should always be thoroughly explored, the top two, medical indications and patient preferences, "trump" the bottom two, quality of life and contextual features.

To illustrate the "clinical ethics" approach at the beginning of this chapter you reviewed "Patient Encounter", which represents one of the four topics, quality of life. Below are two additional cases that involve some ethical dilemmas demonstrating how the application of the clinical ethics "four box" system defines and resolves each case.

## CASE 1

During an annual checkup, a 60-year-old man is found to have an elevated prostate-specific antigen (PSA) level of 5.5 and prostate biopsy reveals cancer with a Gleason score of 3+3. He is referred to a surgeon who recommends a total prostatectomy. He then consults a radiation oncologist who recommends a course of radiation therapy rather than surgery. The patient, confused, returns to his primary physician, who explains that either choice is medically reasonable. Although surgery may increase the patient's long-term survival, it is associated with higher risk of incontinence and impotence.

## CASE 1 DISCUSSION

### A case involving medical indications and shared decision-making model of clinician-patient relationship

In this case, the surgeon and the radiation oncologist each present the patient with a treatment option; each option is based on sound medical evidence. But the patient feels he has to choose between the two options given. Physicians typically formulate recommendations in terms of their best medical judgment in light of the options available. Each physician stated their beliefs about which option seemed best for this particular patient rather than a menu of choices. Ultimately, the best medical decision for an individual patient will depend on how the patient evaluates different risks and benefits. The patient's evaluation of impotence was as integral to the decision as the medical evidence about survival.

## CASE 1 OUTCOME

In this case, the primary care physician and the patient worked together to define the medical and personal goals. Later in the chapter, you will read more about this shared decision-making model of the clinician-patient relationship. After considering the medical indications, risks, and benefits, the patient chose to undergo the radiation therapy instead of the total prostatectomy. This case is based largely on a case from Jonsen et al.[1]

## CASE 2

A 45-year-old man with insulin-dependent diabetes experienced frequent episodes of ketoacidosis and hypoglycemia. In addition, he had traumatic and poorly healing foot ulcers. He has not adhered with a diabetic diet and has begun abusing alcohol after a stormy divorce. He has been hospitalized several times for diabetic and alcohol-related complications. On several admissions he was found to be eating excessively in the hospital cafeteria. His physician and pharmacist wonder if they should withdraw from the therapeutic relationship because it appeared futile—the patient continued to engage in behavior that posed serious risk to health and even life despite many hours of cumulative time given by clinicians regarding recommendations and consequences of his noncompliant and risky behavior. There were some who began to wonder if the patient should continue to be admitted, especially if his situation wasn't critical because his risky behavior was self-imposed and he was "wasting resources" taking up bed space that other patients who did not engage in these behaviors might be able to use.

## CASE 2 DISCUSSION

**A case involving patient preferences and contextual features: failure to cooperate with medical recommendations (patient preferences) and contextual features of resource allocation and the risk of clinician bias/discrimination.**

In this patient's case, and in similar cases of patients who continue to engage in behaviors that result in worsening health (such as patients with emphysema who are repeatedly admitted for respiratory failure or obese patients who overeat with consequent medical complications), the situation is frustrating to healthcare providers and puts great strain on the clinician-patient relationship. It is important to determine whether and to what extent the patient is acting voluntarily or involuntarily. Some noncompliance may be secondary to emotional disturbance. If the clinician judges the noncompliance to be voluntary, efforts should be made at rational persuasion. If these fail, it is ethical for the clinician to adjust therapeutic goals and to do his or her best in the circumstance. In rare cases, it is ethically permissible to withdraw from the case after advising the patient how to obtain care from other sources. However, keep in mind that clinicians swear in their Hippocratic Oath to undertake difficult tasks and even risks in the care of persons in need of medical attention. Inconvenience, frustration, provocation, and dislike are not sufficient reasons to exempt you from that duty. If contextual features such as inability to pay for medicines, inadequate housing, and so on are a source of noncooperation, help should be provided in these circumstances. If noncooperation arises from psychological pathology, the clinician has a strong ethical obligation to remain with the patient, adjusting treatment plans. Professional assistance in treating the pathology should be sought.[1] You may feel frustrated, but the frustration is not, in itself, sufficient to justify leaving the patient.

The issue of distributive justice and resource allocation (also called rationing) that was raised by the bed space argument for nonadmission is not a rare complaint voiced by frustrated health professionals. However, in the context of the current American medical system (which is not socialized), it is very important to avoid making rationing decisions at the bedside. The criteria for deciding good from poor uses of societal resources is impossible and inappropriate to do at the bedside. It is the kind of decision that must be made at the policy level. The overall view of social need and the contribution of particular decisions to that need are not known to clinicians. For example, there is no guarantee that whatever is "saved" by refusing this patient will be used in any better manner. Blame for "wasting resources" is better laid on the system than the patient.[1]

Also, be very careful of clinician bias as far as deciding who "deserves" to be admitted. One of the important ethical tenets is that those in need should be cared for regardless of race, religion, or nationality. However, clinicians may have beliefs and values (maybe even unrecognized) against certain persons or classes of persons, and these attitudes may affect clinical decisions. The Tuskegee Syphilis Study is one example of clinicians in the US Public Health Service, who thought they were doing something valuable and good for humanity in general by withholding penicillin treatment to hundreds of black men with syphilis so that they could study the evolution of syphilis despite the ready availability and known efficacy of penicillin. The study wasn't secret. It took 40 years before the health professionals realized it was unethical, and the study was halted.

Studies have revealed that clinicians are also biased against elderly patients, termed ageism, and may choose to undertreat. Other studies have confirmed bias against gay patients, women, and those of low "social worth" (such as criminals). Singling out socially disapproved behaviors (such as overeating in patients who are obese, or repeatedly drinking alcohol in patients who may be criminals) as less deserving of treatment reflects social prejudices rather than logic (eg, engaging in dangerous sports is socially tolerated, even praised, and is associated with high risk and consequences).

### CASE 2 OUTCOME

In this patient's case, it was determined that he was severely depressed. Psychiatric consultation was obtained. Medications and psychotherapy were begun. Over time, the patient's compliance with medical management improved significantly.

This case is based largely on a case from Jonsen et al.[1]

## CODES OF CONDUCT IN THE PROFESSIONS AND, SPECIFICALLY, CLINICAL ETHICS

A profession is one in which one "professes" or takes an oath. The essence of professionalism is the primary concern for the welfare of those whom the professional serves over his own proprietary interests.[5]

Bernat's *Ethics in Neurology*[5] lists 10 defining characteristics of a learned profession:

1. The profession possesses a circumscribed and socially valuable body of knowledge.
2. The members of the profession determine the profession's standards of knowledge and expertise.
3. The profession attracts high-quality students who undergo an extensive socialization process as they are absorbed into the profession.
4. The profession is given authority to license practitioners by the state, with licensing and admission boards made up largely of members of the profession.
5. There is an ostensible sense of community and mutuality of interests among members of a profession.

6. Social policy and legislation that relate to the profession are heavily influenced by members of the profession through such mechanisms as lobbying and expert testimony.
7. The profession has a code of ethics that governs practice, the tenets of which are more stringent than legal controls.
8. A service orientation supersedes the proprietary interests of the professionals.
9. A profession is a terminal occupation, that is, it is the practitioner's singular and lifelong occupational choice.
10. A profession is largely free of lay control, with its practitioners exercising a high degree of occupational autonomy.

The focus of clinical ethics is set on the duties clinicians owe to their patients. Clinicians also have ethical duties toward families of patients, toward other health-care providers, to society, and in patient research.

The clinician's duty to his or her patients is the cornerstone of clinical medical ethics. Application of moral rules and ethical theories is codified into practice by professional societies. The following are excerpts modified from the American College of Physicians *Ethics Manual*.[11] It incorporates principles of *beneficence*—duty to promote good and prevent harm to patients; *nonmaleficence*—the duty to do no harm to patients; respect for a patient's *autonomy*—the duty to protect and foster an individual's free and uncoerced choices as well as rules for *truth telling, disclosure,* and *informed consent*. It includes the basic tenets of the doctor-patient relationship. The codes of conduct are the same for you in the pharmacy profession:

- The patient's welfare and best interests must be the clinician's main concern. The physician and team should treat and cure when possible and help patients cope with illness, disability, and death. In all instances, the physician and team must help maintain the dignity of the person and respect the uniqueness of each person.
- Confidentiality is a fundamental tenet of medical care. It respects the privacy of patients, encourages them to seek medical care and to discuss their problems candidly, and prevents discrimination based on their medical condition. The clinician must not release information without the patient's consent. Confidentiality, like other ethical duties, is not absolute. It may have to be overridden to protect others or the public—for example, to warn sexual partners that a patient has syphilis or AIDS. Before breaching confidentiality, the clinician should make every effort to discuss the issues with the patient and minimize harm to the patient.
- The physician and team are obligated to ensure that the patient is informed about the nature of the patient's medical condition, the objectives of the proposed treatment, treatment alternatives, possible outcomes, and the risks involved. This doctrine of informed consent must not be coerced.
  - Lack of *decision-making capacity* can usually be determined by the physician when it has been carefully determined that the patient is incapable of understanding the nature of the proposed treatment, the alternatives, the risks and benefits, and the

consequences. When a patient lacks *decision-making capacity*, an appropriate surrogate should make decisions with the physician. Ideally, the surrogate decision makers should know the patient's choices and values and act in the best interests of the patient. If the patient has designated a proxy, as through a durable power of attorney for health care, that choice should be respected. When patients have not selected surrogates, the standard clinical practice is for family members to serve as surrogates. Some states designate the order in which family members will serve as surrogates, and physicians should be aware of legal requirements in their state for surrogate appointment and decision making. Physicians should take reasonable care to assure that the surrogate's decisions are consistent with the patient's preferences. Physicians should emphasize that decisions be based on what the patient would want and not on what surrogates would choose for themselves. In order of priority, decisions should be based on advance directives (competent patients state what treatments they would accept or decline if they lost decision-making capacity), substituted judgments (the surrogate attempts to make the judgment that the patient, if competent, would have made), and best interests of the patient.

- It is unethical for a physician to refuse to care for a patient solely because of medical risk, or perceived risk, to the physician.
- Requests by patients for treatment outside the recognized methods of medical care pit the physician's judgment on optimal medical therapy against the patient's right to choose what care to receive and from whom. The physician should be sure that the patient understands the condition, traditional medical treatment, and expected outcomes. The physician should not abandon the patient who elects to try an unorthodox treatment and should regard the patient's decision with grace and compassion. In general, the physician should not participate in such treatment. When the treatment is clearly harmful to patients, the physician should seek the best means by which to protect the patient and, where possible, have dangerous therapy challenged.
- Physicians should be discouraged from treating close friends or family members. Potential problems include feelings of constraints on time or resources, incomplete disclosure of patient information, or limited physical examination.
- It is unethical for a physician to become sexually involved with a current patient even if the patient initiates or consents to the contact. Issues of dependency, trust, transference, and inequalities of power lead to increased vulnerability of the patient and require that a physician not cross the boundary.
- Financial arrangements should be clarified, and means of payment or inability to pay should be established. Fees for physician services should accurately reflect services provided. As professionals dedicated to serving the sick, physicians should contribute services to the uninsured and underinsured and do their fair share to ensure that all people receive adequate medical care.
- When conflicts of interest arise, the moral principle is clear. The welfare of the patient must at all times be paramount, and the clinician must insist that the

medically appropriate level of care take primacy over fiscal considerations imposed by the physician's own practice, investments, or financial arrangements. Trust in the profession is undermined when there is even the appearance of impropriety.

- Physicians should distinguish among withdrawing life-sustaining treatment, allowing the natural process of death to occur, and taking deliberate actions to shorten a patient's life. Physician involvement in deliberately hastening a patient's death has long been prohibited in professional codes. Uncontrolled pain may lead patients to request assisted suicide. Physicians should make relief of suffering in the terminally ill patient their highest priority as long as this accords to the patient's wishes. In most cases, the patient will withdraw the request for assisted suicide when pain management, depression, and other concerns have been addressed.

- Physicians should obtain consultation when they feel a need for assistance in caring for the patient.

- Patient care must never be compromised because a physician's judgment or skill is impaired. Every physician is responsible for protecting patients from an impaired physician and for assisting a colleague whose professional capability is impaired.

- It is unethical for a clinician to disparage the professional competence, knowledge, qualifications, or services of another clinician to a patient or a third party or to state or imply that a patient has been poorly managed or mistreated by a colleague without substantial evidence, especially when such behavior is used to recruit patients. Of equal importance, it is unethical for a clinician not to report fraud, professional misconduct, incompetence, or abandonment of a patient by another clinician. All clinicians have a duty to participate in peer review.

- Society has conferred professional prerogatives on physicians in the belief that they will use such power for the benefit of patients. In turn, physicians and the health-care team are responsible and accountable to society for their professional actions.

- All physicians must fulfill the profession's collective responsibility to be advocates for the health of the public.

- Decisions on resource allocations must not be made in the context of an individual patient-physician encounter but must be part of a broader social process.

- The physician and pharmacist should help develop health policy at the local, state, and national levels by expressing views as an individual and as a professional.

- The interests of the patient have primacy in all aspects of the patient-physician relationship. All health professionals share a commitment to work together to serve the patient's interests. The best patient care is often a team effort, and mutual respect, cooperation, and communication should govern this effort.

- Ethics committees and consultants contribute to achieving patient care goals primarily by developing educational programs in the institution coordinating institutional resources, providing a forum for discussion among medical and hospital professionals, and assisting institutions to develop sound policies and practices. Although it is generally agreed that neither ethics committees nor consultants should have decision-making authority, they can advise physicians on ethical matters.

- Physicians should remember that all citizens are equal under the law, and being ill does not diminish the right or expectation to be treated equally.
- Although physicians cannot be compelled to participate as expert witnesses, the profession as a whole has the ethical duty to assist patients and society in resolving disputes.
- It is unethical for physicians to withhold medical services through strikes when patients will be harmed or when the strike is for the physician's benefit.
- Advances in the diagnosis and treatment of disease are based on well-designed, carefully controlled, and ethically conducted clinical studies. Subjects must be equitably selected and instructed concerning the nature of the research; consent from the subject or an authorized representative must be truly informed and given freely; research must be planned thoughtfully, so that it has a high probability of yielding significant results; risks to patients must be minimized; and the benefit/risk ratio must be sufficiently high to justify the research effort.
- When there is no precedent for innovative therapy, consultation with peers, an institutional review board, or other expert group is necessary to assess whether the innovation is in the patient's best interest, the risks of the innovation, and probable outcomes of not using a standard therapy.[11]

Notice within the codes of conduct, the clinician has some ethical duties beyond the patient, including to the patient's family, to the medical profession, to society, and in patient research. The patient's family is often a partner in patient care. Duties to other medical professionals include teaching other clinicians as well as the patients and participation in peer-reviewed activities to protect patients from impaired and incompetent physicians. Duties to society include protecting the safety of the general public. This may even override the very important oath of confidentiality. The President's Commission for the Study of Ethical Problems in Medicine and Biomedical and Behavioral Research stipulated five conditions for which a physician may override his ordinary ethical duty to maintain the confidentiality of a patient's clinical information[8]:

1. Reasonable efforts to elicit voluntary consent to disclosure have failed.
2. There is a high probability that harm would occur if the information is withheld.
3. There is a high probability that the disclosed information would avert that harm.
4. There is a high probability that the harm inflicted on the third party would be serious.
5. Appropriate precautions would be taken to ensure that the only information conveyed is that necessary to avert the harm.

Duties to society require physicians and pharmacists to promote measures to improve the public health of all citizens. The physician and pharmacist who conduct clinical research should have the research critiqued and approved by institutional review boards to safeguard patient/subject safety.[8]

## CONCLUSION: THE DOCTOR/CLINICIAN-PATIENT RELATIONSHIP IS THE CORE OF CLINICAL ETHICS

The doctor/clinician-patient relationship is at the core of clinical ethics. Dr. Mark Siegler published an article entitled "Falling off the pedestal: what is happening to the traditional doctor-patient relationship?" in *Mayo Clinic Proceedings* in 1993[12] in which he described the Doctor-Patient Accommodation Model that respected the autonomy of both patients and physicians. This model is a *shared decision-making* model in which both physicians and patients make active and essential contributions. Physicians bring their medical training, knowledge, and expertise, including an understanding of the available treatment alternatives, to the diagnosis and management of the patient's conditions. Patients bring their own subjective aims and values through which the risks and benefits of various treatment options can be evaluated. The Doctor-Patient Accommodation Model relies heavily on communication, discussion, and negotiation. It incorporates Plato's description of "medicine befitting free men" (in Plato's *The Laws*). Plato wrote that the citizen physician "treats a disease by going into things thoroughly from the beginning in a scientific way and takes the patient and his family into confidence. Thus, he learns something from the sufferers. . . . He does not give prescriptions until he has won the patient's support, and when he has done so, he steadily aims at producing complete restoration to health by persuading the sufferer into compliance."[12]

You, as a practicing pharmacist in the outpatient or inpatient setting, make clinical decisions every day. After reading this chapter it is hoped that you now recognize that ethical decision making is involved in every clinical interaction you have with patients. As clinicians with the best intentions of "doing the right thing," you can refer to your professional society, which has codes of conduct, and the legal system, which has statutes and laws, but the core of how to decide what is ethically acceptable and not acceptable is found within yourself, vigilantly keeping in mind the duties and biases you bring to the clinician/doctor-patient relationship. If in the course of clinical decision making you encounter situations in which you find yourself trying to sort out which course of action would have acceptable ethical grounding, this chapter was incorporated into this book to help you think these situations through as thoroughly as possible. Use the information from this chapter. Remember the history of events that led to the development of the field of clinical ethics. Remember the four biomedical principles (*autonomy, beneficence, nonmaleficence,* and *justice*). Then apply the "four boxes" clinical ethics analysis method of Jonsen et al (*medical indications, patient preferences, quality of life,* and *contextual features*) to assist yourself in identifying, analyzing, and resolving ethical issues in your clinical case.

## APPLICATION EXERCISES

1. In Jonsen et al's four boxes of clinical medical ethics decision making, the four are not weighted equally. Which two trump the other two?
2. If conflicts of interest arise, what is the overriding moral principal?
3. What are the four bioethics principles?
4. What are Siegler's four boxes in clinical medical ethics decision making?
5. What is the core of clinical medical ethics?

## REFERENCES

1. Jonsen A, Siegler M, Winslade W. *Clinical Ethics: A Practical Approach to Ethical Decisions in Clinical Medicine.* 6th ed. New York, NY: McGraw-Hill; 2006.
2. Miles S. Translations of the Oath. Presentation at University of Chicago McLean Center for Clinical Medical Ethics Conference. November 2001.
3. American Pharmacists Association. The Oath of a Pharmacist. Available at http://www.pharmacist.com/oath-pharmacist. Accessed March, 2014.
4. American Pharmacists Association. The Code of Ethics for Pharmacists. Available at http://www.pharmacist.com/code-ethics. Accessed March, 2014.
5. Bernat JL. *Ethical Issues in Neurology.* Boston, MA: Butterworth-Heinemann; 1994.
6. Shuster E. The Nuremberg Code: Hippocratic ethics and human rights. *Lancet.* 1998;351(n9107):974–977.
7. Wolinsky H. Steps still being taken to undo damage of "America's Nuremberg." *Ann Intern Med.* 1997;127(4):143–144.
8. The National Commission for the Protection of Human Subjects of Biomedical and Behavioral Research. *The Belmont Report: Ethical Principles and Guidelines for the Protection of Human Subjects of Research.* OPRR Reports. Washington: US Government Printing Office; 1978:1–8.
9. Beauchamp TL, Childress JF. *Principles of Biomedical Ethics.* 3rd ed. New York, NY: Oxford University Press; 1989.
10. Siegler M. Communication during his address to the University of Chicago McLean Center for Clinical Medical Ethics Conference. November 2001.
11. American College of Physicians. Ethics manual. 3rd ed. *Ann Intern Med.* 1992;117:947–960.
12. Siegler M. Falling off the pedestal: what is happening to the traditional doctor–patient relationship? *Mayo Clin Proc.* 1993;68:461–467.

## ANSWERS TO APPLICATION EXERCISES

1. Medical indications and patient preferences.
2. When conflicts of interest arise, the moral principle is clear. The welfare of the patient must at all times be paramount, and the clinician must insist that the

medically appropriate level of care take primacy over fiscal considerations imposed by the clinician's own practice, investments, or financial arrangements. Trust in the profession is undermined when there is even the appearance of impropriety.

3. Autonomy, beneficence, nonmaleficence, justice.
4. Medical indications, patient preferences, quality of life, contextual features.
5. The doctor/clinician-patient relationship is the core of clinical ethics.

CHAPTER

3

# Pharmacy as a Community-Based Profession

*Kevin R. Kearney*

**Objectives: Upon completion of the chapter and exercises, the student pharmacist will be able to**

1. Define service-learning and describe ways that it has been implemented in the education of pharmacists.
2. Explain how service to the community, coupled with appropriate reflection, can lead to relevant learning.
3. Describe the professional and educational potential of community engagement and service-learning.
4. Evaluate outcomes resulting from service-learning in pharmacy education or pharmacist involvement in community programs.
5. Employ reflection in the classroom and following activities in the community.
6. Predict the impact of a community engagement through a student organization, or service-learning in a course on your future practice of pharmacy.

---

### Patient Encounter

### "PHARMACY AS A COMMUNITY-BASED PROFESSION"

### (SERVICE-LEARNING)

Discussion (based on the Patient Encounter from Chap. 2, pages 18–19):

Consider how this tragic situation could be transformed into a positive one, benefiting both the patient and the community. Imagine how you, the pharmacist, could both bring hope to the patient (and his family) and turn this into a "teaching moment" for the community. Specifically: Though it is clear that this young man will most likely never ride a bicycle again, can we find a way for him to channel his energy and drive to benefit others? He may never win another Olympic medal, but might he be able to save lives or improve others' lives? And might this not eventually be an accomplishment at least as significant as winning another gold medal?

*(continued on next page)*

As a pharmacist who understands both the community's needs and some of the resources available to meet those needs, especially in the area of health care, could you suggest some ways that this young man could work to achieve some important goals? Is there a Brain Injury Association or Public Health Department in your community, with which he might work to encourage people to take concrete steps to reduce the risk of brain injuries (such as wearing bicycle helmets)? Could he work with a hospital or rehabilitation center to help people recovering from brain injuries? Could he visit local schools to encourage children to practice "safe cycling?" As an Olympic Gold Medalist, he might be able to attract attention to these important issues—more so than others could. As someone recovering from a severe life-altering injury, he might be able to offer hope to others in similar circumstances. (You might want to read, and tell your patient, about the great African American cyclist Marshall "Major" Taylor—someone who overcame tremendous adversity.)

As a pharmacist grounded in your community, you may be able to benefit both this patient and the community. Deciding whether and how to do this is up to you.

## INTRODUCTION

It is critically important that pharmacists understand, and be prepared to provide service and care for the diverse populations in the communities where they practice. For many people, the pharmacist is the first or primary contact with the health-care system. The way pharmacists are dispersed throughout the community, anyone can walk into the neighborhood pharmacy at almost any time and speak with a pharmacist about health-care or public health issues.

Few people would question the importance of educating pharmacy students in the pharmaceutical sciences or the practice of patient-centered care. However, there are those who would, and do, question why student pharmacists are placed in the community to learn in areas that are on the surface considered unrelated to the practice of pharmacy. Many pharmacy practitioners and others believe that learning about the population of communities where they will practice and the diversity that exists within those communities is as important for students as the basic sciences and therapeutic topics. Some of this knowledge can be acquired from reading, scanning information on the Internet, and in a classroom, but one of the best ways to learn about the community is to link real-world experiences to traditional methods of teaching and learning. Many educators believe that integrating multiple experiences for students in the community throughout the pharmacy curriculum is more effective and long lasting than providing one or two experiences near the end of the curriculum. An integrated curriculum indicates that these educational experiences are vital to the students learning.

## SERVICE-LEARNING

When students' real-world experiences involve providing service to underserved populations in local communities, and these experiences are coupled with educational outcomes designed to help students to learn from the experiences and reflection about the experiences, the result is a teaching and learning methodology called service-learning (SL). Educators and community leaders talk and write about the place of service-learning in health-care education, and specifically in pharmacy education. In fact, theorizing and conversation has been going on for close to 20 years. Connors and Seifer[1,2] have written articles that are quoted by national leaders in health-care education and practice. Community-Campus Partnerships for Health (CCPH) is an organization in the United States that was born from these ideas. The leaders of CCPH support, develop, and promote extensive information on their web site, about service-learning in health-care education and community partnerships.[3] Other US and international organizations also seek to improve health professions and community partnerships and to encourage engagement by university faculty and students. Various authors have written about service-learning in pharmacy education[4-23] and in 2004 the *American Journal of Pharmaceutical Education* published a theme issue on service-learning in pharmacy education.[24-31]

### Community Partnerships

Community engagement, and partnership, means listening to the leaders of the community and meeting their needs, as well as those of a course, an individual faculty member, or a student. Trust is important in partnerships, and even as a student it is essential that you become a part of that trust. Service-learning is the same: it is important that all the parties involved listen to each other to plans for action, and that courses be developed by faculty members who partner with organizations, build trust, and promote communication.

### Courses in the Pharmacy Curriculum

Service-learning has been incorporated into courses as a part of the education of student pharmacists. Across the 100 plus colleges of pharmacy in the United States and Canada, the methodology of service-learning has been integrated into courses in multiple places. Courses using service-learning may appear early in the professional phase of the curriculum,[5,9,15–17,19–23,25,27] across the curriculum, or toward the end,[12,13,14] and/or as part of a residency program.[11] The place in the curriculum, and the desired educational outcomes, guide the selection of partnerships and associated learning activities. In the early part of a curriculum, a wide variety of service activities may be instituted including tutoring, distributing food and clothing in a shelter, working with Habitat for Humanity, and being paired with an individual from the community. All of these activities provide potential for learning when they are attached to curricular goals such as developing communication skills, becoming familiar or comfortable with diverse populations, and learning about public health. Later in the curriculum, more advanced learning objectives such as developing patient counseling skills, and learning about the management of specific disease states, may be part of a course that requires service-learning. The activities in these courses may be connected to the practice of pharmacy as it is in 2013, but they may also help move the practice to what can be imagined for 2020.

The following core questions drive the discussion and move you to place of understanding in order for you to be able to answer them. What can you learn from a course that uses service-learning to teach? What do you need to do to learn from service as a future health-care professional? Who benefits and how is that benefit received from service-learning and partnerships?

## WHAT CAN YOU LEARN FROM SERVICE-LEARNING?

Eyler, Giles, and colleagues have written at length about this topic, with regard to many disciplines and various levels of education.[32,33] These authors provide ample evidence that service-learning can and does lead to relevant curricular outcomes for students who participate. Reading articles and books written by these authors and others will help you better understand and incorporate into your practice the basic information provided in this chapter. The following paragraphs discuss the outcomes from participation in service-learning courses, which are relevant to pharmacy education.

### Communication Skills

Community service experiences offer opportunities for hands-on development and honing of verbal, nonverbal, presentation, and writing skills. For example, you can practice active listening and nonverbal communication with leaders, peers, and clients during this kind of course. You are encouraged to try out new communication techniques during your experiences in the community. You may reflect on your experiences in classroom discussions or by writing about your feelings related to participating in community and service projects. An entire chapter of this textbook is devoted to communication: for more review and application exercises refer to Chapter 4.

## Diverse Populations

It is much easier to be comfortable with people of similar backgrounds, such as members of our families and friends, than with strangers who do not share the same background and values. We are probably also more comfortable with people like those we know in our neighborhoods and communities, than with those who do not come from there. Comfort is primarily due to awareness and similarity of backgrounds. We may have common friends, similar educational experiences, and common interests to draw on when determining how to act in a professional situation. The wider the circle of associations, however, the less comfortable we may feel because we are less familiar with them. A pharmacist, in order to provide quality care to any patient encountered must be comfortable with a wide variety of people and backgrounds, not just those that are like her/his family and neighbors. Comfort and the ability to care for others depend on recognition and respect of the differences of others. One way to increase this understanding is to engage in work with, or to provide help to, people with diverse backgrounds and values. Providing assistance as part of a course that includes service-learning is an excellent way to improve your comfort level with those who do not look like, or have the same values, as you. Appropriate learning exercises will be assigned throughout a course to go along with your experiences in the community. You can increase your knowledge, skills, and ability to care for people of differing backgrounds by maintaining an open mind, being curious, and respectful of tradition and beliefs. There are several good resources that address the issue of understanding diverse populations or improving cultural competence that you or your faculty may use in the classroom.[34-38] An online resource that is easily accessible is Galanti's Cultural Diversity in Health Care web site.[39]

In a course taught at a School of Pharmacy in New England, classroom exercises focused on cultural competence begin with the primary resource available—the students' own diverse cultural backgrounds. A quick survey of the students in the class is conducted to identify backgrounds, family of origin, and living or working experience with diverse populations. Each student is assigned to become an expert on a culture, ideally her/his own, such that all major cultures are represented in the class. Students are required to read a selection of materials about their assigned cultures and health-care issues related to that civilization, and to come to the next classroom discussion prepared to talk about those cultures from the perspective of a member, based on their readings and personal experiences. In a culturally diverse classroom, this typically leads to lively and enlightening discussions. In classrooms with less natural diversity, the potential exists for lively discussion if all the participants take the exercise seriously. This offers students an opportunity to both teach and learn from classmates. If your professor does not assign this type of work for the classroom, you and a group of friends can design your own exercise, assign cultures to each other, and practice improving your cultural competence outside of the classroom.

## How to Assess the Quality of Service

How does one evaluate the quality of service or assistance provided? This is an important question whether the service is provided by students in a course or by a pharmacist in a pharmacy. If the goal is to provide high-quality service, then we need to know what high quality entails. What I propose to students at the beginning of their service-learning course is that they use five criteria identified by Indritz and Hadsall[40] to assess their work. These authors wrote about how pharmacists could evaluate the quality of the service provided in a retail pharmacy. Their evaluation criteria are also applicable to service-learning outcomes. The following describes those criteria in a question format that can be used by you to assess individual quality.

Are you *reliable*? Can people count on you to provide the service they need? Are you prepared for your work? Do you arrive on time?

Are you *responsive* to the people with whom you work? The prerequisite for this is that the student must be attentive to those with whom she/he works. Do you listen to people? Do you do your best to understand and respond to their needs?

Do you provide *assurance* to those you are serving? Do you provide competent advice, encouragement, and assistance? Do you provide it in such a way that people know that they are safe?

Are you *empathetic* in your work? In contrast to empathy, sympathy is feeling sorry for someone. Empathy requires that the provider make a point to know the person she/he is working with well enough to know what it means to identify with that person's feelings. A computer may be able to provide competent technical/clinical information (eg, about drug interactions) but a pharmacist needs to also appreciate (empathize with) patients feelings in order to be able to provide high-quality service.

The last criterion is *tangibles*. In any human interaction, there are physical dimensions which, though may not be the most important aspect of the interaction, still require attention. Most of the time the tangible factors are acceptable, so most of us do not even notice them. It is only when something is askew that we notice it. The task of the provider is to make sure that these tangibles are in order. For example, professional dress and behavior set the stage for professional service. Physical setting is also important: it may be difficult to tutor children in a disordered or noisy environment, just as customers or patients may wonder about the quality of the service they can expect in a disordered or dirty pharmacy. Health-care professionals need to understand the importance of such tangible factors and being attentive to them during a service-learning experience can help you determine what the tangibles are and the extent of their importance.

Using these five criteria to measure the success of your community work may prompt thinking about what it means to be a service- and patient-centered care provider. These behaviors will be a primary focus of the pharmacist in the future. With this in mind, the link between service-learning and pharmacy as a community-based profession should become clear, and this should help launch your plans for future action.

## WHAT DO YOU NEED TO DO TO LEARN FROM SERVICE IN THE COMMUNITY?

Learning does not just happen when one does work in the community. It is possible that you may learn some lessons simply because of your involvement in volunteering or service; but to maximize and optimize learning, it is essential to take certain steps before, during, and after the work. You should engage in a variety of exercises for the best learning outcomes. Individual preparation for, and reflection on, experiences may be the most appropriate learning tool for you. Remember that one of the required components of the service-learning teaching method is reflection. Some will find that the discipline of writing about experiences helps them learn. Others will learn from discussing their experiences, or giving a presentation about their work. Ideally, a service-learning course will involve all of these methods, so that students having a variety of preferred learning styles will be able to learn as much as possible from their activities. Whatever community service you do, there are things to learn that will affect your professional actions.

### Prepare

You may already appreciate that what one learns from an educational experience depends on the amount of effort applied to it. For example, if you are going to tutor a child, you may need to review the subject matter before meeting with the child, and possibly prepare some examples to teach a concept. In this way you also learn something, whether it is the concepts you teach, or how to communicate effectively. If you are going to visit an elder in a nursing home, you may want to bring some stories from recent news to share with her/him in order to engage that person in what is happening outside the walls of the home. In this manner, you may keep up with the local events, or practice a different style of communication than you are used to. If you are going to explain the elements of proper nutrition to a group of people at a community center, you need to review nutrition principles and practice, and devise a plan for presenting the material. Such preparatory work will improve both the quality of the service and what you learn.

### Listen

A professional typically approaches volunteer or service work with the knowledge that she/he has the skills necessary for the job, and a plan for using those skills to benefit others. It is important to have the appropriate skills and plans, but they are not the sole prerequisites if one wants to provide quality service and to learn from it. You must also approach the work with an open mind and a readiness to learn from the experience. The first part of that approach is a readiness to listen. This is both an element of effective communication, and the prerequisite for being a responsive provider.

If you listen to the people you want to serve, you will come to know them better and you will be able to meet their needs more efficiently and effectively. By listening you will learn what the immediate wants of the community are, and what their

strengths and most important needs are at the moment. This approach to engagement applies to a homeless person in a soup kitchen, a child in a recreation program, an elder in a nursing home, or a patient in a pharmacy. Listening will lead to
enhanced learning in a service-learning course placement, and the same skills will
someday make you a better pharmacist.

## Think and Write

Another way to learn from service experiences is to think and write about them.
For optimal learning, this reflective process should be organized in some systematic
way. One system is based on the subjective, objective, assessment, and plan method,
which is used by many health-care professionals and students. This system guides a
student's reflection on experiences based on four areas: subjective, objective, assessment, and planning (SOAP). Questions that you might ask yourself, and things you
might write about, that fit into the format, are the following:

*Subjective*: How did this experience affect you? What was your reaction to the expe-
    rience? What were your impressions of the staff or of the clients—the people you
    served? Did anything surprise you? Encourage you? Disappoint you?
*Objective*: Describe what you observed and did at your service site. Describe any
    people you worked with. What did the site look like? What did people say or do?
    What successes did you have? What problems did you encounter? How did you
    deal with them?
*Assessment*: As you reflect on your experience, what can you learn from it? What did
    you learn about the people you were serving—their strengths, needs, etc? Were
    you successful in your work? If not, how could you do it better?
*Planning*: Based on experiences, what do you plan to do on your next visit to the work
    site? Are there successful activities that you want to repeat? Might you do some
    things differently the next time? How do you plan to prepare for you next visit?

If you keep a journal, making SOAP entries after each session at a site will
enrich the learning associated with the service and provide a record of the service
and learning accomplishments. This also prepares you for the reflective processes
that will be used later in the curriculum to learn from patient-focused experiences.
There is further discussion of the SOAP note in Chapter 5. Refer back to it for more
in-depth discussion.

## Discuss

Some people learn from experiences by talking about them. If you learn like this,
then classroom discussion with its opportunities for face-to-face interaction is an
excellent way to reflect on service to the community and learn. Some topics lend
themselves especially well to this form of reflection. For example, reading and talking about the diversity of cultures can enhance cultural competence, as noted above.

Another topic that can be addressed in a classroom discussion is communication: active listening techniques can be modeled and practiced, and both good and poor body language can be demonstrated. Focused discussions about cultural diversity and communication can help students learn from their outside-the-classroom service work and prepare to improve the processes for the future.

*Tell Someone What You Have Done and Learned*

A good way to learn about a topic is to teach it. One of the most effective ways to guide students to learn from service experiences is to ask them to give presentations to classmates about their service and learning accomplishments. To prepare a presentation, you might first ask yourself some of the following questions: How did I serve people in the community and what were the concrete results of my service? What did I learn about the people I served, the organization with which I worked, and the community where this took place? Finally, how will this service and learning make me a better person, and someday a better health-care professional? The discipline of organizing and distilling one's thoughts about these topics helps both the presenter and the listeners.

## WHO BENEFITS FROM SERVICE-LEARNING AND HOW?

### The People You Work with

By definition, in service-learning all partners should benefit. If only the community benefits then the activities offered to the community were likely not tied to educational goals for those involved. If only the student benefits, then community members were likely not involved in deciding what could be done to meet their needs, or perhaps a partnership and trust were lacking. The beneficiaries of a course involving service-learning must include all involved parties, including students.[1–3] Whether one is tutoring children, supervising a recreation program, serving a meal in a soup kitchen, visiting elders in a nursing home, or performing almost any other form of service, those being served should benefit in some way. Service projects ought to be selected based on actual needs identified by members of the community, and the service activities should be designed to effectively meet those needs. The child who is tutored should do better in a class or overall in school as a result of the tutoring. People served by an organization should thrive with additional help. It may be possible to add new services because there are more service-providers, so more individuals may be served. These are some of the benefits seen for individuals when service-learning courses are implemented with community partners.

### The Organization You Work with

Many nonprofit organizations where students work when involved in a course have limited human and financial resources. Students fill a critical need for such organizations. The addition of students enables the agencies to fulfill their missions, and students provide support and relief to the employees of the organizations while learning important ideals and skills. In some cases, students may have special skills that may benefit an organization in unique ways. For example, a student may have strong computer skills and may be able to teach people within the organization, or clients such as those in a senior center or nursing home. Someone with web design experience may be able to help a nonprofit organization improve its web site. A bilingual student may be able to provide translation services for an organization. It is helpful for students to identify such skills before beginning a course so that their ability can be put to good use if needed.

## Your Community

Communities depend on the individuals and organizations providing critical services, such as education, housing, health care, and social services. One person may have a limited impact on a community, depending on her/his involvement; but a large contingent of students completing a course can have a significant impact on a community, especially if efforts are targeted to reach a specific population or problem. An example of a group impact would be health professions students' involvement with an entire school system or a subsection of a large school district. If pharmacy students serve as tutors, mentors, and classroom aides in the elementary, middle, and high schools, over a period of time it is likely that students in that system will encounter pharmacy students multiple times. These repeated contacts may help some children do better in school, give them an incentive to set high goals in their lives, and even encourage some to consider a career in health care.

## You

Many students find that they gain significantly from service-learning experiences in a course. Students have reported increased self-confidence, development of important people skills that will benefit them later in life, and knowledge gain about service organizations in the community. The community impact may also extend beyond the course and leave an indelible mark upon the community. In addition, the knowledge you gain from your participation in the community as a student may inspire you to do more of such work, not only during your pharmacy school career, but later in life. As a pharmacist, you have a responsibility to improve the health of a community through service, advocacy, and advancement of the profession. These opportunities to participate in community engagement and service-learning courses throughout the curriculum provide you the chance to grow both personally and professionally. There are pharmacists and faculty members who will guide you and support your interests because they will have the same mission.

This chapter has focused on service to the community as part of a course. You can gain many of the benefits of service-learning even if you are not enrolled in a course. Individually, or in a group, you can volunteer to help in your community and combine this work with reflection. By writing down your experiences and emotions in a journal you can develop your knowledge and skills beyond what volunteering alone would do to enhance your learning. If you participate in professional student organizations, you can incorporate ideas suggested in this chapter to learn and to improve the quality of your service while you are participating in specific community projects. You can lead a small group discussion reflecting on the activities of the organization. Another exercise that you may do is to gather a group of classmates together for participation in some of the practice exercises at the end of this chapter. Use your experiences from individual volunteer activities or professional student organizations to reflect and learn, comparing experiences, concerns, and plans for future involvement.

## CONCLUSION

Pharmacies constitute one of the most widely dispersed networks in the health-care system in any community, which places pharmacists on the front line and forefront to lead the future of prevention and wellness in health care. To make the best use of this broad network, it is essential that pharmacy students be educated to know and respect, and be prepared to serve, the diverse populations of people they will encounter as a professional in health care. Courses that incorporate community-based service-learning provide students that opportunity to learn.

## APPLICATION EXERCISES

1. What elements of service-learning are essential for effective learning?
2. What are some of the potential learning outcomes of service-learning, relevant to pharmacists and pharmacy students?
3. What are some criteria for assessing the quality of the service you provide?
4. What issues and questions should be addressed in journal entries to lead to learning from service experiences?
5. What should be included in a written report or oral presentation to explain to a reader or audience the outcomes of service-learning experiences?

## REFLECTIVE EXERCISES

These exercises can be assigned to individuals or small groups or can be altered to fit into a large classroom exercise.

1. To begin, take a few minutes to jot down your thoughts about the following questions related to your work in the community: What successes have you had? What have you learned from your experiences? Would you like feedback from the

others in your group about any issues you have encountered? Next, each member shares with the group what he/she has written. It is best if everyone in the group initially listens to each other as he/she speaks. Finally, the group discusses what the members have said, with the goal of learning from each other's experiences and helping each other by providing constructive feedback.

2. Consider one specific activity from the site where you have been placed—for example, tutoring, developing a presentation, or providing soup to a hungry child. Ask yourself this question: How will doing this improve my knowledge as a health-care provider in a world where the pharmacist's responsibility is to improve public health and individuals' wellness? Write a list of 10 items and then write a paragraph using 5 of those items explaining the practice of pharmacy in the year 2020 in a way that a 10-year-old can understand.

## REFERENCES

1. Connors K, Seifer SD. Service-learning in health professions education: what is service-learning, and why now? *A Guide for Developing Community-Responsive Models in Health Professions Education.* San Francisco, CA: Community-Campus Partnerships for Health; 1997:11–17.

2. Seifer SD. Service-learning: community-campus partnerships for health professions education. *Acad Med.* 1998;73(3):273–277.

3. Community-Campus Partnerships for Health. Service-Learning. Available at http://depts.washington.edu/ccph/servicelearningres.html. Accessed March, 2014.

4. Murawski MM, Murawski D, Wilson M. Service-learning and pharmaceutical education: an exploratory survey. *Am J Pharm Educ.* 1999;63:160–164. Available at http://archive.ajpe.org/legacy/pdfs/aj630207.pdf. Accessed March, 2014.

5. Nickman NA. (Re-)learning to care: use of service-learning as an early professionalization experience. *Am J Pharm Educ.* 1998;62:380–387. Available at http://archive.ajpe.org/legacy/pdfs/aj620404.pdf. Accessed March, 2014.

6. Lamsam GD. Development of a service-learning program. *Am J Pharm Educ.* 1999;63:41–45. Available at http://archive.ajpe.org/legacy/pdfs/aj630106.pdf. Accessed March, 2014.

7. Piper B, DeYoung M, Lamsam GD. Student perceptions of a service-learning experience. *Am J Pharm Educ.* 2000;64:159–165. Available at http://archive.ajpe.org/legacy/pdfs/aj640208.pdf. Accessed March, 2014.

8. Barner JC. Implementing service-learning in the pharmacy curriculum. *Am J Pharm Educ.* 2000;64:260–265. Available at http://archive.ajpe.org/legacy/pdfs/aj640306.pdf. Accessed on March, 2014.

9. Barner JC. First-year pharmacy students' perceptions of their service-learning experience. *Am J Pharm Educ.* 2000;64:266–271. Available at http://archive.ajpe.org/legacy/pdfs/aj640307.pdf. Accessed March, 2014.

10. Carter JT, Cochran GA. Service-learning projects in a public health in pharmacy course. *Am J Pharm Educ.* 2002;66:312–318. Available at http://archive.ajpe.org/legacy/pdfs/aj660316.pdf. Accessed March, 2014.

11. Conrad P, Murphy J, Sketris I. Drug use management and policy residency: a service-learning application. *Am J Pharm Educ.* 2004;69(5):Article 96. Available at http://archive.ajpe.org/aj6905/aj690596/aj690596.pdf. Accessed March, 2014.

12. Kirwin JL, VanAmbaugh JA, Napoli KM. Service-learning at a camp for children with asthma as part of an advanced pharmacy practice experience. *Am J Pharm Educ.* 2005;69(3):Article 49, 321–329. Available at http://archive.ajpe.org/aj6903/aj690349/aj690349.pdf. Accessed March, 2014.

13. Johnson JF. A diabetes camp as the service-learning capstone experience in a diabetes concentration. *Am J Pharm Educ.* 2007;71(6):Article 119, 1–8. Available at http://archive.ajpe.org/aj7106/aj7106119/aj7106119.pdf. Accessed March, 2014.

14. Roche VF, Jones RM, Hinman CE, et al. A service-learning elective in Native American culture, health and professional practice. *Am J Pharm Educ.* 2007;71(6):Article 129, 1–8. Available at http://archive.ajpe.org/aj7106/aj7106129/aj7106129.pdf. Accessed March, 2014.

15. Allen R, Mihm LB, Mihm DJ, Robinson D, et al. Evaluating the impact of a nutrition service-learning course on first-year pharmacy students. Meeting Abstracts: 109th Annual Meeting of the American Association of Colleges of Pharmacy, Chicago, IL, July 19–23, 2008. *Am J Pharm Educ.* 2008;72(3):Article 72. Available at http://www.ajpe.org/doi/pdf/10.5688/aj720372. Accessed March, 2014.

16. Brown B, Heaton PC, Wall A. A service-learning elective to promote enhanced understanding of civic, cultural, and social issues and health disparities in pharmacy. *Am J Pharm Educ.* 2007;71(1). Available at http://www.ajpe.org/doi/pdf/10.5688/aj710109. Accessed March, 2014.

17. Falter RA, Pignotti-Dumas K, Popish SJ, Petrelli HMW, Best MA, Wilkinson, JJ. A service learning program in providing nutrition education to children. *Am J Pharm Educ.* 2011;75(5):Article 85. Available at http://www.ajpe.org/doi/pdf/10.5688/ajpe75585. Accessed March, 2014.

18. Huynh C, Lott A. Lessons from a service-learning trip to Haiti. *American Journal of Health-System Pharmacy.* 2011;68(3):196–200.

19. Kearney KR. A service-learning course for first-year pharmacy students. *Am J Pharm Educ.* 2008;72(4):Article 86. Available at http://www.ajpe.org/doi/pdf/10.5688/aj720486. Accessed March, 2014.

20. Kearney KR. What educational difference does service-learning make? Poster abstract in *Am J Pharm Educ.* 2009;73(4):Article 57. Available at http://www.ajpe.org/doi/pdf/10.5688/aj730457. Accessed March, 2014.

21. Kearney KR. Impact of a service-learning course on first-year pharmacy students' learning outcomes. *Am J Pharm Educ.* 2013;77(2):Article 34.

22. Packard K, Sexson E, Spangler M, Walters R. A novel cardiovascular risk screening and health promotion service learning course. *Curr Pharm Teach Learn.* 2010;2:228–237.

23. Timpe EM, Wuller WR, Karpinski JP. A regional poison prevention education service-learning project. *Am J Pharm Educ.* 2008;72(4):Article 87. Available at http://www.ajpe.org/doi/pdf/10.5688/aj720487. Accessed March, 2014.

24. Kearney KR. Service-learning in pharmacy education. *Am J Pharm Educ.* 2004;68(1):Article 26. Available at http://www.ajpe.org/doi/pdf/10.5688/aj680126. Accessed March, 2014.

25. Peters SJ, MacKinnon GE, III. Introductory practice and service learning experiences in US pharmacy curricula. *Am J Pharm Educ.* 2004;68(1):Article 27. Available at http://www.ajpe.org/doi/pdf/10.5688/aj680127. Accessed March, 2014.

26. Nemire RE, Margulis L, Frenzel-Shepherd E. Prescription for a healthy service-learning course: a focus on the partnership. *Am J Pharm Educ.* 2004;68(1): Article 28. Available at http://www.ajpe.org/doi/pdf/10.5688/aj680128. Accessed March, 2014.

27. Kearney KR. Students' self-assessment of learning through service-learning. *Am J Pharm Educ.* 2004;68(1):Article 29. Available at http://www.ajpe.org/doi/pdf/10.5688/aj680129. Accessed March, 2014.

28. Jarvis C, James VL, Giles J, et al. Nutrition and nurturing: a service-learning nutrition pharmacy course. *Am J Pharm Educ.* 2004;68(2):Article 43. Available at http://www.ajpe.org/doi/pdf/10.5688/aj680243. Accessed March, 2014.

29. Drab S, Lamsam G, Connor S, et al. Incorporation of service-learning across four years of the PharmD curriculum. *Am J Pharm Educ.* 2004;68(2):Article 44. Available at http://www.ajpe.org/doi/pdf/10.5688/aj680244. Accessed March, 2014.

30. Schumann W, Moxley DP, Vanderwill W. Integrating service and reflection in the professional development of pharmacy students. *Am J Pharm Educ.* 2004;68(2):Article 45. Available at http://www.ajpe.org/doi/pdf/10.5688/aj680245. Accessed March, 2014.

31. Surratt CK, Desselle SP. The neuroscience behind drugs of abuse: a PharmD service-learning project. *Am J Pharm Educ.* 2004;68(4):Article 99. Available at http://www.ajpe.org/doi/pdf/10.5688/aj680499. Accessed March, 2014.

32. Eyler JS, Giles DE. *Where's the Learning in Service-Learning.* San Francisco, CA: Jossey-Bass; 1999.

33. Eyler JS, Giles DE, Stenson CM, et al. At a glance: what we know about the effects of service-learning on college students, faculty, institutions and communities, 1993-2000. *Campus Compact.* 3rd ed. Available at http://www.compact.org/wp-content/uploads/resources/downloads/aag.pdf. Accessed March, 2014.

34. Galanti G-A. *Caring for Patients from Different Cultures.* Philadelphia, PA: University of Pennsylvania Press; 2004.

35. Tseng W-S, Streltzer J. *Cultural Competence in Health Care.* New York, NY: Springer; 2008.

36. Rundle A, Carvalho M, Robinson M. *Cultural Competence in Health Care: A Practical Guide.* San Francisco, CA: Jossey-Bass; 2002.

37. CC: Halbur KV, Halbur DA. *Essentials of Cultural Competence in Pharmacy Practice.* Washington, DC: American Pharmacists Association; 2008.

38. CC: Haack S, Phillips C. Teaching cultural competency through a pharmacy skills and applications course series. *Am J Pharm Educ.* 2012;76(2):27. Available at http://www.ajpe.org/doi/pdf/10.5688/ajpe76227. Accessed March, 2014.

39. Galanti G-A. *Cultural Diversity in Healthcare.* Available at http://gagalanti.com/index.html. Accessed March, 2014.

40. Indritz MES, Hadsall RS. An active learning approach to teaching service at one college of pharmacy. *Am J Pharm Educ.* 1999;63(2):126–131. Available at http://archive.ajpe.org/legacy/pdfs/aj630202.pdf. Accessed March, 2014.

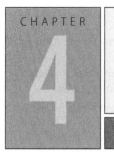
# Communication: An Overview

*Michelle T. Assa-Eley, Ceressa T. Ward*

**Objectives: Upon completion of the chapter and exercises, the student pharmacist will be able to**

1. Articulate the importance of communication skills.
2. Explain the process of communication including the types of messages (verbal or nonverbal), barriers, and the significance of participants' backgrounds.
3. Demonstrate appropriate listening behaviors and responses.
4. Conduct an efficient, effective patient interview and patient education session.
5. Use assertiveness to deal with difficult situations.
6. Explain the dimensions of nonverbal communication.
7. Explain common types of presentations for pharmacists.
8. Properly design presentation visual aids.
9. Identify key information needed when preparing a presentation.
10. Practice effective presentation techniques.
11. Describe the rationale for pharmacists to become effective writers.
12. Cite examples of writing responsibilities within the profession of pharmacy.
13. Develop strategies for improving your writing.

---

### Patient Encounter

### DISCUSSION POINTS: COMMUNICATION

Since you were approached by the patient's wife with her request to cease antibiotic therapy, you decide you need to speak with her in more detail about the situation and her feelings. Following appropriate guidelines for privacy, you take her into a small, unoccupied waiting room to have your conversation. Before you begin, you think about how you would try to structure and guide the conversation you have with her. Specifically, you think of how you would use the techniques presented in this chapter in your conversation with her. As you think about these things, answer the following questions:

*(continued on next page)*

- Considering the education background of your audience, will your responses consist of high-level medical terminology or layman's terms?
- Which types of responses to her concerns will be most effective? Which would not work as well?
- How will you use empathy in your responses?
- Think of responses to the patient's wife who says:

"I can't believe that my husband would want to live this way! These antibiotics are not necessary!"

"Why can't you just tell them not to give the antibiotics?"

"Would you want to live this way?"

"Don't you think this is the right thing to do?"

After your conversation, you must document what you have learned. Where and how will you do this?

While you are speaking with the patient's wife, it comes to mind that you have to present a patient's case at the weekly pharmacy student meeting with your preceptor, the attending pharmacist. You would like to discuss the case at the meeting. You know you would have to present a brief description of the patient's medical history. What format would you use for the presentation? How much time are you allotted for the presentation? How will you structure your materials (eg, handouts, slides etc.)? If handouts are used, how many should be prepared for distribution? Has the preceptor outlined any special requirements or instructions for how this presentation should be delivered? Once your presentation is complete, do you have enough time to practice and fine tune?

## INTRODUCTION

Many people assume that when children learn to talk, they also learn to communicate well. Other people believe that communication competence is something inherent in one's personality; that one can naturally communicate well or not well at all. Both of these are generally misconceptions. In truth, communication skills are learned and honed over time.

Communication skills are also very important to a person's success in his or her chosen profession. Now, as you are learning how to be a pharmacist, is a good time to evaluate your communication skills and to improve them where necessary. Personality is a factor in communication style, but people can certainly learn to be better communicators. Although there are requisite skills to master, you should definitely be yourself when you are talking with others, especially in a professional setting. People can perceive whether or not you are sincere. Trying to fake an interest in someone else is usually transparent. When patients recognize this lack of interest, they are unlikely to cooperate with you or provide you with the information that you need to help them.

As a pharmacist, you will be interacting with many people from different backgrounds, all in the same day. You may have to talk to physicians and nurses more than patients or vice versa, depending on your practice site. This chapter reviews techniques you can use to work with health-care providers, patients, or your employers/employees. The chapter focuses first on interactions with patients and patient-interviewing skills because patient interaction is one of the most significant types of communication for pharmacists. After a discussion of the importance of communication skills and a review of a model of communication, sections in this chapter are devoted to oral communication, barriers to communication, nonverbal communication, patient interviewing, patient education, making presentations, and written communication. You, too, can be an effective communicator even if you do not feel confident in your abilities right now. Some of you may feel you already know everything you need to know. Because applying communication techniques in a pharmacy is different from social settings, you may pick up a few good ideas in this chapter to help you develop professionally. As you read, try to leave your assumptions aside and envision how you can incorporate these skills into your daily communication.

## IMPORTANCE OF COMMUNICATION SKILLS

Communication skills are crucial to helping you develop your practice. Your position as a pharmacist will require you to communicate well verbally, orally, and in writing with health-care professionals and with patients. Writing skills are equally important as presenting a professional image with your oral communication. This section discusses the significance of fostering your good communication skills for yourself, your patients, and the health-care professionals with whom you work.

Early communication research[1] has shown that communication skills play an important role in career advancement. The skills that were identified as crucial included speaking, listening, and working well with groups. You may benefit in your career by improving your communication skills; however, your patients will also benefit. As Ley[2] describes, improving health-care provider communication has been shown to have several positive outcomes for patients. Specifically, better communication with health-care providers leads to a higher level of patient recall of information. This improvement in recall can help patients better manage their medications and their disease state. Further, enhanced communication has been found to be associated with patient satisfaction. Although this may seem trivial, patient satisfaction plays a major role in a patient's decision to return to a health-care provider and in the trust they place in that provider. Improved communication with providers can also have a moderate effect on patients' compliance with their medication regimens. Finally, communication has been shown to reduce the length of hospital stays for some patients. These benefits for patients have been proven repeatedly. Effective pharmacist communication has been shown to ensure optimal therapeutic outcomes and improve patients' medication use.[3–6] Pharmacists' participation in health care can reduce overall costs, reduce medication errors in the ordering stage, reduce length of patients' hospital stays, and reduce rates of hospital readmission.[7–10] Clearly, there are advantages for patients when their pharmacist becomes skilled in the art of communication.

Other health-care providers may benefit from your improved communication because they will be better able to learn from you. Having a pharmacist as part of the health-care team can prove to be extremely valuable for all of the professionals involved. Yet, a pharmacist who is unable to make her points heard and understood will not be an effective member of the team. Conversely, a pharmacist with good communication skills can make valuable contributions to the team. More importantly, these contributions can be made without creating tension among other professionals who may not fully understand the pharmacist's expanding role on the team.

Whether the improvement in your skills makes an impact on patients or other professionals, the benefits of a well-communicating pharmacist are immeasurable. In order to understand the factors that make up an interaction and the skills necessary to make those interactions go smoothly, we now turn to an exploration of a model of communication. By investigating these factors, you are better able to recognize the important points of communication that will help you develop your own approach.

## MODEL OF COMMUNICATION

Many researchers have investigated the nature of human communication by trying to explain and label the components associated with it. Thus, there are many models of communication. A model attempts to explain a phenomenon and lend a structure to an otherwise amorphous concept. Models help us better understand such concepts by allowing us to test the premises of the models and build on them. Even the earliest communication researchers developed models to guide their study.

There are many factors that can influence the process of communication. Think about the last time you had a conversation with a friend. You probably paid attention to the way he or she responded to you, both verbally and nonverbally. However, what you may not have considered are all the background factors that go into your interpretation of other people's behavior and their interpretation of yours. Your experience with them, your experiences in communicating with other people, your personality, your beliefs in general, your beliefs about the interaction you are having,

**Figure 4.1.** Integrated model of communication.

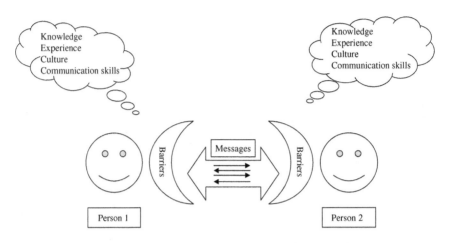

and your desired outcome all affect the way you interact with a friend. Although each of these factors is important, not all models of communication include them. Early models took a more simplistic view of the process, making the assumption that communication flows only in one direction at a time, or that only verbal messages were interpreted.

In our discussion of a model, let us consider the model illustrated in Fig. 4.1. This model includes elements from early models such as the Sender Message Channel Receiver (SMCR) model, Shannon-Weaver model, and the transaction model. Earlier models labeled one person as the "sender" and one as "receiver," but we now know that people are simultaneously sending and receiving messages, whether verbal or nonverbal. Throughout the course of a conversation, the parties may take turns sending verbal messages but are likely to be communicating even when not verbally during the entire exchange. Thus, in our model, the two participants are labeled as "person 1" and "person 2."

From the SMCR model,[11] we know that both people bring to the interaction their past experiences with each other and with other people. It is impossible to separate a person's background from the way he or she will perceive a message. Thus, two people's cultures, including the rules of interaction that they share, will shape their interactions and have been included in our model. For example, in some cultures it is considered rude to interrupt when another person is talking. Yet, in other cultures, the person who talks the loudest over the other is the one who is given the floor. You can see how this may influence the way one talks to another person.

Other examples of factors that may influence how a person interacts include his knowledge in the area being discussed as well as his communication skills. You can imagine a situation in which a pharmacist is sharing information with a physician regarding a new prescription medication. Because the pharmacist has a great deal of knowledge about the topic, she is going to be doing more of the talking. The interaction between pharmacist and physician is also going to be affected by the pharmacist's communication skills. Perhaps the physician is not interested in learning about the new dosing regimen. However, with sufficient skill, the pharmacist may be able to underscore the importance of appropriate prescribing and teach the physician what he needs to know.

Notice that, in the integrated model depicted in Fig. 4.1, messages are flowing back and forth between the two people at the same time. These may be verbal or nonverbal messages. For example, nonverbal messages may be sent via facial expressions while the other person is speaking. Although the model appears linear, communication is in fact a dynamic process. Each interaction helps frame the next. Each interaction provides the participants with experience from which to base expectations regarding future interactions. Finally, notice that messages are subject to barriers that may inhibit their transmission. Barriers may include preconceived ideas about the message, physical barriers such as a high counter, or noise in the area preventing the message from being heard. A further discussion of potential barriers to communication is presented in the next section.

## POTENTIAL BARRIERS TO PHARMACIST'S COMMUNICATION

Much research has been conducted on the barriers to pharmacists' communication with patients, especially in the community setting.[12-14] Pharmacy environment as well as barriers that were pharmacist-related, patient-related, informational/philosophical, and miscellaneous have been addressed.

Herrier and Boyce[14] offer the most comprehensive evidence with results from workshops with nearly 30,000 pharmacists. Participating pharmacists were asked to identify barriers to patient counseling at their practice sites. Common themes emerged in the discussions. Barriers in the pharmacy environment may include the store layout, lack of privacy, workload issues, and a lack of reimbursement for the counseling services. Pharmacists' personal barriers to provision of counseling services in the community setting may include their feelings of competence and their willingness to communicate. Pharmacist-related barriers included lack of formal education in patient counseling or lack of knowledge about the prescribed drug or poor counseling skills.

Patient-related barriers were most frequently identified as the patient being in a hurry or uninterested in receiving information about the medication. Philosophical or information barriers were related to pharmacists' questioning of their abilities to affect patient outcomes through counseling activities. Finally, miscellaneous barriers include concerns over liability and lack of reimbursement as barriers to providing counseling services.

In practice, as in the model of communication, these barriers prove to be a challenge for pharmacists who hope to establish and maintain good communication with their patients in the retail setting. Other practice settings may share similar barriers, or other issues may create problems. Overcoming these barriers is crucial to ensuring that your messages are received and understood by the receiver. Now, let's further explore the types of messages that can be sent from one person to another, including both verbal and nonverbal messages.

## ORAL COMMUNICATION SKILLS

As we can see from the model of communication, there are many components to an interaction with another person. To have an interaction with another, we must be able to act as senders and receivers of messages. In this section, skills necessary to accomplish that end are reviewed, including listening, responding, phrasing questions, and assertiveness.

### Listening

The best way to show your commitment to developing and maintaining relationships with those you work with, whether patients or colleagues, is to listen to them. Listening, like communication in general, does not come naturally to some people. The first step in listening is to stop talking. However, just being quiet does not necessarily qualify as listening. Both nonverbal and verbal communication can give someone the impression that you are in fact listening to them. In order to listen to someone, you must have an environment that is conducive to the interaction. Central to this idea is that you should not be distracted when you are listening. In a busy pharmacy, it can be difficult to stop all tasks in order to listen to a patient, but unless the patient has your undivided attention, you will have a difficult time understanding them. It is imperative that you find a quiet place with some degree of privacy in order to consult with patients. Even in the busiest of pharmacies, there is likely to be a corner of the store that has less traffic and can be used for consultation. Having a private area enables you to listen better and also provides the patient with the sense that he or she is not opening themselves up to the general public when discussing a concern with you.

When listening to another person, one must attempt to truly understand her point of view and then convey that understanding to her. By demonstrating that you have understood, you can communicate that you have in fact heard what she has to say. At times, health-care professionals do not respond to patients in the most appropriate ways. It is common to want to solve problems or to want to tell people how to handle their situations rather than acknowledging what they are feeling.

For example, consider Mr. Nodough, a patient who is picking up a prescription at the pharmacy. During the exchange, he says, "These prescription prices are so high. The pharmacist must be making a mint." As Tindall et al[15] describe, many types of potential responses are possible, yet few will have the desired effect. In Table 4.1, we briefly review less effective response strategies and then discuss better ways to demonstrate that you have heard and understood Mr. Nodough.

Empathy is a very useful tool. It can be most helpful when you feel that you do not know what to say or that you cannot do anything to help the person. By recognizing and responding to the feelings the person has, you are demonstrating

**TABLE 4.1. TYPES OF RESPONSES**

| Response | Example | Description | Result |
|---|---|---|---|
| Judging | "You shouldn't complain, Mr. Nodough. These medications are helping to keep you healthy." | Suggests that someone should not have the feelings she does about a particular situation. | Invalidates the person's feelings and may discourage him from sharing feelings in the future. |
| Reassuring | "Don't worry about it; I'm sure you'll manage to figure out something." | Tends to be given with good intentions to make someone feel better, but offers false reassurance since you do not know how things will work out. Often given when people don't know what to say. | Invalidates the person's feelings. |
| Probing | "How much money do you spend on prescriptions each month?" | Usually in the form of a question designed to elicit additional information. | Does not address the patient's concerns about cost, rather it redirects the interaction taking focus away from the patient. |
| Generalizing | "Everyone feels that way sometimes." Or "I feel the same way when I get a prescription filled." | Generalizes what the patient may be feeling. | Takes focus away from the patient, some may feel that this type of response trivializes their feelings. |
| Distracting | "Well, your prescription is ready now." | Does not acknowledge what the patient has said; can be as drastic as a change of subject. | Takes focus away from the patient, invalidates the person's feelings, discourages patient from sharing feelings in the future. |

*(continued)*

61

**TABLE 4.1. TYPES OF RESPONSES** (*Continued*)

| Response | Example | Description | Result |
|---|---|---|---|
| Advising | "You should find a better health insurance company, one that covers prescriptions." | Suggests what a person should do. | Offering alternatives is one way of helping the patient identify his own solution. Often, there is little you can do to solve their problem, but conveying that you have heard and understood it can go a long way. |
| Understanding | "I understand you feel the prescription prices are too high." | Allows you to convey your understanding of the message you received. | This can be helpful, but you may not completely understand the patient's concern or situation. You will never be able to fully appreciate the patient's experience; to suggest you do may be offensive. |
| Empathy[a] | "It must be very frustrating trying to pay for all your prescriptions and other costs of living." | Goes beyond an understanding response to address the feelings that underlie a statement; demonstrates not only that you heard and understood what the person said, but also that you recognize the emotions that led him to say what he did. | Acknowledges that you have heard the patient's concern and understand how it makes him feel. |

[a]Best type of response to Mr. Nodough. After this you would go on to explore ways to help him.

true listening skills and also caring. It is important to note that empathy is difficult if not impossible to fake. People can easily see through a false attempt at empathy and are likely to respond negatively to it. Unless you are genuine in your willingness to understand and relate to another person, empathy will be difficult to master.

In most cases, an empathic response is a beginning to a dialogue. It is not the only thing you will say to the patient. However, as you first recognize their feelings and demonstrate your understanding, the patient will be reassured of your sincere caring about his or her concern. This will help you foster a helping relationship with the patient and will encourage him to begin a further discussion of the issue. At that point, you may be able to offer additional assistance. For Mr. Nodough, you may be able to suggest financial assistance programs or equivalent medications at a lower cost. If nothing else, you will have made Mr. Nodough feel that you have heard his concern.

Listening to patients and responding empathically to their concerns are both important skills to master. In order to elicit information from them, however, you will need to initiate a dialogue. To do this, appropriate phrasing of questions is essential. The next section focuses on this skill.

## How to Ask a Question

The way a question is phrased influences the amount and type of information one receives in response. A closed-ended question, for example, is a question that is phrased to elicit a "yes" or "no" response. One example of a closed-ended question is "Are you taking your medication as prescribed?" The patient responding to this question may say either "yes" or "no" but is unlikely to provide any additional information. Closed-ended questions are useful in a patient interview when you are following up on information you already have, when probing for additional information, or when you need to have something confirmed. A case in point may be when you check your understanding of information a patient has provided. You might say, "Is it correct that you experience headaches 1 hour after taking your blood pressure medication?" This will tell you if you are right; however, if you are looking for additional information about the type of headache the patient has, you are likely to learn more from an answer to a question that encourages the respondent to elaborate. Contrast this style of question with an open-ended one.

An open-ended question is a question that allows the person responding to elaborate on the topic. This is particularly useful when you are beginning an interview and would like to get as much information as possible. One way to phrase an open-ended question is to begin with the word "how." For example, "How are you taking your medication?" provides a patient with the opportunity to talk about his response to a medication. When asking patients open-ended questions, one should avoid beginning with the word "why." For example, asking a patient "Why isn't your medication working for you?" may put her on the defensive. The patient may feel that you are accusing her of improper use of the medication or suggesting that she is in some way at fault for the ineffectiveness of the medication. There are times when it is appropriate to use the word "why"; however, it should be used cautiously. It can be used in combination with other key phrases such as in the case of the question, "Why do you think you are forgetting to take your medication?" In this example, the pharmacist is eliciting the patient's opinion rather than challenging her.

To follow open-ended questions, probing questions can be used. A probing question helps you gather detailed information along the lines of the open-ended question. Often, these are closed-ended questions, yet they can also be open ended. Consider a situation in which a patient shares with his pharmacist that he has been having difficulty adhering to a medication regimen. He further offers that when he does take his medication properly, he suffers from stomach discomfort. The pharmacist agrees that the stomach problems may be caused by the medication but knows they may also be related to the patient's ulcer. The pharmacist also knows that if the patient takes the medication with food, the stomach discomfort will likely dissipate if it is caused by the medication. In this case, a closed-ended probing question may be "Are you taking the medication with food?" An example of an open-ended probing question may be "Would you describe the discomfort you've experienced?" Both of these questions are probing questions because they both search for additional information based on what the patient has already said. Both will enable the pharmacist to gather the additional information that is needed to make a recommendation for this patient.

One type of question that is common among health-care professionals but is best to avoid is the leading question. A leading question is phrased such that it prompts a patient to answer a certain way. Health-care professionals use these questions, often inadvertently, because they have an idea in mind about what the patient is experiencing. For example, when a pharmacist says, "You're having a hard time sticking with the medication because of the side effects, aren't you?" to a patient who is late for a refill, she is using a leading question. Although there are many other reasons the patient may be late picking up the refill from the pharmacy, the pharmacist has made an assumption about the patient's situation.

In another example, when a pharmacy technician says to a patient, "You don't have any questions for the pharmacist, do you?" he implies that the patient should say that she does not in fact have any questions for the pharmacist. Contrast this with the following way of phrasing the same question. If the pharmacy technician were to say, "Would you like to ask the pharmacist any questions?" the patient is likely to perceive that he or she does have the option of speaking with the pharmacist. It is of particular significance to avoid leading questions when discussing sensitive subjects such as adherence. Consider the following example.

Pharmacist Dexter is speaking with Mrs. Green about her untimely refill of an antihypertensive prescription. In the course of the conversation, Pharmacist Dexter says, "Well, it's not that you can't afford these medications, is it?" Mrs. Green, obviously flustered, responds by saying "No, no, of course not. . . . I guess I'm just forgetful." Although the pharmacist may feel he was asking Mrs. Green if she had financial concerns about her medication, Mrs. Green perceived the question as judgmental and was unable to respond truthfully. Had the pharmacist phrased the question differently, such as "Is it sometimes difficult to pay for the medications all at once?" perhaps Mrs. Green would have felt more comfortable discussing her financial situation with him. This would have potentially allowed the pharmacist to solve the problem of nonadherence by working out a payment schedule for Mrs. Green or by recommending another less expensive therapeutic option to the physician.

In summary, it is generally best to begin by asking open-ended questions. This will enable the person to elaborate on the issue at hand and will give you an insight into her perspective. Following up on the answers with closed-ended questions can help you pinpoint specific information you need or help you better understand the other person's view. Finally, it is better not to phrase questions in a leading manner to ensure that you truly understand their perspective.

### Dealing with Difficult Situations: Assertiveness

Often you will be faced with situations in which people are being difficult. Examples may include a situation in which a patient is upset with something that has happened at the pharmacy, an employee is unhappy with an administrative decision, or a physician chooses to debate a suggestion you have made regarding medication therapy. In each of these cases, in order to keep the situation from escalating into an argument, depending on your personality, you may want to concede your point and allow the other person to have his or her way. In the extreme, this would be considered passive behavior. Although passive behavior is effective in avoiding conflict, it can create other problems by leaving situations unresolved or poorly resolved. Some people may choose to handle the situation by fueling it and allowing it to escalate. This type of behavior would be considered aggressive. A mature, professional approach would be to handle these situations and others like them with assertiveness. Assertiveness allows you to maintain your position without responding aggressively to a situation. The following techniques can help you develop ways to respond assertively. Tindall et al[15] offer a full explanation of the following techniques. Here, each is briefly summarized.

### Fogging

Fogging is a technique with which you acknowledge the truth about a statement yet ignore the implicit value judgment contained within it. For example, a physician who is unfamiliar with the clinical role pharmacists can play on the health-care team says, "In attempting to manage a patient's medications, you pharmacists are crossing the line!" Your response to him may be "Yes, clinical pharmacists are expanding the boundaries of their practices." With this response, you are acknowledging the truth of the physician's comments in that pharmacy has a newly expanded role. What you are not acknowledging, however, is the underlying suggestion that pharmacists are impinging on the physician's role and that they should not participate in the management of a patient's medication therapy.

## Acknowledging the Truth

Another technique is acknowledging the truth in a criticism. When someone confronts you with a criticism or a complaint, the natural tendency is to try to explain why you did what you did. This can sound defensive and may escalate the situation. For example, if a patient complains about the long wait for her prescription, you could respond by explaining that each prescription is processed in the order it was received and that there are several steps involved in filling a prescription. However, it is unlikely that the patient is interested in learning about the processing of a prescription. Rather, she is frustrated by the length of time it will take her to complete her task of picking up the prescription. By acknowledging that the wait is long, you are demonstrating that you understand her concern, but you are neither apologizing for it nor making excuses. In apologizing for the wait, you are behaving less assertively in your attempt to avoid a conflict with this patient. If you begin to explain the entire process of accurately and safely filling a prescription in an attempt to justify your position, it will appear that you are becoming defensive about the situation. This would illustrate a more aggressive response to the patient.

The truth of the matter is that the patient may have to wait a long time for her prescription. In responding to her, acknowledging the truth of the situation will be beneficial. The patient will notice that you are not attempting to disagree with her or change her mind about her perception of the situation. She will also notice that you are not going to be able to do anything to change the situation.

## Disagreeing with Criticism

In contrast to those times when a criticism is valid, when you are confronted with criticism that is unfounded, it is equally important to disagree with it. For example, your employer observes an interaction with a patient in which perhaps you did not provide the patient with all the information he needed and mentions to you that you "never give patients enough time." The implication that you are not practicing pharmacy at the level required by your employer is implicit in her comment to you. If this criticism is untrue or unfounded, it is best to address it immediately. Using an aggressive response is not recommended. However, when you do acknowledge that you did not spend sufficient time with a particular patient, it is appropriate to identify it as an isolated incident rather than a general pattern of behavior. For example, you may say, "You're right. I didn't spend enough time with Mr. Quinn today. I usually take much more time with my patients." In making it clear to your employer that you disagree with her general characterization, you are responding assertively.

## Broken Record Technique

A technique that has many applications is the broken record technique in which your response does not change as long as the person with whom you are speaking repeats the same request. Consider a situation in which a physician wishes to prescribe a medication for a hospitalized patient that is not on that hospital's formulary. It may be the pharmacist's responsibility to review the physician's request and make a decision regarding that prescription. If, in the pharmacist's best professional judgment, that nonformulary medication is not necessary, she may experience resistance from the physician in accepting that decision. In this situation, the pharmacist might respond to the physician by saying, "In my professional judgment, this situation does not call for a nonformulary medication; there are sufficient therapeutic choices on the formulary." For each argument made by the physician, the pharmacist using the broken record technique will respond again that the nonformulary medication is not called for in her professional judgment.

This type of response can be difficult to employ when the other party responds aggressively. With this response, you are merely stating your position; not attempting to escalate the interaction into an argument. Neither are you conceding your point and allowing the physician, in this case, to declare victory. It may be frustrating for the physician to continue to discuss the issue with the pharmacist because it will become clear that she has no intention of changing her mind.

## Getting Useful Feedback

When you find that a criticism is vague, it is best to get a useful feedback in order to understand the nature of the criticism. For example, if your preceptor tells you that you "don't know how to practice pharmacy," it would be easy to get upset and disregard the comment entirely. However, the preceptor probably has something in mind that he would like you to master. By asking the preceptor, "What specifically do I need to work on?" you will get the precise information you need. You may discover that you made an error on a prescription and that you will need to be more careful with your work. You can then utilize one of the other assertive response techniques to deal with the situation. However, without an understanding of the true concerns the preceptor has, you would be unable to respond to the situation in an assertive way. Another situation where this technique would be helpful may occur if a patient accuses a pharmacist of not responding to his concerns. The pharmacist would be better able to respond if she knew what had happened to make the patient feel that way.

## Delaying a Response

On occasions, you may find that someone pressures you for a response. In general, the assertive response to this situation is to delay a reply until you have had sufficient time to ponder on your answer. For example, consider a situation in which a physician demands to know why you recommended a particular medication for a patient.

If you do not have that patient's chart readily available or do not recall the specific situation to which the physician is referring, how can you respond? You could agree to change your recommendation to the physician's choice, yet that would be seen as passive. On the other hand, an assertive response may be to tell him that you will review your notes and meet with him at a later time to discuss the patient's medication therapy. In contrast to passive behavior, which may include bowing to the physician's authority and making the therapeutic change he requests, this assertive technique helps avoid an escalating conflict with the physician as well as giving you the time you need to prepare to have the discussion with him.

In summary, assertive responses, such as the types reviewed in this section, are useful in many situations. They will come naturally to you with practice, and not feel so awkward. Being assertive allows you to avoid conflict and at the same time hold your position. See Table 4.2 for a review of the response options. This section of the chapter has reviewed basic verbal communication skills including listening, responding, phrasing of questions, and assertiveness. These skills can be used to overcome many barriers to communication, both personal and environmental. We now move to a discussion of nonverbal communication skills. As we have seen from the model of communication, these too can play a dramatic role in the way messages are sent and perceived.

## NONVERBAL COMMUNICATION SKILLS

Nonverbal cues help people interpret the meaning behind your words. Whether you are aware of it or not, people routinely consider the words they hear within the context of the accompanying nonverbal communication. Nonverbal communication can be defined as a message or messages that are conveyed without using language. It includes everything from the way you stand to the maintenance of eye contact as you are talking to someone. Consider a pharmacist in a busy community pharmacy asking a patient if he has any questions, while she is simultaneously typing something in the computer and speaking on the telephone. That pharmacist is likely to convey the message that she is too busy to talk to the patient rather than the message that she is sincerely interested in talking to the patient and answering his questions. A similar situation exists when a pharmacist enters a hospital room to conduct discharge counseling, stands near the doorway, and rushes through the information being presented. This pharmacist is likely to give the patient the impression that she is too busy to review the medications the patient will be taking home with him. Sometimes nonverbal cues can give someone an impression about the message you are trying to send that is incongruent with your intentions. Consider the same scenario when the pharmacist comes into the room, sits by the bed, and reviews each medication thoroughly with the patient. The nonverbal act of sitting down gives the patient the impression that the pharmacist is there as long as she needs to be. An important point to remember is that if there is a discrepancy between verbal and nonverbal

**TABLE 4.2.** ASSERTIVENESS TECHNIQUES

| Assertiveness Technique | Description |
| --- | --- |
| Fogging | Allows you to acknowledge the truth about a statement while ignoring value judgment within it. Example: To a physician who tells you not to interfere in her relationships with patients, "I am fulfilling my obligation to our patients." |
| Acknowledging the truth | As implied by the name, agrees with truth in a statement without becoming defensive and escalating the situation. Example: To your manager who accuses you of always being late, "You are right, I was late today. It was the only time in several months." |
| Disagreeing with criticism | Calmly disagrees with what you believe is inaccurate criticism. Example: To a patient who complains about the length of time to fill his prescription, "I am taking my time to ensure all of my patients' safety." |
| Broken record technique | Responds to each argument with a statement of your position. Example: To a patient who repeatedly complains about the cost of his medication, "This prescription is expensive. Your co-payment is $45." |
| Getting useful feedback | Faced with vague criticism, this allows you to gather specific information you can use. Example: To a patient who tells you he will transfer his prescriptions elsewhere, "What happened to make you so upset with the pharmacy technician Mr. Smith?" |
| Delaying a response | When pressured for a response, gives you time to think about it until you feel ready to answer. Example: To the manager who is pressuring you to work on your day off, "After I check my calendar, I'll let you know if I'm available to work on Friday." |

messages, it is the nonverbal cues that are taken as a true reflection of the person's feelings, so pay attention to keeping your nonverbal and verbal signals congruent!

The best way to convey, nonverbally, that you are interested in a patient, or anyone else, and what he is trying to tell you is to face him. Whether you are sitting or standing, unless you are facing the patient and making eye contact, he is likely to perceive you as uninterested in what he is saying. Next, be aware of your arms. Keeping your arms crossed in front of you, folded across your chest, suggests a closed posture. This does not invite patients to share with you; rather, it is telling them that you are either upset or preoccupied and are uninterested in their information. It is also helpful to lean slightly in toward the patient while maintaining relaxed, steady eye contact. When the person is speaking, you may nod your head to indicate that you are paying attention and hearing what is being said. This can also encourage him to continue speaking. This subtly conveys that you are listening and that you care. This technique, when used properly with appropriate verbal techniques, will help you establish a good relationship with patients. It will help patients feel more at ease with you and will ultimately make your job easier by allowing you to find out the crucial information you need. Specific nonverbal cues may be based on posture, distance, time, or touch. Each of these is discussed briefly.

## Posture

*Kinesics* is the method by which messages are conveyed through one's posture. The way one holds one's body sends a message to others with whom we are interacting. Think about going for a job interview. During that interview, you sit straight in the chair and keep your hands folded in your lap. This will generally present a professional, mature image to your prospective employer. Contrast this with a person who slouches down in the chair and is tapping her foot throughout the interview. It is possible that the person slouching is nervous about the interview, but the message that she is sending is that she is not interested in obtaining the position. Another example is the position of your arms. Keeping your arms crossed in front of your body suggests that you are not open to hearing another person's ideas. This is definitely a position to avoid when trying to engage in a dialogue. In your interactions with patients, giving them the impression that your attention is elsewhere can be easy with kinesics. By maintaining eye contact, ceasing other tasks, and maintaining a relaxed but professional posture, you will be sending the desired message of interest and concern for the patient.

## Distance

*Proxemics* refers to the messages that are conveyed by the use of space and distance. Usually, different types of communication occur at different distances. A message that is sent to another person from very far away is likely to be a public one because it is one where the sender will have to shout. One example of such a message may be greeting a classmate who is quite a distance down the hall from you.

Private types of communication occur at closer distances. When you are sharing a secret with your best friend, you are probably quite close to him or her, which enables you to convey quietly your message without being overheard. In between these two extremes is the distance that is comfortable in social or professional situations. This distance varies among cultures. In the United States, a comfortable distance is approximately 2 to 4 ft. Of course, individuals have their own preferences as well. There are no clear-cut guidelines about what is too close or too far away. Distance is generally negotiated during an interaction. If someone feels that you are invading his personal space, he will back away from you. Instead of moving closer to him, allow him to define the distance between you. Finding the comfortable distance from which to talk with patients or other health-care professionals will make productive interactions easier.

## Time

*Chronemics* refers to the messages that are sent by the use of time. This may sound confusing, but the best example of chronemics generally occurs in physicians' offices. Patients are kept waiting until the physician is free to see them. This is often a source of frustration for patients because as anecdotal evidence suggests, appointments are rarely kept on schedule. Thus, patients are left waiting and given the feeling that the physician does not respect their time. Likewise, in the pharmacy, chronemics can play an important role in your relationship with patients. The amount of time patients spend waiting to speak with someone about a prescription, as well as the time they wait for the prescription to be filled, can send a strong message to them about the value you place on their patronage. Although it is not always possible to fill prescriptions as quickly as a patient would like, addressing patients' concerns about these issues can help mitigate potentially frustrating situations for everyone involved.

## Touch

*Haptics* refers to the messages that are conveyed through touch. Touch is an integral portion of human communication. It is the first form of communication that babies sense and is used to show caring and support for those around us. Health-care professionals, for example, on a regular basis offer a handshake as a greeting or a reassuring hand on a patient's shoulder providing comfort during a time of emotional distress. Even a pat on the back or a high five given to a child can help create warmth in a provider-patient relationship. A word of caution is needed, however. Not all patients respond well to touch. Cultural and personal differences will dictate the extent to which you incorporate touch into your practice.

In summary, the use of nonverbal cues can reinforce your verbal messages. Thus, it is essential to be aware of all the messages you are sending to your receiver. Each dimension of nonverbal communication discussed here is important, but the most important seems to be kinesics. That concept will prove to be most true when working with patients. Next, we discuss ways of integrating the skills presented thus far in performing patient consultation.

## PUTTING IT ALL TOGETHER: PATIENT INTERVIEWING

Gathering information from patients is probably one of the most important and most common functions pharmacists perform. It is also one that requires the most awareness of your communication skills. By correctly phrasing questions to the patient within the context of a sincere desire to help, most patients will provide the information you need to know. In this section the phrasing and ordering of questions are explored. It is crucial to prepare and organize when approaching a patient so that you will not inadvertently omit important questions or be surprised at that patient's response to you. It is important to remember that the patient is the only one who has important bits of information you need. It is not sufficient to ask patients how they are doing with their medication. Patients may feel that you are not really interested in how they are doing and will tell you everything is just fine, even when it may not be.

Sometimes it is hard for patients to differentiate between something that is of importance and something that is not. Therefore, it is your job to ask the right questions, to help patients formulate their questions, and to make sure patients understand the information presented. In the real world, pharmacists are often unable to spend as much time with a patient as they would like. In this case, it becomes important to prioritize the information you wish to give. Even more important is developing an ongoing relationship with patients, as some things can wait a month or two until you see the patient again, but others require immediate attention. In the community setting, when a patient is picking up a new prescription, there is a lot of information the patient should receive. For a refill prescription, the type of information you should gather may be different. In this case, perhaps the most important information to assess is how that patient has been taking the medication. Table 4.3 provides a checklist of items to be included in a full initial patient interview. Take a moment to review the components.

## Process

We have already discussed the importance and use of open-ended and closed-ended questions. Prudent use of both types of questions will help the interview flow smoothly. We have also reviewed the concept of empathy and the importance of responding empathically to patients. In this section, we focus on the process of patient interviewing and the order in which questions are asked.

First, you must establish the goal for the interaction. A patient interview may consist solely of gathering information from the patient. Alternatively, following the patient interview, a patient education session may be conducted. By developing your own system for asking questions, you will be less likely to leave out questions inadvertently. You will also be able to guide the interview to flow quickly and smoothly. One way to maximize the time you have with a patient is to address only those issues which are of concern to you or the patient. It is not always necessary to address everything about a patient's drug therapy at one time. Neither you nor the patient is likely to have time for that.

In addition to being prepared to meet with the patient, you can also maximize your time with the patient by eliciting what information the patient already has. You do not need to reiterate information that patient already knows. For example, rather

TABLE 4.3. CHECKLIST FOR THE EVALUATION OF THE CONTENT AND
STRUCTURE OF A PATIENT INTERVIEW[a]

During the patient interview, did the pharmacy student/pharmacist perform the
following:

| | | | |
|---|---|---|---|
| 1. **Identify the patient (or caregiver)** | Yes | No | N/A |
| 2. **Introduce self** | Yes | No | N/A |
| 3. **Explain purpose of the interview** | Yes | No | N/A |
| 4. **Estimate the length of time necessary for interview** | Yes | No | N/A |
| 5. **Explain how patient will benefit from interview** | Yes | No | N/A |
| 6. **Obtain patient consent to proceed** | Yes | No | N/A |
| 7. **Obtain a complete and accurate history of** | | | |
|    *a. present medical problems* | Yes | No | N/A |
|    *b. past medical problems* | Yes | No | N/A |
|    *c. present prescription drug use* | Yes | No | N/A |
|    *d. past prescription drug use* | Yes | No | N/A |
|    *e. present OTC use* | Yes | No | N/A |
|    *f. past OTC use* | Yes | No | N/A |
|    *g. patient compliance with drug regimen(s)* | Yes | No | N/A |
|    *h. social-behavioral factors that may influence medicine use patterns* | Yes | No | N/A |
|    *i. suspected/documented drug allergies or sensitivities* | Yes | No | N/A |
|      (i) date of occurrence | Yes | No | N/A |
|      (ii) type of reaction | Yes | No | N/A |
| 8. **Verify accuracy of the information already in the chart** | Yes | No | N/A |
| 9. **Assess, through open-ended questions, the patient's understanding:** | | | |
|    *a. of medication dosage* | Yes | No | N/A |
|    *b. of dosage frequency* | Yes | No | N/A |
|    *c. of method of administration* | Yes | No | N/A |
| 10. **Assess patient's actual use of medication(s)** | Yes | No | N/A |
| 11. **Obtain from patient information regarding factors that may affect compliance:** | | | |
|    *a. lifestyle* | Yes | Np | N/A |
|    *b. compliance history* | Yes | No | N/A |
|    *c. attitudes toward disease and medication* | Yes | No | N/A |
|    *d. physical and/or mental impairments* | Yes | No | N/A |
|    *e. socioeconomic constraints* | Yes | No | N/A |

*(continued)*

TABLE 4.3. CHECKLIST FOR THE EVALUATION OF THE CONTENT AND STRUCTURE OF A PATIENT INTERVIEW[a] (*Continued*)

| | | | |
|---|---|---|---|
| f. *patient's perception of the severity of the disease(s)* | Yes | No | N/A |
| g. *patient's perception of the importance of the prescribed drug(s)* | Yes | No | N/A |
| 12. **Summarize information gathered from patient to assess accuracy and completeness** | Yes | No | N/A |
| 13. **Gather complete medication history before providing new information** | Yes | No | N/A |
| 14. **Determine appropriate dosage regimen based on prescription directions, drug characteristics, and patient's compliance factors** | Yes | No | N/A |
| 15. **Explain new prescription(s) to patient** | | | |
| a. *Provide the indication(s)* | Yes | No | N/A |
| b. *Explain dosage regimen(s)* | Yes | No | N/A |
| c. *Suggest time(s) of administration* | Yes | No | N/A |
| d. *Explain or demonstrate method of administration* | Yes | No | N/A |
| e. *Instruct patient in what to do if a dose is missed or an extra dose is ingested* | Yes | No | N/A |
| f. *Explain potential side effects* | Yes | No | N/A |
| g. *Explain how to recognize the signs and symptoms of a therapeutic response* | Yes | No | N/A |
| h. *Explain how to recognize the signs and symptoms of therapeutic failure* | Yes | No | N/A |
| i. *Explain what to do if signs and symptoms of therapeutic failure or important side effects occur* | Yes | No | N/A |
| j. *Explain methods by which side effects can be minimized* | Yes | No | N/A |
| 16. **Determine the patient's level of comprehension via open-ended questions such as** | | | |
| a. *How you are going to take this medication?* | Yes | No | N/A |
| b. *How will you be able to tell the medication is working?* | Yes | No | N/A |
| c. *What will you do if you miss a dose?* | Yes | No | N/A |
| 17. **Arrange for follow-up with patient** | Yes | No | N/A |
| 18. **Provide written and/or pictorial information to enhance patient understanding** | Yes | No | N/A |
| 19. **Make self available to answer questions in the future** | Yes | No | N/A |
| 20. **Ask patient's permission to contact physician, when needed** | Yes | No | N/A |

(*continued*)

| TABLE 4.3. CHECKLIST FOR THE EVALUATION OF THE CONTENT AND STRUCTURE OF A PATIENT INTERVIEW[a] (Continued) | | | |
|---|---|---|---|
| **21. Throughout the interview** | | | |
| a. Communicate at the appropriate level for the patient (caregiver) | Yes | No | N/A |
| b. Solicit and encourage questions from the patient (caregiver) | Yes | No | N/A |
| c. Respond empathically to patient's (caregiver's) concerns | | | |

[a]This checklist may be used as an aid in developing your own interview structure. It may also be used as a self-evaluative tool or in a rotation evaluation. The content of this list represents material that may be covered during a complete, initial session. Subsequent sessions with patients may not include each element.

than reviewing how to take each medication, you may simply ask the patient how he or she is taking each one. That way, you can assess if the patient already knows how to take the medication and address any issues that may arise as a result of this. Be careful how your questions are phrased. Which of the following questions do you think will best help you identify potential problems with patient understanding?

1. Are you taking your medications as prescribed?
2. How are you taking your medication?

If you chose question 1, you may be surprised when you hear that all of your patients are in fact taking their medications as prescribed. Question 1 is a closed-ended question, and patients are likely to respond with a "yes" or "no." Most people will not want to admit that they are not following their doctor's instructions, so they will respond affirmatively even if they are not taking their medications as prescribed. Question 2, as an open-ended question, allows patients to tell you how they are taking their medication. At that point, you can determine if they are taking them as prescribed or not. You can then follow up and discuss possible solutions to managing their medication regimens.

## Introduction

The first thing you will say to the patient is likely to be a greeting of some sort. "Good morning, Mr. Simmons," is a nice way to begin. Let's consider other items to include in your opening. Unless the patient already knows you, he will not know what to expect from talking with you. Therefore, at an initial meeting, after you introduce yourself, you should explain to the patient why you would like to speak with him, how long it will take, and what will be accomplished during the session. For example, one pharmacist might say:

> Good afternoon, Mrs. Hope. I am Stacy Student, the pharmacist here at the clinic. I would like to spend about 5 minutes discussing your medications with you so that we may prevent any potential problems and resolve any problems you might be having with your medications.

After obtaining the patient's permission to proceed, you may begin asking the patient questions.

## Phrasing Key Questions

After the introduction, proceed by making sure you have a complete list of all the medications a patient is taking. Even if you have a list of medications from the patient profile, the profile may not be current. In addition, it may not contain all of the medications the patient is taking. Perhaps he has prescriptions filled at another pharmacy, or perhaps he is taking nonprescription items that may interfere with the prescription medications. In asking, "What prescription medications are you currently taking?" you will be sure to have a complete, updated list from which to work. After gathering that list, you may want to ask the following questions for each of the medications on the list. At this point, it is important not to confuse the patient or yourself by discussing more than one medication at a time. Using a transition such as "let's talk about your blood pressure medication first" will help minimize confusion.

In addition to how patients are taking their medications, important areas to explore include what medications they are taking (both prescription and over the counter), what problems they might be having, if they are experiencing side effects that they attribute to their medications, if they are using any alternative therapies to treat their medical conditions, and if they have other health concerns they would like to discuss. When asking about other health concerns, keep in mind that a patient may be experiencing side effects from a medication that he does not attribute to that medication. It will be up to you to help him determine what issues are medication related and what issues are not. In either case, if a concern is revealed, resolution may involve a discussion with the patient's physician. Important points to ask about each and every medication include the following:

> "How did the doctor tell you to take the medication?"
> "How are you taking your medication?"
> "Have you noticed any problems with this medication?"
> "How effective has the medication been?"
> "How can you tell the medication is working?"

Refer again to Table 4.3 for the checklist of items to cover during a patient interview. This may be helpful for you in developing your own interview checklist or for a self-evaluative tool.

## Providing Education

After you have gathered your information, you will likely want to make recommendations to the patient. It is wise to wait until after you have collected all the pertinent information before initiating a patient education session. If you respond to each potential problem before getting a clear, complete picture of the patient's medical and pharmacologic state, you may need to modify the information you have given the patient. In addition to taking longer, it is likely to confuse the patient. Therefore, it is best to wait until you have gathered all the details before providing any information.

Similar to the interviewing process, providing patient education should be done in an organized, systematic way. Begin by addressing the most important issue. Prioritization is essential because it is unlikely that you will be able to address completely all of the necessary issues with a patient at one time. That is why the development of a strong relationship with patients will be helpful. When you see patients on a regular basis, you can cover one topic at a time and know that you will have other opportunities at a future date to refine the patient's understanding of other issues. Certainly, addressing the most pressing first makes sense. Anything that is potentially life threatening should be addressed immediately. As you work in clinical settings, you will hone your ability to recognize the clinical significance of each patient's issues, and you will be able to determine how quickly you need to address them.

You can maximize your time in patient education by providing only new information for them. It is unnecessary for you to review information that the patient already understands. By asking open-ended questions, you can ascertain what information the patient still needs and provide that information to him.

The format of the information you provide is also important. Research has shown that it is not sufficient merely to tell patients about something. It is very helpful for patients to have written information to which they can refer when they are at home.[16,17] Using written information in addition to orally communicating the information reinforces the concepts for patients. This will minimize misunderstandings and will give patients something to refer to if you are not available to answer their questions. Some patients may research on their own and may come to you with a great understanding of their medical conditions and their medications, yet others may rely on you to provide that information to them. You can be of help to both types of patients and to the majority of patients who will lie somewhere in between those two ends of the spectrum. By making yourself available to answer all levels of questions and being willing to provide information at levels appropriate to each patient, you will be fulfilling their needs. Be prepared to provide information at a lower level than the computer-generated patient information leaflets or to provide references to scientific journals for patients who want to read the latest clinical trials.

Your ultimate goal is for the patient to retain and utilize the information you have provided. There are certain things you can do to help patients remember the important points. Tindall et al[15] offer the following suggestions. First, like students in a classroom who are told that something is important for an exam, patients who are told that something is important will better remember what follows. By telling patients that something is important, you cause them to pay more attention. For example, Pharmacist Phillips may say to her patient, "Mr. Brown, what I'm about to tell you is very important. This medication may cause your eyes to change color." Although the mere mention of such a radical side effect may have been enough for Mr. Brown to remember it, preceding that statement with a declaration that the information to come is important helped the patient focus on the upcoming information. This technique is useful, but only if used sparingly. If every other sentence you utter begins with, "now, this is very important," it will lose its effect, and patients will not pay attention to it any longer.

Another way to help patients remember information is to summarize key points after you have given it to them. It is most effective when you have the patient summarize the information for you rather than you summarizing for the patient. By asking the patient to repeat the important points from the education session, you accomplish two things. First, you are able to assess the patient's understanding of the information, and second, you are able to determine if you inadvertently omitted some information. Using probing questions such as "How do you plan to take your medication?" can help you assess patients' understanding of particular portions of the education session. You may also ask the following questions to assess patients' understanding:

"What will you do if you miss a dose?"
"How will you be able to tell if the medication is working?"
"What side effects may you experience from this medication?"

A third way to minimize misunderstandings is by providing clear instructions. Telling a patient to take a medication with food, for example, is rather vague. The patient may have questions about how much food would be sufficient or if the medication should be taken only at mealtimes. By being specific about your instructions, you can prevent this confusion. Telling the patient to take the medication with food, such as a small snack or with meals, depending on the dosing regimen, will help the patient take the medication properly in order to realize its full benefit.

Finally, explaining to patients just why something is important will help them understand and remember the point. In the above example, if a patient understands that not taking the medication with food may cause stomach discomfort, he is more likely to follow those instructions. Conversely, if the patient is not aware of the potential consequences of following the instructions, he may not be as motivated to follow the instructions.

See Table 4.4 for a summary of ways to help patients understand and remember the information you provide them. These five skills will help you optimize the time you have with patients and help you identify areas for exploration and explanation at future encounters with the patient.

| TABLE 4.4. WAYS TO IMPROVE PATIENT UNDERSTANDING |
| --- |
| 1. Advising patients that important information is to follow |
| 2. Explaining to patients why the information is important |
| 3. Giving clear instructions |
| 4. Providing written information to supplement oral information |
| 5. Assessing patient understanding |

The main points in the structure and process of a patient interview include the following:

1. A formal introduction if it is an initial consultation.
2. Gathering of information: This may include making sure your patient profile is complete, assessing how patients are taking medications, and whether they are having any problems with those medications.
3. Provision of information that the patient needs: In order to maximize your time and the patients', only provide information that the patient does not already know.
4. Assessment of patient understanding.
5. Arrangement for follow-up with the patient, if necessary. Also, make yourself available in the future should the patient have additional questions or concerns.

The next section of the chapter will focus on developing and making different types of presentations. As a pharmacy student and as a pharmacist you will be called upon to present information in a variety of settings and formats. Let's explore a few of those now.

## THE WHAT, WHY, AND HOW OF PRESENTATIONS

As a health-care professional, you will be expected to verbalize information to your peers, other health-care professionals, and to patients. Although many of these communications will likely occur on a one-to-one basis, there may be times when you are asked to present at a scientific conference, in a classroom/auditorium, or a more intimate setting such as the nurses' break room. These situations can be stressful and unnerving if you are not experienced in the art of public speaking. As with anything, there are rules: rules on how to prepare the presentation and rules on how to give the presentation. This section is designed to provide a little background on the types of presentations, a few tips on preparing yourself for the presentation and some pointers to help you avoid making common mistakes that we have all made from time to time during a presentation . . . or two.

## Types of Presentations

*Case Presentations*

Case presentations are learning opportunities for you to disseminate information on the management of a specific disease state as it relates to an actual patient. The purpose is not to merely add new information to the clinical repertoire of the audience; it is to illustrate how the audience can readily incorporate this new information into daily clinical practice.

The case patient is typically one that you actively managed during that specific advanced pharmacy practice experience. During the presentation, you are expected to provide a brief review of the primary disease; give a synopsis of the patient's hospital course; discuss the goals of therapy and necessary monitoring parameters; and finally, offer an evidence-based critique of the patient's therapeutic management (see Table 4.5). The patient's hospital course should be detailed in chronologic order, devoid of irrelevant information. For example, a discussion about the patient's hyperglycemic and hyperlipidemic therapies is irrelevant to a case presentation about hospital-acquired pneumonia. Additionally, in accordance with the Health Insurance Portability and Accountability Act (HIPAA), it is imperative that no identifying information (ie, patient initials, date of birth, room number, etc.) is utilized in the presentation.[18,19] Presentations are generally 20 to

---

**TABLE 4.5. FORMAT FOR PATIENT HOSPITAL COURSE**

Patient hospital course should only detail information relevant to the case presentation. The case should include:

- Patient demographics (age, height, weight, sex, and race)
- Chief complaint
- History of present illness
- Past medical history
- Family / social history
- Physical examination (only report the abnormalities)
- Laboratory data (only report the abnormalities)
- Diagnostic procedures
- Allergies
- Comprehensive medication history (name, strength, dosage form, route, dates of administration)
- Daily progress
- Final outcome (continued hospitalization , discharge, or death)

30 minutes in duration and may be delivered as either an informal roundtable or a formal lecture.[20]

*Journal Clubs*

Journal clubs provide a forum in which you and your attendees can be apprised of current and innovative therapeutic strategies. Approximately 40% to 50% of published articles are of poor quality (ie, flawed research methodology).[21,22] Therefore, it is imperative for you to become skilled in literature evaluation. As you gain experience and grow as a pharmacy clinician, you will recognize the importance of critiquing medical literature prior to applying the information to patient care. Most preceptors will require you to present at least one journal article. Presentations are generally limited to 15 minutes and typically conducted in a roundtable format. Journal articles selected for presentation should be current (within 3 months) and written in a research format. Review articles and case reports are not appropriate. See Chapter 13 for an example of the type of information generally covered during journal clubs.

*Instructional Presentations (eg, Formal, In-Services)*

One of the most common methods for presenting information is through lecture. Traditionally, you stand in front of an audience and disseminate information while the audience passively learns. The disadvantage to this method is that the audience may not give you their undivided attention and/or they may have difficulty assimilating this information into clinical practice.

Today, there is an enormous amount of literature that details new, innovative techniques for actively engaging the audience during presentations. Extensive discussion on these techniques is beyond the scope of this chapter. However, one suggestion for encouraging active participation is to insert a few questions within the presentation and poll the audience. The advantage, it gives you a break from speaking; maintains the audience interest in the topic, and improves audience retention of the material.[23]

Think back to how some of your classes were taught. Did you find yourself disengaged with some teaching methods as opposed to others? How would you improve the learning experience? Do you really want to present to others in a way that you found less enjoyable? The answer is no! The presentation can and should be enjoyable for both you and your audience. So unless otherwise specified, be creative and have fun!

*Poster Presentations*

A poster should be designed such that the audience can easily review the overall rationale, methodology, and outcome(s) of a study or topic. In other words, you are painting a portrait of your project.[24] The aesthetics of your poster is as important as what you say. Why, you ask. If the poster does not look good: (1) people will not be compelled to read it and (2) people may question the credibility of the information.

After your audience has had the opportunity to review your poster, you may be asked specific questions or to provide a brief synopsis of the project. This can be effectively accomplished in 3 to 5 minutes when you: (1) are comfortably familiar with the overall project (including poster content/layout) and (2) have practiced the delivery of the synopsis. The synopsis should highlight essential elements of the project. As well, the synopsis should be used to provide information not stated in the poster and/or provide further details on certain points of interest.

## GETTING STARTED

### Presentation Details

Know the directions and vital details needed for a successful presentation. When you are asked or assigned to do a presentation, there is a certain amount of information that you need to collect in advance.

*Topic*

Exactly what are you expected to cover in this presentation?[25] Pretend you are asked to give a presentation entitled "Introduction to warfarin management" to the nursing staff. What specifically are the nurses interested in learning about as it pertains to warfarin? Dosing and monitoring? Drug-drug and drug-food interactions? Tips for patient counseling?

*Logistics*

- Date and time: Being late to your own presentation is unprofessional! It gives the audience a sense that you perceive their time as not being valuable. You lose credibility. In addition, you may become nervous, flustered, and may potentially rush through your well-prepared presentation.
- Time constraints: This is important because if your presentation is longer than expected, the audience will become agitated and disinterested (ie, looking at their watch, gathering up their belongings). Your big finale will be ignored because your audience is now more focused on leaving than your presentation.
- Visual aid requirements: If handouts or other props are to be distributed, you should determine the number of people expected to be in attendance. The last thing you need or want is the stress of trying to please your audience by attempting to make more materials available.
- Evaluation: Review the evaluation form that will be used so that you are fully aware of how your presentation will be graded. If a copy is not available in your syllabus, ask your preceptor for a copy.

*Know Your Audience*

Who will be attending your presentation? Knowing your audience will be helpful as you prepare your presentation. It will help you determine what material you wish to cover, the extent to which you want to discuss this material, and the style you will use for the presentation.

For instance, if you gave a presentation entitled, "Introduction to warfarin management," how would your presentation differ for health-care professionals (eg, physicians, nurses), pharmacists/pharmacy students, or patients? Would you give the exact same presentation? Who in your audience would be interested in hearing about warfarin absorption and metabolism? Would the details of warfarin pharmacokinetics be of the same benefit to nurses as it would be for pharmacists or pharmacy students? When talking to patients about warfarin, would you refer to it as an anticoagulant or a blood thinner?

Knowing your audience can make all the difference between a successful or unsuccessful presentation. When presentations are appropriately designed for the intended audience (ie, based on education level and utility of information provided), you will be more likely to maintain their attention and potentially engage them in discussions.[25]

### Outlining

Similar to when you write a paper, it is a good practice to start with an outline for your presentation. This is a good way to organize your thoughts and identify the main points that you wish to cover. A basic outline for any presentation includes the introduction, objectives, main content, conclusion, and an opportunity for questions and answers.

- Introduction: Provide your name and the title of your presentation.
- Objectives: Provide an agenda of what you intend to discuss during the presentation.
- Main content: The content in this section will vary based on the type and topic of the presentation.
- Conclusion: Provide a synopsis of the key points already discussed and close with your final thoughts (ie, the "take home" message).
- Questions and answers: Give the audience an opportunity to gain clarification or get further explanation.

### Note Preparation

Unless specified, presentations do not have to be memorized or impromptu. A good presenter is someone who takes the time to prepare his or her thoughts prior to the presentation. Although some people do not require the use of notes during their presentation, others may find note preparation useful when attempting to organize their thoughts. Better yet, this is also a great time to determine how you will explain complex material or an intricate graph.

With note preparation, you may discover that your original presentation outline is not the most conducive order for delivery. It is during this time that you can edit and reorganize your audiovisuals as well as delete points that are irrelevant and unnecessary.

If it is your intention to use notes during your presentation, a good practice is to number the cards in the event that you drop them. *Rattled nerves and unnumbered note cards strewn all across the floor are a bad combination!*

**Figure 4.2.** A cohesive presentation includes visual aids and verbal communication.

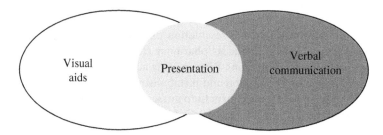

## Visual Aids

When used appropriately, visual aids can greatly enhance a presentation. They can offer visual support to content that is expressed verbally (see Fig. 4.2). The proper visual aid(s) can also be useful in keeping your audience engaged in the topic. On the contrary, misuse of or poorly designed visual aids can disengage your audience just as easily. Refer to the scenarios below.

Scenario 1: Pretend you are giving a presentation on hypertension management and then proceed to show a 5-minute video that details the history of the Joint National Committee (JNC) on Prevention, Detection, Evaluation, and Treatment of High Blood Pressure.

Scenario 2: Pretend you are giving a presentation on hypertension management and then proceed to show a 5-minute video on blood pressure monitoring techniques.

In which scenario is the use of a video more appropriate? Scenario 2. Why? Because although the JNC is an important panel as it relates to hypertension, a 5-minute video about the history of the committee does not add to the presentation. A concise review of the JNC can be sufficiently accomplished with one slide. On the other hand, an explanation on blood pressure monitoring techniques may be better achieved with a video demonstration as opposed to multiple slides with a lot of written instructions and images.

In this chapter, the discussion of visual aids will focus on handouts, PowerPoint, and posters. Other types of visual aids include videos, flip charts, SMART boards, and overhead transparencies.

### Handouts

Handouts are useful for those who wish to take notes and/or have information that they can refer to at a later time. The aim is not to overload your handout with information. By doing so, the audience will read the handout and ignore you. Why should they listen to you when the entire presentation has just been handed to them? If the audience would like a copy of your PowerPoint slides, or if you wish to provide a more detailed handout, consider distributing these items after the presentation.[26]

A good rule of thumb is to make your handout in outline form with significant bullets. Your audience will then rely on your verbal communication to "fill-in" the gaps. Here are a few pointers for developing a successful handout.

- Font size and font style
  - A good, standard font size is 11 or 12 point. However, remember your audience. If you are presenting to an elderly group of patients, you may need to increase your font size slightly to a 14 or 16 point. The handout means nothing if your audience is unable to read it.
  - Keep your font style simple. The rules of sans serif versus serif do not apply to handouts. However, you should avoid script-like fonts such as Lucida Handwriting and Freestyle script.
- Style
  - Your handout should be free from punctuation and grammatical errors. It is annoying to your audience. How many times have you sat in on a presentation loaded with errors? Did you ever wonder if the presenter cared enough to proofread their work (or take advantage of spell check, at the least)? Don't let that be you!
  - Outline structure (ie, tab indentations, bullet types) should be consistent.

*PowerPoint*

Studies have shown that students in colleges and universities prefer educational lectures that utilize PowerPoint. Overall, students believe that course material presented with PowerPoint was more organized and easier to understand.[27] It is likely that you have experienced at least one PowerPoint presentation during your didactic training. From this experience, you may have filed away a list of things that you found to be either good or bad about the way the material was presented. In some cases, you may have even thought of some better or more creative ways in which to deliver the information. Throughout your pharmacy practice experiential training, you may be required to give a PowerPoint presentation. If you are uncomfortable with PowerPoint, or have never used this program to develop a presentation, now is the time to learn and enhance your skills. Many students embark on their advanced pharmacy practice experiences thinking (or at least hoping) that they will never have to give a presentation or use PowerPoint again. More often than not, they are very wrong. During the course of your career, you may be asked to give a presentation to other health-care professionals or present data to a committee. Whatever the case, there are a few rules of PowerPoint etiquette that should be remembered (see Fig. 4.3).

- Font size and font style
  - Ideally, the font size for slide headings should range from 36 to 44 point (minimum 32-point font) and for slide text 32 to 36 point (minimum 28-point font).[18,28]
  - Font styles with minimal curves such as Arial, Helvetica, or other types of sans serif are most effective. Serif font types such as Times New Roman and Garamond have more curves and may be more difficult to read at a distance.[27,28]

**Figure 4.3.** Examples of PowerPoint slides. (A) Example of a poorly designed Power-Point slide. (B) Example of a properly designed PowerPoint slide.

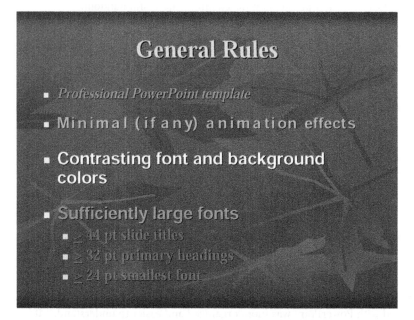

- Avoid using more than two different font styles within the presentation as this can be distracting.[27]
- The use of all lowercase or a combination of uppercase and lowercase letters is preferred. The use of all uppercase, bold, and/or italicized letters can be difficult to decipher and is, therefore, not recommended.[18,27] Instead, reserve this type of lettering to emphasize salient points.[18]
- Color schemes
  - Basic colors with strong contrast between the text and background (eg, white background with black text, dark blue background with yellow text) are preferred.[27,28] In one report, students preferred backgrounds that were not white or brightly colored while another report found blue to be the popular background.[18,27] The color scheme should remain consistent throughout the presentation.
  - The title and text should be in different colors.[18]
- Slide background and layout
  - A simple background (ie, solid color backgrounds) or one with minimal design patterns allows the text to be viewed easily. A busy background can make it difficult for the audience to focus on the material being presented.
  - There should be no more than six words per line and six lines of text on each slide.[18,28]
- Special effects
  - The unnecessary use of multiple colors, sounds, slide transitions (eg, wipe down, wipe right), and animation (eg, spin, zoom) can be very distracting to the audience and shift the focus away from your presentation. These special effects should be used conservatively and should be used at select times to emphasize important points. For instance, colors can be used to highlight an important word, phrase, or concept. In the case of animation (eg, highlight), it can be useful when you wish to reveal and discuss one bullet point at a time. This is referred to as "building."[18,27]
- Style
  - Maintain consistency throughout your PowerPoint slides. The color; font style/size; and the use of bold, italics, or underline to emphasize words or phrases should be uniform from beginning to end.[29]

*Poster Presentation*

As previously mentioned, poster presentations are a great way to interface with others and discuss your work. Successful dialogue can potentially result in both you and your audience walking away with gained knowledge. Your audience learns about your research and you acquire comments and feedback which will be useful for future presentations or if you wish to publish your work.[24] A win-win situation!

First, however, you have to get their attention. Why? Would you stop to smell a flower that you cannot see? Of course not! So how can you expect to capture an audience with a poster that is not clearly visible and appealing to the eye? Below are a few helpful pointers.

- Poster size
  - How large should your poster be? What dimensions should you use to design your poster? To prevent a grade deduction or embarrassment (ie, a poster that is way too large for the cork board that is provided), take time to find this information out *before* designing your poster. If this is a school assignment, read the instructions or ask your instructor if this information in not readily available. Conferences that host poster presentations typically specify the dimensions of the felt/cork boards that will be provided. The last thing that you want to do is spend an enormous amount of time designing a beautiful poster and then have to display it sideways because you failed to read the instructions. Trust me, I have seen this happen.
- Layout
  - Organize your contents in a logical order. How can you effectively tell an entire story with only one poster? (See Fig. 4.4)
  - Keep it simple. Do not attempt to cram every piece of information about your research onto one poster. Keep your background and methods brief. The highlight of any research project is the results. Even then, only present your main findings unless space permits for more information. Again, you are there to answer questions and fill in the gaps when necessary.
- Font size and font style
  - Avoid using a font size less than 24 point.[24]
  - As previously mentioned, select a simple font style. Refer to the font style discussion in the handouts and PowerPoint sections for more details.
- Color scheme
  - Select a color combination with high contrast. See color scheme discussion in the PowerPoint section for more details.

**Figure 4.4.** Standard layout for poster presentations.

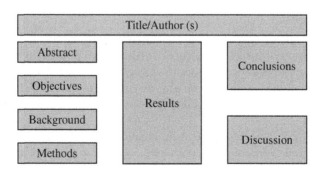

- Title/author(s)
  - Advertise your poster with a short, catchy title. The title should emphasize the focus of your project without being long and overdrawn. It can be stated in the form of a question or could simply answer the question.[24,29] For example, your research project was designed to determine whether or not drug X significantly lowers hemoglobin A1c. A simple title could be "Drug X lowers hemoglobin A1c" or "Does drug X really lower hemoglobin A1c?"
  - The title should be larger than the text used within the body of the poster. Again, you want your title to standout and catch people's attention.
  - Remember to include a byline with all of the authors and their respective institutions. The byline should not be the same size as the title.[29]

## Presentation Skills

*Practice*

Practicing will improve your comfort with the information and thus improve your presentation. Knowing your presentation is just as important as knowing your audience; preparing audiovisuals that are clear to read; and having grammatically correct handouts. In fact, you can have a presentation filled with the most sophisticated charts and graphs that will become worthless to the audience if you are not prepared to explain them in a clear, concise manner. Your audience will have a lot of questions or may simply become disengaged. In addition, your unfamiliarity with the material will be apparent. This will increase your level of nervousness and in some situations, cause you to lose credibility. To prevent this from happening, you want to set aside some time to practice, revise, and ultimately time your presentation. As you practice, you will be able to notice things such as whether your material is organized in a logical fashion; where additional discussion may be required; where some material may need to be removed; and more efficient ways to explain complex charts and graphs. In the end, you will be confident and poised as you deliver your presentation.[25]

## The Dos and Don'ts of Presentations

*Do*

- Practice your presentation. Make sure that you will be able to complete the presentation within the allotted time.
- Dress to impress. Your attire will influence the audience's initial impression/attitude about you.
- Maintain confident body composure. In other words, stand up straight and address the audience (not your note cards and not the presentation screen).
- Stand to the side of the screen or poster and use a laser pointer to direct the audience's eyes to particular details within a slide. Practice using the laser pointer prior to the presentation. When using a laser pointer, maintain a steady hand to aim

at the subject, provide the explanation, and then withdraw the laser beam. Avoid unnecessary use of the laser pointer.

- Spell check your visual aids.
- Maintain good eye contact with the audience.
- Enunciate and project your voice.
- Refrain from saying "uh" or "umm."
- Speak at a normal speed. Do not talk too fast or too slow.
- Avoid any distracting mannerisms such as rocking in the chair, tapping a pencil, jingling keys in your pocket, excessive hand waving, and so on.
- Invite the audience to ask questions and engage in discussion.
- Smile and be enthusiastic about the topic. Remember . . . attitude is contagious!

*Don't*

- Read your presentation. Do not read your note cards, the video screen, or your poster. By doing so, your back will be to the audience. Therefore, you will be talking to your visual aid and not your audience.
- Assume your audience already knows the material. Prepare your presentation in such a way that you are the expert teaching new information to colleagues and/ or patients. Be prepared to give a brief background or overview of the topic, to define certain terminology, and/or to thoroughly explain your graphic material.[29]

## References

Give credit where credit is due. If your presentation contains information derived from any source of literature (eg, primary, secondary, tertiary), it is important that you correctly reference and cite these sources. For information on how to cite references, refer to the *Uniform Requirements for Manuscripts Submitted to Biomedical Journals: Writing and Editing for Biomedical Publications* (www.icmje.org).

In the last section of the chapter, we will focus on written communication and how it impacts pharmacy practice.

## WRITING IN THE PROFESSIONS

Professions and professionals are defined by any number of attributes. The following attribute, while central, rarely shows up on the typical lists; however, professionals are communities of technical writers, who owe part of their ability to succeed in their fields of activity to their ability to construct written messages with care and clarity. Writing is one of the primary tools by which professionals get their jobs done. Pharmacy is no exception.

### Writing's Centrality to Pharmacy Practice

Writing is the vehicle that drives pharmacy practice, regardless of practice type or setting. This assertion may appear oppositional to observed activity in pharmacy practice settings: the most immediately observable communication activity across pharmacy practice settings is that of the spoken word, not the written. Pharmacists are seen talking, face-to-face or via the telephone, to patients, fellow pharmacists, technicians, physicians, other health-care providers, other agents in the larger health-care economy, and other members of the community. However, as with many phenomena, first impressions and/or surface activity can misrepresent reality.

Although oral communication gets the most attention in the education of pharmacists, both as students and as continuing practitioners, writing is the frontline communication medium for three reasons:

1. The health-care activity for which pharmacists are most readily identified and most often reimbursed for involve transactions initiated and mediated by written documents.
2. Writing has strong legal standing; oral communication does not.
3. Emerging technologies' role in patient care and business practice.

*Writing: The Action Catalyst in Health Care*

A thorough look at contemporary health-care systems reveals that writing occupies a central place in all aspects of health-care delivery. From physicians' offices to third-party insurers' claims processing centers, and at nearly every point between, writing is a preferred and, in many cases the mandatory means of recording activity (from historical to diagnostic to therapeutic), justifying decisions and action plans, and initiating therapy, including the joining of multiple health-care providers to specific cases. The national emphasis on electronic patient medical records (even web-based patient records, accessible by all participants in a patient's care) will only enhance the fact that writing is the catalyst that accelerates contemporary health care.

At the simplest level, for pharmacy the ubiquitous written health-care document is the written prescription. Without this document, authored by a credible and authorized health-care provider, pharmacists' ability to engage in the full scope of practice is legally cut off. Pharmacists' roles as professional writers are witnessed in the many, often mundane, day-to-day job-related tasks of updating patient records, interacting with insurers, answering drug information questions for physicians, and dealing with the full range of personnel and business management, as well as regulatory tasks that come along with pharmacy practice regardless of setting.

*Writing: The Legal Coin of the Realm*

As much as pharmacists pride themselves in developing strong oral communication skills, the strength of their written communication skills serves greatly to improve long-term career success. Although oral and interpersonal communication skills are essential tools in direct patient care, when the role of legal compliance and professional liability is considered, it is quickly apparent that the written work carries much more power. More than one health providers have faced the no-win proposition of the "she said, he said" confrontation that results when no written record exists to substantiate either side's claims.

The pharmacy community has responded to this reality of strong legal weight afforded to writing by instating increasingly complex systems of patient records, paralleling in many respects the patient records long maintained by physicians and hospitals. Written documents (including patient charts, e-mail, telephone text message records, etc.) are among the first materials collected and considered materially admissible in malpractice and other civil litigation. While sloppy-written documents often hurt the defense in such litigation, the presence of written records provides stronger positions for exoneration (or settlement) than a reliance on an oral history.

*Writing: The Heart of Computer-Technology-Mediated Practice*

Contemporary professional life (in and out of health-care disciplines) is awash in electronically mediated communication. The pager, once the essential tool for pharmacists practicing in a hospital setting, has been replaced by the web-enhanced cell phone. Paper journals have gone electronic, as have much of the volume and the access processes that drive quality drug- and health-information question-and-answer activity.

E-mail is a constant presence, even allowing one's work activities to intrude on nonwork time. What the next decade holds for expansion of the role of electronic-mediated communication in health care is hard to predict due to the rapid developments in communication technologies and increased public and private interests in the business of managing health information.

Pharmacy is also involved in the next push of computer-mediated health-care activity, the electronic/web-based patient medical record. Electronic medical record (EMR) initiatives will fundamentally shift the realities for pharmacy as a community of writers: clearinghouses of patient care data, such as those envisioned by EMR initiatives in the public and private sector, will result in pharmacy recording more depth and breadth of its patient-care activities. The medium of this activity will be writing, not speech (or, if voice recorded, all entries will be transcribed into written form).

## Range of Writing in Pharmacy

For an activity that occupies practitioner time and comes with very real risks, writing within the daily practice realities of pharmacy has attracted scant attention in comparison to other types of pharmacy-based activity. The first, and currently only, systematic assessment of the types of writing that pharmacists are expected to author within their job functions was published in 2002. Kennicutt et al surveyed 129 pharmacists serving as advanced pharmacy practice experience preceptors and reported a range of 34 documents that they author at least once a year as part of their pharmacist roles (see Table 4.6).[30]

All respondents reported writing on a daily basis within their practice of pharmacy. Of the 23 writing tasks that served as the survey's document base, survey respondents identified 16 as being of "high value" to their practice, regardless of the frequency with which they wrote these documents. These 16 "high value" documents, in order of frequency of occurrence, are: memorandum/letter, progress note, pharmacy-care plan, patient consult note, drug utilization review/evaluation (DUR/DUE),

**TABLE 4.6.** DOCUMENTS AUTHORED BY PHARMACISTS

| Pharmacy Patient Care | Clinical Report | Research | Administration/Other |
|---|---|---|---|
| Patient consult note | Clinical algorithm | Book chapter | Continuous quality improvement (CQI) or quality assurance (QA) plan |
| Pharmacy care plan | Clinical guideline | Book review | Formulary book |
| Pharmacist-to-pharmacist patient-care note | Drug information review | Clinical drug study interpretation | In-service presentation |
| Progress note | Drug utilization review (DUR) or drug utilization evaluation (DUE) | Final drug study report | Letter to editor or letter of recommendation |
| | P&T/formulary review | Grant proposal | Management report |
| | Summary/new drug report | Grant review | Memorandum or letter |
| | | Manuscript review | Newsletter |
| | | Poster/report for publication | Patient education pamphlet |
| | | Survey instrument | Performance evaluation |
| | | | Pharmacy services report |
| | | | Pharmacy legislation review |
| | | | Policies and procedures |
| | | | Position justification |
| | | | Utility analysis report |
| | | | Variance report |

drug information review, pharmacy and therapeutics (P&T) committee/formulary review, policies and procedures, performance evaluation, newsletter, in-service presentation, clinical algorithm, clinical guideline, grant proposal, poster/report for publication, and continuous quality improvement (CQI)/quality assurance (QA) plan.

Kennicutt and his coauthors note that the study was limited by a respondent population situated disproportionately in clinical practices. The reported document range reflects that practice bias. However, similar research into the writing activities of other professional communities, including mental health providers, reveals similar ranges of writing tasks, spanning the spectrum from highly technical to generically administrative, from more- to less-frequently authored, from more- to less valuable to practice.[31–33]

## Pharmacy Student Experiences with Writing

Some anecdotal discussions of pharmacy students' experiences with and perceptions about writing have been published. However, most of these focused on writing activity within classroom contexts.[34–37] For the most part, these authors have focused on how to use writing as a powerful teaching and learning tool, or have offered writing assignments and strategies designed to expand student pharmacists' basic communication skills and heighten their levels of rhetorical sophistication. Even when articles focus on helping students learn to write the types of documents that they should expect to encounter within pharmacy practice settings, the focus remains narrow: learn how to do X.

The less common approach found in the literature that addresses pharmacy student writing is that of Nemire,[38] and Hobson et al,[39] who focused specifically on the types of documents that students author during the experiential components of their education. These should be documents that bear similarity to the types of documents that practitioners report writing as part of their ongoing professional lives. Nemire identified 12 document types that "pharmacy students realize they must write . . . as part of their professional practice."[38] They are listed in Table 4.7.

---

**TABLE 4.7.  DOCUMENTS AUTHORED BY PHARMACY STUDENTS**

| | | |
|---|---|---|
| Medication histories | Progress notes | Peer-reviewed published papers |
| Grant proposals | Student education materials | Consultation reports |
| Teaching materials | Letters to physicians | Discharge summaries |
| Communications to patients | Patient education materials | Physician education materials |

**TABLE 4.8.** DOCUMENT CATEGORIES

| | | | |
|---|---|---|---|
| In-service presentation | Summary | Case write-up | Formulary review |
| Newsletter | Research manuscript | Clinical algorithm | Journal article critique |
| Research methods comparison | Informed-consent form | Adverse drug-reaction report | Drug utilization review/evaluation (DUR/DUE) |
| Student education material | Patient education document | Drug information inquiry write-up | Continuing education program |
| Consultation | Drug-use assessment | Commentary | Retrospective analysis |
| Experimental data | Procedure | Review article | Market analysis |
| Research protocol | Correspondence | Abstract | Survey |

This list's contents reflect less overlap with the range of practitioner writing reported by Kennicutt et al than one would like to see if the projections of practitioner need, offered by thought leaders within the academy, reflect current practice realities.

Hobson et al went further in a study of the writing tasks that pharmacy students carry out during the final experience courses in a doctor of pharmacy program.[39] The team reviewed 200 documents from among hundreds submitted by doctor of pharmacy students as part of their advanced professional practice experience portfolios. Analysis of this sample set identified 28 distinct document categories listed in Table 4.8.

Of these, 5 accounted for over 60% of the documents written by students: in-service presentations (23%), summaries (16%), patient case write-ups (9%), formulary review (8%), and newsletters (8%). Interestingly, of the documents that students wrote, Hobson et al could find few instances where students had been instructed in how to author these documents in coursework leading up to their practice experiences. The authors note, "The belief that 'pharmacists don't write' ignores the presence and value of writing in all aspects of pharmacy practice."[39]

## Pharmacists are Professional Writers . . . Even as Students

Whether or not it makes everyone excited, pharmacists, and those completing their education, are professional writers: they carry out and record significant portions of their professional responsibilities through the generation of written documents. As seen in studies of this reality, practicing pharmacists and pharmacy students can expect to write a wide range of document types in the course of their regular job and patient-care functions. While this reality can be daunting, the following six admonitions provide a generally agreed upon set of base perspectives upon which to build one's effectiveness as a writer. Remember, effective professional writing is about your audience and its needs, accuracy, clarity, concision, correctness, and credibility or confidence in the author.

*Strategies for Developing Strong Professional Writing Skills*

Five general tips to improving one's writing as a professional:

1. Accept the following truth: There are now two writers in your head—general and professional.
2. Invest in planning time.
3. Develop and use trusted colleagues as proofreaders.
4. Let the document sit before sending it.
5. Adequacy can be a sufficient standard.

*Pitfalls to Avoid as a Professional Writer*

Five general tips to avoiding embarrassment, or worse, as a professional writer:

1. Always give your readers enough credit/high-enough expectations.
2. Don't rush important/key tasks.
3. Don't cut corners.
4. Don't believe the mundane tasks are not important.
5. Don't lower your own standards of ethical practice.

## SUMMARY

The authors in this chapter reviewed basic communication skills that may be used in various areas of interaction. The careful consideration of nonverbal communication, the phrasing of questions, appropriate use of empathy, and assertiveness are all useful tools when interacting with employers, colleagues, and patients. A systematic way to conduct patient medication interviews and patient education sessions was presented. Following a structured format will allow you to make best use of the time that you have with each patient.

Pharmacists and pharmacy students are called upon to make various presentations, including case presentations, journal clubs, in-services, and poster presentations. Suggestions for preparing and presenting in a clear, professional manner were outlined. Specific tips were given for generating effective handouts, slides, and posters. Finally, a list of "dos and don'ts" for presentations detailed the best ways to ensure your presentation is a success.

In the writing section, an overview of the importance of writing to the profession of pharmacy was argued. Examples of the numerous writing opportunities for pharmacists and pharmacy students were supplied. Suggestions for becoming a successful professional writer are also provided for your further reflection and practice.

Any new knowledge or skill requires practice. Communication skills require a lot of practice. As mentioned at the beginning of the chapter, few people are able instinctively to conduct an efficient patient interview. With time and practice, you will become both effective and efficient in your role as a patient educator, health-care professional educator, and pharmacy professional. As you practice pharmacy and grow in experience, you will also gain insight into communicating with patients and colleagues. You will develop your own style and gain confidence in your ability to communicate effectively with others. To practice communicating, turn to the role-playing scenarios at the end of this chapter.

## APPLICATION EXERCISES

The answers are not provided for the exercises in this chapter. This is a good opportunity for you to work out the answers for these questions and then discuss them with faculty in the appropriate courses.

1. What nonverbal cues send a positive message to others?
2. What components make up communication?
3. How would you respond to a patient who says, "This medication isn't working at all. I don't know what else to try?" What techniques would you use?
4. How would you respond to a nurse who says, "It took way too long to get this laxative. We ordered it STAT!" What assertiveness technique would you use?
5. Explain the usage of open-ended and closed-ended questions in a patient interview.
6. What types of presentations are pharmacy students and pharmacists likely to make?
7. Design a sample handout for a presentation using PowerPoint.
8. Why is writing of such importance to the profession of pharmacy?
9. What can you do to improve your writing?

## ACKNOWLEDGMENT

The authors wish to acknowledge the contributions of Eric H. Hobson to this chapter.

## REFERENCES

1. Muchmore J, Galvin K. A report of the task force on career competencies in oral communication skills for community college students seeking immediate entry into the work force. *Commun Ed.* 1983;32:207–220.
2. Ley P. *Communicating with Patients: Improving Communication, Satisfaction and Compliance.* New York, NY: Croom Helm; 1988.
3. Ali F, Laurin MY, Lariviere C, et al. The effect of pharmacist intervention and patient education on lipid-lowering medication compliance and plasma cholesterol levels. *Can J Clin Pharmacol.* 2003;10:101–106.
4. Davis NM, Cohen MR. Counseling reduces dispensing accidents. *Am Pharm.* 1992;NS32:22.
5. Zillich AJ, Sutherland JM, Kumbera PA, et al. Hypertension outcomes through blood pressure monitoring and evaluation by pharmacists (HOME study). *J Gen Intern Med.* 2005;20:1091–1096.

6. Bell S, McLachlan AJ, Aslani P, et al. Community pharmacy services to optimize the use of medications for mental illness: a systematic review. BioMed Central Australia and New Zealand Health Policy. 2005;2:29. Available at http://www.anzhealthpolicy.com/content/2/1/29. Accessed March, 2014.

7. Zermansky AG, Petty DR, Rayno DK, et al. Randomised controlled trial of clinical medication review by a pharmacist of elderly patients receiving repeat prescriptions in general practice. *BMJ.* 2001;323:1–5.

8. Dooly MJ, Allen KM, Doecke CJ, et al. A prospective multicentre study of pharmacist initiated changes to drug therapy and patient management in acute care government funded hospitals. *Br J Clin Pharmacol.* 2003;57(4):513–521.

9. Kucukarslan SN, Peters M, Mlynarek M, et al. Pharmacists on rounding teams reduce preventable adverse drug events in hospital general medicine units. *Arch Intern Med.* 2003;163:2014–2018.

10. Scarsi KK, Fotis MA, Noskin GA. Pharmacist participation in medical rounds reduces medication errors. *Am J Health Syst Pharm.* 2002;59:2089–2092.

11. Berlo DK. *The Process of Communication.* New York, NY: Holt, Rinehart and Winston; 1960.

12. Nelson AR, Zelnio RN, Beno CE. Clinical pharmaceutical services in retail practice II. Factors influencing the provision of services. *Drug Intell Clin Pharmacy.* 1984;8(12):992–996.

13. Raisch DW. Barriers to providing cognitive services. *Am Pharmacy.* 1993;33(12):54–58.

14. Herrier R, Boyce R. Why aren't more pharmacists counseling? *Am Pharmacy.* 1994;34(11):22–23.

15. Tindall WN, Beardsley RS, Kimberlin CL. *Communication Skills in Pharmacy Practice.* Malvern, PA: Lea & Febiger; 1994.

16. Kimberlin CL, Berardo DH. A comparison of patient education methods used in community pharmacies. *J Pharm Market Manag.* 1987;1(4):75–94.

17. Gotsch AR, Liguori S. Knowledge, attitude, and compliance dimensions of antibiotic therapy with PPIs. *Med Care.* 1982;20(6):581–595.

18. Harolds JA. Tips for giving a memorable presentation, part IV: using and composing PowerPoint slides. *Clin Nucl Med* 2012;37:977–980.

19. Cohen H. How to write a patient case report. *AJHP* 2006;63:1888–1892.

20. Boh LE, Beck D. Professional practice experiences: goals, objectives, and activities. In: Boh LE, Young LY, eds. *Pharmacy Practice Manual: A Guide to the Clinical Experience.* 2nd ed. Baltimore, MD: Lippincott Williams & Wilkins; 2001:12–44.

21. Khan KS, Gee H. A new approach to teaching and learning in journal club. *Med Teach.* 1999;21(3):289–293.

22. Mosdell KW. Literature evaluation I: controlled clinical trials. In: Malone PM, Mosdell KW, Kier KL, et al., eds. *Drug Information: A Guide for Pharmacists.* 2nd ed. New York, NY: McGraw-Hill; 2001:133–172.

23. Harolds JA. Tips for giving a memorable presentation, part I: the speaker as an educator. *Clin Nucl Med* 2012;37:669–670.

24. Erren TC, Bourne PE. Ten simple rules for a good poster presentation. *PLoS Comput Biol.* 2007;3(5):e102.

25. Bourne PE. Ten simple rules for making good oral presentations. *PLoS Comput Biol.* 2007;3(4):e77.

26. Harolds JA. Tips for giving a memorable presentation, part III: composing an important formal presentation. *Clin Nucl Med* 2012;37:872–873.

27. Apperson JM, Laws EL, Scepansky JA. An assessment of student preferences for PowerPoint presentation structure in undergraduate courses. *Comput Educ.* 2008;50:148–153.

28. Kennedy DH, Ward CT, Metzner MC. Distance education: using compressed interactive video technology for an entry-level Doctor of Pharmacy program. *Am J Pharm Educ.* 2003;67(4):Article 118.

29. Block SM. Dos and don'ts of poster presentation. *Biophys J.* 1996;71(6):3527–3529.

30. Kennicutt JD, Hobson EH, Briceland LL, Waite NM. On-the-job writing tasks of clerkship preceptors. *Am J Health-Syst Pharm.* 2002;59:63–67.

31. Winsor DA. *Writing Like an Engineer: A Rhetorical Education.* Mahwah, NJ: Erlbaum; 1996.

32. Matalene CB, ed. *Worlds of Writing: Teaching and Learning in Discourse Communities of Work.* New York, NY: Random House; 1989.

33. Reynolds JF, Mair DC, Fischer PC. *Writing and Reading Mental Health Records.* 2nd ed. Mahwah, NJ; Erlbaum: 1995.

34. Hobson EH, Schafermeyer KW. Writing and critical thinking: writing-to-learn in large classes. *Am J Pharm Educ.* 1994;58:423–427.

35. Prosser TR, Burke JM, Hobson EH. Teaching pharmacy students to write in the medical record. *Am J Pharm Educ.* 1997;61:136–140.

36. Ranelli PL, Nelson JV. Assessing writing perceptions and practices of pharmacy students. *Am J Pharm Educ.* 1998;62:426–432.

37. Ranelli PL. Using student-written book reviews as a teaching tool. *J Pharm Teach.* 1991;2(4):42–52.

38. Nemire RE. Writing across the curriculum: an introduction to the pharmacy classroom. In: Holiday-Goodman M, Lively BT, eds. *Writing Across the Curriculum for Colleges of Pharmacy: A Sourcebook.* Toledo, OH: The University of Toledo College of Pharmacy & American Association of Colleges of Pharmacy; 1992:5.1–5.7.

39. Hobson EH, Waite NM, Briceland LL. Writing tasks performed by doctor of pharmacy students during clerkship rotations. *Am J Health-Syst Pharm.* 2002;59:58–62.

## ROLE-PLAYING SCENARIOS

The following pages contain 15 examples of pharmacy-related communication scenarios. These scenarios were developed by Dr. Ruth Nemire and Dr. Michelle

Assa-Eley for a class at Nova Southeastern University. They are designed for pharmacy students to practice their communication skills through role playing.

For each scenario, two alternative approaches are proposed for the exchange. We suggest you try them both ways and get feedback from your friends. Additionally, discussion questions for each scenario are included. Reviewing such situations before you encounter them will be helpful.

The exercises may also be used as learning tools for study groups or for exercises to practice with your preceptor. In addition to the discussion questions, for each scenario, consider what communication tools would be most helpful in working through the issues presented. It will be helpful to have others provide feedback on the interactions and offer suggestions for improvement; a discussion of different perspectives can reveal new methods of approaching communication. It may also be appropriate for you to write a reflective journal entry to determine your responses and learning from the activity.

## SCENARIO I

While the pharmacist (student 1) is busy filling a prescription for a surgical patient waiting at the counter, another patient (student 2) comes into the pharmacy to ask for advice concerning her medications. She has started taking a new drug called Euphoravil for the treatment of depression. In addition to this prescription, she wants to take St. John's Wort because she knows that it worked for a neighbor. This patient is older and just wants to feel better; she has diabetes and is already on many medications. She is impatient and interrupts you many times while you are trying to finish filling the surgical patient's prescription.

### Version 1

The pharmacist drops everything to help the patient and counsels her immediately. Complicating the interview is the patient's confusion about her medications and inability to fully answer the pharmacist's questions. This counseling session requires patience on the part of both parties.

### Version 2

The patient is in a hurry and wants the pharmacist to answer her questions before finishing with the surgical patient. The pharmacist asks the patient to wait for a moment, at which point the patient begins to get belligerent. The pharmacist agrees to counsel her at that point.

### Discussion Questions

1. As the patient, how did you feel?
2. As the pharmacist, what were your frustrations?
3. What could have improved the communication better in each scenario?

## SCENARIO II

The pharmacist (student 1) in a really slow pharmacy is talking on the phone with her boyfriend. A patient (student 2) comes to the counter and wants to have a prescription filled. The pharmacist hangs up and comes to help the patient, but the drug is not in stock.

### Version 1

The pharmacist tries to be helpful, but the patient is very upset because the prescription is for a baby. Further, the patient does not know what to do because he came to the pharmacy by bus and does not have enough money for transportation to another pharmacy.

### Version 2

The pharmacist hangs up the phone and comes to the counter to help. The patient cannot find the prescription but is certain he has it. After receiving the prescription from the patient, the pharmacist reviews it and says it is not available. The patient wants to know what it is for (antibiotic) and what is he supposed to do now. It is now 8:45 PM, and the pharmacy closes in 15 minutes.

### Discussion Questions

1. How might you improve the communication in each version?
2. What factors are important to recognize in dealing with this type of situation?
3. What might the pharmacist be feeling that interferes with her communication with this patient?
4. What might the patient be feeling?

## SCENARIO III

A physician (student 1) calls the pharmacy to ask for advice. The physician has a patient who needs to be started on two inhalers, but does not have sufficient time to teach the patient how to use them. The doctor wants the pharmacist (student 2) to fill the prescriptions and teach the patient how to use the inhalers, with an aerochamber (device to help use inhalers) if necessary. The pharmacist is working alone today because the pharmacy technician called in sick. It is early in the day, and he has already filled 40 prescriptions. The doctor is a friend of the pharmacist and is always asking for favors such as this. The pharmacist has been considering asking the physician for a fee for providing these services and decides to do that today.

## Version 1

The pharmacist agrees to spend time with the patient today.

## Version 2

The pharmacist says it cannot be done today.

## Discussion Questions

1. What feelings does the physician need to validate for the pharmacist?
2. Should the pharmacist have asked for a fee from the physician, or should the pharmacist provide the education at the physician's request for free?
3. Is the physician taking advantage of his friendship with the pharmacist?

## SCENARIO IV

A patient (student 1) comes to the pharmacy seeking advice regarding the choice of a vitamin supplement. The patient is elderly and is living on a fixed income. The patient confides in the pharmacist (student 2) that she has lost 20 lb in 1 month and attributes this weight loss to an improper diet. In addition to the weight loss, she is thirsty all the time and has spells when she cannot remember where she has been. The pharmacist listens patiently and then offers suggestions to the patient.

## Version 1

The patient is hard of hearing.

## Version 2

The pharmacist is hard of hearing.

## Discussion Questions

1. What advice would you offer the pharmacist to improve the communication?
2. As the patient, what information did you want from the pharmacist? Did you get it?
3. As the pharmacist, what information would have been helpful to have from the patient?
4. What did this conversation look like from the perspective of a customer waiting to pick up a prescription?

## SCENARIO V

A nurse (student 1) calls the pharmacy to find out the store's hours and if the pharmacy offers a delivery service. She also tells the pharmacist (student 2) she wants to call in a prescription for a patient. The patient, who does not have transportation, is the physician's mother. The prescription is for Nopain, a schedule II medication for which a hard copy of the prescription is required by law. The nurse tells the pharmacist she will mail the prescription today. The pharmacist must handle this. Both times, the pharmacist will not fill the prescription.

### Version 1

The rationale for not filling the prescription is that the pharmacy does not offer a delivery service for anyone.

### Version 2

The rationale for not filling the prescription is that, legally, the pharmacist cannot fill a prescription for Nopain without a valid prescription in hand.

### Discussion Questions

1. What communication skills are important to utilize in such situations?
2. What is of particular concern for the pharmacist in either scenario?
3. What should be expected of the pharmacist in this situation? What should be expected of the nurse in this situation?

## SCENARIO VI

A patient (student 1) calls the pharmacist (student 2) requesting a refill of a heart medication but cannot recall its name. The profile in the computer says that she is on Heartache once daily. The patient usually gets a 30-day supply, but has not had a refill for 90 days. The patient is still on the phone. There are no other medications on file. The patient does not speak English very well, and the pharmacist speaks only English. The pharmacist needs to know why the patient has not been taking the Heartache and/or if there is a new medication.

### Version 1

The patient has a prescription for another medication that was filled by a mail-order company. Unfortunately, the prescription was lost in the mail. When the pharmacist tries to fill this prescription with the patient still on the phone, it is rejected by the insurance company as an early refill. The pharmacist will have to call the insurance company.

### Version 2

The patient was feeling better, so she stopped the medication. Now she feels bad and thought she should start again because she has a doctor's appointment in 2 days and has to get a blood level drawn.

## Discussion Questions

1. What is the problem for the pharmacist in either case?
2. What is the problem for the patient?
3. What should the pharmacist do?

## SCENARIO VII

It is 5:30 PM on Sunday afternoon, and the pharmacy will close in half an hour. A cardiologist (student 1) calls in a prescription for an allergy medication for a patient who is the son of one of the physician's friends. The doctor mentions that the parent cannot get to the pharmacy until after 6:00 PM. Because the manager will not allow the pharmacist (student 2) to leave the pharmacy open even 1 minute after 6:00 PM, the pharmacist must explain to the doctor that the parent must get there before 6:00 PM or the pharmacy will be closed.

## Version 1

The cardiologist gives the wrong directions for the allergy medication because it is not something she normally prescribes. She then asks you about the hours. The cardiologist tells you that you will have to stay open past closing because you are a health-care professional. The pharmacist thinks that this should have been taken care of earlier in the day and that it is not an emergency situation. Based on this, the pharmacist refuses to stay open.

## Version 2

The cardiologist gives wrong directions for the medication and then adds that the patient also needs an antibiotic. Because the physician does not know the patient but does know that the child has some allergies, the physician tells the pharmacist to give the patient the same prescription as the antibiotic bottle the mother brings in. The pharmacist must explain why she will not do this. The cardiologist reminds the pharmacist that she is the doctor and that the pharmacist has to do what she is told.

## Discussion Questions

1. What is the problem here, and what makes communication so difficult?
2. What suggestions do you have for improving the potential outcomes of the scenarios?
3. What are you going to do when this happens to you?
4. Did the pharmacist or physician get defensive, abusive?
5. How should those issues be dealt with?

## SCENARIO VIII

A pharmacist (student 1) is working in a hospital. There is a survey team coming from the accreditation body, and all you can think about is all the work and paperwork that there is to do. Because the other clinical pharmacist called in sick, you have to cover rounds on the internal medicine floor and the intensive care unit (ICU). In the ICU, a medical student (student 2) asks you to tell him how to mix total parenteral nutrition (TPN). You do not do that routinely in your practice, so you are unsure yourself. The pharmacist believes that the medical student should have to do this as an exercise, but the student thinks it is the pharmacist's job to take care of this.

### Version 1

The medical student is a brash, overconfident person who believes the other healthcare professionals at the hospital are there to serve the needs of the medical students. The pharmacist is a responsible professional who will not have patients suffer as a result of the lack of involvement from the medical student.

### Version 2

The pharmacist believes the medical students are in the hospital for learning and will not do the TPN orders.

### Discussion Questions

1. What is happening when these two health-care professionals communicate?
2. When power struggles occur, is there always a communication problem?
3. Who will suffer if this is not worked out?
4. What do you think should occur in the scenario?

## SCENARIO IX

A patient (student 1) with diarrhea comes to the pharmacy in distress. The patient wants the pharmacist (student 2) to make a recommendation for an over-the-counter product. The patient tells the pharmacist that it is bloody diarrhea, and because it is Saturday night, she cannot see her doctor. This patient should be seen by a doctor, so the pharmacist attempts to suggest that the patient go to the emergency room (ER). The patient does not have insurance and will not go to the ER because it costs too much. The pharmacist must make a decision about whether to tell the patient to get Imodium AD or not.

### Version 1

The patient plans to buy an over-the-counter product such as Pepto Bismol. The pharmacist knows that it may not really help the diarrhea and that a bloody stool is a sign of a larger problem because the patient says it is bright red blood. The patient is wishy-washy and reluctantly agrees to go to the ER.

## Version 2

After the pharmacist learns that the diarrhea is tinged with bright red blood, she insists that the patient seek medical attention. The patient says she will die before going to the ER.

### Discussion Questions

1. Were there any problems in communication in either scenario?
2. What do you think is the best way to handle this?
3. Did the patient feel she was being counseled well in either scene?
4. What could have made the interaction better?

## SCENARIO X

The pharmacist (student 1) at this pharmacy has just started charging for counseling sessions for patients who want to know about their medications that have been purchased elsewhere (ie, mail order). The usual fee for "brown bag" counseling is $10.00 per half-hour. A patient (student 2), who had been a regular patron of the pharmacy until insurance required her to receive her prescriptions by mail order, enters the pharmacy with a bag of pills. She mentions that she has several questions about each of the medications. The patient has not been in the pharmacy for over a year and hopes the pharmacist will take the time necessary to counsel her. The pharmacist is upset because the insurance company will not pay him to dispense the medications, and yet the patient wants to discuss them.

## Version 1

The patient does not understand how health care has come to this. The patient argues with the pharmacist, saying that it is the responsibility of pharmacists everywhere to help anyone with questions free of charge.

## Version 2

The pharmacist tells the patient about the fee, and the patient agrees to pay for the counseling session.

### Discussion Questions

1. What dilemma does the pharmacist face?
2. What dilemma does the patient face?
3. Did both pharmacists communicate effectively? What improvements could be made in each case?

## SCENARIO XI

A pharmacist (student 1) is working in a nursing home reviewing charts. A patient's family member (student 2) demands to know why his 98-year-old relative is on Tranquil. He understands that it is an awful drug and that it is very addicting. The pharmacist feels that although the drug is addicting, the addiction potential is irrelevant when the patient is 98 years old. The patient was prescribed Tranquil because she has been getting out of bed in the middle of the night and wandering the halls of the nursing home. The drug was given in hope that it would keep the patient from waking up during the night and wandering to where she should not. The family member is screaming at the pharmacist to get her off of the drug.

### Version 1

The family member does not calm down until the pharmacist does something to get his attention such as yelling back. After that, the pharmacist can explain her perspective, and the family member asks questions appropriately.

### Version 2

The family member is willing to listen to the pharmacist, but the pharmacist seems glib about the entire situation because of the patient's age. The family member threatens to report the pharmacist to her supervisor.

### Discussion Questions

1. What did the first pharmacist do that was effective? What was not effective?
2. What happened in the second version that was probably not an effective form of communication?
3. What important factors should be considered when communicating with any family member or patient?

## SCENARIO XII

A person (student 1) telephones the pharmacy to ask a question about the prescription drug Nodrinky. She asks the pharmacist (student 2) what will happen if one drinks alcohol with the prescription. Drinking with this drug will cause her to vomit and to have flu-like symptoms, a high fever, and a rapid heart rate. She tells the pharmacist that she has already had a drink and now feels quite sick. The person blames the pharmacist. The pharmacist clearly recalls telling a patient earlier in the day about Nodrinky's interaction with alcohol.

### Version 1

The person who calls the pharmacy is not the patient. By law, the pharmacist cannot discuss the patient's medications with anyone but the patient. After some discussion, the patient (student 3) gets on the phone and is angry that the pharmacist would not talk to her friend. This issue should be resolved with the patient agreeing to go to the hospital.

## Version 2

The person on the phone is the patient. She wants to drink and attempts to get the pharmacist to agree that it is okay to have a drink and that nothing will happen. The pharmacist tells the patient the potential outcome of consuming alcohol while taking the medication and that she should not drink. The pharmacist resorts to trying to scare the patient.

## Discussion Questions

1. What could help the pharmacist more effectively convey the message?
2. What should the pharmacist have done when the prescription was picked up?
3. Does the pharmacist have a responsibility to make sure the patient does not drink, or does the pharmacist's responsibility end with counseling?
4. What was good about the communication that went on? What could be improved?

## SCENARIO XIII

A busy pharmacist (student 1) in the hospital notices that an order has been written for a dose of Apedrug that will kill a child. The pharmacist knows that the physician (student 2) is always hard to get hold of and has a reputation for being rude and disrespectful. The pharmacist places a call to the physician, who happens to be in the hospital on the floor writing orders and answers right away.

## Version 1

The pharmacist asks the doctor if what has been written is really what the doctor wants. The pharmacist repeats the dose and the age of the patient, says that the patient will die, and refuses to fill the prescription. This is said in such a way as to anger the doctor. Tempers flare, but the pharmacist still refuses to fill the prescription. The doctor hangs up.

## Version 2

The pharmacist reaches the doctor as in scene 1, but finds a better way to tell the doctor the dose is wrong. The doctor, who starts out the conversation abruptly, thanks the pharmacist in the end.

## Discussion Questions

1. What elements of Version 1 and Version 2 made a difference in the outcome?
2. What else could the pharmacist have done?

3. How can pharmacists change other health-care professionals' perception of their role on the health-care team from watchdog to team member?
4. How might the pharmacist best approach the physician: on the phone, in person, or ask the nurse?

## SCENARIO XIV

A patient (student 1) brings in 10 prescriptions and tells the pharmacist (student 2) that he will return in 15 minutes exactly to pick them up. This patient is a young person who does this every month. The patient also wants the pharmacist to fill out insurance paperwork in that amount of time.

### Version 1

The pharmacist tells the patient that it will be at least 2 hours or more before the prescriptions are filled, and the paperwork will not be done until the next day. The pharmacist is able to present this information in such a manner that the patient accepts the answer readily.

### Version 2

The patient is not willing to accept anything the pharmacist says and insists that the prescriptions and paperwork be ready in 15 minutes.

### Discussion Questions

1. In the first scene, did the pharmacist really appease the patient with the answer? Or did the patient just accept it because he thought he had to?
2. What if the patient started screaming and yelling? How would that be handled?
3. Is there ever a time when it is okay to tell the patient that the pharmacist is a professional and deserves some courtesy?
4. What about the pharmacist's actions made the patient accept that the prescription would not be available right away?

## SCENARIO XV

A patient (student 1) arrives in the pharmacy with a question about a prescription she received. The bottle says Artemis 10 mg; take one tablet daily. The problem is that the pill on the inside is usually green with yellow stripes. The pill inside now is red with white dots. The patient wants to know what has happened. The pharmacist (student 2) looks at the bottle and notices that it was not filled at this particular pharmacy. The pharmacist does not recognize the pill in the bottle, but does recognize that it is not Artemis 10 mg.

## Version 1

The patient is very upset to learn that the prescription was misfilled. She is not screaming but is on the verge of yelling. The pharmacist is very calm and explains that he does not recognize the pill in the bottle. Ultimately, the pharmacist makes a comment about the pharmacist who filled the prescription and tells the patient to get a lawyer.

## Version 2

The patient is not yelling or screaming, but wants to know the number of the Board of Pharmacy because she is going to file suit against the pharmacist who filled the prescription. The pharmacist is careful not to comment on the misfill. Further, the pharmacist is helpful in determining what is in the bottle. After some investigation, it is revealed that the medication in the bottle is one of the patient's vitamin supplements.

## Discussion Questions

1. What is the appropriate way to handle a prescription when it has been misfiled?
2. What communication techniques would be the most appropriate and professional for handling this situation?
3. How would you improve on the pharmacist's communication in either version?

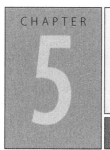

# Rounding, Documentation, and Patient Education

*Jacquelyn L. Bainbridge*

**Objectives: Upon completion of the chapter and exercises, the student pharmacist will be able to**

1. Identify members of an interprofessional team and define their roles. This includes the role of a student pharmacist.
2. Describe three important concepts for documenting patient care.
3. When given a patient case, document patient information using the subjective, objective, assessment, and plan (SOAP) format.
4. Discuss barriers to patient care as they pertain to the practice of pharmacy.

---

### Patient Encounter

You read online about a 26-year-old African American male Gold Medal Olympic bicyclist training for his second Olympic trial, who has been hospitalized due to an accident. You remember that about a week ago he came into the pharmacy with his wife. He stated that he was experiencing a lot of itching, a burning sensation, and redness in his groin area. Symptoms started 3 days earlier and had gotten worse. He noticed that the skin was starting to flake and peel. He stated that he has had this problem before and used an over-the-counter product, but could not remember the name of the product.

After asking several questions you obtained the following information from the patient: he had no known medical conditions or allergies; father has high blood pressure controlled by medication and his mother had breast cancer. He stated that he does not drink alcohol or use tobacco. The only supplements he was taking were a

*(continued on next page)*

---

multivitamin daily, calcium twice a day, and vitamin D once a day. He did not remember the strength but was able to point out the specific products on the shelf. You note that he is using calcium carbonate 500 mg and vitamin D 1000 IU. Patient estimated that his height is 5 ft 10 in and weight is 142 lb. Blood pressure and heart rate were measured at 118/74 mm Hg and 62 bpm, respectively.

The following is what you have last documented in your pharmacy charts.

### Example SOAP Note:

Subject: 26 y/o AA male athlete presents to pharmacy with a chief complaint of itching, redness, and burning in the groin area for the last 3 days. He also states that the skin is starting to flake and peel. He said that he has had this problem before and used an over-the-counter product but could not remember the name of the product.

PMH: Tinea cruris
FH: Father has hypertension, mother had breast cancer
Soc Hx: Married, Denies tobacco and ETOH use, Olympic athlete

### Objective:

Allergies: NKDA
Medications: Multivitamin daily, Calcium carbonate 500 mg orally twice daily; Vitamin D 1000 IU orally once daily
VS: Ht: 5'10", Wt: 142 lb, BP: 118/74, HR: 62

**Assessment:** Suspected Tinea cruris as evidenced by patient reports of burning, itching, flaking, peeling and redness in the groin area.

**Plan:** Recommend terbinafine (Lamisil AT) 1% cream. Apply once daily to affected and surrounding areas for 7 days. Educate on preventative measures. If signs/symptoms not resolved after 7 days, follow-up with your primary care physician.

## INTRODUCTION

The purpose of this chapter is to familiarize you with expectations and challenges that you may encounter during advanced practice courses. Topics that will be discussed include how to prepare for these educational experiences, the interprofessional team, documentation, writing SOAP notes, general goals for treatment, and the importance of providing patient education. During your advanced practice course you will be challenged to take knowledge learned from the classroom or online environment to the next level and practice patient-centered care. In 1990, Hepler and Strand defined pharmaceutical care as the responsible provision of drug therapy for the purposes of achieving definite outcomes.[1] In 1993, the American Society of Health-System Pharmacists (ASHP) issued a statement that "Pharmaceutical care is the direct, responsible provision of medication-related care for the purpose of achieving definite outcomes that improve a patient's quality of life."[2] In 1998, the International Pharmaceutical Federation (FIP) adopted the definition of pharmaceutical care as the responsible provision of pharmacotherapy for the purpose of achieving definite outcomes that improve or maintain a patient's quality of life.[3] The definition of pharmaceutical care has been modified over time but the root of the definition has essentially remained unchanged. Rather than continuing with the term pharmaceutical care, as the public has not adopted the terminology, patient-centered care will be used throughout this textbook. It is important to individualize the care provided to each patient and have a clear understanding of the diagnosis, goals of therapy, risks, benefits, and barriers to patient care.

You will encounter many different styles of practice throughout your education. With the knowledge and confidence you gain through each practice experience you will develop your own unique style of practice. This is achieved by integrating pieces from the styles of others.

## ADVANCED PRACTICE EXPERIENCES

Advanced practice courses enable you to take the knowledge gained in the classroom or from online courses and apply them to patient-centered care. Initially, you may feel uncomfortable or out of place. The following suggestions are provided to help you make the most of your advanced practice experiences, in addition to the information contained in Chapter 1 of this textbook.

1. Make a great first impression.
2. Use your time wisely.
3. Be familiar with and take advantage of all the resources available.
4. Maintain a positive and enthusiastic attitude.

Schools and colleges of pharmacy faculty members have worked closely with the sites, pharmacists, and other health-care professionals who will be the preceptors for the advanced practice experience. The educational institution and the site for practice will have mutually defined the coursework, goals, and objectives. It is important for you to contact your preceptor ahead of time and discuss the role you will have at the site and general expectations of your practice as a student pharmacist. Preceptor expectations will vary based on the practice setting but may include the following[4]:

- Rounding with an interprofessional team
- Writing SOAP notes and/or documenting in patient charts or electronic health information (EHI)
- Provision of drug information to other health-care providers
- Medication order evaluation and modification
- Work-up of new patients
- Therapeutic drug monitoring
- Selective monitoring for patients with renal or hepatic disease
- Patient education
- Literature evaluation
- Pharmacokinetic consultation
- Educational programs for pharmacists or other health-care providers
- Adverse drug reaction identification and reporting
- Medication reconciliation

## Interprofessional Team Membership and Rounds

The interprofessional team approach may be functional in many hospitals, nursing homes, and private practices. Individual members bring different approaches and expertise to patient care. As a student pharmacist, you bring knowledge of drug therapy and medication safety. You may be asked questions regarding mechanism of action, metabolism, duration of action, duration of therapy, dosing, and adverse events in addition to a host of other questions. You are responsible for identifying potential drug interactions, dosing errors, and performing medication therapy management. Incorporating your knowledge and skills as part of the team approach optimizes patient therapy and helps identify and prevent medication errors. Team members will vary depending on the institutional setting but may include those listed in Table 5.1.

Participating in patient care rounds is an excellent opportunity to learn and teach. Patient care rounds are part of clinical experiences in many large teaching hospitals.[1] Rounding is defined as traveling to each patient room with the interprofessional team for discussion of disease and therapies, monitoring patient progress, and to determine patient outcomes. This may also be accomplished through chart review and team discussion. Rounds are an opportunity to evaluate the patient's response to therapeutic interventions and make changes as necessary. Interprofessional teams will function differently depending on the setting. It is important to be respectful and professional when participating in rounds. Some basic guidelines for practicing professionalism include[1]:

- Introduce yourself and state you are a student pharmacist.
- Know the dress code and dress appropriately.
- Be on time.

- Be prepared—bring your Smartphone which is maintained on silent or vibrate/ tablet, pocket reference books/cards, note cards, and a pen.
- Review the patient charts ahead of time (take notes if necessary).
- Respect and maintain patient confidentiality.
- Listen and observe.
- Ask questions.
- Answer questions.
- Speak up and articulate your knowledge.
- Follow up with all drug information responses in a timely manner.
- Go from "Good to Great," look up an article to support your discussion on rounds of a specific disease state or drug therapy to educate your rounding team. It is always positive when you can educate your preceptor on new mechanism of disease or drug therapy for a given topic.

When reviewing a patient's chart consider questions such as:

- Does the patient have any drug allergies?
- What are the patient's current medications? Is the dose appropriate?
- Are there any significant laboratory values that could affect drug therapy (impaired renal or liver function)?
- What are the comorbid disease states?
- Are there any clinically significant drug interactions?
- Is there any therapeutic duplication?
- Can patient be switched from IV to PO?

---

**TABLE 5.1. INTERPROFESSIONAL TEAM MEMBERS**

- Attending physician
- Pharmacist
- Nurse or nurse practitioner
- Physician assistant
- Dietician or nutritionist
- Respiratory therapist
- Physical therapist
- Social worker
- Chaplain or ethicist
- Radiologist
- Surgeon
- Pathologist
- Medical residents
- Students

- Is the patient experiencing any symptoms that could be related to an adverse event?
- Are the medications appropriate for treating the medical condition?

The size of the institution and location will influence the availability of experiences such as rounding. It is important to have an appreciation for how patient care is provided in large teaching institutions versus small, urban, or rural hospitals or clinics.

## Writing

An essential form of communication is writing. As a health-care provider, it is important that you communicate effectively and be skilled in writing and diligent at documenting. It is important to make a habit of documenting your actions and communicating essential elements of the conversations. Documentation can be a beneficial way to assess your progress as a professional and chart academic growth as assessed by the experiential committee. Additionally, your ability to document appropriately can serve as a beneficial way to demonstrate your skills to your future employer or residency director.[5] Appropriate writing skills and documentation are key to providing evidence of quality patient-centered care. General rules for writing:

- Be clear and concise.
- When writing notes, use permanent ink and write legibly.
- Use correct spelling and grammar.
- Know your audience.
- Have a clear understanding of the topic.
- Organize your thoughts and determine the main point.
- Avoid redundancy and bias.

First, let us focus on documenting activities in a permanent medical record (PMR), which is now widely available in the digital format commonly referred to as electronic medical record (EMR) or electronic health information (EHI). Information in an EMR has many purposes. First and foremost, it is a legal, permanent health record that conveys information for use in patient care. In addition, it can serve as a tool for drug use evaluation, justification for reimbursement, a method to improve continuity of care, and a quality assurance tool for practice.[6,7] An EMR note ought to include the patient's medical and medication history, a list of existing and potential patient care problems, including drug-related problems, interventions and referrals that were made, goals of therapy and plans for follow-up. Do not assume that the next health-care provider is familiar with the patient. When documenting a note in an EMR there are several rules or good practices to guide your writing:

1. Indicate the date, time, and patient's name on each record (include a birth date and medical record number, if appropriate).
2. Use as few words as possible.
3. Use objective rather than subjective language.
4. Be objective and state the facts. Do not insert personal opinions or feelings.
5. Always sign and date your note.

6. If you make an error, bracket the erroneous portion of the entry and draw a single line through it. Label it as an "error," include the date and your initials.
7. If there is more than one entry on a page, do not leave blank lines between entries.
8. Use data that supports your recommendations.
9. Word all recommendations so that the prescriber does not feel that their judgments are coming under attack or are exposed legally.
10. When making recommendations, use statements that describe specific actions with check boxes, which allow the provider to accept or reject recommendations in a clear manner.
11. Avoid using judgmental words to describe the patient or medication (unreasonable, stubborn, lazy, inappropriate, wrong, senseless).
12. Avoid using abbreviations.

Table 5.2 provides examples of words that can be used to write a clear and concise note.[8]

**TABLE 5.2.** WORDS/PHRASES TO AVOID WHEN WRITING IN A PMR[8]

| Avoid | When You Mean |
| --- | --- |
| In case of | When, if |
| At the same time as | During |
| Make an exception for | Except for, or when, exceptions include |
| At the time | From (specific times, dates, etc.) |
| Adequate quantity | >100 cc's (be precise) |
| In spite of the fact that | Despite |
| Due to the fact that | Because |
| At a later date | Later (include specific date and time if known) |
| A majority of | Nearly all, most |
| Accounted for by the fact | Justified by |
| As a consequence of | The result of |
| Has the ability to | Can |
| In order to . . . | To |
| In some cases | Occasionally |
| It is clear that | Obviously |
| It is apparent | Clearly |
| It was written by Smith | Smith noted |
| Take into consideration | Consider |
| In case that | If |
| It is common knowledge that | I haven't bothered to look up the reference |

The following are several examples of how to use objective language when documenting in a PMR/EHI.

Subjective: "I find the patient to be distraught and feeling a bit overwhelmed."
Objective: "I found the patient screaming at the top of her voice and threatening to jump out of the window."
Subjective: "Patient does not use herbals."
Objective: "Patient denies use of herbals." This statement indicates the pharmacist actually assessed and questioned the patient.

| TABLE 5.3. DO NOT USE ABBREVIATIONS[9,10] | | |
|---|---|---|
| **Abbreviation** | **Potential Problem** | **Solution** |
| $MgSO_4$ or $MSO_4$ | Can be interpreted as magnesium sulfate or morphine sulfate | Write "magnesium sulfate" or "morphine sulfate" |
| MS | Can be interpreted as magnesium sulfate or morphine sulfate | Write "morphine sulfate" |
| IU | Mistaken for IV (intravenous) or the number 10 | Write "international unit" |
| QD, Q.D., q.d., qd QOD, Q.O.D., q.o.d, qod | Mistaken for each other, period after the Q mistaken for "I" and the "O" mistaken for "I" | Write "daily" or "every day" Write "every other day" |
| U (unit) | Mistaken for 0 (zero) the number 4 (four) or "cc" | Write "unit" |
| X.0 mg (trailing zero) or .X mg (lack of leading zero) | Decimal point is missed, can result in overdose or under dosing of medication | Write "X mg" Write "0.X mg" |
| > (greater than) or < (less than) | Misinterpreted as the number "7" (seven) or the letter "L", confused for one another | Write "greater than" or "less than" |
| Abbreviations for drug names | Misinterpreted due to similar abbreviations for multiple drugs | Write drug names in full |
| Apothecary units | Unfamiliar to many practitioners, confused with metric units | Use metric units |
| @ | Mistaken for the number "2" (two) | Write "at" |
| Cc | Mistaken for U (units) when written poorly | Write "mL" or "milliliters" |
| μg | Mistaken for mg (milligrams) resulting one thousand-fold overdose | Write "mcg" or "micrograms" |

Individual institutions may have other abbreviations that are prohibited for use and you will want to be cognizant at each institution of the policies regarding abbreviations. Table 5.3 shows the list of abbreviations that are on the official "Do Not Use" or recommended for the "Do Not Use" list developed by the Joint Commission of Hospital Accreditation.[9]

The Institute for Safe Medication Practices publishes a list of error-prone abbreviations, symbols, and dose designations, which is available at: http://www.ismp.org/Tools/errorproneabbreviations.pdf. Some abbreviations can have multiple meanings that vary among settings. The incorrect use could prove embarrassing and dangerous rather than fashionable. Consider the commonly used abbreviation WNL. It might mean, "within normal limits" or it could be construed to mean, "we never looked." The term "within normal limits," is subjective and can be interpreted in various ways by other professionals and so it is good practice not to use WNL. Another example is the abbreviations DC and dc.[11] The first abbreviation usually is interpreted to mean "discharge," and the second may mean "discontinue." The easiest way to circumvent this problem is to avoid using abbreviations altogether. It is always best to write exactly what you mean when documenting information in charts.

What to document includes[12]:

1. Routine activities that are required (drug review, patient counseling).
2. Unusual or out of the ordinary events.
3. Therapeutic notation and drug recommendations that may affect future treatment decisions.
4. Extraordinary measures taken on behalf of the patient (extra time spent training a patient).
5. Routine matters that can be quickly documented.
6. Procedures that may need to be replicated (compounding).
7. Medication notes necessary for other health-care providers or caregivers (drug-drug interactions, drug-food interactions, monitoring).
8. Potential or foreseeable future problems that may need a special alert (major drug interactions, patient history may show potential for abuse-monitor refills).
9. Whenever the pharmacist questions a prescription or feels it necessary to contact the prescriber (include question/concern, date, time, response, and name of person that responded).
10. Patient counseling on a potential interaction, allergy, or dangerous side effects.
11. Any situation in which professional judgment suggests that future proof of facts be known or reasons for judgment may be required.

Standardized formatting for documentation is important. It provides completeness and consistency to the PMR. There are several types of standardized formatting. The most commonly used format is the SOAP note. Other formats include the title, introduction, text, recommendation, and signature (TITRS) and the findings, assessment, recommendations or resolutions, and management (FARM) note. The SOAP note is an interventionist approach, TITRS is an assessment approach, and FARM focuses on monitoring. The SOAP note is the one you will most likely encounter during your educational experiences and will be the focus of the next section.

## SOAP Notes

SOAP is an acronym that stands for *Subjective, Objective, Assessment,* and *Plan.* Each section is distinctive. You will want to write as follows:

1. The subjective section will include the patients' complaint or reason for the visit and a description of the problem (onset of symptoms, pain intensity, location, duration, and what makes symptoms better or worse). This information is elicited from interviewing the patient. It is imperative to investigate past episodes of similar symptoms and treatment received on prior occasions. An example of questions to ask the patient includes:
   - Why are you here today? (This is the chief complaint, presented in quotation marks)
   - How are you feeling today?
   - How long has this been going on? Tell me exactly when you felt this start? Is it better at some times than others? Is there anything that makes this better or worse?
   - Is there a family situation that may be contributing to your health/illness?
   - What do you do for work?
   - Is there anything else you would like to add?

   This section is where you would document past medical history, social history, and allergies. This list is not inclusive. You will need to develop your own style of interview, as discussed in Chapter 4. (See Table 4.3 also.)

2. The objective section is for documenting measurements that are observed (seen, heard, touched, smelt) by the clinician. Examples include blood pressure, pulse, temperature, skin color, and important laboratory values. If a physical examination is completed, it will be documented here as well. Information in this section is based on diagnostic and monitoring measurements. Current medications will be listed in this section, including start dates if available and last refilled.

3. The assessment section is for documenting and prioritizing the patient's problems. Be sure to assess the level of therapeutic efficacy, include pertinent labs that define differential diagnosis with relation to drug problems, potential confounders to efficacy or adherence, pertinent positive or negative signs, and symptoms related to the patient's condition. You will also want to identify the goal(s) of therapy.

4. The plan section is where recommendations based on your assessment are documented. This includes therapy additions, deletions, or modifications, lifestyle changes; requests for laboratory and diagnostic assessments; standards of care; special directions; referrals; possible toxicity and efficacy; self-monitoring recommendations; medical personnel emergency contacts; and time to follow up appointments. If medication counseling is recommended, it will be documented here and provided before the patient leaves the office.

The assessment and plan are the most important aspects of your clinical note. Some clinicians will combine the assessment and plan into one section. If you would like more information on documenting patient care, refer to American Society of Health-System Pharmacist Guidelines on Documenting Pharmaceutical Care in Patient Medical Records and Guidelines on a Standardized Method for Pharmaceutical Care.[13,14]

## Role of the Patient in the Interprofessional Team

Once you have developed a plan, you will want to discuss your plan with your preceptor and then other members of the interprofessional team. After the team has decided on a plan of action, the next step is to bring the patient into the decision-making process, if possible. Patient involvement in the health-care decision-making process allows the patient to have more control over their health and treatment, which could potentially impact their satisfaction with the quality of care and improve adherence with treatment recommendations. It also provides an opportunity to identify potential barriers, such as those listed in Table 5.4 and develop solutions to overcome those barriers.[15,16]

The amount of time that you have to develop and implement a plan will vary depending on the practice setting. For example, if working in a hospital setting the goal may be to treat the acute problem until a patient is stabilized and can return home safely. In an ambulatory setting, patients with chronic disease states can be managed on a long-term basis when conditions are not life threatening.

## Patient Education

Patient counseling and education are large components of patient-centered care. The World Health Organization (WHO) projects that only 50% of patients typically take their medications as prescribed on a world-wide basis.[17] Noncompliance or lack of adherence has an estimated cost of $177 billion annually, in direct and indirect costs.[18] The annual cost to the US health-care system is approximately $100 billion, drug-related hospitalizations account for an estimated $47 billion of that.[19-21] Medication noncompliance is not only costly but it can also lead to unnecessary disease progression, disease complications, reduced functional abilities, lower quality of life, and premature death.[17] Lack of adherence increases the risk of developing resistance to needed therapies, more intense relapses, and withdrawal and rebound effects.[17] There is a growing body of evidence that indicates compliance leads to improved outcomes and reduced costs.[22]

The goals of patient counseling are to:[23]

1. Establish a relationship with the patient and to develop trust.
2. Demonstrate concern and care for the patient.
3. Help the patient manage and adapt to their illness.
4. Help the patient manage and adapt to their medication(s).

---

**TABLE 5.4.  BARRIERS TO PATIENT-CARE MANAGEMENT[15,16]**

- Cost of medication/co-payment
- Complexity of treatment (dosing frequency, administration)
- Compliance (missed appointments, refills, follow-up, etc.)
- Poor provider-patient relationship
- Lack of a primary care provider
- Lack of knowledge regarding illness/denial of illness
- Lack of belief in treatment
- Belief that natural treatments are better and safer
- Side effects
- Asymptomatic disease/condition
- Cognitive impairment
- Psychological problems
- Support system
- Social stigma
- Media influence regarding safety or risk issues
- Duration of therapy (short term vs. long term)
- Health literacy
- English language proficiency
- Influence of media

---

5. Identify and minimize factors that contribute to noncompliance.
6. Empower the patient to be an active participant in their health care.
7. Minimize poor patient outcomes due to medication misuse (OTC/herbal drug interactions, injectable administration mistakes, etc.).

A survey commissioned by the National Community Pharmacists Association (NCPA) found that[24]:

- Three out of four American consumers report not always taking their prescription medicine as directed.
- Thirty-one percent had not filled a prescription they were given.
- Twenty-nine percent stopped taking a medication before the supply ran out.
- Twenty-four percent took less than the recommended dosage.

Other research findings:

- From 12% to 20% of patients take other people's medicines.
- Adherence among patients in developed countries with chronic conditions averages 50%.[17]

- One-third of patients fully comply with recommended treatment, one-third sometimes comply, and one-third never comply.[25]
- Even the potential for serious harm (loss of vision, organ rejections, even death) may not be enough to motivate patients to comply.[26-28]

Tailoring a therapeutic regimen to an individual patient will increase the likelihood that the patient will comply and that the therapy will be effective. There are many reasons a patient may appear to be noncompliant or nonadherent which include:

1. Cannot afford the medication
2. Confused about the prescribed dose
3. Intolerable side effects
4. Lack of response to medication
5. Inconvenient dosing schedule
6. Inconvenient dosage form

Many of these factors (see Table 5.4) can be identified and minimized by patient counseling and communication. When counseling an individual about medications there is a lot of information that needs to be communicated in an organized and concise fashion and usually with limited time available. The information provided will vary depending on the institutional setting as well. It is up to you, as the student pharmacist, to identify the information that is relevant to the patient at the time of the encounter.

When counseling a patient you will want to *always*:

1. Use appropriate language throughout the session.
2. Maintain control of the session.
3. Organize information in an appropriate manner.
4. Respond to patient with appropriate empathy, listening, and attention to concerns.
5. Maintain good eye contact with the patient.
6. Don't dominate the conversation. Allow the patient to engage in an active discussion with open-ended questions.
7. Provide follow-up care.

Below are some general guidelines to follow when counseling a patient.

1. Introduce yourself and identify the patient by name.
2. Ask patient if it is a convenient time to discuss their medications.
3. Explain the importance of discussing their medications.
4. Verify what medications they are taking, known disease states, drug allergies, and so on.
5. Ask what they know about the medication and their illness.
6. Tell patient the name (brand and generic) of medication, dosage, frequency, and route of administration.
7. Explain how long it will take for the medication to show an effect.
8. Emphasize the benefits of the medication.

9. Describe potential side effects (common and serious).
   a. Tell patient what signs to look for.
   b. Recommend ways to minimize side effects or identify if the side effects will go away (including possible time frame).
   c. If side effects do not go away or become intolerable, tell patient to notify the prescriber.
   d. Discuss rare but serious side effects (emphasize rare) and when to seek immediate medical attention.
10. Discuss lifestyle modifications when appropriate (exercise, diet, smoking cessation).
11. Identify drug-drug, drug-food, and drug-disease interactions.
12. Discuss how to store medication.
13. Discuss how to handle a missed dose.
14. Discuss how to properly dispose of used or expired medications.
15. Ask patient to repeat information back to you to verify their understanding.
16. Ask if patient has additional questions or concerns.
17. Provide written instructions in addition to verbal instructions.

The time spent educating and counseling is not just an opportunity to give information, but also an opportunity to get information. As a student pharmacist you are the expert in drug therapy, but the patients are the experts on themselves. You can develop the most effective pharmacological plan for a patient, but if the routine does not match the patient's lifestyle then it will not be effective. For example, frequency of the dosing schedule has been shown to impact adherence. Cramer et al. reports that compliance rates are 87% for once daily dosing, 81% for twice-daily dosing, 77% for three-times-a-day, and only 39% for four-times-a-day dosing.[8,9] Cognitive impairment may make the patient appear to be noncompliant, especially if the medication regimen is confusing and has multiple dosing or dosing adjustments.[7] Suggestions to overcome these barriers include using a pill box, providing written instructions for the patient or care giver and making the individual pill bottles easily identifiable, such as using a color code or numbering system.

Most community and hospital pharmacies have electronic resources that can print generic patient information sheets about medications, disease states, and check multiple medications for drug interactions. These are valuable resources that ought to be used. At some point you may be asked to design and implement a version of a patient-teaching sheet that allows provision of specific information that has been individualized to the patient. For example, if the individual needs to titrate a medication, write out the specific titration schedule. Written information reinforces important recommendations and serves as a reference for the patient if they later forget or have other questions. Individuals find written instructions from their practitioner or pharmacist more personal than the generic instructions and precautions provided by outpatient and ambulatory pharmacies and they are probably more likely to read them.[30] Copies of these educational sheets will be placed in the EHI. This is an easy and effective way to document education and often required by law.

## Practicing as a Professional Pharmacist

Professionalism is not learned from a textbook or classroom lecture. It is learned through mentorship and socialization.[31] It is important to observe the positive behaviors and attitudes that are presented by your educators, peers, and colleagues as these will help you to define your style of professionalism. You will want to seek out and attach yourself to mentors who are professional and caring health-care providers.

Finally, it is important to be aware that the classroom experiences do not simulate in most cases the real-life situation. The classroom experience gives you the knowledge to operate in ideal situations, while the advanced practice courses give you the real-life experience. The goal of the advanced practice course is to enable you to take the knowledge learned and apply it to the patient care practice setting. Your knowledge, skills, judgment, and values will be tested, challenged, and reshaped constantly. Professionalism is a continuum.[32] It is not achieved in a day, in a week, in a month, but in a life time. It is important to understand that you will make errors. As a professional, you need to take responsibility and immediately take the necessary action to correct and prevent errors. Professionalism is not about having the right answer all the time. Professionalism is showing respect for yourself and earning the respect of others. This is done through the attitudes and behaviors that you display when interacting with other people and will improve your credibility with other health-care providers who will be participants in your education.[33] A demonstrated professional image enhances the confidence others have in you and you have in yourself.

## APPLICATION EXERCISES

1. What are the benefits of a interprofessional team for you and for the patient?
2. What is the purpose of rounding? Why is rounding important?
3. Predict five types of questions you may be asked on rounds.
4. Why is a patient chart so important? What are three issues that might arise from an incomplete patient chart?
5. Explain the importance of writing what you mean instead of using abbreviations.
6. Compare and contrast SOAP, TITRS, and FARM notes. Be sure to include when it is appropriate to use each.
7. How does involving a patient in the plan improve patient adherence?
8. Why is it important to counsel patients on length of treatment, storage, and expiration of medication?
9. What are three strategies you can use to improve patient adherence?
10. Compare patient-centered care and education in a hospital setting versus an ambulatory care setting.

## ACKNOWLEDGMENT

The authors wish to acknowledge the contributions of Sarah L. Johnson, Ruth C. Taggart, and Janina Z. P. Janes to this chapter.

## REFERENCES

1. Hepler CD, Strand LM. Opportunities and responsibilities in pharmaceutical care. *Am J Hosp Pharm.* 1990;47:533–543.
2. ASHP Council on Professional Affairs. American Society of Hospital Pharmacists. Draft statement on pharmaceutical care. *Am J Hosp Pharm.* 1993;50:126–128.
3. FIP Statement of Professional Standards in Pharmaceutical Care. *FIP Guidelines for Dissolution Testing of Solid Oral Products (1997, Vancouver) Joint report of the OLMCS and Industrial Section.* The Hague, The Netherlands: International Pharmaceutical Federation (FIP) Council meeting; 1998.
4. Sauer BL, Heeren DL, Walker RG, et al. Computerized documentation of activities of Pharm.D. clerkship students. *Am J Health Syst Pharm.* 1997;54:1727–1732.
5. Stevenson TL, Fox BI, Andrus M, Carroll D. Implementation of a school-wide clinical intervention documentation system. *Am J Pharm Educ.* 2011; 75(5): 90, June 10.
6. Zierler-Brown S, Brown TR, Chen D, et al. Clinical documentation for patient care: models, concepts, and liability considerations for pharmacists. *Am J Health Syst Pharm.* 2007;64:1851–1858.
7. Monarch K. Documentation, part 1: principles for self-protection. Preserve the medical record and defend yourself. *Am J Nurs.* 2007;107:58–60.
8. Day RA, Gastel B. *How to Write & Publish a Scientific Paper.* 6th ed. Westport, CT: Greenwood Press; 2006.
9. Joint Commission on the Accreditation of Healthcare Organizations. The Official "Do Not Use" List. Available at http://www.jointcommission.org/about_us/patient_safety_fact_sheets.aspx. Accessed March, 2014.
10. Christensen AJ. *Patient Adherence to Medical Treatment Regimens: Bridging the Gap between Behavioral Science and Biomedicine.* New Haven, CT: Yale University Press; 2004.
11. Taber CW. *Taber's Cyclopedic Medical Dictionary.* 17th ed. Philadelphia, PA: FA Davis Co; 1993:2352–2355.
12. Baker KR. Documentation in pharmacy practice: a pharmacist-lawyer's perspective. In: Boh LE, Young LY, eds. *Pharmacy Practice Manual: A Guide to the Clinical Experience.* 2nd ed. Philadelphia, PA: Lippincott Williams & Wilkins; 2001:627–638.
13. American Society of Health-System Pharmacists. ASHP guidelines on a standardized method for pharmaceutical care. *Am J Health Syst Pharm.* 1996;53:1713–1716.
14. ASHP guidelines on documenting pharmaceutical care in patient medical records. *Am J Health Syst Pharm.* 2003;60:705–707.
15. Osterberg L, Blaschke T. Adherence to medication. *N Engl J Med.* 2005;353:487–497.
16. Ashar BH. Complementary and alternative medicine. In: Fiebach NH, Kern DE, Thomas PA, et al, eds. *Principles of Ambulatory Medicine.* 7th ed. Philadelphia, PA: Lippincott Williams & Wilkins; 2007:61–73.

17. De Geest S, Sabate E. Adherence to long-term therapies: evidence for action. *Eur J Cardiovasc Nurs*. 2003;2:323.

18. Ernst FR, Grizzle AJ. Drug-related morbidity and mortality: updating the cost-of-illness model. *J Am Pharm Assoc (Wash)*. 2001;41:192–199.

19. Berg JS, Dischler J, Wagner DJ, et al. Medication compliance: a healthcare problem. *Ann Pharmacother*. 1993;27:S1–S24.

20. Johnson JA, Bootman JL. Drug-related morbidity and mortality: a cost-of-illness model. *Arch Intern Med*. 1995;155:1949–1956.

21. McDonnell PJ, Jacobs MR. Hospital admissions resulting from preventable adverse drug reactions. *Ann Pharmacother*. 2002;36:1331–1336.

22. Dunbar-Jacob J, Erlen JA, Schlenk EA, et al. Adherence in chronic disease. *Ann Rev Nurs Res*. 2000;18:48–90.

23. Rantucci MJ. Pharmacists talking with patients: a guide to patient counseling. Baltimore, MD: Williams & Wilkins; 1997.

24. Take as Directed: A Prescription Not Followed [press release]. Alexandria, VA: National Community Pharmacist Association; December 15, 2006.

25. Fedder DO. Managing medication and compliance: physician-pharmacist-patient interactions. *J Am Geriatr Soc*. 1982;30:S113–S117.

26. Butler JA, Roderick P, Mullee M, et al. Frequency and impact of nonadherence to immunosuppressants after renal transplantation: a systematic review. *Transplantation*. 2004;77:769–776.

27. Gallant JE, Block DS. Adherence to antiretroviral regimens in HIV-infected patients: results of a survey among physicians and patients. *J Int Assoc Physicians AIDS Care*. 1998;4:32–35.

28. Vincent P. Factors influencing patient noncompliance: a theoretical approach. *Nurs Res*. 1971;20:509–516.

29. Cramer JA, Mattson RH, Prevey ML, et al. How often is medication taken as prescribed? A novel assessment technique. *JAMA*. 1989;261:3273–3277.

30. Kern DE. Patient compliance with medical advice. In: Barker LR, Burton JR, Zieve PD, eds. *Principles of Ambulatory Medicine*. 4th ed. Baltimore, MD: Williams & Wilkins; 1994:49.

31. American Pharmacists Association. Academy of Students of Pharmacy—American Association of Colleges of Pharmacy Council of Deans Task Force on Professionalism. White paper on pharmacy student professionalism. *J Am Pharm Assoc (Wash)*. 2000;40:96–102.

32. Ahmadi K, Hassali MAA. Professionalism in pharmacy: a continual societal and intellectual challenge. *Am J Pharm Educ*. 2012;76(4):72, May 10.

33. Rosowski PG, Spunt AL. Standards of professional conduct. In: Boh LE, Young LY, eds. *Pharmacy Practice Manual: A Guide to the Clinical Experience*. 2nd ed. Philadelphia, PA: Lippincott Williams & Wilkins; 2001:44–67.

# Monitoring Drug Therapy

*Chasity M. Shelton, Kelly C. Rogers*

**Objectives: Upon completion of the chapter and exercises, the student pharmacist will be able to**

1. Recognize the role of deductive reasoning in the drug monitoring process.
2. Know what a patient database is and how it is used to monitor drug therapy.
3. Be able to extract appropriate patient information and integrate it with drug information to formulate a process for monitoring drug therapy.
4. Utilize common calculations when monitoring drug therapy in a patient, for example, creatinine clearance, modification of diet in renal disease (MDRD), body mass index (BMI).
5. Discuss the importance of a chief complaint (CC) and history of present illness (HPI) in monitoring drug therapy.

---

### Patient Encounter

Back at the hospital the attending pharmacist has collected additional information.

One week since his accident, the patient is in the ICU and mechanically ventilated. You are preparing for rounds with the ICU service and notice in the chart an order for levofloxacin 500 mg IV q24h, first dose stat. You obtain the following information from the chart:

Height 70 in.

Weight 70 kg

Scr 1.7 (baseline on admission 1.0 mg/dL)

WBC = 12% neutrophils

$T_{max}$ = 101°F

BP = 100/60

HR = 85

*(continued on next page)*

---

## PATIENT ENCOUNTER: DISCUSSION

There are a number of questions that the student should ask about the patient's medication regimen.

1. Is the drug being used for an appropriate diagnosis or indication? Knowing the diagnosis establishes a basis for selection of an appropriate medication.
   - You determine from the chart that the patient is being treated empirically for ventilator-associated pneumonia (VAP).
2. Is the dose of the medication appropriate for this specific patient? Take into account patient characteristics such as age, weight, sex, ethnic background, and allergies as well as concurrent disease states and medications used.
   - You know nothing about VAP or how to treat it. What resources should you access to determine if the treatment with levofloxacin 500 mg IV q24h is appropriate?
   - How will you determine if the dose of levofloxacin is appropriate for patient X, especially since his Scr is increasing? What calculation should you use to determine patient X's renal function?
3. What are the most likely adverse effects caused by this medication? Does the patient exhibit any of these adverse effects?
   - What if your patient began to experience an erythematous rash 2 days after starting levofloxacin? What would you do?
4. Are there any patient-specific barriers to taking this medication?
   - How would you address the family's concerns about withholding antibiotics?
5. What proof do you have that the medication is effective?
   - What objective measures will you follow to determine if the antibiotic is working?

---

## INTRODUCTION

The purpose of this chapter is to provide some direction primarily for the student who will be beginning his or her first exposure to direct patient care. It will also be helpful for those individuals who already have some experience in this area.

To get the most out of this chapter, prepare yourself to learn to integrate and use your therapeutic and pathophysiology knowledge. Those classroom drug facts along with an understanding of laboratory and diagnostic tests are required to assess and monitor the appropriateness of patient-specific therapeutic regimens. The facts you know must now be used to determine whether the therapeutic regimen is achieving the intended outcome, that is, modification of a disease state to promote cure or mitigation. You must understand the reasons behind treatment failures and what impact this may have on future modifications of the therapy.

Students frequently ask, "What should I read to prepare for your advanced practice course; a therapeutics text, a pharmacology text, national guidelines, or perhaps specialty journals?" The usual response is none of the above. Your best preparation for this or any other pharmacy practice experience course is to read any Sherlock Holmes story. Although this may seem implausible at first, it is actually very sound advice that will stand you in good stead throughout your career. The author of the Sherlock Holmes stories was a physician by training. The methods by which the detective reached his conclusions are illustrative of the type of reasoning taught in medical schools. Sherlock Holmes was a fictional detective in 19th century London, who was a proponent of deductive reasoning. This process involves drawing conclusions from general observations. In a clinical venue, this is accomplished by combining laboratory and physical data to provide a response to a therapeutic question. For example, it may be observed that a patient with a rising blood urea nitrogen (BUN) and serum creatinine is being treated with an aminoglycoside antibiotic. With the foregoing information, it could be reasoned that the changes in renal function may be an adverse event produced by the antibiotic. The response is therefore either to make some modification in the dose or frequency of administration of the aminoglycoside or to change to a different class of antibiotic that has the same antibacterial spectrum but does not cause nephrotoxicity.

Monitoring drug therapy is an organized process that provides information necessary to determine whether a patient's therapeutic regimen is achieving the expected outcome or must be changed or adjusted because of a lack of response or undesirable or dangerous adverse drug reactions. Pharmacists must acquire skills in order to interpret certain specific monitoring parameters. These assessment skills combined with pharmacists' knowledge of pharmacokinetics, pharmacotherapeutics, pharmacogenetics, and pharmacoeconomics enhance the ability of the pharmacist to monitor patient outcomes. An understanding of the application and interpretation of laboratory and other diagnostic procedures, such as X-rays, magnetic resonance imaging (MRI), or electrocardiograms (ECG), improves the ability of the pharmacist to assess the patient's condition and provide care. Pharmacists may also be able to enhance patient participation by educating patients on the risks of medication-related problems and how frequent monitoring of key clinical indicators may help reduce those risks.

## STEPS FOR MONITORING DRUG THERAPY

When faced with monitoring a patient, the student pharmacist must go through a process of fact finding and collecting data, analyzing the information, drawing conclusions from the information collected, and making recommendations. In order to collect information effectively, you should work to create a patient database (see Profile 6.1). Creation of a database helps the student determine what information is pertinent. Using a standardized form helps to organize data in a manner that can be readily retrieved. Information can be obtained from a variety of sources including interviewing the patient, patient's family or caregiver, patient's chart (written and/or electronic), past medical records, and/or medication profile. Information can be found as either a hard copy or stored on a computer file in a data bank. Also, there

---

**PROFILE 6.1.** PATIENT MONITORING FORMAT

**Current Medications**

| Start Date | Medication/Route | Dose/Schedule | Stop Date | Start Date |
|---|---|---|---|---|
| 1/20 | EC ASA po | 81 mg daily | | |
| 1/20 | Simvastatin po | 20 mg qhs | | |
| 1/20 | NTG patch transdermal | 5 mg/24 h daily | | |
| 1/20 | Metoprolol XL po | 100 mg daily | | |
| 1/20 | NTG SL | 0.4 mg prn | | |
| 1/20 | APAP 325 mg | 1-2 tabs prn | | |
| 1/20 | Enoxaparin SQ | 100 mg bid | | |

**Vital Signs**

| Date | 01/20 | | | | | | | |
|---|---|---|---|---|---|---|---|---|
| Wt (kg) | 96 | | | | | | | |
| Temp (°F) | 98.1 | | | | | | | |
| HR/RR | 79/18 | | | | | | | |
| BP | 160/92 | | | | | | | |
| I/O | | | | | | | | |

*(continued)*

**PROFILE 6.1.** PATIENT MONITORING FORMAT (*Continued*)

Chemistry Lab Values

| Date | 1/20 | | | | | | |
|---|---|---|---|---|---|---|---|
| Na | 138 | | | | | | |
| K | 3.6 | | | | | | |
| Cl | 103 | | | | | | |
| HCO$_3$ | 26 | | | | | | |
| BUN | 14 | | | | | | |
| SCr | 1.1 | | | | | | |
| Glucose | 132 | | | | | | |
| Ca | 9.1 | | | | | | |
| Phos | 2.6 | | | | | | |
| Mg | 1.3 | | | | | | |
| Anion gap | | | | | | | |
| Uric acid | 3.4 | | | | | | |
| Total protein | 7.0 | | | | | | |
| Albumin | 4.0 | | | | | | |
| Alkphos | 102 | | | | | | |
| T. Bili | 0.8 | | | | | | |
| D. Bili | 0 | | | | | | |
| ALT | 33 | | | | | | |
| AST | 41 | | | | | | |
| Amylase | | | | | | | |
| Lipase | | | | | | | |
| WBC | 9.8 | | | | | | |
| Segs | 62.9 | | | | | | |
| Bands | 0 | | | | | | |

*(continued)*

**PROFILE 6.1. PATIENT MONITORING FORMAT** (*Continued*)

**Chemistry Lab Values**

| Date | 1/20 | | | | | | |
|---|---|---|---|---|---|---|---|
| Lymphs | 33 | | | | | | |
| Monos | 3 | | | | | | |
| Eosinophils | 1 | | | | | | |
| Basophils | 0.1 | | | | | | |
| Atypicals | 0 | | | | | | |
| RBC | 4.7 | | | | | | |
| Hgb | 12.8 | | | | | | |
| Hct | 44 | | | | | | |
| MCV | 92 | | | | | | |
| MCH | 29 | | | | | | |
| Plts | 254 | | | | | | |
| PTT | 36.6 | | | | | | |
| PT | 11.1 | | | | | | |
| INR | 1.01 | | | | | | |
| Warfarin dose | N/A | | | | | | |

**Miscellaneous Lab Values**

| Date | 1/20 | 1/21 | 1/22 | | | | |
|---|---|---|---|---|---|---|---|
| Troponin I | 0.5 | 0.5 | 0.5 | | | | |
| Total Chol | | 280 | | | | | |
| Triglycerides | | 380 | | | | | |
| HDL | | 30 | | | | | |
| LDL | | 174 | | | | | |

(continued)

**PROFILE 6.1.** PATIENT MONITORING FORMAT (*Continued*)

Cultures and Sensitivities

| Date | | | | | | |
|------|--|--|--|--|--|--|
| Source | | | | | | |
| Organisims | | | | | | |
| Sensitivities | | | | | | |

is wide use of electronic medical records or computerized records where information is stored on a server. From this patient's database, the student pharmacist can make rational decisions about the patient's outcomes, course of treatment, and the medication regimen.

The student pharmacist uses administrative and demographic information as a means of identifying and locating a patient (Fig. 6.1). It will also be used as a means of differentiating patients from each other in case of identical names.

**Figure 6.1.** Administrative and demographic information.

Account number: 2000-001        Medical record: MR-149360

Physician: I. M. Well, MD

Room: 401      Date of admission: 02/20/2009

Patient name: Doe, John Q.        Birthday: 07/01/1948

Telephone: (555) 555-5555

Address: 400 Elm St.      City: Anywhere        State: USA

Zip code: 00000

Age: 60      Gender: Male      Race: Caucasian

Ht (in): 71      Wt (kg): 96

IBW (kg): 75      BMI (kg/m$^2$): 29.5

Religion: Protestant        Occupation: Shipyard worker (retired)

Allergies: Penicillin (rash), ibuprofen (causes stomach pain)

*Account number or medical record number* serves as a means of locating information about the patient, such as a patient's older medical record. This is similar to locating a prescription drug profile in the community drug store by using a prescription or account number.

*Physician or care provider* is identified in case the student has questions or recommendations about treatment.

TABLE 6.1. AGE-RELATED CHANGES IN DRUG PHARMACOKINETICS

| Pharmacokinetic Phase | Pharmacokinetic Parameter | |
| --- | --- | --- |
| | Adults | Pediatrics |
| Gastrointestinal absorption | Unchanged passive diffusion and no change in bioavailability for most drugs | Gastric pH ↑ in neonates ↑ Bioavailability for acid-labile drugs |
| | ↓ Active transport and ↓ bioavailability for some drugs | ↓ Bioavailability for drugs requiring |
| | ↓ First-pass extraction and ↑ bioavailability | acid to be absorbed |
| Distribution | ↓ Volume of distribution and ↑ plasma concentration of water-soluble drugs | ↑ Volume of distribution and ↓ plasma concentration of water-soluble drugs |
| | ↑ Volume of distribution and ↑ terminal disposition half-life $(t_{1/2})$ for fat-soluble drugs | ↓ Volume of distribution for fat-soluble drugs |
| | ↑ or ↓ free fraction of highly plasma protein-bound drugs | ↓ Circulating plasma proteins in neonates |
| Hepatic metabolism | ↓ Clearance and ↑ half-life for some oxidatively metabolized drugs | ↓ CYP450 activity (initially then ↑ during early childhood) |
| | ↓ Clearance and ↑ half-life of drugs with high hepatic extraction ratios | ↓ Glucuronidation (initially then ↑ during early childhood) |
| Renal excretion | ↓ Clearance and ↑ half-life of renally eliminated drugs and active metabolites | ↑ Clearance and ↓ half-life of renally eliminated drugs and active metabolites |

*Demographic information* including items such as name, address, and telephone number may be helpful in identifying and contacting the patient.

*Age and gender* are useful to distinguish male from female patients. It is helpful to identify the patient as being either pediatric or geriatric. These patients may have altered pharmacokinetics and pharmacodynamics (Table 6.1).

Health professionals are practicing in global societies and recognition of cultural, ethnic, and religious differences are important to providing patient-centered care. Ideally, practitioners will want to work toward developing cultural awareness and addressing diverse patient issues not just those used as examples in this chapter.

*Religion and occupation* may be important in cases where religious beliefs conflict with medical treatment (ie, Jehovah's Witness patients will not receive a blood transfusion). Occupational information may be an important part of the patient's history, as it may reveal exposure to toxins (eg, ship-builder's exposure to asbestos, painter's exposure to lead, etc.).

*Race* is relevant because certain medications may not work in specific ethnic groups. For example, β-blockers have been shown to be less effective in African Americans. Certain ethnic groups have been shown to be poor metabolizers; they are deficient in their ability to oxidize a substrate. Poor metabolizers will not be able to metabolize certain medications well and accumulate medication, resulting in elevated serum concentrations and an increased risk of adverse effects. Extensive metabolizers are persons able to metabolize certain medications rapidly and therefore do not respond to normal doses.

*Weight and height* permit calculation of ideal body weight (IBW), BMI, or body surface area (BSA) (Table 6.2). IBW and BSA may be important in calculation of the appropriate dose of medication for a patient. BMI is a measurement that estimates a person's body fat. In general, a person is considered obese if he has a BMI of 27 or more.

*Allergy information* describes both drug and nondrug items that the patient cannot tolerate or that produces a reaction. Allergy can range from minor symptoms such as nasal stuffiness or mild rash to more serious symptoms such as anaphylaxis.

---

**TABLE 6.2. CALCULATION OF BODY WEIGHT, MASS, AND SURFACE AREA**

Ideal body weight (IBW)

| | |
|---|---|
| Male | IBW (kg) = 50 kg + (2.3 kg × height in inches over 60 in) |
| Female | IBW (kg) = 45.5 kg + (2.3 kg × height in inches over 60 in) |

Body mass index (BMI)

$$BMI\ (kg/m^2) = (\text{weight in kilograms})/(\text{height in meters})^2$$

Body surface area (BSA)

$$BSA\ (m^2) = \sqrt{\text{height in centimeters} \times \text{weight in kilometers}/3600}$$

---

**TABLE 6.3.** CHIEF COMPLAINT AND HISTORY OF PRESENT ILLNESS

**CC:** "My chest is hurting, and it is hard to breathe."

**HPI:** John Doe is a 60-year-old Caucasian man who presents to the emergency department with substernal chest pain that feels as if someone is squeezing his chest. The pain is also radiating down his left arm. The pain began approximately 2 hours ago, while he was raking his yard. Pain was not relieved with rest or nitroglycerin 0.4 mg tablets × 2, which he swallowed with a glass of water. The patient states, "I always keep these pills with me" and points to a small metal container, which he keeps in his shirt pocket.

---

It is important for the student to inquire not only about the causes of an allergic reaction but a description of the patient's reaction after exposure to the allergen. You must be able to distinguish between a true allergic reaction and an intolerance or adverse effect to medication.[1] For example, a patient with a true allergy to a medication may break out in a rash, experience swelling, complain of itching of the skin, or describe a difficulty in breathing. This is different from a patient who describes having intolerance to or experiences an adverse effect of medication. In Figure 6.1, the administrative and demographic information, patient John Doe has listed a true allergy to penicillin. However, the ibuprofen problem is not to be considered a true drug allergy because stomach pain is considered a side effect.

The *chief complaint* (*CC*) is the primary problem that the patient is experiencing. It is usually written in the patient's own words. The student needs to interview the patient, family, or caregivers to ask specific questions about the patient's symptoms (Table 6.3).

The *history of present illness* (*HPI*) (Table 6.4) describes when the symptoms started, quality, location, concurrent symptoms, what causes the symptoms to

---

**TABLE 6.4.** QUESTIONS CONCERNING PATIENT SYMPTOM(S)

**1.** Have the symptom(s) occurred before?

**2.** When did the symptom(s) begin?

**3.** How long have the symptom(s) been going on?

**4.** Can you identify where the symptom(s) occur most frequently or have the most pain associated with them?

**5.** Does anyone else in the household have similar symptom(s) or is there a history of any relatives having these symptom(s)?

**6.** Does anything cause the symptom(s) to occur or worsen?

**7.** Does anything cause the symptom(s) to lessen or go away (including medication therapy)?

**8.** Are there any other associated signs or symptoms (eg, radiating pain, numbness, nausea/vomiting)?

---

**TABLE 6.5. PAST MEDICAL HISTORY**

**PMH:** Hypertension (15 years' duration), hyperlipidemia (7 years' duration), myocardial infarction (3 years ago)

**SH:** Cardiac catheterization 3 years ago with drug-eluting stent in right coronary artery

---

worsen, what causes the symptoms to be lessened or relieved, and what the patient has done to relieve the symptoms (including prescription or OTC medication).

The chief complaint and the history of present illness are essential in helping to determine the diagnosis. Appropriate diagnosis aids in selection of appropriate therapy, including medication. In addition, problems with the medication therapy may be uncovered. From the information contained in Table 6.3, the student will want to make a note to counsel the patient on proper use of the nitroglycerin tablets. Counseling includes the proper placement of the medication (sublingual not oral), proper dosing (use one tablet, if no pain relief in 5 minutes seek emergency care), the need for proper storage, and when to seek emergency treatment.

The *past medical history (PMH) and surgical history (SH)* (Table 6.5) lists past and present medical conditions, including any surgeries performed. You must be aware of what concomitant conditions may cause or worsen the patient's acute problem. For example, John Doe has a past history of hypertension, hyperlipidemia, and myocardial infarction that may cause or worsen the chest pain. In addition, you now have a list of diagnoses, and drug regimens and goals of therapy can be formulated. You may increase efficiency by targeting multiple diagnoses with a single-drug treatment.

Chronic illnesses may have a *genetic influence* resulting in higher incidences of disease within a family. You will want to investigate the patient's history or interview the patient, family, or caregiver about any significant past illness or cause of death in any primary family member (Table 6.6). It is important to include the age at which a family member died because it may constitute a risk factor for a disease and therefore be of significance in determining drug therapy.[2] For example, John Doe has an additional risk factor for coronary heart disease (CHD) because of his father's death at age 54 from an acute myocardial infarction.

The *social history or lifestyle* section (Table 6.7) contains information about the patient's living environment, social habits, and financial information, including insurance and prescription drug plan information. This section identifies nondrug treatments that have been tried in the past. Social habits that may improve or worsen

---

**TABLE 6.6. FAMILY HISTORY**

**FH:** Father died of acute myocardial infarction at the age of 54. Mother, 82, has a history of hypertension, hyperlipidemia, and heart failure. Patient has two brothers, both with a positive history of atherosclerosis and coronary heart disease. One brother with myocardial infarction at the age of 62.

---

**TABLE 6.7.** LIFESTYLE AND SOCIAL HISTORY

| Social history | Patient lives with wife of 36 years. Has two children no longer living at home. Retired from local shipyard, where he was employed as a welder. Patient has insurance and prescription plan through former employer. |
| --- | --- |
| Diet | 2-g low-sodium, low-cholesterol diet |
| Alcohol use | Three to four 12-oz beers per day |
| Tobacco use | Cigarette use 40-pack-year history (1 pack per day × 40 years) |
| Caffeine use | Eight to ten cups of coffee per day; two to three glasses of iced tea with meals |
| Exercise | Occasional yard work |

the patient's condition such as diet, exercise, use of alcohol, tobacco, caffeine, illicit drugs, and sexual history may be identified in this section. Remember that drug therapy is only a part of the patient-monitoring process. Pharmacists play a key role in prevention of disease as well as treatment.

The social history and lifestyle section noted in Table 6.7 shows that John Doe is retired; however, he does have health insurance and a prescription drug plan through his old employer. This patient is on a low-sodium and low-cholesterol diet for treatment of his hypertension and hyperlipidemia. Exercise is minimal, with only occasional yard work. In addition, John Doe continues to use alcohol, tobacco, and caffeine in excess amounts. The student pharmacist will want to counsel this patient on the identified problems. John Doe may have improvement in his illnesses with adherence to a planned schedule of diet, exercise, cessation of smoking, and moderate use of caffeine and alcohol (see Profile 6.1).

The *physical examination* (Table 6.8) notes any physical findings that serve as objective evidence of a disease or condition.

Clinical laboratory tests along with other monitoring examinations, such as the physical examination, X-rays, ECG, and MRI, are important monitoring indicators

**TABLE 6.8.** PHYSICAL EXAMINATION

| General | Moderately obese WM, somewhat anxious, A&O × 3 |
| --- | --- |
| Heart | RRR, w/o MRG; c/o SOB, denies orthopnea, DOE, or PND, no JVD |
| Lungs | CTA bilaterally; no rales or rhonchi, c/o nausea associated with CP, denies N/V |
| CXR | Heart is slightly enlarged; clear lung fields |
| ECG | NSR, HR 75, nonspecific ST segment changes in inferior leads |
| ECHO | — |

---

**TABLE 6.9.** REASONS FOR USING CLINICAL LABS AS MONITORING TOOLS

1. **Diagnostic:** Indicates the presence of disease or health problem. For example, elevated fasting glucose levels may indicate the presence of diabetes.

2. **Baseline:** Measurements before initiation of drug therapy. For example, hepatic liver enzyme measurement before starting antihyperlipidemic therapy with HMG-CoA enzyme inhibitors (such as simvastatin).

3. **Monitor:** Indicates the progress toward therapeutic goals. For example, decreased total cholesterol and low-density lipoprotein and increased high-density lipoprotein, elevated INR with warfarin.

4. Adjustment of medication dose indicated by decreased renal or hepatic functioning.

5. Toxic or subtherapeutic concentration of medication.

---

(Table 6.9).[3] This information is an important source of objective information. It is important for the student pharmacist to recognize and understand the consequences of abnormal laboratory values in order to make sound decisions concerning medication therapy. In addition, findings from other diagnostic examinations, such as X-rays, ECG, and MRI, may indicate a need for medication therapy, track the progress of drug therapy in treating disease, and serve as a monitor for any toxic or adverse effects of medication.

Timing of the laboratory sample may be important; it does make a difference to know when a laboratory sample is drawn. Timing may be critical to the validity of the examination. Laboratory tests are usually drawn fasting or nonfasting. Fasting describes a laboratory sample that is taken from a patient who has not had anything to eat or drink (except water) for at least 9 to 12 hours. A fasting laboratory sample is usually taken in the morning after a patient awakens. For example, a fasting lipid profile would be more valuable than a nonfasting laboratory sample in determining elevated serum cholesterol. A fasting glucose would be used as a diagnostic tool for diabetes mellitus.

Timing of a laboratory sample is especially critical when sampling drug serum concentrations and may be crucial when a patient is taking a medication with a narrow therapeutic index.[4] A peak level describes a drug serum concentration that is taken after the dose is given and represents the medication's maximum serum concentration. A trough level describes the lowest point of serum concentration of a medication and is taken just before the next dose of medication.

The use of serum concentrations to monitor drug therapy and make predictions about the absorption, distribution, metabolism, and excretion of a medication is identified as pharmacokinetics. Therapeutic drug monitoring is performed on medications that have a narrow therapeutic index and thus a narrow margin of safety (Table 6.10). Drugs considered to have a narrow therapeutic index must be monitored more frequently than medications that have a wide margin of safety.

| TABLE 6.10. SELECTED THERAPEUTIC RANGES | |
|---|---|
| **DRUG** | **THERAPEUTIC RANGE** |
| Digoxin | 0.5–2 ng/mL |
| Amikacin | 20–30 µg/mL (peak) |
| | < 5 µg/mL (trough) |
| Gentamicin, tobramycin | 5–10 µg/mL (peak) |
| | < 2 µg/mL (trough) |
| Vancomycin | 30–50 µg/mL (peak) |
| | 10–20 µg/mL (trough) |
| Lithium | 0.6–1.4 mEq/L |
| Carbamazepine | 4–12 µg/mL |
| Phenobarbital | 15–40 µg/mL |
| Phenytoin | 10–20 µg/mL |
| Primidone | 5–12 µg/mL |
| Valproic acid | 50–100 µg/mL |
| Theophylline | 10–20 µg/mL |
| Cyclosporine | 150–400 ng/mL (blood) |
| Tacrolimus | 5–20 ng/mL (whole blood) |

Use of specific laboratory tests will also aid in making decisions about proper dosing. Assessment of renal function can be performed using chemistry tests of BUN and serum creatinine. Determining the creatinine clearance helps select the proper dosing for medications that are eliminated primarily by renal mechanisms.[3]

Likewise, review of laboratory tests that are specific for hepatic function would indicate a need for dosage adjustment for medications that are primarily eliminated by hepatic mechanisms. Laboratory tests that are specific for hepatic function include lactate dehydrogenase (LDH), aspartate aminotransferase (AST), alanine aminotransferase (ALT), and bilirubin.

### CASE EXAMPLE: PROFILE 1

John Doe (Profile 6.1) was admitted to the emergency department with a tentative diagnosis of unstable angina. Several laboratory and diagnostic tests aid in clarifying the diagnosis and rule out other potential causes. In this case, acute myocardial infarction is a condition that must be ruled out. In order to help clarify the diagnosis, an electrocardiogram was performed, which showed signs of ischemia but no evidence of myocardial infarction. A serum marker that is necessary to rule out myocardial infarction is cardiac troponin I or T.

Renal function is estimated using the BUN and serum creatinine. In the case example, estimation of the creatinine clearance using the Cockcroft-Gault formula (see Table 6.11) for John Doe would be approximately 97 mL/min using his actual body weight. This creatinine clearance value represents adequate renal function and no need for adjustment of any medication that is renally eliminated.

Calculation of the low-density lipoprotein (LDL) fraction using the Friedwald equation (Table 6.12) and laboratory values obtained from the lipid profile reveals a calculated LDL of 174 mg/dL.

According to the Third Report of the National Cholesterol Education Program (NCEP) Expert Panel on Detection Evaluation, and Treatment of High Blood Cholesterol in Adults (Adult Treatment Panel III),[1] John Doe has multiple risk factors for CHD (ie, previous history of myocardial infarction, cigarette smoking, positive family history, hypertension, low HDL, age). Treatment for hyperlipidemia is necessary because his LDL is greater than or equal to 160 mg/dL. Due to his history of CHD, John Doe's LDL goal for treatment with medication needs to be at least less than 100 mg/dL. In addition, his HDL is low (< 40 mg/dL) and his triglycerides are 380 mg/dL (goal is < 150 mg/dL).

### TABLE 6.11. ESTIMATED CREATININE CLEARANCE:(ADULTS & PEDIATRICS)

Estimated creatinine clearance ($Cl_{cr}$) (mL/min):

COCKROFT AND GAULT FORMULA – Adults

$$Male = \frac{(140 - age) \times ABW\,(kg)}{(72 \times serum\,creatinine)}$$

Female = estimated creatinine clearance ($Cl_{cr}$) for male × 0.85

Estimated creatinine clearance ($CL_{cr}$) (mL/min/m$^2$):

SCHWARTZ EQUATION – Pediatrics

$$\frac{k \times height\,(cm)}{SCr\,(mg/dL)}$$

k = 0.33 in pre-term infants < 1 year

k = 0.45 in full-term infants < 1 year

k = 0.55 in age 1–12 years and adolescent girls

k = 0.7 in adolescent boys

---

**TABLE 6.12.** LDL CHOLESTEROL CALCULATION

Calculation of LDL cholesterol using the Friedwald equation:

$$LDL = total\,cholesterol - \left(HDL + \frac{TGL}{5}\right)$$

---

Vital signs are used to:

1. Help diagnose disease. Abnormal vital signs such as elevated blood pressure, temperature, pulse, respiration rate, or body weight may indicate the presence of disease.
2. Track progression of a patient toward his or her therapeutic goal. Decreased blood pressure, temperature, pulse, or respiratory rate may indicate an improvement in a patient's condition. This may indicate that the patient is responding to the prescribed treatment.

---

**CASE EXAMPLE: PROFILE 1**

A review of the patient's vital signs indicates that John Doe has a blood pressure that is slightly elevated. Because this patient has a history of long-standing hypertension, monitoring the blood pressure is in order for you to determine if the current antihypertensive medication regimen is effective. The student may note the elevated blood pressure on a list of potential problems. In establishing a patient-specific monitoring plan, the student pharmacist must make sure that patients are receiving the most rational, appropriate, and cost-effective form of therapy. A review of the patient's medication regimen (Fig. 6.2) is important in establishing any problems that the patient may have.

---

There are a number of questions you will want to ask about the patient's medication regimen.

1. Is the drug being used for an appropriate diagnosis or indication? Knowing the diagnosis establishes a basis for selection of an appropriate medication. Some medication is used for off-label purposes. You will want to review scientific literature for evidence of efficacy.
2. Is the dose of the medication appropriate for this specific patient? Take into account patient characteristics such as age, weight, sex, ethnic background, and allergies as well as concurrent disease states and medications used. Is the duration of treatment appropriate?
3. What are the most likely adverse effects caused by this medication? Does the patient exhibit any of these adverse effects?
4. Are there any interactions with other medications or diseases that the patient may have? Is the patient taking each medication at the appropriate time?

**Figure 6.2.** Medication profile review.

**Current Medications**

| Start Date | Medication/Route | Dose/Schedule | Stop Date | Diagnosis |
|---|---|---|---|---|
| 06/15/01 | EC Aspirin/po | 81 mg daily (7 AM) | | Post-MI/platelet inhibitor |
| 06/15/01 | Simvastatin/po | 20 mg daily (7 AM) | | Hyperlipidemia/Post-MI |
| 06/15/05 | Nitroglycerin transdermal patch | 5 mg/24 h (7 AM) | | Angina |
| 06/15/98 | Metoprolol | 100 mg daily | | Hypertension/Post-MI |
| 06/15/05 | Nitroglycerin/SL | 0.4 mg prn chest pain | | Angina |
| | Acetaminophen | 500 mg 2 tabs prn | | Pain/HA |

Time Line—circle actual administration times and record appropriate medications and meals below

AM

6 7 8 9 10 11 12 1 2 3 4 5 6 7 8 9 10 11 12 1 2 3 4 5

noon    PM    midnight    AM

E C aspirin, simvastatin, nitroglycerin patch, metoprolol

5. Are there any patient-specific barriers to taking this medication? Is the medication affordable? Are the instructions for use easy to understand? Are there devices that must be used with the medication (syringes, inhalers) about which the patient must be counseled?

6. What proof do you have that the medication is effective? Medication effectiveness can be determined by subjectively asking the patient if their disease has improved, such as pain relief. Objective evidence would include assessment tests or instruments, or improvement of vital signs, diagnostic tests, or laboratory parameters.

Drug interactions and adverse effects present a health risk to patients and a challenge to pharmacists. Patients at high risk for drug interactions and adverse effects include the chronically ill, older, and frail patient, patients with multiple medications, critical-care patients, and patients undergoing high-risk surgery. Adverse effects can be caused by several factors:

1. Characteristic of the medication or drug class, as in gastrointestinal bleeding caused by nonsteroidal anti-inflammatory drugs (NSAIDs), hyperglycemia associated with niacin therapy.

2. Characteristic of a toxic effect of a medication. Inhibition of the cytochrome P-450 hepatic enzyme system (Table 6.13) will result in increased concentration of medication and a greater risk for toxic adverse effects, as in bradycardia caused by a serum digoxin concentration greater than 2 ng/mL.

3. Decreased concentration of the medication. For example, worsening seizures caused decreased seizure control by a low serum phenytoin concentration.

4. Induction of the cytochrome P-450 hepatic enzyme system (Table 6.13), resulting in decreased concentrations of the medications. For example, decreased carbamazepine serum concentration resulting in worsening seizures. Carbamazepine induces its own metabolism in the liver, resulting in lower serum concentrations of the medication.

5. Interference with one medication by another medication. This includes effects such as protein binding, chelation, interference with absorption, interference with elimination, or one medication counteracting another medication.

6. Drugs with similar adverse effects act synergistically to increase the risk of an adverse effect. For example, combined use of a nonsteroidal anti-inflammatory agent and aspirin that results in symptoms of gastrointestinal ulceration.

## Timing of Medication

Changing the dose of simvastatin 20 mg daily from 7 AM to bedtime (9 PM) will increase the effectiveness of lowering the total cholesterol and LDL. John Doe will want to be counseled on appropriate use of the nitroglycerin patch. Application of the nitroglycerin patch for 10 to 12 hours with a nitrate-free interval of 12 to 14 hours will improve this patient's exercise tolerance by decreasing the risk of nitrate tolerance. The enteric-coated aspirin may need to be scheduled at mealtime in order to decrease the risk of abdominal discomfort (Fig. 6.2).

**TABLE 6.13.** CYTOCHROME P-450 ENZYME FAMILY AND SELECTED SUBSTRATES

| CYP1A Substrates | | CYP2C Substrates | | CYP2D6 Substrates | |
|---|---|---|---|---|---|
| Acetaminophen | Olanzapine | Amitriptyline | Irbesartan | Amitriptyline | Fluphenazine |
| Amitriptyline | Ondansetron | Celecoxib | Lansoprazole | Captopril | Haloperidol |
| Caffeine | Propafenone | Citalopram | Losartan | Carvedilol | Imipramine |
| Clarithromycin | Propranolol | Clomipramine | Mephenytoin | Citalopram | Labetalol |
| Clomipramine | Prostaglandins | Cyclophosphamide | Naproxen | Chlorpheniramine | Maprotiline |
| Clozapine | R-warfarin | Dapsone | Nelfinavir | Chlorpromazine | R-methadone |
| Cyclobenzaprine | Ritonavir | Diazepam | Nifedipine | Clomipramine | Methamphet- |
| Dantrolene | Tamoxifen | Diclofenac | Omeprazole | Clozapine | amine |
| Desipramine | Theobromine | Ethosuximide | Pantoprazole | Codeine | Metoclopramide |
| Diazepam | Theophylline | Fluoxetine | Phenytoin | Desipramine | Metoprolol |
| Estradiol | Verapamil | Fluvastatin | Piroxicam | Dextromethorphan | Mexilitine |
| Fluvoxamine | Zileuton | Glipizide | Primidone | Doxepin | Morphine |
| Haloperidol | Zolmitriptan | Glyburide | Progesterone | Encainide | Nelfinavir |
| Imipramine | | Ibuprofen | Propranolol | Flecanide | Nortriptyline |
| Lidocaine | | Imipramine | Ritonavir | Fluoxetine | Omeprazole |
| Methadone | | Indomethacin | Rosiglitazone | Fluvoxamine | Ondansetron |
| Naproxen | | | S,R-warfarin | | Paroxetine |
| | | | Sulfinpyrazone | | |
| | | | Sulfaphenazole | | |
| | | | Sulfonamides | | |
| | | | Tamoxifen | | |
| | | | Taxol | | |
| | | | Testosterone | | |
| | | | Tetrahydrocanabinol | | |
| | | | Tolbutamide | | |
| | | | Torsemide | | |
| | | | Tricyclics | | |
| | | | Valproic Acid | | |

## CYP2D6 Substrates

| | |
|---|---|
| Perphenazine | Trifluperidol |
| Phenformin | Trimipramine |
| Propafenone | Venlafaxine |
| Propranolol | Vinblastine |
| Quinidine | Zonisamide |
| Risperidone | |
| Ritonavir | |
| RU486 | |
| Tamoxifen | |
| Taxol | |
| Teniposide | |
| Testosterone | |
| Thioridazine | |
| Timolol | |
| Tramadol | |
| Trazodone | |
| Triazolam | |

## CYP3A Substrates

| | | | | |
|---|---|---|---|---|
| Alfentanil | Dantrolene | Flutamide | Nelfinavir | Simvastatin |
| Alprazolam | Dapsone | Gleevec | Nicardipine | Sirolimus |
| Amiodarone | Delavirdine | Haloperidol | Nifedipine | Tacrolimus |
| Amlodipine | Dextromethorphan | Hydrocortisone | Nisoldipine | Tamoxifen |
| Antipyrine | Diazepam | Indinavir | Omeprazole | Taxol |
| Astemizole | Digitoxin | Irinotecan | Ondansetron | Testosterone |
| Atorvastatin | Diltiazem | Itraconazole | Paclitaxel | Trazodone |
| Buspirone | Disopyramide | Ketoconazole | Pimozide | Triazolam |
| Caffeine | Enalapril | Lidocaine | Prednisone | Verapamil |
| Carbamazepine | Erythromycin | Lopinavir | Progesterone | Vinblastine |
| Chlorpheniramine | Estradiol | Loratidine | Propranolol | Vincristine |
| Chlorpromazine | Estrogen | Lovastatin | Quinidine | Zaleplon |
| Clarithromycin | Ethosuximide | Mephenytoin | R-warfarin | Zolpidem |
| Cocaine | Etoposide | Methadone | Ritonavir | |
| Cortisol | Felodipine | Miconazole | Saquinavir | |
| Cyclophosphamide | Fentanyl | Midazolam | Sertraline | |
| Cyclosporine | Finasteride | Nefazodone | Sildenafil | |

Taken with permission & modified from Dipiro 6th ed. Table 87-5, p. 1624.

As the number of medications used to treat disease in a patient increases, the risk of drug–drug interactions also increases. Anticipation of adverse effects and educating the patient or caregiver about adverse effects and drug–drug interactions will result in increased awareness and correction or avoidance of any potential problems. Make every effort to counsel the patient and caregivers extensively about the most common side effects and less common side effects that may require alteration of the drug regimen.

### CASE EXAMPLE: PROFILE 1

A review of John Doe's medication profile indicates a need for adjustment of his drug therapy. (See Fig. 6.2)

## Adverse Effects

John Doe should be monitored for the following adverse effects:

Enteric-coated aspirin: signs or symptoms of gastrointestinal bleeding or abdominal pain, increased bleeding or bruising
Simvastatin: gastrointestinal upset, headache, dizziness, muscle pain
Nitroglycerin transdermal patch: rash, dizziness, hypotension, increased heart rate
Metoprolol succinate: decreased heart rate, hypotension, dizziness, fatigue, constipation, cardiac arrhythmia, edema, heart failure
Acetaminophen: rash, hypersensitivity reactions

John Doe will want to be counseled on the most common adverse effects of the medication and ways to prevent these adverse effects.

## Proper Use of Medication

Counsel the patient on how to store and use the sublingual nitroglycerin tablets and when to seek medical assistance. Warning the patient not to take more than 4 g of acetaminophen daily will decrease his risk of hepatic injury.

## Monitoring Parameters

Monitoring parameters include vital signs, episodes of chest pain, and exercise tolerance.

## PUTTING IT ALL TOGETHER

Use of multiple medications requires the integration of individual drug-monitoring plans. This can be achieved by creation of a master flow sheet. A flow sheet specifies a parameter (such as blood pressure) and notes all the medications with the potential for causing a problem.

---

**TABLE 6.14.** POSSIBLE OUTCOMES FOR THERAPEUTIC MONITORING

**1.** Therapeutic regimen provides the expected outcome for the patient. Therapeutic regimen is continued.

**2.** Therapeutic regimen does not provide the expected clinical outcome.

   **a.** Dose of current regimen must be increased.

   **b.** Adjunctive agent is added to current drug regimen.

   **c.** Current drug regimen is stopped and an alternative agent is started.

**3.** Therapeutic regimen produces an adverse or unwanted condition. Reduction or discontinuation of current dose or use of an alternative agent can be considered.

---

You will want to monitor a patient's response to drug therapy continuously by assessing both subjective and objective data. If the patient's response to drug therapy is appropriate, then no alteration of the drug regimen is indicated. Sometimes, a reduction in the dose of medication may be warranted. If the drug regimen does not achieve the desired therapeutic goal or is associated with adverse side effects or toxicities, then an alteration of the therapeutic regimen is indicated (Table 6.14).

Failure of a patient to obtain a therapeutic goal can be related to numerous factors: noncompliance to the drug regimen, inadequate dose of medication, drug-drug interactions, or drug-disease interactions. Each of these aspects needs to be considered. It is important that the pharmacist investigate all pharmacologic and nonpharmacologic reasons why a patient's therapeutic outcome is not achieved.

Decisions to alter the therapeutic regimen are indicated by the response of the patient. Once a new therapeutic plan is decided on, the process of monitoring drug therapy is started over with new monitoring parameters being set for each patient. Remember that monitoring is based on each individual case. Every patient will have different characteristics and circumstances surrounding him or her. Understanding the process of how to monitor a patient will lessen the chance of missing key information.

Following are a couple of cases for you to use as practice for all of the aforementioned principles.

### PATIENT CASE 1

RN is an 18-month-old WF who presents with a 2-day history of cough and rhinorrhea. Her mother says she "feels warm and has a fever." On examination, she is noted to be fussy and irritable. Vital signs are: temperature 38.9°C, respiratory rate 24, pulse 88. Pneumatic otoscopy findings include decreased excursions and a red and inflamed tympanic membrane. She had been treated with amoxicillin for acute otitis media (AOM) 6 months ago. Mom denies that she has been pulling at her ears.

## Determine the Therapeutic Goal

### Cure of the Infection (AOM)

The American Academy of Pediatrics developed evidence-based clinical practice guidelines to provide recommendations to clinicians for the diagnosis and management of acute otitis media.[5] This is the easy part—cure the child, and all else resolves. Because the only way to definitively determine the cause of the infection is to culture a sample from the site of the infection (which in this case would require a myringotomy to obtain middle-ear fluid), the decision about treatment in this case is based on clinical judgment. Although most episodes of acute otitis media are not bacterial, her prior history of AOM would suggest that it would be prudent to treat with antibiotics. The question is, which antibiotic? The Ersatz Pharmaceutical representative was just in the office and left samples of Gorillacillin that treats 75 different organisms. How do you decide between it and amoxicillin?

1. What are the most likely organisms that cause AOM?
2. What are the adverse effects of potential agents?
3. What are the costs (not just acquisition cost)?
4. What dosage forms are available?
5. How often must the drug be given?
6. How palatable is the drug or can the taste be altered?
7. What patient factors need to be considered?
   a. Are immunizations up-to-date?
   b. Is the parent likely to give the drug appropriately?
   c. Is there a history of allergy to antibiotics?
   d. What antibiotics have been used in this patient in the past to treat AOM?
   e. Would it be possible to provide observation therapy for 48–72 hours if the patient has nonsevere illness (mild otalgia, fever < 39°C) and is of the appropriate age?

### Relief of Symptoms (Pain, Fever, Cough)

Cough and fever are natural responses to irritants and infections. Both are innate protective mechanisms designed to help the host get rid of the offending agent. It is probably preferable not to treat these symptoms separately, as they will resolve with cure of the infection. However, from a purely practical standpoint, most parents (or health-care providers) are not willing to *not* relieve the cough and fever. What considerations are involved in selecting therapy?

1. Is the cough severe enough that it keeps the child or parents awake?
2. Is the cough dry or productive?
3. Is the fever causing the child to be in great discomfort?
4. Is one antipyretic more effective than another?
5. Are there nonpharmacologic alternatives?

**6.** Should a combination product be used?

**7.** What is the age of the child (newer Food and Drug Administration recommendations on avoiding in children <4 years of age due to lack of safety/ efficacy data)?

The symptoms produced by AOM are not specific to the disease state. Instead, they are really clinical signs as noted above. The best indicator in this case is the child herself. If the antibiotic therapy is effective, she will return to her normal personality and routine.

## What Is the Patient's Response to Therapy?

*Evaluate in 48 to 72 hours*

**1.** Getting better
   **a.** Make no change in therapy.
   **b.** Continue full course of therapy—this is dependent on the specific antibiotic chosen, usually 10 days but may be less.
**2.** No change—reassess
   **a.** Is it nonadherence?
   **b.** Improper device to accurately measure dose (teaspoon vs. dosing spoon)?
   **c.** Inadequate dose?
      **i.** Not high enough
      **ii.** Not administered frequent enough
   **d.** Natural history of the disease, for example, it takes a little longer to resolve
   **e.** Wrong drug or resistance?
   **f.** Improper storage (does it require refrigeration or not)?

Your response depends on what you believe to be the reason for the lack of response. Education of the caregiver (course of AOM, necessity for accurate dosing, frequency of dosing), adjustment of dosage, or change in therapy may be warranted.

**3.** Getting Worse
   **a.** Ask the same questions as for no change
   **b.** Possible concurrent, unrelated illness

The modification of therapy is based on the assessment. The most likely cause of drug failure is nonadherence. This must not be taken to imply child abuse or indifference. It is almost always a consequence of incomplete understanding of the purpose of the treatment and the consequences of not completing the full course of therapy. It could also be the result of a misunderstanding of the proper storage and administration of the drug. In both cases, the pharmacist is in the best position of health-care professionals to address these issues. The importance of adequate education of patients and their caregivers cannot be overstressed. It may also be necessary to change therapy by adjusting the dose or frequency of the current drug or changing or adding another drug.

*Adverse Effects*

Adverse effects associated with antibiotic therapy can be broken into two primary categories. The first and of most concern is an allergic reaction. The most common presentation is an urticarial rash. Fortunately, this is very uncommon and may not require any intervention. However, it is often difficult to distinguish between nonallergic and allergic rashes, so it may be better to discontinue the antibiotic and change to another chemically unrelated agent, especially since there are many alternatives.

The second and far more likely adverse effects are related to the GI tract and include diarrhea and diaper rash. In many cases they may be self-limited, and no change is necessary, or in the case of diaper rash topical therapy may be sufficient. Diarrhea is an undesirable but not catastrophic consequence and is best left untreated. The administration of a lactobacillus preparation, or eating yogurt with active yeast cultures, although of no proven benefit, is innocuous and provides some comfort to the parents.

*How Is the Therapy Modified as a Consequence of the Assessment?*

Modification of the therapy as related to lack of efficacy in this case consists of selecting alternative antibiotic therapy. The same principles of selection that apply to the primary therapy will be applied here. If adverse effects are a consequence of a possible allergic reaction, antibiotics from a different chemical class for which cross-sensitivity is unlikely ought to be selected. Modification to decrease or eliminate the GI effects could include giving the drug with food or administering a lactobacillus preparation as cited earlier. The use of yogurt addresses both approaches.

---

**PATIENT CASE 2**

HL is a 48-year-old WM who presents to his primary care physician for a routine check-up and receives a cholesterol screening. He has no significant past medical history. He smokes ½ ppd but does not drink alcohol. He does not take any routine scheduled medications. His family history is significant for a father who died of a myocardial infarction (MI) at 50. His mother is alive and well at 70 and none of his siblings are known to have heart disease at this time. Pertinent physical findings include a weight of 104 kg, height of 71 in, BP 140/85, HR 75, RR 12, carotid pulses symmetric bilaterally without bruits, no abdominal pain or bruits, no evidence of xanthomas, xanthelasma, or corneal arcus. His laboratory data reveal normal kidney and liver function. His fasting cholesterol panel shows total cholesterol of 240 mg/dL, triglycerides 180 mg/dL, high-density lipoprotein (HDL) 30 mg/dL, and calculated LDL 174 mg/dL.

## What Is Your Initial Assessment of This Patient?

According to the NCEP/ATP III guidelines, serum cholesterol ought to be monitored in all adults 20 years of age and older at least once every 5 years.[6] Once hyperlipidemia is identified, a full evaluation of the patient should take place and include a thorough history, physical examination, and baseline laboratory assessments. The initial history and physical examination will include an assessment of any cardiovascular (CV) risk factors, family history of premature CV disease or lipid disorders, the presence or absence of secondary cause of hyperlipidemia, and the presence or absence of xanthomas, pancreatitis, renal or liver disease, peripheral vascular disease, or cerebral vascular disease. Therefore, your initial assessment of this hyperlipidemic patient is that he has three positive risk factors that increase his risk for CHD which are male greater than 45, low HDL cholesterol defined as less than 40 mg/dL, smoker, and a family history of premature CAD. His 10-year risk for CHD is 25%.

## What Is Your Therapeutic Goal for This Patient?

Again, according to the NCEP guidelines, this patient has high blood cholesterol defined as greater than or equal to 240 mg/dL, and his lipoprotein analysis reveals high LDL cholesterol defined as between 160 and 189 mg/dL. Therefore, a clinical evaluation is warranted. Based on the findings previously stated, this patient is an ideal candidate for diet therapy, as well as drug therapy aimed to lower his high cholesterol to a goal LDL of less than 100 mg/dL to reduce long-term risk. There have been numerous clinical trials showing the morbidity and mortality benefits of primary prevention with drug therapy in a patient with hypercholesterolemia.[7-11] Most would agree that use of statins in a patient with a 10-year risk for CHD that is >20% is reasonable and appropriate.[12] Therefore, he ought to be started on the TLC diet as recommended by the NCEP ATP III, as well as a pharmacologic agent to lower his cholesterol. To choose an appropriate agent, you need to be aware of the effects on the lipid panel and adverse drug effects of each class, as well as each agent within the class. The class of drugs most clinicians would choose to treat this patient would be an HMG-CoA reductase inhibitor, or statin. Which statin to choose is ideally based on three things: (1) the percentage lowering of LDL required to achieve the goal, (2) the agent and dose to achieve this goal without significant adverse effects or drug interactions, and (3) which agent can achieve this in the most cost-effective manner. This patient needs at least a 25% reduction in his LDL, and one will want to look at the reported lowering of LDL for each dosage form and determine which agent would be the most cost-effective. For example, statin A may lower LDL up to 40% with a starting dose of 10 mg daily and cost the patient $75 for a month's supply. However, statin B may lower LDL only 20% with a starting dose of 20 mg daily and 30% with a dose of 40 mg daily. The 40-mg dose of statin B costs the patient $65 a month. Which statin is more cost-efficient for this patient? Although statin B 40 mg daily doesn't lower cholesterol as much as statin A 10 mg daily, it is more cost efficient in our patient who requires only a 25% reduction in his LDL.

### The Next Question You Will Want to Ask Yourself Is How Do I Monitor This Patient?

Monitoring parameters (MPs) are divided into two categories, therapeutic and adverse effect MPs. Considering therapeutic MPs first, it might seem obvious that the first therapeutic MP for this patient is an LDL less than or equal to 130 mg/dL. However, do not forget that another important therapeutic MP for our patient is the primary prevention of CAD. An important decision is how often to obtain a lipid panel in a patient being treated for hypercholesterolemia? Usually, a lipid panel will be drawn every 6 weeks after initiation of therapy until the goal is achieved. Then a lipid panel may be reviewed every 6 months thereafter. If a patient is not having the desired therapeutic effects, you may need to adjust his therapy. You may need to increase or decrease the dose or add another agent. After making any changes in a therapeutic regimen, you must continually reassess your patient and determine new therapeutic MPs if necessary.

Adverse MPs may seem more involved. Assuming a statin is chosen to treat this patient's hypercholesterolemia, baseline and follow-up assessments of laboratory parameters are required. Baseline liver function tests (LFTs), mainly ALT and AST, can be done before initiation of therapy with a statin to ensure that the patient has no existing liver dysfunction. Different statin manufacturers may have slightly different recommendations for follow-up assessments of LFTs however most recommend periodic assessments when clinically indicated. If a patient complains of new-onset or unexplained muscle pain, a creatinine phosphokinase (CPK) can be ordered and assessed to rule out rhabdomyolysis.

If a patient is experiencing an adverse effect, it is always important to determine if it is clinically relevant or not. You may have a patient present withnew-onset muscle pain who, on questioning, reveals that he has recently started a new vigorous workout regime. Certainly, it would be prudent to check a CPK to be safe, but it may also be advisable to counsel the patient on exercise moderation and appropriate stretching and cooling-off techniques. Additionally, a patient with an elevated AST is not automatically excluded from receiving a statin. The important question is how much the AST is elevated. Generally, if the LFTs are greater than or equal to three times the upper limit of normal, you may want to find the reason for the elevation (recent MI, for example). Determining clinical relevance is something that comes with time and years of practice, but it is an important aspect of clinical practice. If an adverse effect is deemed clinically relevant, you may need to adjust the therapy appropriately by decreasing the dose or changing to a different drug class altogether. Again, after making any changes in a therapeutic regimen, you must continually reassess your patient and determine new adverse MPs if necessary.

### If a Patient Is Having No Adverse Effects and Has Reached His Therapeutic Goal, Can You Simply Send Him off and Never See Him Again?

Of course you would never do this. Patient care and monitoring are a continual process and occur for as long as the patient needs a therapeutic intervention, either pharmacologic or nonpharmacologic. For example, in this patient who achieves a goal LDL of less than or equal to 130 mg/dL and is experiencing no adverse effects, a conceivable monitoring assessment could take place every 6 to 12 months. This patient will probably need to be assessed for the rest of his life. Each patient and each clinical scenario is unique and will require different approaches to determining therapeutic goals and monitoring parameters.

## DEDICATION

In memory of Dr. Bruce Parks who originated the idea for this chapter. Your memory lives with all who knew your kind and gentle spirit.

## APPLICATION EXERCISES

1. The process of drawing a conclusion from given information and reasoning from the general to the specific is called
   A. inductive reasoning
   B. hypothesizing
   C. regeneration
   D. deductive reasoning

2. If the primary adverse effect of a drug is bone marrow suppression, which of the following would be the most appropriate laboratory test for monitoring of toxicity?
   A. Liver panel
   B. Complete blood count
   C. Serum glucose
   D. BUN and creatinine

3. A patient has a BUN of 42 mg/dL and a serum creatinine of 2.1 mg/dL. His estimated creatinine clearance is determined to be 19 mL/min. This information would be important for drugs that
   A. are eliminated by the liver
   B. are eliminated by the kidney
   C. are poorly absorbed from the GI tract
   D. have a high first-pass effect

4. A patient taking a nonsteroidal anti-inflammatory drug (NSAID) complains of frequent abdominal pain and GI upset. This is an example of
   A. drug allergy
   B. drug sensitivity
   C. drug intolerance
   D. drug variable

5. Which of the following are appropriate questions concerning the chief complaint and the history of present illness?
   A. How long have the symptoms been occurring?
   B. Does anything lessen these symptoms or make them go away?

   **C.** Are there any associated signs or symptoms?
   **D.** All of the above.
**6.** An example of subjective information would be
   **A.** X-ray report
   **B.** laboratory test result
   **C.** physical examination
   **D.** patient symptoms

## ACKNOWLEDGEMENT

The authors wish to acknowledge the contributions of Joel R. Pittman to this chapter.

## REFERENCES

1. Roden D. Chapter 5. Principles of clinical pharmacology. In: Longo D, Fauci A, Kasper, SL DH, Jameson J, Loscalzo J, eds. *Harrison's Principles of Internal Medicine*. 18th ed. New York, NY: McGraw-Hill; 2012. Available at http://www.accessmedicine.com/content.aspx?aID=9092427 (subscription required). Accessed March, 2014.

2. Blaha MJ KK, Ndumele CE, Gluckman TJ, Blumenthal RS. Chapter 51. Preventive strategies for coronary heart disease. In: Fuster V, Walsh RA, Harrington RA, eds. *Hurst's The Heart*. 13th ed. New York, NY: McGraw-Hill; 2011. Available at http://www.accessmedicine.com/content.aspx?aID=7817557 (subscription required). Accessed March, 2014.

3. Gomella LG. HSCLDC, immunology, serology. In: Gomella LG, Haist SA, eds. *Clinician's Pocket Reference: The Scut Monkey*. 11th ed. New York, NY: McGraw-Hill; 2007. Available at http://www.accessmedicine.com/content.aspx?aID=2699454 (subscription required). Accessed March, 2014.

4. Nicoll D LC, Pignone M, McPhee SJ. Chapter 4. Therapeutic drug monitoring and pharmacogenetic testing: principles and test interpretation. In: Nicoll D, Lu CM, Pignone M, McPhee SJ, eds. *Pocket Guide to Diagnostic Tests*. 6th ed. New York, NY: McGraw-Hill; 2012. Available at http://www.accessmedicine.com/content.aspx?aID=56993957. Accessed March, 2014.

5. Diagnosis and management of acute otitis media. *Pediatrics*. 2004;113(5):1451–1465, May.

6. Expert Panel on Detection Evaluation, Treatment of High Blood Cholesterol in Adults. Executive summary of the third report of the national cholesterol education program (ncep) expert panel on detection, evaluation, and treatment of high blood cholesterol in adults (adult treatment panel iii). *JAMA : the journal of the American Medical Association*. 2001;285(19):2486–2497.

7. Shepherd J, Cobbe SM, Ford I, et al. Prevention of coronary heart disease with pravastatin in men with hypercholesterolemia. West of Scotland Coronary

Prevention Study Group. *The New England Journal of Medicine.* 1995;333(20): 1301–1307, November 16.

8. Downs JR, Clearfield M, Weis S, et al. Primary prevention of acute coronary events with lovastatin in men and women with average cholesterol levels: results of AFCAPS/TexCAPS. Air Force/Texas Coronary Atherosclerosis Prevention Study. *JAMA : the journal of the American Medical Association.* 1998;279(20):1615–1622, May 27.

9. Collins R, Armitage J, Parish S, Sleigh P, Peto R. MRC/BHF Heart Protection Study of cholesterol-lowering with simvastatin in 5963 people with diabetes: a randomised placebo-controlled trial. *Lancet.* 2003;361(9374):2005–2016, June 14.

10. Colhoun HM, Betteridge DJ, Durrington PN, et al. Primary prevention of cardiovascular disease with atorvastatin in type 2 diabetes in the Collaborative Atorvastatin Diabetes Study (CARDS): multicentre randomised placebo-controlled trial. *Lancet.* 2004;364(9435):685–696, August 21–27.

11. Ridker PM, Danielson E, Fonseca FA, et al. Rosuvastatin to prevent vascular events in men and women with elevated C-reactive protein. *The New England journal of medicine.* 2008;359(21):2195–2207, November 20.

12. Taylor F, Ward K, Moore TH, et al. Statins for the primary prevention of cardiovascular disease. *Cochrane Database Syst Rev.* 2011(1):CD004816.

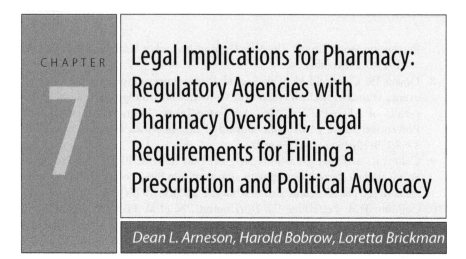

CHAPTER

7

# Legal Implications for Pharmacy: Regulatory Agencies with Pharmacy Oversight, Legal Requirements for Filling a Prescription and Political Advocacy

*Dean L. Arneson, Harold Bobrow, Loretta Brickman*

**Objectives: Upon completion of the chapter and exercises, the student pharmacist will be able to**

1. Define *drug* according to the FDA.
2. Identify and discuss information that is required to be included on a prescription.
3. Examine a prescription label to determine the appropriate information.
4. Identify the factors that make a prescription legal.
5. Define and distinguish the difference between controlled substances.
6. List and explain the pharmacist's responsibilities for implementing Omnibus Budget Reconciliation Act of 1990 (OBRA 1990).
7. List and explain the pharmacist's responsibilities for implementing the Poison Prevention Packaging Act.
8. Define and differentiate between risk assessment and risk management.
9. Describe the impact of the 2007 FDA Amendment Act on pharmacy.
10. Describe the pharmacists' legal responsibility when providing medication therapy management to patients.
11. Define political advocacy and its importance for the profession of pharmacy.
12. Plan a course of action for successful political advocacy.

---

**Patient Encounter**

The responsibility for attending pharmacist has fallen to you this month in the ICU. The pharmacy director has always been supportive of the decisions made by the attending pharmacists in conjunction

---

*(continued on next page)*

with the ethics team in the ICU. The legal issues of this situation may be different depending on where you practice. For the purposes of this case, let's say that the laws in the Country or State do not address this issue specifically.

The patient's family has not asked for the pain medications to be withheld. They have not asked for the ventilator to be stopped. How did the wife come to the decision to stop the antibiotics? How will you approach the family in order to gain the following outcome?

### Outcome

In this patient's case, he is temporarily in need of proxy decision makers, but will ultimately be able to state his own patient preferences. It is appropriate to continue antibiotics until the patient is able to communicate his own preferences. Because the patient had not communicated his wishes beforehand (and because you know that people, once disabled, often accept their disability), you are able to convince the family to wait until his speech therapy is successful and he is able to communicate his wishes.

What are the laws concerning practice of the pharmacist that take precedence in this scenario?

Do legal and ethical questions coincide here, is there a point where legal and ethical diverge?

## INTRODUCTION

To fill a prescription a pharmacist must be aware of all the legal requirements. The pharmacist must also keep in mind that his or her actions may be open to civil liability if he or she makes an error in filling a prescription and causes harm to a patient. This chapter discusses the Federal law and briefly touches on some state requirements for filling a prescription. The learning objectives outline the areas to be covered.

This chapter is designed to describe the legal aspects of filling a prescription systematically. One of the first steps is to define a *drug* and then discuss what makes a prescription a legal prescription. The information that must appear on the prescription is also outlined. Information that appears on the label is explained with a discussion of the differences between federal and state requirements. The legal requirements for the container in which the medication is dispensed are also discussed, with the requirements and exemptions presented. Finally, the requirements for the information that the pharmacist must provide to the patient are presented and discussed.

## ADMINISTRATIVE AGENCIES

### The Food and Drug Administration

The federal government has established an administrative agency, the Food and Drug Administration (FDA, www.fda.gov), to oversee the area of pharmaceuticals. The FDA oversees all aspects of the pharmaceutical market. One of the most important duties it performs is to approve new medications for use in the United States. In overseeing this function, it has established the procedures manufacturers must follow to perform pharmacologic/toxicologic studies on new chemical entities. These methods determine the potential benefit the entity may have versus the risk of harm it may cause. This is accomplished through the clinical testing of medications on human subjects. The FDA also approves and monitors the manufacturing process established by the drug company. The company must file the exact process they use to manufacture the drug with the FDA, and if the company decides to change the process in any way, they must notify the FDA and obtain approval. The FDA defines a drug as "articles intended for use in the diagnosis, cure, mitigation, treatment, or prevention of disease" and "articles (other than food) intended to affect the structure or any function of the body of man or other animals" [FDCA, §201(g)(1)].

Among the parameters the FDA monitors are the absorption, distribution, metabolism, and elimination of the medication by the body; these comprise its pharmacokinetics. The FDA uses this parameter to approve generic medications. The decision to approve a generic medication is based on the comparison of the bioavailability of the generic medication to the brand-name product. Because the FDA has the authority over the manufacturing process, the federal government has also given them the right to inspect any facility where medication is held.

Other areas that are regulated by the FDA include the approval of all drug advertising to health-care professionals, such as in the package insert. They also approve advertising to the public. They regulate the distribution of drug samples. Pharmacists are not allowed to be in possession of sample products except in very structured situations.

The primary goal of the FDA is to protect the safety of the public, and they do this by requiring testing for the safety and efficacy of medicinal products. They monitor the products even after they have been approved and are on the market. The FDA has the authority to require pharmaceutical manufacturers to perform drug recalls to retrieve any product that may pose a danger to the public.

## The Drug Enforcement Administration

A second administration agency that is involved with medications is the Drug Enforcement Administration (DEA, www.justice.gov/dea). It is a branch of the US Justice Department, and its main purpose is to administer the federal Controlled Substances Act (CSA). The CSA (21 U.S.C. §§801-970) regulates a particular set of medications (controlled substances, which are defined later in the chapter) that have a high potential for physical and/or psychological addiction (http://www.deadiversion.usdoj.gov/21cfr/21usc/).

The DEA has the authority to perform inspections on pharmacies where controlled substances are held. The inspectors have the authority, through permission of the pharmacist or an administrative warrant, to inspect any pharmacy where they feel illegal activity is taking place. The inspectors have the authority to audit the pharmacy's invoices, inventory, and prescription files to determine if there are any discrepancies between what has been purchased, what is presently in inventory, and what has been dispensed by the pharmacy. If a pharmacist is found in violation of the federal CSA, his or her license may be revoked, and he or she may be incarcerated in a federal prison.

## DRUG LAWS

### The Food, Drug, and Cosmetic Act of 1938

A major piece of federal legislation that regulates the pharmaceutical industry now is the Food, Drug, and Cosmetic Act (FDCA) of 1938 (http://www.fda.gov/RegulatoryInformation/Legislation/FederalFoodDrugandCosmeticActFDCAct/). It was enacted to protect the public's safety and was passed in response to a tragedy involving sulfanilamide (an antibiotic) and diethylene glycol (commonly used in antifreeze). A pharmaceutical company desired to make an elixir of the antibiotic and discovered that sulfanilamide easily dissolved in the diethylene glycol. The product was never tested for toxicity before marketing. One hundred and seven deaths were caused by the drug. Thus, the FDCA of 1938 was passed to set guidelines for the definition of a drug or a cosmetic and to establish methods to determine their safety.

Presently a drug is defined as the following:

1. Articles recognized in the official United States Pharmacopoeia, official Homeopathic Pharmacopoeia of the United States, or official National Formulary.
2. Articles intended for use in the diagnosis, cure, mitigation, treatment, or prevention of disease in man or other animals.
3. Articles (other than food) intended to affect the structure or any function of the body of man or other animal.

**4.** Articles intended for use as components of any articles specified in Clause A, B, or C, FDCA §201(g)(1), 21 U.S.C. §321(g)(1). (Chap. 21 of the Code of Federal Regulation[1] may be accessed through the FDA web site, www.fda.gov).

Certain medications, because of their physical and/or psychological addictive nature, are classified as controlled substances. This means that the prescribing, acquisition, dispensing, and inventorying of these medications is more tightly controlled than other medications. The definition, prescribing, acquisition, dispensing, and inventorying of these medications are outlined in the CSA. The CSA defines the controlled substances in the following schedules:

**Schedule I:** High potential for abuse; no currently accepted medical use in treatment in the United States; lack of accepted information on the safety of their use, even under medical supervision (21 C.F.R. §1300.11). Examples include heroin, marijuana, peyote, mescaline, and dihydromorphine.

**Schedule II:** High potential for abuse; does have a currently accepted medical use in treatment in the United States or a currently accepted medical use with severe restrictions; abuse of the drug or other substance may lead to severe physical or psychological dependence (21 C.F.R. §1300.12). Examples include cocaine, morphine, meperidine, codeine, and methadone.

**Schedule III:** The drug has a potential for abuse less than that of the drugs or other substances in schedules I and II; does have a currently accepted medical use in treatment in the United States; abuse of the drug or other substance may lead to moderate physical or psychological dependence (21 C.F.R. §1300.13). Examples include acetaminophen with codeine, anabolic steroids, and paregoric.

**Schedule IV:** The drug has a low potential for abuse relative to the drugs or other substances in schedule III; does have a currently accepted medical use in treatment in the United States; abuse of the drug or other substance may lead to limited physical or psychological dependence relative to the drugs or other substances in schedule III (21 C.F.R. §1300.14). Examples include diazepam, chloral hydrate, phenobarbital, and diethylpropion.

**Schedule V:** The drug has a low potential for abuse relative to the drugs or other substances in schedule IV; does have a currently accepted medical use in treatment in the United States; abuse of the drug or other substance may lead to limited physical or psychological dependence relative to the drugs or other substances in schedule IV (21 C.F.R. §1300.15). A schedule V drug cannot contain more than 200 mg of codeine per 100 mL or 100 g, 100 mg of dihydrocodeine per 100 mL or 100 g.

## Poison Prevention Packaging Act

Another requirement that governs the practice of pharmacy is that a pharmacist must dispense prescriptions according to the Poison Prevention Packaging Act (PPPA) (16 C.F.R. §1700) (http://www.cpsc.gov/Regulations-Laws--Standards/Statutes/Poison-Prevention-Packaging-Act/). This law requires that prescriptions

---

**TABLE 7.1.** PARTIAL LIST OF PRODUCTS SUBJECT TO THE POISON PREVENTION PACKAGING ACT (16 C.F.R. §1700.14)

- Oral prescription drugs (exemptions noted in Table 7.2)
- Controlled substances in dosage forms intended for oral human administration
- Liquid preparations containing more than 5% by weight of methyl salicylate
- Oral aspirin preparations containing more than 5% by weight of methyl salicylate
- Oral aspirin preparations (exemptions noted in Table 7.2)
- All drugs and dietary supplements that provide iron for therapeutic or prophylactic purposes and contain a total amount of elemental iron from any source in a single package that is equivalent to 250 mg or more elemental iron in a concentration of 0.025% or more w/v, and 0.05% or more on w/w for nonliquids
- Oral dosage form of acetaminophen in containers holding more than 1 g
- Ibuprofen in oral dosage forms containing 1 g or more of the drug in a single package
- Diphenhydramine HCl in oral dosage forms containing more than the equivalent of 66 mg of the diphenhydramine base in a single package
- Loperamide in oral dosage forms containing more than 0.045 mg of the drug in a single package
- Mouthwash preparations for human use containing 3 g or more of ethanol in a single package

---

be dispensed in child-resistant closures. A child-resistant container is defined as a container that 80% of children less than 5 years of age cannot open and 90% of adults can. Table 7.1 lists the products that are subject to the PPPA. Because the containers can lose their integrity with use, a new container must be used each time a prescription is filled, whether it is new or a refill.

Patients or their physicians may orally or in writing request that a prescription be dispensed in non-child-resistant containers. To protect themselves from liability, if the request is oral, a pharmacist should document this request in writing with the patient signing a statement to the effect:

I, ___(patient's signature)___, request that my prescription be dispensed in a non-child-resistant container.

This statement should be stamped on the back of each prescription, and the patient should sign each time. Alternatively, a comprehensive blanket statement requesting non-child-resistant containers signed one time by the patient and kept on file is acceptable. If the patient's physician makes the requests, it must be on a per-prescription basis.

Products that are exempt from the PPPA are listed in Table 7.2.

---

**TABLE 7.2.** PARTIAL LIST OF PRODUCTS EXEMPT OF THE POISON PREVENTION PACKAGING ACT [16 C.F.R. §1700.14(A)(10)]

- Sublingual dosage forms of nitroglycerin
- Sublingual and chewable forms of isosorbide dinitrate in strengths of 10 mg or less
- Anhydrous cholestyramine in powder form
- Sodium fluoride products containing not more than 264 mg of sodium fluoride per package
- Methylprednisolone tablets containing not more than 84 mg of the drug per package
- Mebendazole tablets containing not more than 600 mg of the drug per package
- Betamethasone tablets containing not more than 12.6 mg of the drug per package
- Potassium supplements in unit dose forms, including effervescent tablets, unit dose vials of liquid potassium, and powdered potassium in unit dose packets containing not more than 50 mEq per unit dose
- Erythromycin ethylsuccinate granules for oral suspension and oral suspensions in packages containing not more than 8 g of the equivalent erythromycin
- Pancrelipase preparations
- Preparations in aerosol containers intended for inhalation therapy
- Colestipol in powder form up to 5 g in a packet
- Prednisone tablets not containing more than 105 mg per package
- Cyclically administered oral contraceptives, conjugated estrogens, and norethindrone acetate tablets in manufacturer's mnemonic dispenser packages
- Medroxyprogesterone acetate tablets

---

## Omnibus Budget Reconciliation Act of 1990

When dispensing the prescription, the pharmacist must follow a law that was part of the Omnibus Budget Reconciliation Act of 1990 (OBRA 1990) (P.L. 101-508). The law requires each state that provides Medicaid benefits to establish pharmacy requirements. However, that would create two levels of care for residents of the state. Because of legal and/or ethical standards, most states will not allow that to happen. Therefore, what applies to the Medicaid patient must apply to all citizens of the state.

One requirement under this act is that the state must perform a retrospective drug utilization review (DUR). To complete this, the state must establish a panel to review medication use to determine that the medication prescribed is therapeutically appropriate and medically necessary and compare the treatment to predetermined standards. They must also look for adverse drug results and monitor for potential abuse. The state must also watch for underutilization and overutilization and be vigilant for any fraud that may be taking place. If it is determined by the panel that there is a problem in any of these areas, an "educational process" for the prescriber or pharmacist is implemented to address and correct the situation.

A second requirement is that pharmacists perform prospective DUR in which he or she is to monitor for:

Drug-drug interactions
Therapeutic duplications
Adverse drug-drug interactions
Incorrect dosages
Incorrect duration
Drug-allergy interactions
Clinical abuse/misuse
Drug-food interactions

In order to perform the prospective DUR, the pharmacist must have certain information and is required to make a reasonable effort to obtain a medical history on patients. The minimal information that should be obtained from the history includes name, address, telephone number, date of birth, gender; individual history, including disease state(s), known allergies, and drug reactions; and a comprehensive list of medications and relevant devices.

The pharmacist must also (depending on the state) make an offer to council patients who are having prescriptions filled or answer any questions that the patient may have. Depending on the state, the pharmacist's offer to council may need to be extended on both new and refill prescriptions. The minimal requirements for counseling must include:

• Name and description of the medication
• Dosage, dosage form, route of administration, and duration of drug therapy
• Special directions and precautions for preparation, administration, and use by the patient
• Common severe side effects, or interactions and therapeutic contraindications that may be encountered, including ways to prevent them and the action required if they do occur
• Techniques for self-monitoring of drug therapy
• Actions to be taken in case of a missed dose

Each state is required to establish its own statutes pertaining to OBRA 1990, and they vary considerably across the country. A pharmacist must become familiar with his state's requirements before dispensing prescriptions. With the enactment of OBRA 1990, the state boards and courts are determining that pharmacists are responsible for patient education and are accountable for counseling.

OBRA 1990 implicates the pharmacist in risk management. The pharmacist must help the patient manage the drug therapy that has been prescribed by the practitioner.

The practitioner performs a risk assessment in deciding which treatment is the best for the patient. He will compare the risk versus the benefits for the patient and decide on an approved drug therapy. The pharmacist must then assist the patient in managing aspects of the therapy. This includes side effects or indications that the treatment is not working. The courts are increasingly recognizing the pharmacist's responsibility in risk management by upholding OBRA 1990 requirements.

## 2007 FDA Amendment Act

This legislation will have the greatest impact on pharmacy for the next 10 years. FDA Amendment Act (FDAAA, http://www.fda.gov/RegulatoryInformation/Legislation/FederalFoodDrugandCosmeticActFDCAct/SignificantAmendmentstotheFDCAct/FoodandDrugAdministrationAmendmentsActof2007/default.htm) is the name for legislation that adds many new provisions to the FDCA. In addition, the Prescription Drug User Fee Act (PDUFA) and the Medical Device User Fee and Modernization Act (MDUFMA) have been reauthorized and expanded. This amendment provides the FDA with authority to really evaluate and focus on drug safety as a priority. Yes, drugs will still need to show that they are efficacious, but this now provides a much greater emphasis on protecting the public from unwanted side effects. As with other amendments, changes in the medical environment have stimulated the need for this additional protection. Since 2001, the world has had patients experience serious postmarketing adverse events such as drug-induced stroke, cardiovascular disease, and death. This increase in morbidity and mortality was the driving force behind the approval of this act. The law also provides for the creation of the Reagen-Udall Foundation to modernize product development, accelerate innovation, and enhance product safety. It also provides for additional requirements for food safety as well as drug safety. The FDAAA also provides for provisions for better clinical trial registries. In addition, the act includes the Best Pharmaceuticals for Children Act (BPCA), which encourages more studies in children and promotes the development of treatments for children. Likewise, it also includes the *Pediatric Research Equity Act (PREA)*, which continues the FDA's authority to require studies in children concerning certain medical products and under other specific circumstances.


## THE PRESCRIPTION

### The Practitioner

A practitioner is the person who is legally entitled to prescribe medications as determined by each state. It is the state and not the federal government that determines who is entitled to prescribe medication. The states then generally require that the practitioner be licensed and/or registered in that state. This is usually accomplished by having the practitioner pass a competency exam, which evaluates his or her knowledge of the diagnosis and treatment of diseases. Examples of practitioners are allopathic physicians, osteopathic physicians, dentists, veterinarians, and nurse practitioners. Veterinarians are allowed to prescribe only for animals. Nurse practitioners may be allowed to prescribe only under certain protocols or limited to a particular formulary. In the ambulatory setting, the practitioner then writes a prescription for the patient to have filled at a community pharmacy. This does not apply in a hospital or institutional setting, where the patient's chart serves as the medication order record.

Another area that pharmacists must consider when filling a prescription is the scope of practice of each practitioner. Practitioners are generally allowed to prescribe only in their area of expertise. An example of this is a surgeon prescribing analgesic medications and antibiotics. This is within the scope of practice of a surgeon: his patients may need analgesics for any pain they may be suffering, and antibiotics to prevent or treat infection. On the other hand, a dentist prescribing birth control pills will generally be considered beyond the scope of practice. The pharmacist can and should refuse to fill the prescription until he or she has contacted the dentist. In some cases, a pharmacist must use his or her professional judgment when making a decision about the scope of practice. If there is a question, the pharmacist should contact the practitioner to determine if the prescribed medication may be for a new indication.

## Presentation of the Prescription to the Pharmacy

Nonscheduled and schedule III, IV, and V prescriptions may be presented in the pharmacy either by the patient or her agent, or it may be telephoned or faxed to the pharmacy by the practitioner or his agent (21 C.F.R. §1306.21). Schedule II prescriptions must be physically presented to the pharmacy unless it is an emergency. The DEA defines an emergency as:

Immediate administration of the controlled substance is necessary for the proper treatment of the patient.
No appropriate alternative treatment is available.
It is not reasonably possible for the prescribing physician to provide a written prescription to the pharmacist before dispensing (21 C.F.R. §290.10).

If the situation is deemed to be an emergency:

The quantity prescribed and dispensed is limited to the amount necessary to treat the patient for the emergency period.
The prescription must be immediately reduced to writing by the pharmacist and shall contain all required information except the signature of the prescriber. If the prescriber is not known to the pharmacist, the pharmacist must make a reasonable, good-faith effort to determine that the oral authorization came from a registered individual practitioner. This reasonable effort could include a call back to the prescriber using the telephone number in the telephone directory rather than the number given by the prescriber over the telephone.

Within 7 days after authorizing an emergency oral prescription, the prescriber must deliver to the dispensing pharmacist a written prescription for the emergency quantity prescribed. The prescription must have written on its face "Authorization for Emergency Dispensing" and the date of the oral order. The written prescription may be delivered to the pharmacist in person or by mail. If delivered by mail, it must be postmarked within the 7-day period. On receipt, the dispensing pharmacist shall attach this prescription to the oral emergency prescription previously reduced to writing. If the prescriber fails to deliver the written prescription within the 7-day period, the pharmacist must notify the nearest office of the DEA. Failure of the pharmacist to do so will void the prescription [21 C.F.R. §1306.11(d)].

Also, in general, schedule II prescriptions cannot be faxed to pharmacies; all schedule II prescriptions must be dispensed pursuant to an original signed prescription. The schedule prescription may be faxed to a pharmacy, but the original must be received before the medication can be dispensed. There are three situations in which a faxed schedule II prescription may be used as the original:

1. If the prescription is faxed by the practitioner or practitioner's agent to a pharmacy and is for a narcotic schedule II substance to be compounded for the direct administration to a patient by parenteral, intravenous, intramuscular, subcutaneous, or intraspinal infusion [21 C.F.R. §1306.11(e)].
2. If the prescription faxed by the practitioner or practitioner's agent is for a schedule II narcotic substance for a resident of a long-term care facility (LTCF) [21 C.F.R. §1306.11(f)].
3. If the prescription faxed by the practitioner or practitioner's agent is for a schedule II narcotic substance for a patient residing in a hospice certified by Medicare under Title XVIII or licensed by the state, the practitioner or agent must note on the prescription that the patient is a hospice patient [21 C.F.R. §1306.11(g)].

## Legitimacy

A prescription is generated for a patient, who is in need of medical attention and seeks out a practitioner who determines that the patient needs to have medication, thus creating the patient-practitioner relationship. A prescription must be generated from a valid patient-practitioner relationship. This patient-practitioner relationship must be established so that a prescription is generated for a legitimate medical condition. If it is not a legitimate medical condition, then the prescription is not valid and cannot be filled [21 C.F.R. §1306.04 (a)]. It is the pharmacist's professional judgment to try to determine if the prescription is valid. The DEA has a suggested list of questions for pharmacist to help him or her determine the legitimacy of a prescription.

1. Does the prescriber write significantly larger numbers of prescriptions orders (or in larger quantities) than other practitioners in your area?
2. Does the prescriber write for antagonistic drugs, such as depressants and stimulants, at the same time? Drug abusers often request prescription orders for "ups" and "downs" at the same time.
3. Do patients appear to be returning too frequently? In numerous cases drug abusers have been found to have been receiving prescription orders that ought to have lasted for a month in legitimate use, on a biweekly, weekly, or even a daily basis.
4. Do patients appear presenting prescription orders written in the names of other people?
5. Do a number of people appear simultaneously, or within a short time, all bearing similar prescription orders from the same practitioner?
6. Are numerous "strangers," people who are not regular patrons or residents of community, suddenly showing up with prescription orders from the same physician? Typically, you will find that these individuals are in the 18- to 25-year-old age group, although drug abuse does not necessarily end with the achievement of chronological maturity.
7. Are your purchases of controlled substances rising dramatically? If so, it is time to look at your prescription counter policies. Drug abusers may have found a "vendor" who dispenses prescription orders mechanically, without using professional judgment (Pharmacist's Manual, pp. 30–31).[2]

These are some of the questions that a pharmacist must ask himself or herself when trying to determine if a prescription is legitimate, and she will have to rely on her professional judgment when presented with a questionable situation.

### Information That Must Be Present on the Prescription

The prescription paper must contain certain information, depending on whether it is a controlled substance or a noncontrolled medication. An example of a prescription is depicted in Figure 7.1. A prescription for a noncontrolled substance must contain the following information: (1) patient's name, (2) date on which the prescription was written, (3) name of the medication, (4) dosage form, (5) strength of the medication, (6) quantity to dispense, (7) directions for use, (8) number of refills, and (9) practitioner's signature in ink or indelible pencil. If the prescription is for a controlled substance (see below), it also requires (10) the patient's address, (11) the practitioner's address, and (12) DEA registration number [21 C.F.R. §1306.05 (a)].

The DEA registration number is a number issued to a practitioner to identify persons authorized by the state and Drug Enforcement Agency to prescribe controlled substances. It consists of nine characters; the first two are letters, and the next seven are numbers. Originally, the first letter was A and the second letter was the first letter of the registrants last name. For example, Dr. Margaret Brown's number

**Figure 7.1.** Prescription information.

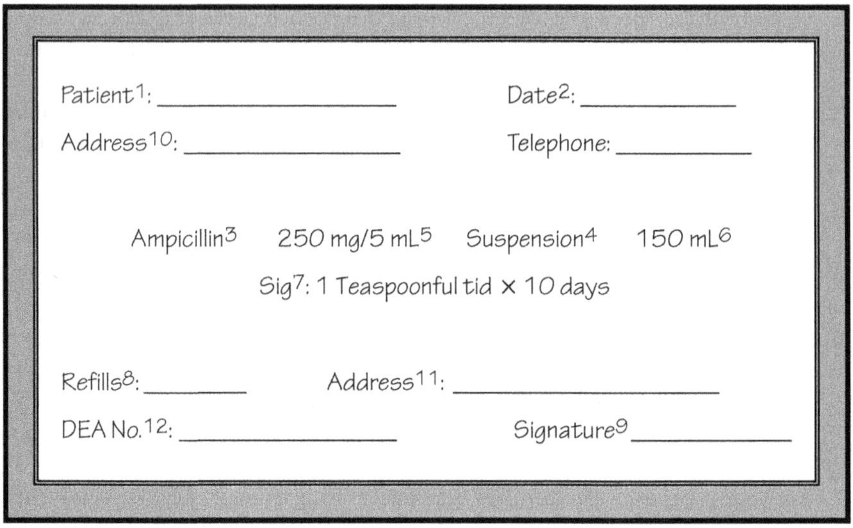

Patient[1]: _____          Date[2]: _____

Address[10]: _____          Telephone: _____

Ampicillin[3]     250 mg/5 mL[5]     Suspension[4]     150 mL[6]

Sig[7]: 1 Teaspoonful tid × 10 days

Refills[8]: _____          Address[11]: _____

DEA No.[12]: _____          Signature[9] _____

begins with the characters AB. Subsequently, the DEA has used all the available A numbers and has started using the Bs, and it is assumed that they will continue with the Cs when necessary. The second character may be a number if the registrant is registered as a business and the business's name begins with a number. The second group of characters consists of a set of numbers that are unique to each registrant. The last digit is a check number that can be validated by performing three steps:

1. Add the first, third, and fifth digits.
2. Sum the second, fourth, and sixth digits, multiply this sum by 2, and add the results to the first sum.
3. The last digit of the sum should correspond to the ninth character of the DEA number.

As an example, check the DEA number for Dr. Natasha Jones, DEA registration number AJ 1234563:

1. Add the first, third, and fifth digits: $1 + 3 + 5 = 9$.
2. Sum the second, fourth, and sixth digits, then multiply by 2: $(2 + 4 + 6) \times 2 = 24$.
3. Next, sum the two results: $9 + 24 = 33$.

Compare the last digit of step 3 with the last digit of the DEA registration number; because they match, it is an indication that the prescription may be from a legitimate practitioner. Individuals who are attempting to obtain controlled substances by forged prescriptions often know this validation check, so it is not an absolute guarantee.

## Medications

There are two types of medications to be considered, the type that needs to be prescribed and the type that the person can purchase over the counter (OTC). The 1951 Durham-Humphrey amendment (§503:21 U.S.C. §3 53) to the 1938 Food Drug and Cosmetic Act created these two categories of drugs. This amendment created what is referred to as "legend" drugs by requiring the statement "Caution: Federal law prohibits dispensing without a prescription." [Recently changed to "Rx only" U.S.C. 21 §353 (4) (a).] Legend medications can be dispensed only via a prescription, and the practitioner must authorize refills of the prescription. OTC medications do not require a prescription to be purchased. These medications are proven able to be used safely by patients without a prescription and are often sold in nonpharmacy settings such as grocery or mass merchandising stores.

## Drug Product Selection

State law may allow a pharmacist to select drug products and dispense a generic medication that is bioequivalent to a brand name product. There is no federal law that governs this arena; it is left to the state to determine if pharmacists are allowed to perform this activity. The federal government (FDA) does provide some guidance for the pharmacist in making the decision of what is bioequivalent by publishing the *Approved Drug Products with Therapeutic Equivalence Evaluations.*[3] This book rates the bioequivalence of drugs. Bioequivalence is defined as the rate and extent of absorption of a test drug as compared to the rate and extent of absorption of a reference drug, when administered at the same molar dose of the therapeutic ingredient under similar experimental conditions in either a single or multiple dose (*Approved Drug Products with Therapeutic Equivalence Evaluations,* 20th ed., p. ix)[3] of all FDA-approved generic products against the brand name product. Products are given a rating that consists of two letters, the first of which can be either A or B. If the rating is an A designation, the product is considered therapeutically equivalent to the brand name product. If the rating is a B designation, the product is considered not to be bioequivalent, or the product has not been tested against the brand name product. The second letter designates the dosage form of the product; examples include the following:

AA: Drugs that are available in conventional dosage forms and have no bioequivalence problems.

AB: Drugs meeting necessary bioequivalence requirements.

BC: Drugs in extended-release dosage forms with bioequivalence issues.

BP: Active ingredients and dosage forms with potential bioequivalence problems.

B: Drugs for which no determination of therapeutic equivalence will be made until certain questions have been resolved.

## Refills

The number of refills or length of time the prescription is valid is legislated by the states. The number of refills will be limited by federal law, depending on whether the medication is a controlled substance. If it is a schedule III, IV, or V drug (21 C.F.R. §1306.22), it can only be refilled a maximum of five times in a 6-month period from the day it was written, if so indicated by the practitioner. A schedule II medication cannot be refilled under any conditions (21 C.F.R. §1306.12).

Although schedule II prescriptions cannot be refilled, and the total amount is to be dispensed at the time it is presented at the pharmacy, there are certain circumstances when the prescription may have to be partially filled. For example, when the pharmacist is presented a prescription for 60 meperidine tablets and he or she has only 30 on hand, what is the proper procedure? It is permissible to supply the quantity that the pharmacy has available and then fill the balance within 72 hours [21 C.F.R. §1306.13(a)]. If the balance of the prescription cannot be filled within the 72-hour period, the pharmacist is to notify the prescriber and, if needed, have the patient obtain a new prescription. The pharmacist is not allowed to supply any more from the first prescription. There are two other situations where partial filling of a schedule II prescription is allowed, and that is for patients in LTCFs or patients with a documented terminal illness. Then individual dosage units may be dispensed, however, only up to a 60-day supply from the date of issuance [21 C.F.R. §1306.13(b)], and no partial fillings can exceed the original quantity prescribed. The pharmacist must document that the patient is either terminally ill or an LTCF patient, and it must be recorded on the prescription. If it is not recorded, the pharmacist is considered to be in violation of the CSA.

## Labeling of the Prescription Vial

The label of the prescription vial must contain certain information according to the Federal Law. The information to be included on the label is the pharmacy's name and address, serial number or prescription number, date the prescription is written or dispensed, prescriber's name, and, if stated in the prescription, the patient's name, directions for use, and cautionary statements, if any. State law may require other additional information to be on the label. That added information may include the drug name, strength and quantity, expiration date, and pharmacy's telephone number. The labeling requirements apply only to prescriptions dispensed in a community setting; they do not apply to medications dispensed to an institutionalized patient [21 U.S.C. §356 (b)(2)].

## Medication Therapy Management

In 2003, the US Congress passed the Medicare Modernization Act (http://www.gpo.gov/fdsys/pkg/BILLS-108hr1enr/pdf/BILLS-108hr1enr.pdf) which requires each

Part D sponsor to provide a medication therapy management program (MTMP) to patients participating in the program. The requirements are outlined in Title 42 section § 423.153 of the Code of Federal Regulations.[4] Medication Therapy Management (MTM) is defined as the "systematic process of collecting patient-specific information, assessing medication therapies to identify medication-related problems, developing a prioritized list of medication-related problems, and creating a plan to resolve them."[5]

The goals of MTM are to optimize the medication therapy for targeted patients in the program. This includes the reduction of risk and risk management of the treatment that is prescribed.

The requirements specify that the program must aim at the patients who are enrolled in Medicare Part D who have multiple chronic diseases (examples would be diabetes, arthritis, hypertension, dyslipidemia); are taking multiple medications covered by Part D; and will prospectively exceed the predetermined annual costs for covered medications. The legislation also requires that the provider establish a quality assurance program that is aimed at reducing the number medication errors and adverse drug interactions while also improving medication usage by[4]:

   i. Screening for potential drug therapy problems due to therapeutic duplication.
   ii. Age/gender-related contraindications.
   iii. Overutilization and underutilization.
   iv. Drug-drug interaction.
   v. Incorrect drug dosage or duration of drug therapy.
   vi. Drug-allergy contraindications.
   vii. Clinical abuse/misuse.

The program will also include a retrospective DUR system, policies and procedures intended to "identify patterns of inappropriate or medically unnecessary care among enrollees in a sponsor's Part D plan, or associated with specific drugs or groups of drugs" [42 § 423.153 (B)(c)(3)]. The legislation requires a comprehensive medication review with written summary that should be a person to person interactive process performed by a pharmacist or other qualified provider which may result in a recommendation on a medication action plan. This review would also include at least quarterly follow-up interventions when necessary. Targeted patients[6] must also have their MTM coordinated with a care management plan for individuals under chronic care improvement program (CCIP) with the drug utilization claims. Targeted patients include members with diabetes, hypertension with comorbid obesity and/or coronary artery disease, or congestive heart failure.[6]

## SUMMARY

The pharmacist may be held criminally and/or civilly liable if any laws are violated and harm comes to a patient. The physician who prescribes the medicine must perform risk assessment on the patient to determine the best course of treatment for the particular disease. The physician will perform a risk versus benefit analysis on all possible treatment for a patient and determine which is the best for the patient. As long as the treatment that the physician decides on is an accepted medical treatment, he is generally safe from civil liability. The pharmacist, on the other hand, must perform risk management. The pharmacist must help the patient manage the risk of the treatment. For example, if the treatment requires a medication that may cause drowsiness, the pharmacist needs to council the patient about this possibility and ways to control it or to avoid situations that may cause harm. In this way, the pharmacist is helping the patient manage the risk of this treatment.

So far, this chapter has covered the functions of the FDA and DEA agencies and the federal rules and regulations for filling prescriptions. You should now work to learn more about the rules and regulations upheld by these federal agencies. The federal laws discussed here are only a portion of the information you need to practice pharmacy, but they are a good start for your early career. As you advance through the pharmacy program, each piece of information you learn about the laws regulating the practice of pharmacy will add to the basic premises discussed in this chapter. Filling a prescription requires more than putting the right drug in the right bottle. As a pharmacy student/intern you must practice according to the law now, so that when you alone are responsible, you will be able to make the right decisions.

## POLITICAL ADVOCACY

In addition to providing patients with the best care possible, pharmacists can have an impact on patients by becoming involved in political advocacy. Political advocacy is defined as; the act of pleading or arguing a case or a position; forceful persuasion.[7] Political advocacy can also help the profession of pharmacy itself evolve and flourish. With the rapid restructuring of health care in the twenty first century and pharmacy in particular, the need for increased grassroots involvement in political action becomes increasingly important. If pharmacists are to succeed in enhancing their position as valued professionals in the health-care system, they must understand and participate in the political process. It is critical to inform our policy makers in government, both state and federal, on what pharmacists do as well as what we are capable of doing to improve the health care and quality of life of our patients.

The best pharmacy legislation will never occur without perceptive, knowledgeable, persistent, and creative champions of pharmacy. The best way to achieve these goals is to equip pharmacists with the tools they need to make a difference. These tools include identifying representatives that tend to be supportive of pharmacy issues, recognizing the need for and the process of building coalitions within and outside of the health-care profession, and developing appropriate talking points.

One of the critical first steps in advocacy is developing relationships with legislators, persons in government agencies and influential individuals before you need anything from them. This can be accomplished by working on campaigns, donating monies and attending political events. After this relationship has been solidified, you can make yourself available and become a resource on pharmaceutical care. Also volunteering to work on legislation; testifying before committees, and developing coalitions. Always keep in mind that the improving patients' lives is the primary goal. This will lead to a position of trust between pharmacists, legislators, agency executives, and other influential people in your state.

There are several goals for pharmacists serving as advocates. First, pharmacists can better serve their patients by enhancing the conditions in which they practice. Advocacy can also help to ensure the survival of the profession, and guarantee that the pharmacist's role is not usurped by others. The pharmacist's position as a valued professional functioning as an integral part of the new health-care system can be enhanced. Advocacy can play a major role in determining the profession's future and can expand the profession through changes in the pharmacy practice act. Finally, pharmacists can be adequately recognized and compensated as a health care provider.

To identify legislative issues, pharmacists can look to their own practice settings as a source of information. Watch for the way the laws affecting pharmacy practice are followed in your practice setting. Is patient care suffering because of the way a law is written? Are there things a pharmacist legally cannot do that they should be doing to improve patient care? If so, once more information is gathered, it may be time to begin advocating for a change. Additional sources include other health-care providers and their respective associations, both state and national pharmacy associations, state boards of pharmacy (a list with links to State Boards of Pharmacy can be found on the National Association of Boards of Pharmacy (NABP) web site at http://www.nabp.net/boards-of-pharmacy), Colleges of Pharmacy (see the American Association of Colleges of Pharmacy School Locator at http://www. aacp.org/resources/student/pages/schoollocator.aspx), patients, manufacturers (see DrugInfo.net at http://www.druginfonet.com/manufacturers.htm for manufacturer contact information), government agencies and both state and federal legislators (find contact information at http://www.usa.gov/Contact/Elected.shtml). These sources can help identify issues that go beyond the scope of one pharmacy practice. Once an issue has been identified, learning more about it is imperative. Sources of information include pharmacy association web sites (see http://www.pharmacy. org/association.html for a comprehensive list of pharmacy associations), pharmacy journals and magazines (http://www.pharmacy.org/journal.html), state and federal government web sites, private political web sites and the news media.

## Understanding Politics

A review of the legislative process can be found elsewhere (http://www.whitehouse. gov/our-government/legislative-branch). In state governments power is concentrated in the hands of the Governor, the leader of each house and key committee chairpersons. Most action happens only with the consent of the leadership. At different stages of the process, in trying to influence the outcome, the pharmacist will need to contact the sponsor of the bill, the committee chairperson, Assembly/House Speaker, Senate Majority/President, staff members, Governor's counsel, agency director, etc. Introduce yourself to members of the committee with jurisdiction over the bill, staff members, and other legislators who may share or be persuaded to your point of view. The better informed the legislators are, about your position on the issue the greater the chance of passing the legislation you desire. Interest groups exert tremendous power over "their" issues by providing in-depth knowledge. Knowing the origin of legislation assists you in determining the strategy needed to change or defeat it.

## The Art of Advocacy: Important Points for Influencing Legislation

- Know your issue. Be prepared by knowing the facts. Do your homework and know where legislators, their constituencies, and special interest groups stand on issues.
- Be honest and accurate. Those are essential points when building the foundation for a relationship. Do not let your emotional involvement in the issue cloud your facts.
- Plan for contact. A face to face meeting is preferable. Make an appointment. You may want to bring 2-3 allies (no more) with you.
- Be businesslike. You set the tone of the meeting. Limit issues and focus on your goal.
- Be friendly and have your opener planned. Be brief. Know pertinent information including the bill number, title, and description. Be courteous and maintain confidentiality.
- Identify the opposition. Do not argue. Try to avoid a completely negative response.
- Leave an opportunity for you to return another time. You do not want to lose a good working relationship.
- Listen carefully. You can glean much information from what your legislator tells you about your issue.
- Be positive. Do not speak in negative terms. If you do not have an answer to a question, say so and offer to find the answer. If you promise to follow up, keep your promise.
- Thank the legislator for meeting with you. Thank legislators for their support once you have gained it.

If the meeting does not go as well as you would have liked, do not be discouraged. Persistency is important because this communicates how important the issue is to you and therefore it should be important to the legislature. Getting to know the legislator's staff and building a relationship with them is important because you may not always be able to speak with the legislature but their staff can relay important information. You can join forces with other like-minded people (coalition building). Maintain a good working relationship with the legislator. Remain on friendly terms. Write a note of thanks. Your adversary today may be your best advocate tomorrow.

When communicating via telephone, there are a few additional ways to have a positive effect. As with a face-to-face meeting, be prepared. Have pertinent information written down: your positions, bill number, title, description, etc. Place a call at crucial time for issue, for example, before a key vote. Address the legislator appropriately (congressman, congresswoman, senator, representative). Present your position briefly. Identify yourself and where you live (constituency is very important). Present one issue per call. Be factual and honest. Use your own words. Mention how the issue will affect their district or community—their constituents. Ask for their views. Try to ascertain their position and how they will vote. Keep the tone of the conversation friendly. End the conversation politely. Thank the legislator and offer to send information on your issue. If you cannot reach your legislator, do not refuse to speak with a staff person. You may gain useful information and find a helpful source for future reference.

When you e-mail your legislator, address the legislator appropriately. Keep it short and to the point. Let the legislator know what you expect. Only discuss one issue per e-mail. Outline essential information including the bill number, title and description. Use your own words. Describe personal experiences and local impact. Be sure to include your name, address, and telephone number. Include links when appropriate.

## Summary

Be persistent. Don't give up! When your cause is worthy, it is worth the extra effort and the wait. Be positive. Don't contact your legislators just to complain or push an issue. Let them know you support them when they have done a good job. Be polite: say "thank you." Be a part of the process. Don't stop with one issue. Keep an ongoing dialogue with your legislators. Keep working for the betterment of your patients and your profession. After all, as Yogi Berra said, "It's not over till it's over!"

Build relationships and coalitions. Work in conjunction with administration, agencies, and state boards. Know your advocates and adversaries (individuals and groups). Know the background of legislators/representatives. Know the impact of legislation (professional, financial, social).

By learning some tools, you will feel confident that you can make a difference! Create politically astute grassroots healthcare advocates. Use coalition building. Understand the necessity for joining professional associations. It is necessary for pharmacy to speak with one voice.

The three most important things in politics are money, money and money (time in kind is money). Three rules for the betterment of patients, the pharmacy profession and the future. Be an active participant in the political process. Strengthen our associations through membership and active participation. Vote! Encourage others to vote as well. Voter registration is essential.

"We have a very competitive special-interest democracy today. If you fail to speak up or take action (advocacy), you leave it to others to do so. Democracy only works if you play the game." Rick Miller, VP Michael B. Dunn and Associates, spoken at a workshop sponsored by the NCPA Political Action Committee and the NCPA Legislative Defense Fund.

## Anecdotes

In one case, due to fraud and abuse of schedule II medications, legislation was enacted in New Jersey that had an unanticipated negative consequence for patients in long-term care facilities and hospice. According to the new state requirements, physicians were required to provide schedule II prescriptions on a new, official prescription blank that was now required in a timely manner to satisfy the statute (law). However, most physicians only see these patients once a month. This resulted in patients not being able to receive the appropriate medication and dosage to control their pain. In order to adhere to the law, physicians started to prescribe schedule III medications as an alternative. As a result, many patients experienced uncontrolled pain. Since no pharmacists including members of the State Board of Pharmacy were asked for their comments, the resulting unforeseen consequence of this legislation was not allowing residents in long-term care facilities and hospice patients to receive the proper pain management medications in a timely manner.

It was clear this legislation had to be amended. After informing the legislator of the situation, she agreed to work on an amendment. The amendment was passed, and the patients in need were once again able to receive their proper pain medication in a timely manner.

In another situation, millions of dollars of perfectly good repackaged solid dosage form medications were unnecessarily being destroyed due to state regulations and USP (The United States Pharmacopeia) guidelines which mandated the medications' disposal. This not only negatively impacted patients, but all tax payers as well, so an investigation into the rationale behind these regulations and guidelines was initiated. At one time, the beyond use dating (expiration date) guidelines made sense due to environmental conditions. However, those conditions were no longer valid.

New technologies and environmental controls ensure that the medications are safe for a longer period of time so it was time to advocate for a change. After doing some research, the individual at the FDA who actually wrote the original guidelines was identified. Not wanting to do anything that would adversely affect patients, a meeting was held with the gentleman and the concerns were raised. He was extremely cooperative and realized that there were valid arguments for change. Realizing himself that these guidelines should be addressed, he advised approaching the USP staff.

Individuals at the USP referred the issue to members on the working subcommittee for repackaging of solid dosage forms, with the main issue being beyond use dating. After attending meetings for two years and seeing no progress being made, another approach was needed. In the US Congress there are standing committees that have the responsibility of oversight over various governmental agencies, one of which is the FDA. The members of the working subcommittee were provided with the information regarding the great waste caused by the discarding of in date efficacious medications and the enormous waste of tax payer monies. The issue was then taken to the chairman of the Congressional Oversight Committee. After hearing this, the chair of our working subcommittee thought it would be prudent to invite the gentleman from the FDA who originally wrote the guidelines.

At the following meeting, the gentleman from the FDA was introduced by the committee chairman and immediately acknowledged hearing of this previously. After being questioned by the members of the committee, he explained the validity to change these guidelines. The committee reevaluated their opinion and voted to change the guidelines to more accurately reflect the new and improved environmental conditions which maintain the stability/shelf life of the medications. As a result of political advocacy, the guidelines were changed for the entire western hemisphere and billions of dollars are currently being saved.

These two examples prove that with knowledge of how the legislative system works and the desire to make a difference for patients and the pharmacy profession; you can do the same!

## APPLICATION EXERCISES

1. A patient enters your pharmacy and requests that her prescriptions be dispensed in containers with no lids. Is it legal to do this, and if not what could you as the pharmacist do?

2. A gentleman walks into your pharmacy and tells you he has a product that can cure the common cold and wants you to sell it in your pharmacy. Should you do this? Why or why not?

3. A patient brings a prescription for Tylox (a schedule II—controlled substance) into your pharmacy with just the patient's name, the medication's name, the quantity to dispense, and the prescriber's signature. What additional information do you need if any?

4. A new patient brings a prescription into your pharmacy. What types of information do you need to perform a prospective DUR?

5. Is informing a patient that a medication may cause drowsiness risk assessment or risk management, and why?

6. How does the FDA Amendment Act of 2007 differ from the previous legislation? What additional authority does it provide to the FDA?

7. A patient enters your pharmacy for their annual MTM comprehensive review, what type of personal medication information do you need to obtain?
8. Discuss political advocacy with pharmacists at various practice sites. Identify potential areas for improving legislation at each site.
9. After meeting with a legislator, she decides not to follow your recommendation in voting. What will your next steps be?

## ACKNOWLEDGMENT

The authors wish to acknowledge the contributions of Karen L. Kier and Ruth E. Nemire to this chapter.

## REFERENCES

1. *Code of Federal Regulations.* Washington DC: Office of the Federal Register, National Archives and Records Administration, US Government Printing Office; annual.
2. *Pharmacist's Manual: An Informational Outline of the Controlled Substance Act of 1970.* Washington DC: Drug Enforcement Agency; 1995.
3. Food and Drug Administration. *Approved Drug Products with Therapeutics Equivalence Evaluations.* Washington DC: Government Printing Office; 1979 and annual updates.
4. Available at http://www.ecfr.gov/cgi-bin/text-idx?tpl=/ecfrbrowse/Title42/42cfr423_main_02.tpl. Accessed March, 2014.
5. Medication Therapy Management in Pharmacy Practice: Core Elements of and MTM Service Model Version 2.0 March 2008 American Pharmacist Association.
6. Chronic Care Improvement Program (CCIP) Project Completion Report, Instructional Guide. Prepared by the Medicare Advantage Quality Review Organizations for the Centers for Medicare & Medicaid Services (CMS) September 2007.
7. Available at http://www.legal-dictionary.thefreedictionary.com/Political+advocacy. Accessed March, 2014.

## BIBLIOGRAPHY

Curtis JR, Rubenfeld GD. Improving palliative care for patients in the intensive care unit. *J Pall Med.* August 1, 2005;8(4):840–854. doi:10.1089/jpm.2005. 8.840.

Richard A. Mularski RA, Curtis JR, et al. Proposed quality measures for palliative care in the critically ill: a consensus from the Robert Wood Johnson Foundation Critical Care Workgroup. *Crit Care Med.* 2006;34(11):S404.

Wingfeld J, Bissell P, Anderson C. The scope of pharmacy ethics—an evaluation of the international research literature, 1990–2002. *Soc Sci Med.* 2004;58:2383–2396. doi.org/10.1016/j.socscimed.2003.09.003.

# Patient Care
# Tool Box

CHAPTER

8

# A Brief Look at the Construction of Medical Terminology and Common Definitions of Words That are Part of the Pharmacy Vernacular

*Ruth E. Nemire, Karen L. Kier*

**Objectives: Upon completion of the chapter and exercises, the student pharmacist will be able to**

1. Identify the four elements of a medical word.
2. Combine a prefix, root, and/or suffix to form a medical term.
3. Given a medical terminology word, analyze the meaning of the word by defining the prefix, root word, and suffix.
4. Identify words that are commonly used in pharmacy and medicine and have a basic understanding of why and how the profession uses these terms.

---

### Patient Encounter

This patient has urosepsis. This is the first time that you as a student have seen that terminology. Based on the information in the following chapter, what is urosepsis? Is it just a UTI?

The attending physician assigns the student pharmacist to educate the nursing staff about the causes of urosepsis, and treatment.

You have the following information.

Patients with structural or functional obstruction, as well as those with biomaterials or foreign bodies in the urinary tract, are at greater risk for urosepsis.

*(continued on next page)*

Goal-directed resuscitation should be initiated within the first 6 hours after a patient presents with urosepsis.

Adherence to sanitary measures, early removal of indwelling catheters, and preoperative culture-specific antibiotics are some ways to help prevent urosepsis.

Sepsis is characterized by at least two of the following findings:

Temperature less than 36°C or greater than 38°C

Heart rate greater than 90 beats per minute

Respiratory rate greater than 20 breaths per minute or a partial $CO_2$ pressure less than 32 mm Hg

White blood cell (WBC) count greater than 12,000/mm$^3$ or less than 4000/mm$^3$, or more than 10% immature neutrophils[2]

What terminology do you need to know to properly educate the nursing staff and student physicians on the team? What are the intricacies of understanding a disease state, once you know the terminology?

Source:
http://www.ncbi.nlm.nih.gov/pmc/articles/PMC2840933/

## INTRODUCTION

This chapter is included to assist you in understanding the medical terminology that you will be exposed to during classes and your experiences as a pharmacy student. As you start your introductory practice courses, you will be exposed to medical terminology as it pertains to disease states as well as words that are part of a medical vernacular that describes processes in medicine and pharmacy. Many of the medical words we use are derived from Greek and Latin languages. You do not have to speak either of these languages to understand the terminology spoken on a daily basis. Once you learn a few common root words, prefixes, and suffixes, you will be able to sound out a word for pronunciation and determine its meaning.

This chapter is not meant to be inclusive of all terms; it is included to help you begin to find your way around medical terminology. This manual contains two tables, one listing prefixes and root words with their meaning and one that names common suffixes. Following the tables is a list of words, many which are used in this textbook and some that are not. If you are looking for the meaning of a term, refer to the alphabetical list of terminology. If you do not find the word there, see if you can piece together the meaning from the word parts listed in the tables. Putting the words together yourself will help you remember the meaning later. In the beginning check a dictionary to make sure you are correct.

We suggest for in-depth study that you invest in a good medical terminology text, as it will include pictures and many exercises to aid in improving your vocabulary.

## WHAT IS IN A WORD?

Each medical term used has a *root* word. It establishes the basic meaning and is the part to which the prefix and/or suffix are added. You must be always mindful, for a root word can have more than one meaning in different fields of study. Not all roots are complete words; for example, *cardi* is a root word meaning heart. You will not use the word "cardi" alone, but, when combined with the suffix "logy," the word becomes *cardiology* and means the study of the heart. You might wonder why it is spelled with an extra letter "o"; it is to make the word easier to say. A vowel that is inserted between a root and a suffix to ease pronunciation is called a *combining vowel*. In many medical terms this is the letter "o." If you are trying to put word parts together and you can't say it, or it does not sound right, try adding an "o" or other vowel. The example of "cardi" and "logy" is a perfect use for the combining vowel.

A *prefix* is added to the beginning of a word to modify the meaning. For example, if you add the prefix "pre," meaning *before*, to the word surgical, you get presurgical, meaning before surgery.

You will find a list of prefixes and root words with combining vowels and examples of their use in Table 8.1.

The *suffix* is added at the end of the root word to modify the meaning or enhance the meaning. The suffix *itis* means inflammation. When added to the root word *arthr*, meaning joint, you form the word arthritis, meaning inflammation of the joint (Table 8.2).

With a little practice in identifying word parts and putting them together, you will soon be speaking the language of the health-care professional.

## DEFINITIONS OF COMMON TERMS WITHIN THE PHARMACY VERNACULAR

**Accreditation.** Accreditation programs give an official authorization or approval to an organization by comparing it with a set of industry-derived standards. Accreditation Council for Pharmacy Education (ACPE) is the accrediting body for colleges of pharmacy in the United States as an example.

**Adherence.** (Formerly referred to as compliance.) The patient taking the right drug as prescribed, including the prescribed dose of medication at the prescribed frequency for the prescribed length of time.

**TABLE 8.1.** PREFIX AND ROOT WORDS[1-3]

| Root | Meaning | Example |
|------|---------|---------|
| A/an~ | Without, out | Aphonia (without word or speech) |
| Ab, apo, de~ | Away from | Abnormal (pertaining to away from normal) |
| Abdomin~ | Abdomen | Abdominal (pertaining to abdomen) |
| Actino~ | Radiated structure, ray | Actinodermatitis (skin inflammation caused by exposure to radiation) |
| Ad~ | To, toward, near | Adhesion (to sick to) |
| Adip/o~ | Fat | Adiposis (abnormal condition pertaining to fat) |
| Aerlo~ | Air, gas | Aerobic (pertaining to air) |
| Alb, albumin Leuklo~ | White | Albumen (white of egg) |
|  |  | Leukocyte (white blood cell) |
| Alge~ | Pain | Algesia (supersensitivity to pain) |
| Allo~ | Not normal | Allophasis (incoherent speech) |
| Alveo~ | Hollow | Alveolus (small hollow socket of a tooth; air sac of the lungs) |
| Amaur~ | Dark | Amaurosis (complete loss of vision) |
| Ambi, amphi, ampho~ | Both | Ambidextrous (dexterity in both hands) |
| Ambly~ | Dim, dull | Amblyacousia (dullness of hearing) |
| Ambulo~ | Walk about | Ambulatory (able to walk) |
| Aneurysm/o~ | Localized abnormal dilatation of a vessel | Aortic aneurysm (an aneurysm affecting any part of the aorta from the aortic valve to the iliac arteries) |
| Aniso~ | Unequal, dissimilar | Anisocoria (inequality of the size of the pupils) |
| Ankyl~ | Attached, crooked | Ankylodactylia (adhesion of two or more fingers or toes) |

186

| Ante, fore, pre, pro~ | Before, forward | Antepartum (before labor) |
|---|---|---|
| Anter/o~ | In front of | Anterograde (moving frontward) |
| Anti, contra, counter~ | Against, opposite | Anticoagulant (against clotting), contraception (opposed to becoming pregnant) |
| Astro~ | Combining form indicating relationship to a star | Astrocyte (a neuroglial cell of the central nervous system that supports neurons and contributes to the blood-brain barrier) |
| Atel~ | Imperfect | Atelocephaly (incomplete development of the head) |
| Auto~ | Self | Autocytolysis (self-digestion or self-destruction of cells) |
| Bi; bin, di, diplo, dis~ | Two, twice | Bilateral (pertaining to two or both sides) |
| Bio~ | Life | Biology (science of life) |
| Blast~ | Germ | Blastolysis (destruction of a germ cell) |
| Brachy, brevi~ | Short | Brachydactylia (abnormal shortness of the fingers and toes) |
| | | Brevicollis (shortness of the neck) |
| Brady~ | Slow | Bradycardia (condition of slow heart) |
| Bucc~ | Cheek | Buccinator (muscle of the cheek) |
| Caco~ | Bad, ill | Cacosmia (unpleasant odor) |
| Calori~ | Heat | Calorie (unit of heat) |
| Cardio~ | Heart | Cardiologist (one who specializes in treatment of the heart) |
| Cata~ | Down | Catatropia (condition in which both eyes are turned downward) |
| Centi~ | One-hundredth | Centigram (one-hundredth of a gram) |
| Cervico~ | Neck | Cervicodynia (pain or cramp of the neck) |
| Chir~ | Hand | Chiroplasty (plastic surgery on the hand) |

*(continued)*

187

**TABLE 8.1.** PREFIX AND ROOT WORDS[1-3] (Continued)

| Root | Meaning | Example |
|---|---|---|
| Chlor, verdin~ | Green | Chloroplast (green cell organelle found in the leaves of plants) |
| Chroma~ | Color | Chromatism (unnatural pigmentation) |
| Chron~ | Time | Chronological (occurring in natural sequence according to time) |
| Ciner, glauc, polio~ | Gray | Cinerea (gray matter of the brain or spinal cord) |
| Circum, peri~ | Around | Circumvascular (pertaining to around a vessel) |
| Cirrh, flav, lute, xanth~ | Yellow | Cirrhosis (a chronic liver disease), xanthoderma (yellowness of the skin) |
| Clas~ | Break, smash | Clastogenic (capable of breaking chromosomes) |
| Clin~ | Bedside | Clinician (a health-care professional with expertise in patient care rather than research or administration) |
| Co, com, con, sym, syn~ | Together, with | Congenital (pertaining to being born with) |
| Cry~ | Cold | Crymodinia (pain from cold) |
| Cryo~ | Cold | Cryogenic (pertaining to low temperatures) |
| Crypt~ | Hidden | Cryptic (having a hidden meaning) |
| Cyano~ | Blue | Cyanopia (vision in which all objects appear to be blue) |
| Cycl~ | Round, circular | Cyclooxygenase (one of several enzymes that make prostaglandins from arachidonic acids) |
| Cyt~ | Cell | Cytology (study of cell) |
| Deca~ | Ten | Decagram (mass equal to ten grams) |
| Deci~ | One-tenth | Decimeter (one-tenth of a meter) |
| Demi, hemi, semi~ | Half | Hemiplegia (paralysis of one side of the body) |

188

| Dextro~ | To the right | Dextrocardia (condition of the heart on the right side) |
| Di, dis~ | Apart from | Disinfect (to free from infection) |
| Dia, per, trans~ | Across, through | Dialysis (dissolution across or through a membrane transmission to send across or through) |
| Dolicho~ | Long | Dolichofacial (having a long face) |
| Dorsi, dorso~ | Back | Dorsosacral (pertaining to the lower back) |
| Dys~ | Difficult, painful | Dysphonia (condition of difficult voice or speech, hoarseness) |
| E, ec, ex~ | Out from | Edentia (condition of teeth out) |
| | | Eccentric (pertaining to away from center) |
| | | Excise (to cut out) |
| Ecto, extra, extro~ | Outside | Ectopic (pertaining to a place outside) |
| | | Extravascular (pertaining to outside vessel) |
| Em, en, im, in~ | In | Encapsulate (within little box) |
| Endo, ento, intra~ | Within | Endoscope (instument for examination within) |
| | | Entotic (pertaining to the interior of the ear) |
| | | Intracardiac (within the heart) |
| Epi~ | Over, upon | Epidermal (pertaining to upon the skin) |
| Erythr, rube~ | Red | Erythrocyte (red cell) |
| Eso~ | Inward | Esophoria (inward turning of the eye) |
| Eu~ | Easily, well | Eugenic (pertaining to good production) |
| Eury~ | Broad | Eurycephalic (having a broad or wide head) |

(continued)

**TABLE 8.1.** PREFIX AND ROOT WORDS[1-3] (*Continued*)

| Root | Meaning | Example |
|------|---------|---------|
| Extra, hyper, per, pleo, super~ | Outside of, excessive, more | Extracellular (outside the cell) |
| | | Hyperalgesia (an excessive sensitivity to pain) |
| Febri~ | Fever | Febrifacient (producing fever) |
| Gen~ | Producing | Generation (act of reproducing offspring) |
| Gero~ | Aged | Gerontology (the scientific study of the effects of aging) |
| Glyco~ | Sweet, sugar | Glycogeusia (a sweet taste) |
| Gony~ | Knee | Gonyoncus (tumor of the knee) |
| Gust~ | Taste | Gustation (the sense of taste) |
| Haplo~ | Single, simple | Haplopia (single vision) |
| Hecto~ | Hundred | Hectoliter (one hundred liters) |
| Hept, sept~ | Seven | Heptaploidy (having seven sets of chromosomes) |
| Heter~ | Different, other | Heterography (writing different words from those that the writer intended) |
| Hex, sex~ | Six | Sextuplet (one of six children born of a single gestation) |
| Hidro~ | Sweat | Hidrosis (excessive sweating) |
| Histo~ | Tissue | Histoblast (tissue cell) |
| Holo~ | Entire, complete | Holophytic (having plant-like characteristics) |
| Homo~ | Same | Homoblastic (developing from a single type of tissue) |
| Hydro~ | Water | Hydrophobia (exaggerated fear of water) |
| Hyper~ | Above, over | Hyperlipidemia (excessive fat in the blood) |

| Hypno~ | Sleep | Hypnogenic (producing sleep) |
| Hypo~ | Below, beneath, under | Hypothermia (condition of below the normal temperature) |
| Ictero~ | Jaundice | Icterogenic (causing jaundice) |
| Im, in, ir, non, un~ | In, within, not | Nondominant (in neurology, the hemisphere that does not control the speech or preferential use of hand) |
| Infra~, Sub~ | Deficient, less | Infraumbilical (pertaining to under the naval) |
| | | Sublingual (pertaining to under the tongue) |
| Inter~ | Between | Intercostal (pertaining to between ribs) |
| Intra~ | Within | Intraabdominal (within the abdomen) |
| Ipsi, iso~ | Equal, same | Ipsilateral (on the same side) |
| Iso~ | Equal | Isopia (equal vision in the eyes) |
| Juxta~ | Near | Juxtaarticular (situated close to a joint) |
| Kilo~ | Thousand | Kilogram (1000 g) |
| Kinesio~ | Movement | Kinesia (sickness caused by motion) |
| Lapar~ | Flank, loin | Laparocele (abdominal hernia) |
| Latero~ | To the side | Lateroposition (displacement to one side) |
| Leio~ | Smooth | Leiodermia (dermatitis characterized by abnormal glossiness and smoothness of the skin) |
| Lepto~ | Slender, thin | Leptophonia (weakness of the voice) |
| Levo, sinistro~ | To the left | Sinistromanual (left-handed) |
| Lip~ | Fat | Lipoid (resembling fat) |
| Litho | Stone | Lithiasis (presence of a stone) |

(continued)

**TABLE 8.1.** PREFIX AND ROOT WORDS[1-3] (*Continued*)

| Root | Meaning | Example |
|------|---------|---------|
| Lysis | Suffix: dissolving or loosen | Cardiolysis (an operation that seperates adhesions constricting the heart) |
| | Combining form: relief of or reduction | |
| Macro~ | Large, long | Macrocyte (large cell) |
| Mal~ | Bad, ill, poor | Malignant (growing worse) |
| Malaco~ | Soft | Malacosteon (softening of the bones) |
| Medi; mes, mid~ | In the middle | Midline (line that bisects a structure that is bilaterally symmetrical) |
| Medule~ | Marrow | Medullitis (inflammation of marrow) |
| Megalo~ | Large | Megalencephaly (abnormally large size of the brain) |
| Melan, nigro~ | Black | Melanoma (black tumor) |
| Mero~ | Part | Meromelia (partial absence of a limb) |
| Meta~ | After, changes, over | Metastasis (beyond stopping or standing, spread of disease from one part of the body to another) |
| Micro~ | Small | Microlith (small stone) |
| Micro~ | One-millionth | Microgram (one-millionth of a gram) |
| Milli~ | One-thousandth | Milliliter (one-thousandth of a liter) |
| Mis~ | Bar, improper, wrong | Misinformation (data or information concerning a patient that may be assumed erroneously to be accurate) |
| Mono, uni~ | One | Monochromatic (pertaining to one color), unilateral (pertaining to one side) |
| Muco, myx~ | Mucus | Mucocele (mucous cyst), myxadenitis (inflammation of mucous gland) |

| Prefix | Meaning | Example |
|---|---|---|
| Multi, poly~ | Many | Polyphobia (condition of many fears), multicellular (pertaining to many cells) |
| Myco~ | Fungi | Mycoid (fungus-like) |
| Necro~ | Death | Necrocytosis (condition of cell death) |
| Noct~ | Night | Nocturia (excessive or frequent urination after going to bed, typically caused by excessive fluid intake, etc.) |
| Noso~ | Disease | Nosophyte (disease-causing plant microorganism) |
| Octa~ | Eight | Octaploid (having eight pairs of chromosomes) |
| Oligo~ | Few | Oligospermia (condition of deficient sperm) |
| Omo~ | Shoulders | Omodynia (pain in the shoulder) |
| Omphalo~ | Umbilicus | Omphalorrhexis (rupture of the umbilicus) |
| Oneir~ | Dream | Oneirodynia (painful dreaming) |
| Opistho, poster, reto~ | Backward, behind | Opisthotic (located behind the ear) |
| Oxy~ | Keen, sharp | Oxyecoia (abnormal sensitivity to noises) |
| Pachy~ | Thick | Pachycephally (pertaining to thick head) |
| Paleo~ | Old | Paleontology (branch of biology dealing with ancient plant and animal life) |
| Pan~ | All | Panacea (a cure-all) |
| Papilla~ | Pustule, a small protuberance or elevation | Papillomavirus (any group of viruses that cause papillomas or warts in humans and animals) |
| Para~ | Beside, near | Paramedic (pertaining to alongside of medicine) |
| Patho~ | Disease | Pathology (study of disease) |
| Pedia~ | Child | Pediatrics (treatment of child) |
| Pedo~ | Foot | Pedal (pertaining to the foot) |

*(continued)*

193

**TABLE 8.1.** PREFIX AND ROOT WORDS[1-3] (*Continued*)

| Root | Meaning | Example |
|------|---------|---------|
| Penta, quinqu, quinti~ | Five | Quintuplet (one of five children born to one mother during the same birth), quintapara (a woman who has had five pregnancies that have gone beyond the 20th week of gestation) |
| Pero~ | Deformed | Peropus (individual with congenitally deformed feet) |
| Phago~ | Devour, eat | Phagocytosis (a three-staged process where neutrophils, monocytes, and eosinophils engulf and destroy microorganisms, other foreign cell debris, and antigens) |
| Photo~ | Light | Photalgia (pain produced by light) |
| Phren~ | Diaphragm | Phrenospasm (spasm of the diaphragm) |
| Physio~ | Nature | Physiological (concerning body function) |
| Phyt~ | Plant | Phytoid (plantlike) |
| Platy~ | Flat | Platycephaly (flattening of the skull) |
| Pod~ | Foot | Podiatry (treatment of the foot) |
| Poly~ | Many, much | Polyadenous (involving or relating to many glands) |
| Post~ | After, behind | Postoperative (after operation [surgery]) |
| Presby~ | Old | Presbyatric (geriatric) |
| Primi, prot~ | First | Primordial (existing first) |
| Proso~ | Anterior, forward | Prosopoplegia (facial paralysis) |
| Prosop~ | Face | Prosopectasia (abnormal enlargement of the face) |
| Proto~ | First | Protoplasia (primary formation of tissue) |

| Prefix/Root | Meaning | Example |
|---|---|---|
| Pseudo~ | False | Pseudocyst (dilation resembling a cyst) |
| Psychr~ | Cold | Psychroalgia (painful sensation of cold) |
| Puri~ | Pus | Puriform (resembling pus) |
| Purpur~ | Purple | Purpura (any rash in which the blood cells leak into the skin or mucous membranes) |
| Pyro~ | Fever, heat | Pyrogenic (producing fever) |
| Quad, tetra~ | Four | Quadrilateral (having four sides) |
| Radio~ | Ray | Radiolucent (penetrable by X-rays) |
| Re~ | Again | Reactivate (to make active again) |
| Schisto~ | Divide, split | Schistoglossia (a cleft tongue) |
| Sclero~ | Hard | Sclerosis (a condition of hardness) |
| Scoli~ | Crooked, curved | Scoliosis (lateral curvature of the spine) |
| Somni~ | Sleep | Somniferous (sleep-producing) |
| Sphygmo~ | Pulse | Sphygmomanometer (an instrument for measuring aterial blood pressure indirectly) |
| Splanchna~ | Viscera | Splanchnic (pertaining to the viscera) |
| Staphylo~ | Grapelike structure | Staphylococcus (gram-positive bacteria; under a microscope it looks round and clustered like grapes) |
| Stear/steat~ | Fat | Steatosis (fatty degeneration) |
| Steno~ | Contracted, narrow | Stenosis (a condition of narrow) |
| Strepto~ | Curved, twisted | Streptococcus (gram-positive cocci occuring in chains) |

*(continued)*

195

**TABLE 8.1.** PREFIX AND ROOT WORDS[1-3] *(Continued)*

| Root | Meaning | Example |
| --- | --- | --- |
| Super, supra, ultra~ | Above, excessive | Supernumerary (excessive numbers, too small to count), suprarenal (pertaining to above the kidney) |
| Tachy~ | Fast | Tachycardia (a condition of fast heart) |
| Tel, tele, telo~ | Distance, end | Teleceptor (distance receptor) |
| Ter, tri~ | Three, third | Tertiary (third in order or stage) |
| | | Triangular (having three sides) |
| Thermo~ | Heat | Thermotherapy (therapeutic application of heat) |
| Thrombo~ | Clot | Thrombosis (formation or presence of a blood clot within the vascular system) |
| Top/topo~ | Topical | Toponarcosis (local anesthesia) |
| Torsi~ | Twist | Torsive (twisted) |
| Trachy~ | Rough | Trachyphonia (roughness or hoarseness of the voice) |
| Trans~ | Across, through | Transocular (across the eye) |
| Ul~ | Gingiva, scar | Ulitis (gingivitis) |
| Varico~ | Swollen, twisted | Varicose (distended, swollen, knotted veins) |
| Ventro~ | Anterior | Ventrodorsal (in a direction from the front to the back) |
| Viscer~ | Organ | Viscera (internal organs inclosed within a cavity) |
| Vita~ | Life | Vitality (state of being alive) |
| Xeno~ | Foreign, strange | Xenogeneic (obtained from a different species) |
| Xero~ | Dry | Xeroderma (dryness of the skin) |

**TABLE 8.2. SUFFIXES[1-3]**

| Suffix | Definition | Example |
|--------|-----------|---------|
| ~algia, dynia | Pain | Myalgia or myodyni (muscle pain) |
| ~ac | Means pertaining to and forms an adjective when combined with a root | Cardiac (pertaining to the heart) |
| ~al | Means pertaining to or concerning and forms an adjective when combined with a root | Pedal (pertaining to the foot) |
| ~an, ar, ic, ical, ory, tic, eal | Pertaining to | Cyanotic (pertaining to blue), toxic (pertaining to poison) |
| ~oid | Like or resembling | Toxoid (resembling a toxin) |
| ~e, er, icing, ist, or | Agent or noun maker or one who specializes in | Pharmacist |
| ~ia, iasis, id, ism, ity, osis, tia, tion | Abnormal condition, state | Abnormal condition |
| ~cle, cule, culun, culus, et, ium, ole, olum, olus | Small | Ventricle (small belly or pouch) Bronchiole (small airway) Macula (small spot) |
| ~lysis | Breaking down or dissolution | Hemolysis (breakdown of blood) |
| ~megaly | Enlargement | Splenomagaly (enlarged spleen) |
| ~spasm | Involuntary condition | Vasospasm |

**Adjudication.** The process of completing all validity, process, and file edits necessary to prepare a claim for final payment or denial.

**Adjustment.** A credit or debit amount appearing at the carrier/group level on claims
and administrative fee invoices sent to plan sponsors or at a claim level on adjustment advice sent to pharmacies. An adjustment can result from claims processing
and/or billing errors (eg, incorrect dispensing fee paid, incorrect pharmacy paid,
incorrect administration fee billed, wrong carrier/group billed). An adjustment
can also be processed against a general ledger account (eg, bad debt or error).

**Administrative Costs.** The costs assumed by a managed care plan for administrative
services such as claims processing, billing, and overhead costs.

**Adverse Selection.** A particular health plan, whether indemnity or managed care, is
selected against by the enrollee, and thus, an inequitable proportion of enrollees
requiring more medical services are found in that plan.

**Agency for Health-Care Research and Quality (AHRQ).** Created by Congress
in 1989 to conduct federal research into technology assessment and outcomes
management and to develop practice guidelines for public dissemination. The
AHRQ is perhaps best known for funding patient outcome-based research trials
that form the basis for its practice guideline efforts.

**Alkylating Agents.** Drugs used to treat certain kinds of cancers/malignancies.

**American Association of Preferred Provider Organizations (AAPPO).** The
national trade association for PPOs, founded in 1983. There are currently over
1200 members. The vision statement of the AAPPO is in part to "support the
access, choice, and flexibility-the hallmark of preferred provider network (PPN)
and PPO benefit products-that purchasers, employers and consumers value in
expanding affordable health-care coverage to all Americans where regulation is
measurable and equitable, and competition is allowed to flourish."

**Analgesic.** Relieves pain. Acetaminophen (Tylenol®) (aka APAP), aspirin (aka
ASA), nonsteroidal anti-inflammatory drugs (NSAIDs) like ibuprofen (Advil®,
Motrin®), and narcotics are examples of analgesics.

**Angiography.** (1) A description of blood vessels and lymphatics. (2) Diagnostic or therapeutic radiography of the heart and blood vessels using a radiopaque contrast medium.
Types include magnetic resonance, interventional, and computed tomography.

**Antibiotic.** Inhibits growth or destroys microorganisms whose overgrowth causes
infection. Penicillins, quinolones, β-lactams, and cephalosporins are all examples.

**Anticoagulant.** (1) Delaying or preventing blood coagulation. (2) An agent that
prevents or delays blood coagulation, for example warfarin sodium (Coumadin®)
or dabagatrin (Pradaxa®).

**Antidepressant.** Any medicine or other mode of therapy that acts to prevent, cure,
or alleviate mental depression.

**Antihistamine.** A drug that opposes the action of histamine. Although there are
two classes of histamine-blocking drugs, the term antihistamine is typically used
to describe agents that block the action of histamines on the $H_1$ receptors. These
agents are used to treat allergies, hives, etc.

**Anti-inflammatory.** Counteracting inflammation. An agent that counteracts inflammation.

**Apparent Volume of Distribution ($V_z$).** A hypothetical volume calculated using the elimination rate constant. It is considered to be equivalent to $V_{ss}$ in most cases.

**Arthroscopy.** Direct joint visualization by means of an arthroscope, usually to remove tissue such as cartilage fragments or torn ligaments.

**Aspiration.** Withdrawal of fluid from a cavity by suctioning with an aspirator. The purpose of aspiration is to remove fluid or air from an affected area or to obtain specimens.

**Astringent.** Drawing together, constricting, binding. An agent that has a constricting or binding effect.

**Audiometry.** Testing of the hearing sense.

**Authorization.** As it applies to managed care, authorization is the approval of care, such as hospitalization. Preauthorization may be required before admission takes place or care is given by non-Health Maintenance Organization (HMO) providers.

**Average Wholesale Price (AWP).** The published average "cost" of a drug product paid by the pharmacy to the wholesaler. This price is specific to drug strength or concentrating dosage form, package size, and manufacturer or labeler. The AWP of each drug is maintained on the National Drug Code (NDC) master file. This price is used to calculate the upper limit of payment available under a plan.

**Average Wholesale Price Discount.** A cost-containment program implemented to reduce drug program costs for plan sponsors without influencing cardholders. The AWP no longer always equals the actual cost of a drug to the pharmacy, so applying a discount to AWP allows a new upper limit of payment to be established, and savings are realized by the plan sponsors. An example is a plan sponsor with a plan that allows average wholesale price less 10% (AWP 10%).

**Beneficiary (Insured).** The primary person receiving the benefit coverage. This information is maintained on the eligibility file of the plan sponsor. If the client can provide the information, dependent names are also maintained.

**Benefit Package.** Services an insurer, government agency, health plan, or an employer offers under the terms of a contract.

**Bioavailability ($F$).** The fraction of given drug that reaches the systemic circulation. It will be reported as a percentage or fraction.

**Brand-Brand Interchange.** Dispensing one brand name product for another brand name product marketed by another manufacturer.

**Brand Drug.** The drug manufacturer whose name is listed on the application to the FDA for approval of a new drug.

**Brand Name.** The trademarked name of the drug that appears on the package label.

**Bronchoscopy.** Examination of the bronchi through a bronchoscope.

**Capitation.** A per-member monthly payment to a provider that covers contracted services and is paid in advance of its delivery. In essence, a provider agrees to provide specified services to HMO members for this fixed, predetermined payment for a specified length of time (usually a year), regardless of how many times the member uses the service. The rate can be fixed for all members, or it can be adjusted for the age and sex of the member, based on actuarial projections of medical utilization.

**Cardholder (Insured or Beneficiary).** The primary person receiving the benefit coverage in whose name the card is issued. This information is maintained in the eligibility file. If the client can provide the information, dependent names are also maintained.

**Cardiac Catheterization.** Percutaneous intravascular insertion of a catheter into any chamber of the heart or great vessels for diagnosis, assessment of abnormalities, interventional treatment, and evaluation of the effects of pathology on the heart.

**Carrier/Group.** The combination used to signify both the plan sponsor (carrier) and the specific group under it. An example of a carrier/group would be 0007/0023: 0007, Carrier, ABZ Insurance Co.; 0023, Group, The Marley Company.

**Carrier Name.** This term is used to identify any plan sponsor—the underwriter of an insured account or the company name of a self-administered account. This name is often used on management reports sent to the plan sponsor.

**Carrier Number.** An assigned four-digit number that identifies the plan sponsor (insurance company, self-administered account, third-party administrator [TPA], multiple employer trust, HMO). A plan sponsor may have more than one carrier number.

**Case Management.** The process whereby a health-care professional supervises the administration of medical or ancillary services to a patient, typically one who has a catastrophic disorder or who is receiving mental health services. Case managers are thought to reduce the costs associated with the care of such patients while providing high-quality medical services.

**Central Volume of Distribution ($V_c$).** The volume of blood and highly perfused tissues where a drug will initially distribute. It is used to calculate loading doses.

**Certification.** Certification is the official authorization for use of services.

**Claim.** Information submitted by a provider or covered person to establish that medical services were provided to a covered person, from which processing for payment to the provider or covered person is made.

**Claims Adjudication.** See Adjudication.

**Claims Review.** The method by which an enrollee's health-care service claims are reviewed before reimbursement is made. The purpose of this monitoring system is to validate the medical appropriateness of the provided services and to be sure the cost of the service is not excessive.

**Clearance (CL).** The amount of blood that can have all the drug eliminated from it per unit time. Therefore, the units for clearance are volume per time. It is a determinant of $C_{ss,avg}$, $k$, $t\frac{1}{2}$, and peak-to-trough ratio.

**Consolidated Omnibus Budget Reconciliation Act of 1985 (COBRA).** Legislation that requires group health plans of covered employers to give employees and family members the opportunity to continue their health-care coverage at their own expense at group rates in circumstances where coverage would otherwise end.

**Coinsurance.** The percentage of the costs of medical services paid by the patient. This is a characteristic of indemnity insurance and PPO plans. The coinsurance usually is about 20% of the cost of medical services after the deductible is paid.

**Compliance.** (More accurately referred to as adherence.) The ability of a patient to take medication or follow treatment protocol according to the directions for which it was prescribed; patient taking prescribed dose of medication at the prescribed frequency for the prescribed length of time.

**Continuous Quality Improvement (CQI).** A comprehensive philosophy of continuously improving the quality of a product or service by constantly monitoring operations, correcting problems, and implementing systems to better assist customers. It is a comprehensive approach for improving overall organizational performance and challenges the traditional way of doing business. It contends that most quality problems involve procedures and strategies (ie, the process) and are not the fault of individuals.

**Contraceptive.** Any process, device, or method that prevents conception. Categories of contraceptives include steroids, chemical, physical, or barrier or combinations of these.

**Copayment.** A nominal fee charged to an insured member to offset costs of paperwork and administration for each office visit or pharmacy prescription filled.

**Corticosteroid.** Any of several steroid hormones secreted by the cortex of the adrenal gland or manufactured synthetically for use as a drug. Examples would be prednisone, dexamethasone, methylprednisolone.

**Cost-Benefit Analysis.** Cost-benefit analysis expresses the outcomes of therapies (eg, the benefits) in monetary rather than physical units.

**Cost Containment.** A program to decrease the overall costs of a drug, medical benefit, or health care.

**Cost Effectiveness.** Usually considered as a ratio, the cost effectiveness of a drug or procedure, for example, relates the cost of that drug or procedure to the health benefits resulting from it. In health terms, it is often expressed as the cost per year per life-year saved or as the cost per quality-adjusted life-year saved.

**Cost Shifting.** The redistribution of payment sources. Typically, cost shifting occurs when a discount on provider services is obtained by one payer and the providers increase costs to another payer to make up the difference.

**CPT.** Physician's current procedural terminology.

**Cytochrome P-450 Enzymes (CYP).** Phase I enzymes responsible for much of the intestinal and hepatic metabolism of drugs.

**Dispense as Written (DAW).**[4] A notation used by a physician, pharmacy, or cardholder that will determine whether or not generic substitution occurs. There are 10 DAW codes defined as follows (numeric values are assigned to each code for computer entry for online claims adjudication systems):

No product selection indicated.

0—This is the field default value used for prescriptions when product selection is not an issue. Examples include prescriptions written for single-source brand products and prescriptions written using the generic name, and a generic product is dispensed.

1—Substitution not allowed by prescriber.

This value is used when the prescriber indicates, in a manner specified by prevailing law, that the product is to be dispensed as written.

2—Substitution allowed, patient-requested product dispensed.

This value is used when the prescriber has indicated, in a manner specified by prevailing law, that generic substitution is permitted, and the patient requests the brand product. This situation can occur when the prescriber writes the prescription using either the brand or generic name and the product is available from multiple sources.

3—Substitution allowed, pharmacist-selected product dispensed.

This value is used when the prescriber has indicated, in a manner specified by prevailing law, that generic substitution is permitted, and the brand product is dispensed because a currently marketed generic is not stocked in the pharmacy. This situation exists as a result of the buying habits of the pharmacist, not because of the unavailability of the generic product in the marketplace.

4—Substitution allowed, generic drug not in stock.

This value is used when the prescriber has indicated, in a manner specified by prevailing law, that generic substitution is permitted, and the brand product is dispensed because a currently marketed generic is not stocked in the pharmacy. This situation exists as a result of the buying habits of the pharmacist, not because of the unavailability of the generic product in the marketplace.

5—Substitution allowed, brand drug dispensed as a generic.

This value is used when the prescriber has indicated, in a manner specified by prevailing law, that generic substitution is permitted, and the pharmacist is utilizing the brand product as the generic entity.

6—Override.

This value is used by various claims processors in very specific instances as defined by that claims processor and/or its client(s).

7—Substitution not allowed, brand drug mandated by law.

This value is used when the prescriber has indicated, in a manner specified by prevailing law, that generic substitution is permitted, but prevailing law or regulation prohibits the substitution of a generic product even though generic versions of the product may be available in the marketplace.

8—Substitution allowed; generic drug not available in marketplace.

This value is used when the prescriber has indicated, in a manner specified by prevailing law, that generic substitution is permitted, and the brand product is dispensed because the generic is not currently manufactured or distributed or is temporarily unavailable.

**9—Other.**
This value is reserved and currently not in use. NCPDP does not recommend use of this value at the present time. Please contact NCPDP if you intend to use this value and document how it will be utilized by your organization.

**Decongestant.** Reducing congestion or swelling, or any agent that reduces congestion or swelling.

**Deductible.** A fixed amount of health-care dollars of which a person must pay 100% before his or her health benefits begin. Most indemnity plans feature a $200 to $500 deductible and then pay up to 100% of money spent for covered services above this level.

**Dependent Coverage Code.** Allows the plan sponsor to control the type of coverage each cardholder receives.

**Drug Efficacy Study Indicator (DESI).** A study of drugs by the Food and Drug Administration (FDA) that rates certain drugs as not safe and effective and experimental or investigational in nature.

**Diagnostic-Related Groups (DRGs).** A program in which hospital procedures are rated in terms of cost, taking into account the intensity of services delivered. A standard flat rate per procedure is derived from this scale, which is paid by Medicare for its beneficiaries, regardless of the cost to the hospital to provide that service.

**Direct Costs.** Direct costs are those that are wholly attributable to the service in question, for example, the services of professional and paraprofessional personnel, equipment, and materials.

**Disease State Management (also known as Medication Therapy Management, MTM).** A philosophy toward the treatment of the patient with an illness (usually chronic) that seeks to prevent recurrence of symptoms, maintain high quality of life (QOL), and prevent future need for medical resources by using an integrated approach to health care. Pharmaceutical care, CQI, practice guidelines, and case management all play key roles in this effort, which should result in decreased health-care costs as well.

**Dispensing Fee.** Contracted rate of compensation paid to a pharmacy for the processing/filling of a prescription claim. The dispensing fee is added to the negotiated formula for reimbursing ingredient cost.

**Diuretic.** Increasing urine secretion, an agent that increases urine output.

**Doppler Ultrasonography.** The use of ultrasound to produce an image or photograph of an organ or tissue. Doppler effect is the shift in frequency produced when an ultrasound wave is echoed from something in motion. The use of the Doppler effect permits measuring the velocity of that which is being studied.

**Dose Interval ($\tau$ or Tau).** How often the patient is receiving the drug. The units are in time. It is a determinant of peak-to-trough ratio.

**Dose Rate (DR).** The amount of drug the patient is receiving per time. The units will be amount/time. It is a determinant of $C_{ss,avg}$.

**Dullness.** Refers to a sound heard upon physical examination. (This could be a normal or abnormal finding depending on the area being examined.) It is heard over solid organs like the liver and muscles.

**Drug Utilization Evaluation (DUE).** An evaluation of prescribing patterns of physicians to specifically determine the appropriateness of drug therapy.

**Drug Utilization Review (DUR).** A system of drug use review that can detect potential adverse drug interactions, drug-pregnancy conflicts, therapeutic duplication, drug-age conflicts, and so on. There are three forms of DUR: prospective (before dispensing), concurrent (at the time of prescription dispensing), and retrospective (after the therapy has been completed). Appropriate use of an integrated DUR program can curb drug misuse and abuse and monitor quality of care. DUR can reduce hospitalization and other costs related to inappropriate drug use.

**Echocardiogram.** The graphic record produced by echocardiography.

**Electrocardiograph.** A device for recording changes in the electrical energy produced by the action of heart muscles.

**Electroencephalography.** Amplification, recording, and analysis of the electrical activity of the brain. The record obtained is called the electroencephalogram (EEG).

**Elimination Rate Constant ($k$).** Represents the fraction of drug eliminated per time. The units are inverse time. It is a dependent variable determined by clearance (CL) and volume of distribution ($V_d$).

**Endoscopy.** Inspection of body organs or cavities by use of an endoscope.

**Employee Retirement Income Security Act of 1974 (ERISA).** This law mandates reporting and disclosure requirements for group life and health plans.

**Enterohepatic Cycling.** A cycle through which absorbed drug is reintroduced to the intestine. After absorption and exposure to the liver, the drug is stored in the gallbladder and then secreted into the bile to reenter the intestine.

**Exclusive Provider Organization (EPO).** The EPO is a form of a preferred provider organization (PPO) in which patients must visit a caregiver who is on EPO's panel of providers. If a visit to an outside provider is made, the EPO will offer limited or no coverage for the office or hospital visit.

**Expectorant.** An agent, such as guaifenesin, that promotes the clearance of mucus from the respiratory tract.

**Fee for Service.** Traditional provider reimbursement, in which the physician is paid according to the service performed. This is the reimbursement system used by conventional indemnity insurers.

**Fee Schedule.** A comprehensive listing of fees used by either a health-care plan or the government to reimburse physicians and other providers on a fee-for-service basis.

**First-Dollar Coverage.** A feature of an insurance plan in which there is no deductible, and therefore, the plan's sponsor pays a proportion or all of the covered services provided to a patient as soon as he or she enrolls.

**Formulary.** A specific list of drugs included with a given plan for a client. Types include closed formulary, negative formulary, and open formulary.

**Fraction Absorbed ($f_a$).** The fraction of orally administered drug that is absorbed from the gut lumen to the gut wall.

**Fraction Escaping Gut Metabolism ($f_g$).** The fraction of orally administered drug not metabolized or effluxed from the gut wall back into the gut lumen.

**Fraction Escaping Hepatic First Pass ($f_{fp}$).** The fraction of drug presented to the liver that is not metabolized. It has an inverse relationship with hepatic extraction ratio.

**Free Average Concentration at Steady State ($C_{ss,avg,free}$).** The average concentration of only the pharmacologically active unbound drug during a dosing interval at steady state. It is often the parameter that we are trying to maintain within a given therapeutic range. The units are amount per volume.

**Gatekeeper.** Most HMOs rely on the primary-care physician, or "gatekeeper," to screen patients seeking medical care and effectively eliminate costly and sometimes needless referral to specialists for diagnosis and management. The gatekeeper is responsible for the administration of the patient's treatment, and this person must coordinate and obtain authorization for all medical services, laboratory studies, specialty referrals, and hospitalizations. In most HMOs, if an enrollee visits a specialist without prior authorization from his or her designated primary-care physician, the enrollee must pay for medical services.

**Generic Substitution.** In cases in which the patent on a specific pharmaceutical product expires and drug manufacturers produce generic versions of the original branded product, the generic version of the drug (which is theorized to be identical to the product manufactured by a different firm) is dispensed, even though the original product is prescribed. Some managed care organizations and Medicaid programs mandate generic substitution because of the generally lower cost of generic products. There are state and federal regulations regarding generic substitutions.

**Half-Life ($t_{1/2}$).** The time required for the serum concentration to decrease by 50%. It is in units of time. Half-life also is important in determining time to steady state and $P{:}T$ ratio. Volume of distribution ($V_d$) and clearance (CL) determine half-life.

**Health-Care Financing Administration (HCFA).** The federal agency responsible for administering Medicare and overseeing states' administration of Medicaid.

**Health Alliances.** Also known as regional health alliances, these entities are purchasing pools that are responsible for negotiating health insurance for employers and employees. Alliances use their leverage as large health-care purchasers to negotiate contracts.

**HEDIS.** Health education data information system.

**Health Maintenance Organization (HMO).** A form of health insurance in which its members prepay a premium for the HMO's health services, which generally include inpatient and ambulatory care. For the patient, it means reduced out-of-pocket costs (ie, no deductible), no paperwork (ie, insurance forms), and only a small copayment for each office visit to cover the paperwork handled by the HMO. There are several different types of HMOs.

- *Group Model.* In the group-model HMO, the HMO contracts with a physician group, which is paid a fixed amount per patient to provide specific services. The administration of the group practice then decides how the HMO payments are distributed to each participating physician. This type of HMO is usually located in a hospital or clinic setting and may include a pharmacy. These physicians usually do not have any fee-for-service patients.

- *Hybrid Model.* A combination of at least two managed care organizational models that are melded into a single health plan. Because its features do not uniformly fit one model, it is called a hybrid.
- *Individual Practice Association (IPA) Model.* The IPA contracts with independent physicians, who work in their own private practices and see fee-for-service patients as well as HMO enrollees. They are paid by capitation for the HMO patients and by conventional means for their fee-for-service patients. Physicians belonging to the IPA guarantee that the care needed by each patient for whom they are responsible will fall under a certain amount of money. They guarantee this by allowing the HMO to withhold an amount of their payments (usually about 20% per year). If, by the end of the year, the physician's cost for treatment falls under this set amount, then the physician receives his entire "withhold fund." If the opposite is true, the HMO can then withhold any part of this amount, at its discretion, from the fund. Essentially, the physician is put "at risk" for keeping down the treatment cost. This is the key to the HMO's financial viability.
- *Network Model.* A network of group practices under the administration of one HMO.
- *Point-of-Service (POS) Model.* Sometimes referred to as an "open-ended" HMO. The POS model is the one in which the patient can receive care either by physicians contracted with the HMO or by those not contracted. Physicians not contracted with the HMO, who see an HMO patient, are paid according to the services performed. The patient is incentivized to utilize contracted providers through the fuller coverage offered for contracted care.
- *Staff Model.* The staff-model HMO is the purest form of managed care. All of the physicians in a staff-model HMO are in a centralized site, in which all clinical and perhaps inpatient services and pharmacy services are offered. The HMO holds the tightest management reigns in this setting because none of the physicians traditionally practices on an independent fee-for-service basis. Physicians are more likely to be employees of the HMO in this setting because they are not in a private or group practice.

**Holter Monitor.** A portable device small enough to be worn by a patient during normal activity. It consists of an electrocardiograph and a recording system capable of storing up to 24 hours of the individual's ECG record.

**Horizontal Integration.** Affiliation of firms (eg, drug manufacturers) or providers (eg, physicians, pharmacists, etc.) on the same level to expand distribution systems, or multichannel systems in which manufacturers diversify in selecting channels to cover different markets.

**Hospice.** A health-care facility that provides supportive care for the terminally ill.

**ICD-9 Code.** International classification of diseases, ninth edition.

**Indemnity Insurance.** Traditional fee-for-service medicine in which providers are paid according to the service performed.

**Indirect Costs.** Indirect costs are usually termed overhead costs; they are the costs shared by many services concurrently. For example, maintenance, administration, equipment, electricity, and water.

**Insulin.** A hormone secreted by the β-cells of the pancreas that controls the metabolism and cellular uptake of sugars, proteins, and fats. As a drug it is used principally to treat diabetes mellitus.

**Insurance Company (Plan Sponsor).** A client, also referred to as a carrier, who underwrites the insurance for individual groups. The insurance company signs the contract and is financially responsible for all bills incurred by groups insured by them. Each insurance company is assigned a unique insurance code and can generally tailor the program for their individual groups.

**Integrated Health-Care Systems.** Health-care financing and delivery organizations created to provide a "continuum of care," ensuring that patients get the right care at the right time from the right provider. This continuum of care from primary care provider to specialist and ancillary provider under one corporate roof guarantees that patients get cared for appropriately, thus saving money and increasing the quality of care.

**Intervention.** Educational, directive (eg, formulary or prior authorization), or consultative communications between providers, especially pharmacists to physicians.

**Intradermal.** Drug route of administration by injection into the skin.

**Intramuscular.** Drug route of administration by injection into a muscle.

**Intrathecal.** Drug route of administration by injection into the meninges around the spinal cord.

**Laryngoscopy.** Visual examination of the interior of the larynx to determine the cause of hoarseness, obtain cultures, manage the upper airways, or take biopsies.

**Long-Term Care.** Services ordinarily provided in a skilled nursing, intermediate-care, personal-care, supervisory-care, or elder-care facility.

**Maximum Allowable Cost (MAC).** A cost management program that sets upper limits on the payment for equivalent drugs available from multiple manufacturers. It is the highest unit price that will be paid for a drug and is designed to increase generic dispensing, to ensure the pharmacy dispenses economically, and to control future cost increases.

**Magnetic Resonance Imaging (MRI).** A type of diagnostic radiography that uses the characteristic behavior of protons (and other atomic nuclei) when placed in powerful magnetic fields to make images of tissues and organs.

**Managed Health Care.** The sector of health insurance in which health-care providers are not independent businesses run by, for example, the private practitioner, but by administrative firms that managed the allocation of health-care benefits. In contrast with conventional indemnity insurers, which did not govern the provision of medical services but simply paid for them, managed care firms have a significant say in how the services are administered so that they may better control health-care costs. HMOs and PPOs are examples of managed care organizations.

**Managed Services Organization (MSO).** A type of integrated health care plan in which the hospital provides administrative services to a physician group and the physician group provides patients to the hospital.

**Medicaid.** An entitlement program run by both the state and federal government for the provision of health-care insurance to patients younger than 65 years of age, who cannot afford to pay private health insurance. The federal government matches the states' contribution on a certain minimal level of available coverage. The states may institute additional services, but at their own expense.

**Medicaid Prudent Pharmaceutical Purchasing Act (MPPPA).** Enacted as part of the Omnibus Budget Reconciliation Act of 1990, MPPPA provides that Medicaid must receive the best discounted price of any institutional purchaser of pharmaceuticals. Thus, drug companies provide rebates to Medicaid that are the difference between the discounted price and the price at which the drug was sold.

**Medical Protocols.** Medical protocols are the guidelines physicians are asked to follow to achieve an acceptable clinical outcome. The protocol provides the caregiver with specific treatment options or steps to follow when faced with a particular set of clinical symptoms or signs or laboratory data.

**Medicare.** An entitlement program run by the Health Care Financing Administration of the federal government by which people aged 65 years or older receive health-care insurance. Medicare Part A covers hospitalization and is a compulsory benefit. Medicare Part B covers outpatient services and is a voluntary service.

**Medication Therapy Management (MTM).** MTM is a distinct service or group of services that optimizes drug therapy with the intent of improved therapeutic outcomes for individual patients.

**Member.** A participant in a health plan who makes up the plan's enrollment.

**Miotic.** An agent that causes the pupil to contract, such as pilocarpine.

**Mydriatic.** Causing pupillary dilation. A drug that dilates the pupil such as atropine, cocaine, and ephedrine.

**Mucolytic.** Pertaining to a class of agents that liquefy sputum or reduce its viscosity.

**National Council for Prescription Drug Programs (NCPDP).** An organization that promotes standardization and efficiency within the third-party prescription drug program industry and provides accurate and reliable information as to third-party prescription drug programs.

**National Drug Code (NDC).** A unique seven-digit character code given to a drug that identifies the labeler, product, and package size.

**Nitrates.** Salts of nitric acid. Agents in the class include isosorbide dinitrate or monohydrate and nitroglycerin. They are arteriovenous dilators and are used to treat angina, hypertension, and congestive heart failure.

**Outcomes Management.** A clinical outcome is the result of medical or surgical intervention or nonintervention. Managed care is now attempting to better manage the clinical outcomes of their enrollees to increase patient and payer satisfaction while holding down costs. It is thought that a database of outcomes experience will help caregivers see which treatment modalities result in consistently

improved outcomes for patients. Outcomes management will, as a natural consequence, lead to medical protocols.

**Outcomes Research.** Studies that evaluate the effect of a given product, procedure, or medical technology on health or costs. Outcomes research information is vital to the development of practice guidelines.

**Out-of-Pocket Costs.** The share of health services payments paid by the enrollee.

**P-glycoprotein (P-gp).** A drug efflux system that is a member of the ABC cassette family of transporters. P-gp has been found in the cells lining the blood-brain barrier, kidney, adrenal glands, and lungs as well as the gut.

**Palpation.** Examination by application of the hands or fingers to the external surface of the body to detect evidence of disease or abnormalities in the internal organs.

**Parenteral.** Drug administration by other than the oral route, specifically by injection.

**Patient Centered Medical Home (PCMH).** The Agency for Healthcare Research and Quality (AHRQ) defines a medical home not simply as a place but as a model of the organization of primary care that delivers the core functions of primary health care. The PCMH includes five functions and attributes: Patient-centered, comprehensive care, coordinated care, superb access to care, and a systems-based approach to quality and safety.

**Per member per month (PMPM).** Often used in the context of pharmacy or medical costs.

**Pharmacy Benefit Management Companies (PBM).** Firms used by plan sponsors to design and administer pharmaceutical benefit plans.

**Peak-to-Trough Ratio ($P{:}T$).** Ratio describing the variation between the highest and lowest achieved concentrations within a dosing interval.

**Per Diem Reimbursement.** Reimbursement of an institution, usually a hospital, based on a set rate per day rather than on charges. Per dime reimbursement can be varied by service (eg, medical/surgical, obstetrics, mental health, and intensive care) or can be uniform regardless of intensity of services.

**Performance Measures.** Methods or instruments used to estimate or monitor how a health-care provider's actions conform to criteria and standards of quality.

**Pharmaceutical Care.** A fairly new concept in providing health care defined by Hepler and Strand in 1990; it is a strategy that attempts to utilize drug therapy more efficiently to achieve definite outcomes that improve a patient's QOL. A pharmaceutical care system requires a reorientation of physicians, pharmacist, and nurses toward effective drug therapy outcomes. It is a set of relationships and decisions through which pharmacist, physicians, nurses, and patients work together to design, implement, and monitor a therapeutic plan that will produce specific therapeutic outcomes.

**Pharmacy Services Administrative Organization (PSAO).** An organization that is dedicated to providing prescription benefits to enrollees of managed care plans by using existing community pharmacies. The PSAO contracts as a provider group with the managed care organization so that the individual pharmacies receive negotiating representation in numbers and the prepaid health plan does not have to provide the capital necessary to start, own, and operate its own pharmacy department.

**Physician-Hospital Organization (PHO).** A type of integrated health-care system that in its simplest form is an organization that collectively commits both physicians and the hospital to payer contracts. They sometimes use existing IPA structures or individual physician contracting. In its most effective form, the PHO must commit the entire physician and hospital panel, without an opt out, to the PHO organization.

**Plan Sponsor.** The company that assumes financial responsibility for an insured group. A plan sponsor can be an insurance company, third-party administration, or the company itself, if the company is self-insured.

**POS.** Point of sale or point of service.

**Preadmission Certification.** The practice of reviewing claims for hospital admission before the patient actually enters the hospital. This cost-control mechanism is intended to eliminate unnecessary hospital expenses by denying medically unnecessary admissions.

**Preferred Provider Organization (PPO).** A managed care organization in which physicians are paid on a fee-for-service schedule that is discounted, usually about 10% to 20% below normal fees. PPOs are often formed as a competitive reaction to HMOs by physicians who contract out with insurance companies, employers, or TPAs. A patient can use a physician outside of the PPO providers, but he or she will have to pay a greater portion of the fee.

**Preferred Providers.** Physicians, hospitals, and other health-care providers who contract to provide health services to persons covered by a particular health plan.

**Premium.** The amount paid to a carrier for providing coverage under a contract.

**Preventive Care.** Health care emphasizing priorities for prevention, early detection, and early treatment of conditions, generally including routine physical examination, immunization, and wellness care.

**Primary Care Physician (PCP).** Sometimes referred to as a "gatekeeper," the primary care physician is usually the first doctor a patient sees for an illness. This physician then treats the patient directly, refers the patient to a specialist (secondary care), or admits the patient to a hospital when necessary. Often, the primary care physician is a family physician or internist.

**Prior Authorization (PA).** The process of obtaining certification or authorization from the health plan or pharmacy benefit manager for specified medications or specified quantities of medications. Often involves appropriateness review against preestablished criteria. Failure to obtain prior authorization often results in a financial penalty to the subscriber.

**Private-Sector Health-Care Programs.** Signifies health-care companies not directly affiliated with any federal, state, or local government. Normally, they are enterprises that perform services for a profit.

**Provider.** Any supplier of services (ie, physician, pharmacist, case management firm, etc.).

**Pulmonary Function Tests (PFT).** One of several different tests used to evaluate the condition of the respiratory system. Measures of expiratory flow and lung volumes and capacities are obtained.

**Quality-Adjusted Life-Year (QALY).** This unit of measure is one way to quantify health outcomes resulting from some types of intervention. The number of quality-adjusted life-years is the number of years at full health that would be valued equivalently to the number of years of life experienced in a less desirable health state.

**Quality Assurance (QA).** QA or quality assessment is the activity that monitors the level of care being provided by physicians, medical institutions, or any health-care vendor in order to ensure that health plan enrollees are receiving the best care possible. The level of care is measured against preestablished standards, some of which are mandated by law.

**Quality Improvement (QI).** A continuous process that identifies problems in health-care delivery, examines solutions to those problems, and regularly monitors the solutions for improvement.

**Quality of Life (QOL).** A patient's perceptions of how he or she deals with a disease or with everyday life when suffering from a particular condition. It is subjective because information cannot be measured objectively; however, it has been in the health-care literature for at least 20 years.

**Quality-of-Life Measures.** An assessment of the patient's perceptions of how he or she is dealing with a disease or with everyday life when suffering from a particular condition.

**Radiography, Roentgenography.** The process of obtaining an image for diagnosis using a radiologic modality. The most common example would be an X-ray.

**Resonance.** A normal physical assessment sound heard over lung tissue

**Risk Contract.** Also known as a Medicare risk contract. A contract between an HMO or CMP and the HCFA to provide services to Medicare beneficiaries under which the health plan receives a fixed monthly payment for enrolled Medicare members and then must provide all services on an at-risk basis. This type of contract may be between physicians and an HMO, placing the physician at risk for costs of services provided.

**Screening.** The method by which managed care organizations limit access to health care for unnecessary reasons. In most HMOs, a phone call to the physician or his or her medical office staff is required before an office visit can be arranged. "Gatekeepers" and concurrent review are other methods of screening patients.

**Self-Insured.** Clients who obtain benefits on a self-funded basis. The company assumes all of the financial risk and liability that would normally be covered by an insurance company.

**Skilled Nursing Facility (SNF).** Typically an institution for convalescence or a nursing home, the SNF provides a high level of specialized care for long-term or acute illnesses. It is an alternative to extended hospital stays or difficult home care.

**Standards of Quality.** Authoritative statement of minimum levels of acceptable performance, excellent levels of performance, or the range of acceptable performance.

**Subcutaneous.** A drug route of administration in which it is injected just beneath the skin.

**Sublingual.** A drug therapy that is placed under the tongue. An example would be sublingual nitroglycerin used to manage chest pain.

**Surgicenter.** A separate, free-standing medical facility specializing in outpatient or same-day surgical procedures. Surgicenters drastically reduce the costs associated with hospitalizations for routine surgical procedures because extended inpatient care is not required for specific disorders.

**Tertiary Care.** Tertiary care is administered at a highly specialized medical center. It is associated with the utilization of high-cost technology resources.

**Therapeutic Substitution.** A drug that is believed therapeutically equivalent (ie, will achieve the same outcome) to the exact drug prescribed by a physician is substituted. Therapeutic substitution is generally mandated by formulary adherence programs.

**Third-Party Administrator (TPA).** Clients who handle the administration of the program for a group or insurance company. The TPA is considered the plan sponsor and is therefore financially responsible.

**Third-Party Payer.** A public or private organization that pays for or underwrites coverage for health-care expenses.

**Total Average Concentration at Steady State ($C_{ss,avg,tot}$).** The average concentration of both bound and unbound drug during a dosing interval at steady state. It is often the parameter that we are trying to maintain within a given therapeutic range. The units are amount per volume.

**Transdermal.** A medication that is applied to the skin so that the drug can be absorbed through the skin. Examples would include nitroglycerin patches, clonidine patches, estrogen patches, and nicotine patches.

**Triage.** The evaluation of patient conditions for urgency and seriousness, and establishment of a priority list for multiple patients. In the setting of managed care, triage is often performed after office hours on the telephone by a nurse or other health professional to screen patients for emergency treatment.

**Triple Option.** A type of health plan in which employees may choose from an HMO, a PPO, and an indemnity plan, depending on how much they are willing to contribute to cost.

**Tympany.** A normal physical assessment sound heard over most portions of the abdominal cavity.

**Usual and Customary (U&C) Pricing.** The amount that a pharmacist would charge a cash-paying customer for a prescription.

**UCR Pricing.** Usual, customary, and reasonable.

**Ultrasonography.** The use of ultrasound to produce an image or photograph of an organ or tissue. Ultrasonic echoes are recorded as they strike tissues of different densities.

**Unique Physician Identification Number (UPIN).** A unique identification number assigned to a physician that is used for prescribed drug claims.

**Utilization Review (UR).** Performed by the HMO to discover if a particular physician-provider or other provider (eg, pharmacy) is spending as much of the HMO's money on treatment or any specific portion thereof (eg, specialty referral, drug prescribing, hospitalization, radiologic or laboratory services) as his or her peers.

**Volume of Distribution ($V_d$).** Parameter that relates the amount of drug in the body to the measured plasma concentration. The larger the volume of distribution, the higher the amount of tissue binding and the slower the elimination from the body. Elimination rate is dependent on the volume of distribution and the clearance of a drug.

**Volume of Distribution at Steady-State ($V_{ss}$).** A physiologic volume describing the determinants of distribution. It is very difficult to measure and is reported in units of volume. It is primarily dependent on plasma and tissue protein binding.

## APPLICATION EXERCISES

For the following terms, separate prefixes, combining forms, and suffixes. Define each term.

a. Acrodynia
b. Pediatrics
c. Microscope
d. Orthopedic
e. Epigastrium
f. Hemodialysis
g. Vasospasm
h. Podiatry
i. Angiomegaly
j. Tachycardia
k. Cardiograph
l. Dysphonic
m. Urologist
n. Oliguria
o. Gastrostomy
p. Laparotomy
q. Ultrasonography
r. Pancytopenia
s. Cyanosis
t. Pyretic

| SELECT THE COMBINING FORM THAT MATCHES THE MEANING OF EACH OF THE FOLLOWING TERMS: | | | |
|---|---|---|---|
| glia | phasia | a | myel/o |
| itis | thromb/o | oma | Dys |
| mening/o | vascul/o | osis | Rrhagia |
| scler/o | oid | | |

a. Without
b. Abnormal condition
c. Blood clot
d. Blood vessel
e. Glue or gluelike
f. Hardening
g. Inflammation
h. Resembling
i. Softening
j. Speech
k. Spinal cord, bone marrow
l. Tumor

Write the meaning of each word part

a. –dynia
b. –ectomy
c. –edema
d. –logist
e. –malacia
f. –ptosis
g. –scope
h. –spasm
i. –stenosis
j. –aden/o
k. blephar/o
l. dipl/o
m. ophthalmo
n. retin/o
o. scler/o
p. encephal/o
q. neuro/o
r. a
s. adip/o
t. holo

## ACKNOWLEDGMENT

The authors wish to acknowledge the contributions of Pat Parteleno to this chapter.

## REFERENCES

1. Cohen BJ. *Medical Terminology: An Illustrated Guide*. Philadelphia, PA: Lippincott Williams & Wilkins; 1998.
2. Gylys BA, Masters RM. *Medical Terminology Simplified: A Programmed Learning Approach by Body Systems*. Philadelphia, PA: FA Davis; 1998.
3. Medical Terminology Online Version 2.0. 2001, 2003 SweetHaven Publishing Services. Available at http://www.free-ed.net/sweethaven/medtech/medterm/default.asp. Accessed March, 2014.
4. Express Scripts, Inc. Pharmacy Network Manual Guidelines, Policies and Procedures for Express Scripts, Inc. Network Pharmacies, 2005. Available at ftp://ftp.ihs.gov/rpms/POS/Payer%20Pharmacy%20Manuals/Express%20Scripts%20PharmacyNetworkManual.pdf. Accessed March, 2014.

CHAPTER

9

# Pharmacy Calculations

*A. Timothy Eley*

**Objectives: Upon completion of the chapter and exercises, the student pharmacist will be able to**

1. Interpret a prescription or medication order.
2. Convert between the metric and common systems of measurement.
3. Calculate an appropriate dose.
4. Prepare, concentrate, or dilute compounded medications accurately.
5. Interpret osmolarity, isotonicity, and milliequivalents.
6. Prepare isotonic solutions.
7. Reconstitute dry powders to appropriate concentration.
8. Utilize the aliquot method for solids and liquids.

---

### Patient Encounter

In the accident, patient X, suffered a deep abrasion on his leg and may eventually need a skin graft. Signs of infection are present and the decision has been made to irrigate the wound daily with modified Dakin's (diluted sodium hypochlorite) solution and use it on the wound dressing. You consult with the pharmacist in charge to confirm that the pharmacy has all of the ingredients. They are as follows:

Clorox bleach (standard 5.25% strength, not "ultra")
Sodium bicarbonate (1/2 tsp per quart)
Sterile water

The hospital order merely says the following:
Modified Dakin's solution 1/4%, gal #1
Use daily for wound cleansing and dressing on right leg

*(continued on next page)*

216

Questions to follow up in this case include:

1. How many milliliters of Clorox would be needed to make a gallon of this irrigation?

2. Who do you need to go to in the pharmacy to see that this order is correctly processed?

3. What are the procedures in the pharmacy for double check on the calculations?

4. Why did you choose this over an antibiotic?

Solution follows:

$$(5.25\%)(X) = (0.25\%)(3785 \text{ mL})$$
$$X = [(0.25\%)(3785 \text{ mL})]/5.25\%$$
$$= 180 \text{ mL}$$

## INTRODUCTION

The profession of pharmacy is one in which mathematics is used extensively. With the exception of some pharmacokinetic expressions, most of the calculations you will be expected to perform will be simple arithmetic. That being said, *the importance of not making errors in your arithmetic cannot be overemphasized.* An error in a calculation by a pharmacist could easily be the difference between life and death. You should develop several methods to check your work as you go. Estimate the final answer before beginning the work. Anything quite different from your approximation should cause you to reexamine your work. As you progress further into your pharmacy education and your career, you will become more comfortable with estimating what these answers should be in a given situation and for a given patient, such that you can identify an unreasonable solution relatively easily.

In order for this chapter to be brief, basic math is not reviewed. There are a multitude of reliable resources for such material. You are expected to be able to perform basic arithmetic (addition, subtraction, division, and multiplication) and to do so not only with whole numbers or integers but with fractions as well. Last, you are expected to be able to interpret Roman numerals.

This chapter is not meant to be an exhaustive review of the subject matter and should not be considered a substitute for a full course or text on the material. If you are interested in reviewing this subject in more detail, there are several suitable texts available. The latest edition of *Pharmaceutical Calculations* by H. C. Ansel[1] is a valuable resource, as this text could be considered the apparent gold standard for this material. The latest edition of *Remington: The Science and Practice of Pharmacy*[2] has a chapter on calculations that includes information about the history of different weights and measures that pharmacists are expected to be able to use.

## Dimensional Analysis and Ratio/Proportion

In everyday practice you will be expected to convert a value expressed in a certain way (more formally a "denomination") into a value expressed a different way because circumstances dictate it. For instance, a physician has ordered an administration rate for an intravenous drug to be 5 mg/min. You have prepared an intravenous (IV) solution of that drug to have a concentration of 2 mg/mL. The nursing staff needs to know how to administer the IV solution in terms of flow rate (ie, volume per unit time) in order to achieve the administration rate desired by the physician. In order to provide the nursing staff with this answer, you need to determine the volume of the solution you have prepared that contains 5 mg of the drug and direct the nursing staff to administer that volume every minute. You could do this computation by using ratio and proportion or dimensional analysis, but dimensional analysis allows you to do the same calculation in a stepwise approach and be more cautious in the process. Dimensional analysis tends to be safer for the beginner. The calculation would be as follows:

$$\frac{5\ mg}{min} \times \frac{1\ mL}{2\ mg} = \frac{2.5\ mL}{min}$$

Most of the conversions you have to deal with are rather straightforward, like the one above. Frequently we have somewhat uncomplicated problems to solve, for example, "What amount of active ingredient X will give us a 5% ointment when incorporated into ointment base Y," and so on. Prescriptions requiring compounding with several ingredients tend to be more difficult.

## Significant Figures

The purpose of significant figures is to indicate how exact a measurement is. For example, the *absolute number* 54,021.3 has a value of exactly 54,021.3, but the *measurement* 54,021.3 g means exactly 54,021 and approximately 3/10 of a gram. The measurement has six significant figures. If you **add or subtract** a number with more or fewer significant figures, what you need to be worried about is how many digits there are behind (ie, to the right of) the decimal place. For instance, if I want to add 3.222 g to 54,021.3 g, the answer cannot have more than one digit behind the decimal place because 54,021.3 g has only one (the three). The sum cannot be reported as 54,024.522 g; rather it is reported as 54,024.5 g. Because the 0.3 in 54,021.3 g was only approximate, that means that now the 0.5 at the end of 54,024.5 g is only approximate. When **multiplying or dividing**, the answer will have the same number of significant figures as the value with the fewest significant figures in the problem. For example, if you multiply 3.222 by 54,021.3, the answer will have only four significant figures, even though the number of digits in the answer may exceed that value. The product of these two numbers is 17,410 to the nearest ten, which has only four significant figures (the zero is not significant in this case). The only exception to this rule is when you multiply or divide by an absolute number, such as 3. If you are compounding three suppositories that each need to have 125 mg of active ingredient, the quantity you need to prepare them properly is not 400 to the nearest 100 (one significant figure) but 375 mg to the nearest 1 because all three significant figures are retained. The absolute number 3 is not an approximate figure; it is treated as three followed by the decimal place and an infinite number of zeroes, so the number of significant figures in the other number are the only ones of importance. Significant figures in the practice of pharmacy are primarily related to how much accuracy we need to have when measuring out one or more ingredients for compounding in a prescription. If multiple ingredients are listed, each measurement is expected to have the same accuracy as the ingredient listed with the greatest number of significant figures.

For example, you need to compound a cough preparation with 0.125 g of active ingredient A and 0.5 g of active ingredient B. It is implied that the amount of ingredient B that is required is 0.500 g because three significant figures were used to signify the desired amount of ingredient A. Furthermore, it is implied for any prescription requiring compounding that the ingredients be measured to at least three-figure accuracy. To summarize, you should be prepared to measure anything to three-figure accuracy unless greater accuracy is required. Now that you are aware of the accuracy required, you have to assess whether you are able, when asked, to measure with that level of accuracy, and if not, find ways to work around those limitations.

## THE PRESCRIPTION OR MEDICATION ORDER

Interpretation of prescriptions is a skill that most students pick up rapidly. It is usually more difficult to read the physician's handwriting than it is to interpret what is written. There will be occasion for you to accurately assess the meaning of abbreviations used. These abbreviations tell you what commercially available or to-be-compounded medication is requested by the physician and the directions to pass along to the patient. Due to medication errors resulting from misinterpreted prescriptions, there are several groups that have promoted moving away from not only abbreviations but hand-written prescriptions as well. Thus, you may find that more and more prescriptions you encounter are typed or electronically transmitted to the pharmacy, depending on the regulations in your jurisdiction. Chapter 7 discusses the legal requirements of filling prescription orders.

Selected abbreviations that are in frequent use appear in Table 9.1.

**TABLE 9.1. EXAMPLES OF PHARMACY ABBREVIATIONS AND INTERPRETATIONS**

| Abbreviation | Meaning | Abbreviation | Meaning |
| --- | --- | --- | --- |
| aa | Of each | o.d. | Right eye |
| a.c. | Before meals | o.s. or o.l. | Left eye |
| Ad | Up to | o.u. | Each eye |
| a.d. | Right ear | $O_2$ | Both eyes, oxygen |
| a.s. or a.l. | Left ear | p | After |
| a.u. | Each ear | p.c. | After meals |
| b.i.d. | Twice a day | p.o. | By mouth |
| c$^a$ | With | p.r.n. | As needed |
| dil. | Dilute | q.d. | Every day |
| disp. | Dispense | q.h. | Every hour |
| div. | Divide | q.i.d. | Four times a day |
| d.t.d. | Give of such doses | q.o.d. | Every other day |
| Et | And | q.s | A sufficient quantity |
| ft. | Make | q.s. ad | A sufficient quantity to make |
| gr or gr. | Grain | s$^a$ | Without |
| gtt. | Drop or drops | ss$^a$ | One half |
| h.s. | At bedtime | s/s or s&s | Signs/symptoms |
| M. | Mix | tid | Three times a day |
| mEq | Milliequivalent | u.d. or ut dict | As directed |
| N&V or N/V | Nausea and vomiting | ung. or oint. | Ointment |
| non rep or N.R. | Do not repeat | w/a or w.a. | While awake |
| NPO | Nothing by mouth | | |

$^a$These may appear with or without a horizontal line over them. Either way, the meaning is unchanged.

**TABLE 9.2. APOTHECARY WEIGHT**

| Pounds | Ounces | Drams | Scruples | Grains |
|--------|--------|-------|----------|--------|
| 1 | 12 | 96 | 288 | 5760 |
| | 1 | 8 | 24 | 480 |
| | | 1 | 3 | 60 |
| | | | 1 | 20 |

**TABLE 9.3. AVOIRDUPOIS WEIGHT**

| Pounds | Ounces | Grains |
|--------|--------|--------|
| 1 | 16 | 7000 |
| | 1 | 437.5 |

## COMMON SYSTEMS OF MEASUREMENT AND CONVERSION

In the past, pharmacists were required to use the apothecary and avoirdupois systems of measurement. You are still expected to be able to work with these systems of measurement because you may receive prescriptions written in such terminology. Understanding them will allow you to convert rapidly to the metric system and proceed accordingly. It is not necessary for you to memorize these tables in their entirety to work effectively with these systems of measure. The apothecary and avoirdupois system of weights appear in a useful format in Tables 9.2 and 9.3, respectively.

The grain measure in either of these systems is equivalent, but the weight of the pound and the ounce differs between the systems. The avoirdupois system of weight is the one in general use in the United States (eg, at the grocery store). The dram and scruple do not exist in the avoirdupois system. Do your best not to confuse these two systems of weights. Fortunately, the apothecary system of volume is the only system to learn. The gallon, ounce, pint, and quart are familiar measurements of volume seen routinely in the United States. One would rarely have occasion to use the fluidram or minim outside the practice of pharmacy. Like the dram and the scruple, these terms are probably new to you. The apothecary system of volume appears in Table 9.4, in the same format previously used for weights.

### Conversion to the Metric System

If you receive a prescription using a common system of measure, you will probably find it easiest to convert to metric units before preparing it. Table 9.5 contains those metric conversions that tend to be most useful.

**TABLE 9.4.** APOTHECARY VOLUME

| Gallons | Quarts | Pints | Fluidounces | Fluidrams | Minims |
|---------|--------|-------|-------------|-----------|--------|
| 1 | 4 | 8 | 128 | 1024 | 61,440 |
|   | 1 | 2 | 32 | 256 | 15,360 |
|   |   | 1 | 16 | 128 | 7,680 |
|   |   |   | 1 | 8 | 480 |
|   |   |   |   | 1 | 60 |

**TABLE 9.5.** USEFUL METRIC CONVERSIONS

| Common weight/measure | Metric equivalent |
|-----------------------|-------------------|
| 1 fluid ounce | 29.57 mL |
| 1 pint | 473 mL |
| 1 gallon (US) | 3785 mL |
| 1 pound (avoirdupois) | 454 g |
| 1 pound (apothecary) | 373 g |
| 1 ounce (avoirdupois) | 28.35 g |
| 1 ounce (apothecary) | 31.1 g |
| 1 grain | 64.8 mg |
| 2.2 pounds (avoirdupois) | 1 kg |

*Conversions of Convenience*

For ease of use, several *approximate* conversions are in widespread use by pharmacists and physicians. These are: 1 teaspoonful = 5 mL = 1 fluidram, 1 tablespoonful = 15 mL = ½ fluid ounce, and 30 mL = 1 fluid ounce. Of these, the teaspoonful is the farthest from the fluidram, both in absolute value and in relative value. For the vast majority of drugs, the difference in effect will be negligible because most drugs are safe within a wide range of concentrations in the body.

## CALCULATION OF DOSES

The most basic calculation you will perform will be the calculation of a reasonable dose for a patient. The "normal" or "usual" dose for any drug is one that produces the desired response in *most* individuals. It is important to note that the normal dose or dosing interval (once daily, twice daily, etc.) is not always appropriate for everyone. Drug distribution and elimination—covered in more detail in Chapter 12—can usually be related to a patient's body weight or body surface area (BSA) such that the most appropriate dose is tied to those patient demographics (eg, 5 mg/kg or 250 mg/m$^2$ of drug X). The normal or average adult individual is considered to weigh 70 kg or have 1.73 m$^2$ of BSA. Although calculating a dose using the previous method focuses on body size, a patient's age can further influence the selection of an appropriate dose because body composition (in terms of water, fat, and muscle) and organ function (especially liver and kidney) vary with age. These differences in body composition and organ function can affect drug distribution and elimination, which in turn alters the most appropriate dose. Other factors may affect your final recommendation, depending on your area of practice. You will find yourself considering some or all of these things repeatedly in practice, and your preceptors will familiarize you with any specialized calculations they use when optimizing a dosing regimen.

## RATIO STRENGTH AND PERCENTAGE

Several of the active ingredients in products you prepare, dispense, and use will not be pure substances. Rather, they will be diluted in something else (eg, water, syrup, one inactive ingredient, or more). The strength of these products may be represented as a percentage or ratio strength, such as 5% dextrose in water. Percentage is a term that implies "out of a hundred" such that 5% dextrose in water means 5 g dextrose in every 100 mL of water. Percentage and ratio strength may be represented as weight/weight (w/w), volume/volume (v/v), or weight/volume (w/v). If it is not obvious which one of these three applies, it should be noted. Weight/weight is probably the most difficult to use. Percentage really is a ratio strength as well, but think of ratio strength as ratios always represented as 1 to some other quantity that is 1 or larger. Examples of these kinds of ratios are 1:1, 1:5, 1:14, 1:1000, and 1:15,000. A ratio of 1:1 would indicate equal parts. Ratio strength not represented in percentage terms can be changed to percentage and vice versa. You may find it easier when doing ratio and proportion calculations to alter any ratio strength notations to percentages. For example, the 5% dextrose in water above is 1:20 ratio strength because 5 out of 100 simplifies to 1:20. When you need to convert ratio strength to percentage, you have to find out how many parts out of 100 it represents. As another example, 1:1000 represents 0.1% because for every 100 total parts, there is 0.1 part of the ingredient that is in this ratio strength.

## Dilution/Concentration

If you are not starting with basic active elements, you should be able to handle using a concentrated stock solution/compound to make a more dilute solution/compound. Let us say you have an aqueous stock solution that is 25% (w/v) of some drug and we need to dilute it such that the final solution will be 1:2000. We need to know how much of the stock solution and water we need to produce the 1:2000 solution. Basically, you need 1 g in 2 L of water in the final product (1:2000), so you need to figure out how much of the stock solution gives you 1 g of the drug. The difference between that volume and 2 L is the additional water to add to make 1:2000.

$$1\,g \times \frac{100\ mL}{2.5\ g} = 4\ mL$$

Therefore, 4 mL of the stock solution contains 1 g of the active ingredient. We should measure out 4 mL of the stock solution and dilute to 2000 mL with water.

An alternative way to do this calculation is to find out what the percentage strength is of the 1:2000 solution and use mass balance to solve for the quantity of stock solution. In the following equation, $x$ is the percentage strength of the 1:2000 solution:

$$\frac{1\,g}{2000\ mL} = \frac{x}{100\ mL}$$

The percentage strength is 0.05% because $x = 0.05$ g. Next we can set the percentage strength and the volume of the stock and dilute solutions equal to one another, knowing that the amount (mass) of drug in each of them is equivalent, with the volume of the stock solution as the unknown, $y$:

$$(0.05\%)\,(2000\ mL) = (25\%)\,(y)$$

The answer is 4 mL, the same as with the other method of calculation.

Another example using an ointment might be that we have a supply of an ointment in which the active ingredient is found to be 10% (w/w), and we need to make 60 g of 0.25% (1:400) ointment from that supply. Again the process is that you need to figure out how much of the active ingredient is required to complete the compound and then how much stock ointment contains that amount. After you know the amount of the stock compound to use, make up the remainder with ointment base.

$$60\ g\ \text{final product} \times \frac{0.25\ g\ \text{active ingredient}}{100\ g\ \text{final product}} = 0.15\ g\ \text{active ingredient}$$

$$0.15 \text{ active ingredient} \times \frac{100 \text{ g stock ointment}}{10 \text{ g active ingredient}} = 1.5 \text{ g stock ointmemt}$$

You would weigh out 1.5 g of the stock ointment and 58.5 g of the ointment base and mix well in an appropriate manner such as geometric dilution. Similar calculations are useful in making a more concentrated stock solution or similar compound. These sorts of calculations can be simplified if we use alligation methods.

Alligation is especially useful if we have two stock compounds of different ratio strengths and we need to make a third. Note that an ointment base has ratio strength of zero. We can use the alligation to tell us how many parts of each are required (relative proportions) to make any quantity of the final product. Once the desired final quantity is known, you divide the total quantity of the final product by the total number of parts required in the alligation to find the weight or volume of one part. Then multiply the number of parts required by that weight or volume. Let us reuse one of the above problems to illustrate this method.

| Concentration of Drug in Ointment | Concentration of Drug in Final Compounded Product | Number of Parts | Weight of Material |
|---|---|---|---|
| 10% | | 0.25 | 1.5 g |
| | 0.25% | | |
| 0% (ointment base) | | 9.75 | 58.5 g |
| | | 10 parts total | 60 g total |

Because 60 g of the final product is desired, 60 g is equivalent to 10 parts. Therefore, one part is 6 g. To find the amount of 10% ointment to use, you multiply 0.25 parts by 6 g to get 1.5 g of the 10% ointment, which is the same answer we generated above. For the ointment base, you multiply 9.75 parts by 6 g to get 58.5 g of the ointment base, which, again, is the same answer as before. The number of parts of each component required for the final compound is the difference in percentage concentration between the concentration of drug in the final compound and that of the *other* component. You can see above that the difference between 10% and 0.25% is 9.75, but you represent the answer in parts, not percentages. This answer is the number of parts of the ointment base (0%). The opposite calculation supplies you with the figure 0.25 parts, which is the obvious difference between 0.25% and 0%. This method is extremely useful because of its relative speed once you master the process. In order to make a stock solution/compound or to concentrate one you have, you must know what the desired concentration is and from where you are starting. Suppose you want to make a stock ointment more concentrated, to contain, for example, 40% (w/w) of active ingredient instead of 30% (w/w). The final quantity desired is 2000 g. With alligation (illustrated below), the difference between the concentration of pure drug (100%) and the final stock ointment (40%) is 60. The difference between concentration in the present stock (30% w/w) and final stock (40% w/w) ointments is 10. The total number of parts to make 2000 g of ointment is 70, or 28.57 g/part.

| Concentration of Drug in Ointment | Concentration of Drug in Final Compounded Product | Number of Parts | Weight of Material |
|---|---|---|---|
| 30% | | 60 | 1714.3 g |
| | 40% | | |
| 100% (pure drug) | | 10 | 285.7 g |
| | | 70 parts total | 2000 g total |

You would use 60 parts × 28.57 g/part or 1714.3 g of the 30% w/w ointment, and 10 parts × 28.57 g/part or 285.7 g of pure drug. Once properly incorporated, you will have 2000 g of the 40% w/w ointment you wanted.

## ALIQUOTS

When you get into a situation where you need to measure an amount of material that is too small to measure accurately with the equipment you have, you may be forced to use the aliquot method. The standard pharmacy balance has a sensitivity requirement of 6 mg, and the maximum acceptable error in our measurement is 5%. These two figures generate the least weighable amount (LWA) of 120 mg on these balances. This amount is a number that will be repeated to you frequently in your pharmaceutics compounding laboratory. The LWA is the smallest quantity that can be measured with acceptable error. Electronic balances have become much more common. If you are using an electronic balance, you should consult the documentation that came with it to determine the LWA.

When using the aliquot method, we weigh out an amount of the substance in question that is equal to or in excess of the LWA for the balance. Then, you dilute that amount with a known quantity of inert material, mix well, and weigh out the portion of the mixture that contains the desired amount of the substance.

You must remember that everything you weigh on the balance must be equal to or in excess of the LWA. For example, you could not weigh out 120 mg of active ingredient, 120 mg of inert substance, mix well, and weigh 80 mg to take the desired quantity of the active ingredient. Eighty milligrams is less than the LWA, so this measurement is not acceptable. There are multiple keys to doing an aliquot properly. First, you have to choose an amount of the active ingredient you want that is at least the LWA. If at all possible, this amount should be a whole-number multiple of the amount you truly need. Second, you must weigh out a quantity of an appropriately chosen inert substance that is more than or equal to the LWA. The inert substance should be compatible with the active ingredient and all other ingredients of the final product. You must weigh out enough inert substance such that the amount of the mixture to be weighed in the end will be at least the LWA. This decision will take some forethought so as to prevent the example given previously in which the final amount to be weighed was not at least the LWA. The advantage of weighing out a whole-number multiple of the desired quantity makes it easier to select this amount and compute the final amount to be weighed. If you need 50 mg of diphenhydramine, it makes your life much easier to weigh out 150 mg (three times the needed quantity). Here's how: no matter how much inert substance you mix with the 150 mg of diphenhydramine, one-third of it will contain 50 mg of diphenhydramine, assuming uniform mixing (if you had measured out four times the needed amount or 200 mg of diphenhydramine, one-fourth of the eventual mixture will contain 50 mg of diphenhydramine; if you measured out five times what you need, one-fifth of the mixture has the desired quantity and so on). Knowing that you need one-third of the eventual mixture and that this amount must be at least 120 mg, you know that you must make a total quantity of the mixture that is not less than 360 mg. In order to proceed, you could weigh out 210 mg of the inert substance (360 mg – 150 mg), mix well with a mortar and pestle, and 120 mg of the mixture should contain 50 mg of diphenhydramine. Third, the quantity of inert substance selected must be reasonable and typically as little as necessary. For example, you would not make an aliquot with 2 g of inert substance if it could be reasonably performed with 200 mg. In other words, you would not want to have an aliquot that is excessively large. Within reason, conserve the raw materials as best you can and waste only what you must in order to prepare the prescription properly. Costs of compounding are passed along to the consumer (typically including the costs of any waste), so minimize waste, especially when the cost of these materials is high.

Another way to measure a small quantity of a solid could be to measure out a quantity at least the LWA and dissolve it in a suitable solvent. Once it has dissolved, you may be able to measure the solution more reliably, depending on what fluids you have to measure. The proper portion of the solution would contain the right amount of drug. The process is the same. An aliquot method of measuring also exists for volumes that cannot be measured reliably. A good general rule is that one cannot measure accurately a volume that is less than 20% of the total volume of the vessel (eg, 2 mL is the smallest volume measured reliably in a 10 mL graduate). You should measure any volume in the smallest vessel available so as to minimize the potential error in the measurement. If calibrating a dropper is not a reasonable option, measure out a volume accurately using what volumetric tools you have available and dilute in an inert, miscible fluid that is compatible with all other materials in the prescription. Once the fluids are in solution, an aliquot of the mixture can be measured accurately, if properly prepared. These steps are similar to those used in the aliquot method of weighing. The use of a dropper may be indicated if the dropper is properly calibrated for the liquid in question. Remember that a dropper must be calibrated for every liquid to be used; the volume of one drop will vary based on the liquid. There are several references you could refer to for instructions on how to calibrate a dropper.

## TONICITY AND OSMOLARITY

### Isotonic Solutions

There may come a time when you are asked to prepare an isotonic solution. An isotonic solution has the same osmotic pressure as the body fluid it is to be mixed with. Such a solution will be easy to tolerate by the patient, as hypertonic or hypo-tonic solutions may cause discomfort or other unwanted effects. Ophthalmic (for the eye), parenteral (by injection), nasal (for the nose), and some enema (per rectum) preparations are those for which you would most likely see the condition of isotonic-ity placed on your compounding. Normal saline is 0.9% sodium chloride in water, or 9 g of NaCl in 1000 mL of water. This solution is considered to be isotonic with the body fluids. Through extensive work, a table of relationships of tonicity between other substances and sodium chloride has been established. These relationships are collectively called "sodium chloride equivalents." One gram of each of the substances listed has the same tonicity as the number of grams of sodium chloride listed. For instance, 1 g of silver nitrate is equivalent to 0.33 g of sodium chloride because in solution silver nitrate does not have the same tonicity as NaCl. Approximately 3 g of silver nitrate would have the same tonicity as 1 g of sodium chloride in solution (3 × 0.33 g = 0.99 g). The availability of these tables enables us to quickly calculate the appropriate preparation of an isotonic solution with the components listed. For example, the physician writes for 1 oz of 1% pilocarpine nitrate in purified water made isotonic with sodium chloride. If you use 30 mL for 1 oz to make it easier, we know that we need 0.3 g of pilocarpine nitrate. One gram of pilocarpine nitrate is equivalent to 0.23 g sodium chloride, so

$$0.3 \text{ g pilocarpine nitrate} \times \frac{0.23 \text{ g sodium chloride}}{1 \text{ g pilocarpine nitrate}} = 0.069 \text{ g sodium chloride}$$

Therefore, 0.3 g pilocarpine nitrate has the same tonicity as 0.069 g sodium chloride. Now, we need to know how much total sodium chloride would make 30 mL isotonic and subtract 0.069 g from that figure to solve for how much NaCl to add to the bottle.

$$30 \text{ mL} \times \frac{9 \text{ g}}{1000 \text{ mL}} = 0.27 \text{ g sodium chloride}$$

$$0.27 \text{ g} - 0.069 \text{ g} = 0.201 \text{ sodium chloride}$$

To properly compound these eye drops, we need to add 0.3 g pilocarpine nitrate and 0.201 g sodium chloride to an eyedropper bottle and dissolve it in enough purified water to make 30 mL of the solution. *Remington's Pharmaceutical Sciences* has an exhaustive list of sodium chloride equivalents, or you may find a table on the Internet. Obviously, use only resources you are sure you can trust.

## Electrolyte Solutions

A discussion of electrolyte solutions is really a continuation of the previous section on isotonicity. Compounds in solution that dissociate to some degree are called electrolytes. Good examples of electrolytes are sodium chloride and hydrochloric acid. This dissociation leads to the presence of ions that have positive (cations) or negative (anions) electric charges. Those compounds that do not dissociate are called nonelectrolytes. A good example of a nonelectrolyte is glucose. For a more comprehensive review of dissociation, electrolytes, and ions, consult your chemistry textbooks from past courses. You should remember from your chemistry background that concentration can be represented in many ways. In chemistry, you are more likely to use molarity or the number of moles of solute per liter of solution. Its formula or molecular weight gives the number of grams in a mole ($6.02 \times 10^{23}$ molecules) of a compound. A millimole (mmol) is 1/1000 of the molecular or formula weight of the compound in question. For example, the molecular weight of NaCl is 58.5 g. That means that 58.5 g of NaCl makes 1 mol of sodium chloride, and a millimole is 58.5 mg of NaCl. An equivalent weight is the mass of the species in question that is capable of providing 1 mol of positive or negative charge. Like the millimole, the milliequivalent (mEq) is 1/1000 of that weight. So in the case of NaCl, 1 mmol of NaCl is 1 mEq of NaCl because it is capable of providing 1 mol of positive or negative charge. Furthermore, there is 1 mEq of $Na^+$ and 1 mEq of $Cl^-$ in 1 mEq of NaCl. To get the number of milliequivalents, you multiply the number of millimoles present by the total number of positive or negative charges, not both. That's why the number of mEq of NaCl is the same as the number of mEq of $Na^+$ and $Cl^-$ because they are all multiplied by 1. In 1 mmol of $Na_2HPO_4$ there are 2 mEq of $Na_2HPO_4$ and 2 mEq of Na+ and 2 mEq of $HPO_4^{2-}$. In this case, the number of millimoles of sodium (2) and the number of millimoles of hydrogen phosphate (1) do not match up, but the numbers of milliequivalents do. The total number of positive charges should match up with the total number of negative charges, so the number of milliequivalents will as well. The concentration of electrolytes in the blood is likely to be represented in mEq/L or mEq/dL.

Next, the terms osmolarity and osmolality are introduced. Their importance to pharmacy is in the preparation of isotonic solutions and the proper addition of a certain number of equivalents to intravenous fluid or nutrition. Osmotic pressure is proportional to the number of particles in solution. Osmolarity refers to the number of *separate* particles in solution. One millimole of NaCl in a liter of solution represents 2 milliosmoles (mOsm) of NaCl because the sodium and the chloride will dissociate almost completely in solution. One millimole of a nonelectrolyte such as glucose will be 1 mOsm because it does not dissociate. The difference between osmolarity and osmolality is that osmolality is the number of species per kilogram of solution. It is important to remember all of these ways to represent concentration because you may find yourself changing from one to another depending on the situation. As suggested previously, osmolarity will be used frequently when isotonic preparations are being made. For example, you should know that normal saline (0.9% NaCl in water) is isotonic. Assuming complete dissociation, normal saline is 308 mOsm of NaCl per liter of water. The concentration is high enough that at each instance a few NaCl molecules are intact, so the true osmolarity is more like 286 mOsm/L. You should note whether the value being reported on any products you use or prepare is actual or ideal (assuming complete dissociation) osmolarity.

## RECONSTITUTION AND INTRAVENOUS ADMIXTURES

In order to increase the shelf life of a product, it may be produced by the manufacturer in dry powder form (constituted). If you need to dispense the medication or use it to prepare an intravenous medication for someone, you will be faced with having to reconstitute the drug. Reconstitution may produce a solution or a suspension. The most important factor to consider in reconstitution is the contribution of the dry powder to the volume of the reconstituted preparation. For example, if a vial of drug for intravenous use has a very small amount of drug; it will be unlikely that the drug contributes significantly to the volume once reconstituted. Therefore, the concentration of the constituted drug in the vial will simply be the amount of drug in the vial divided by the volume of the appropriate solvent (purified water, sterile water for injection, $D_5W$, NS, etc.). However, if the amount of drug is large enough that it will displace solvent, the volume you must add cannot be the total volume you want in the end. For example, several oral antibiotics come as dry powders in bottles ready for reconstitution. They have directions on the side indicating how much water to add to make the final volume correct. If 250 mL is the final volume, the amount the pharmacist is expected to add will typically be less than 250 mL and may be on the order of 200 mL. The drug itself and any other inactive ingredients (such as flavorings for oral medications) increase the volume of the final preparation, and in order to get the appropriate amount of medication per dose, the final volume must be correct. It is imperative that you follow the directions for reconstitution that accompany a medication requiring it.

With intravenous admixtures, you must make every effort to ensure that the correct amount of medication is in the intravenous solution. Not only is it important that you correctly calculate the amount to add to the IV fluid, but you must be sure to correctly make the addition as well. Suppose you have a 1 g vial of an IV drug that must be reconstituted. To properly reconstitute the drug, 8 mL of sterile water for injection must be added to the vial. Proper mixing produces 10 mL of solution.

If you want 250 mg of the drug, you must take one-fourth of the *final volume* of the drug in solution (2.5 mL)—not one-fourth of the volume you added (2 mL).

You have to take extra steps with intravenous admixtures because the drug will be administered into the circulation. Drugs administered IV need to be in solution if at all possible. Precipitation of drug in the veins can be disastrous. You will be faced with compatibility issues repeatedly: can this drug be reconstituted with solvent A? Is the drug stable in $D_5W$? Does the addition of potassium cause precipitation? Work with your professors, drug information resources, and preceptors to learn about these incompatibilities. Once an IV solution is prepared, as discussed earlier, you may be asked to calculate a flow rate based on either the desired rate of drug administration or based on the time over which the entire volume of the IV solution is to be administered. In another example, if there is 100 mg of drug in the IV solution and the physician wants the patient to receive 10 mg/h, then the drug can be administered for 10 hours before a new IV solution is needed to replace this one. Based on that figure, 1/10 of the volume in the solution must be administered per hour to provide the desired administration rate. You may also be asked to convert the flow rate to volume per minute. If that 100 mg is in a 1 L bag of normal saline (assuming no volume expansion by the drug), the flow rate (mL/min) can be calculated as follows:

$$\frac{10\,mg}{h} \times \frac{1000\,mL}{100\,mg} \times \frac{1\,h}{60\,min} = 1.67\,mL/min$$

If the IV solution with all of its contents is to be given over an 8-hour period, you divide the total volume of IV solution by the time period. If it were a 500 mL solution, the flow rate would be 62.5 mL/h or approximately 1 mL/min. Nurses are frequently responsible for calculating a drip rate that correlates to the desired flow rate. Gravity helps drive the IV solution into the circulation, and a device attached to the IV line can be adjusted to allow a certain number of drops of the IV solution to fall per minute through a small chamber. Just as in calibrating a dropper, you must find out how many drops are in a milliliter using the given equipment and solve accordingly. You may never be asked to do this calculation, but some practice settings may have the pharmacist calculate the drip rate as well.

## SUMMARY

The diversity and frequency of the calculations you will be asked to perform will depend greatly on your practice site and any specialty on which you choose to focus. When you chose to become a pharmacist, mathematics became a much larger part of your life. Regardless of the calculation and the presence of electronic devices to assist you, work carefully; someone's life depends on it.

## APPLICATION EXERCISES

The answers are not provided for the exercises in this chapter. This is a good opportunity for you to work on these exercises and then discuss the answers with your faculty members in the appropriate courses.

1. Interpret each of the following prescription or medication orders:
   A. gtts. iv o.u. q.i.d.
   B. M.ft. ung. Disp. 30 g
   C. tab ss b.i.d. u.d.
   D. cap i tid p.c. et h.s.
2. Convert between the metric and common systems of measurement for each of the following:
   A. How many milliliters are in a pint? A quart? A gallon?
   B. How many milligrams are in 7 gr?
   C. How many grams are in an apothecary ounce?
   D. When can you interpret the fluidram as 5 mL?
3. Calculate an appropriate dose for each of the following problems:
   A. If the normal adult dose is 5 mg/kg/day, how many milligrams will the average adult receive in a day?
   B. If we must compound and dispense 4 oz fluid of syrup that has 15 mg of drug/tsp, how many milligrams are in 4 oz? If we dispense 8 oz at a strength of 5 mg/tsp, how many milligrams are in 8 oz?
   C. Assume that a drug is administered orally once daily at an approximate dose of 5 mg/kg of total body weight to adult patients but is only available in 150 mg tablets that cannot be split or crushed. For a person who weighs 320 lbs, what is the calculated daily dose in mg for this person? Under the limitation of the single strength of tablet available, what will be the most appropriate actual dose to administer?
4. Prepare, concentrate, or dilute compounded medications accurately in the following directions:
   A. An adult patient does not like solid dosage forms and requests an antibiotic suspension from the doctor that is not commercially available. If 500 mg of drug needs to be in each tablespoonful, how many milligrams of drug is needed for the suspension if the directions are to take 1 tablespoonful three times daily for 10 days?
   B. How many milligrams of drug are needed to make 200 g of a 30% (w/w) ointment? A 40% (w/w) ointment?
   C. Use the alligation method to determine how much of each stock solution is needed to make a 40% (w/v) solution? Stock solution A: 70% (w/v). Stock solution B: 20% (w/v).
   D. How many milliliters of water are needed to dilute 100 mL of a 10% (w/v) solution to a ratio strength of 1:200? To a ratio strength of 1:500?

  **E.** How many milliliters of water are needed to dilute 4 oz of 30% (w/v) to a strength of 2% (w/v)?

  **F.** Use the alligation method to determine how much of each stock ointment is needed to make a 20% (w/v) ointment? Stock ointment A: 5% (w/v). Stock ointment B: 25% (w/v). Solve the same problem with the 25% stock ointment and ointment base.

5. Interpret osmolarity, isotonicity, and milliequivalents for each of the following problems:

  **A.** How many milliosmoles are in 1 mmol of aluminum chloride?

  **B.** How many milliequivalents of sodium are in 300 mg of sodium chloride?

  **C.** What is the osmolarity of 0.45% NaCl? Of 0.9% NaCl?

  **D.** What is the osmolarity of $D_5W$ (5% dextrose in water)?

  **E.** How many milliosmoles are in 100 mg of $Na_2HPO_4$?

  **F.** How many milliequivalents are in 100 mg of sodium citrate?

6. Prepare isotonic solutions in the following cases:

  **A.** How many grams of sodium chloride are required to make the following prescription?

| | |
|---|---|
| Physostigmine sulfate | 1% |
| Sodium chloride | q.s. |
| Purified water | ad 30 mL |
| M. isotonic solution | |
| Sig: gtts ii o.d. b.i.d. | |

  **B.** How many grams of boric acid is required to make the following prescription?

| | |
|---|---|
| Cromolyn sodium | 2% |
| Boric acid | q.s. |
| Purified water | ad 60 mL |
| M. isotonic solution | |
| Sig: gtts. iv o.u. q.i.d. | |

7. Reconstitute dry powders to appropriate concentration for each of the following problems:

  **A.** The directions for reconstitution of an antibiotic are to add 188 mL of water to the bottle in order to achieve 250 mL of a 250 mg/5 mL solution. What volume of water would be required to make a 150 mg/5 mL solution?

  **B.** The directions for reconstitution on a 500-mg injection vial are to add 9 mL of normal saline for injection to make 10 mL of solution. What is the concentration of the drug in the vial after reconstitution? How many milliliters would you extract from the vial to get 125 mg?

  **C.** You have appropriately reconstituted 1 g of a drug and placed it in a 500-mL-IV bag of normal saline. What rate of flow (in mL/min) will deliver (1) 25 mg/h of the drug (2) 100 mg/h?

8. Utilize the aliquot method for solids and liquids to complete the answer to the following problems:
   A. Explain how you would use the aliquot method of weighing to obtain 10 mg of codeine sulfate if you have a standard pharmacy balance. Use lactose as an inert diluent.
   B. Explain how you would use the aliquot method of weighing to obtain 5 mg of sodium phenobarbital if you have a standard pharmacy balance. Use lactose as an inert diluent.
   C. Explain how you would use the aliquot method for measuring volume if you need 0.5 mL of a 10 mg/mL solution and the smallest graduate cylinder you have is 10 mL (use 20% least measurable volume rule here). Use water as a diluent.

## REFERENCES

1. Ansel HC. *Pharmaceutical Calculations.* 14th ed. Philadelphia, PA: Lippincott Williams & Wilkins; 2012.
2. *Remington: The Science and Practice of Pharmacy.* 22nd ed. London: Pharmaceutical Press; 2012.

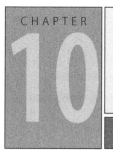

CHAPTER

# Physical Assessment Skills

*Cristina E. Bello-Quintero*

**Objectives: Upon completion of the chapter and exercises, the student pharmacist will be able to**

1. Communicate the importance of physical assessment skills for pharmacists.
2. Name four skills involved in the physical examination.
3. Describe and demonstrate the technique for taking an accurate blood pressure.
4. Explain the process and procedures used to complete a thorough physical examination.

---

### Patient Encounter

Physical Assessment Skills for Pneumonia

*Discussion for the Introductory Pharmacy Practice Experience*

1. State why physical assessment skills are important in evaluation of pneumonia.

2. List information to obtain from medical record that may complement the physical examination.

3. How could physical assessment be used to monitor clinical improvement or deterioration of pneumonia?

*Discussion for the Advanced Pharmacy Practice Experience*

1. What clues does the sputum color give as to the cause of the pneumonia?

2. How may sepsis present on physical examination?

Physical findings for 26-year-old African American with pneumonia:
*RR: 28*
Tachypnea: an increased respiratory rate with normal depth of breathing

---

*(continued on next page)*

*Positive whispered pectoriloquy*

Whispered pectoriloquy is the sound of whispered words by the patient while the chest is being auscultated. The patient is asked to whisper "ninety nine" while the lung fields are auscultated. When a consolidation is present, such as with pneumonia, the whispering is transmitted through the chest wall more clearly. Radiographs and computed tomography have led to a decrease in the use of this physical assessment skill.

*Positive egophony*

Egophony is the increased resonance of voice sounds, with a high-pitched or nasal quality of normal voice tones heard through the chest wall during auscultation. An "E" spoken by the patient should sound like an "E" in the absence of underlying lung pathology. In the presence of a consolidation, the "E" sound will change to an "A" sound.

*Positive tactile fremitus*

Fremitus is a palpable vibration. It may be created by the vocal cords during speech. To assess for tactile fremitus, ask the patient to repeat the word "ninety nine" while you palpate the thorax with the ulnar sides of your hands. Increased fremitus is caused by any condition that increases the density of the lung as with consolidation that occurs in pneumonia.

*Dullness to percussion*

Percussion of the chest wall produces a sound useful in evaluating the underlying lung tissue. Percussion over normal lung is described as normal resonance. Decreased resonance is due to increase lung tissue density such as pneumonia.

*Bronchial breath sounds and inspiratory crackles*

Auscultation

Auscultation of the lungs should include all lobes on the anterior, lateral, and posterior chest. It is best to compare side-to-side and evaluate at least one full ventilatory cycle at each stethoscope position. Bronchial breath sounds are harsh and higher pitched with approximately equal

*(continued on next page)*

inspiratory and expiratory components. This is the sound heard over a major bronchus during normal breathing. Adventitious breath sounds are not normal sounds and include wheezes, rhonchi, and crackles. Crackles are probably produced by the bubbling of air through the airway secretion or by the sudden opening of the small airway.

The examination of a patient with pneumonia involves inspection of the chest, palpation, percussion, and auscultation. The observant student may begin their assessment from the patient's doorway prior to entering the room. Is the patient coughing? What is the patient's respiratory rate? What is the patient's breathing pattern? Are there any signs of shortness of breath? In addition, the student should evaluate the overall patient including assessment of vital signs, skin examination for cyanosis and edema, and mental status changes.

## INTRODUCTION

Pharmacy practice is returning to its roots as a patient-centered care profession. This change in scope of practice provides pharmacists with the opportunity to advance their knowledge and be able to use physical examination skills as part of daily practice. The advent of pharmaceutical care as a philosophy augmented the role of the pharmacist charging them with provision of responsible drug therapy.[1] Unfortunately, even though the term was widely used in pharmacy circles, outside of the profession pharmaceutical care never caught on, perhaps because the public did not understand what it meant. The term medication therapy management has been regulated, and despite the fact that it does not cover the entire scope of a pharmacist's practice, it does seem to be recognized as a term associated with a pharmacist by the lay public and insurance providers. Medication therapy management legislation in the United States expanded the role of the pharmacist. The scope of pharmacy practice continues to evolve in many states and other countries. This expanded responsibility includes the use of physical assessment knowledge and skills for disease management, immunization, and drug therapy evaluation and monitoring.[2] Knowledge and practice in physical assessment can lead to improved dialogue between pharmacists and other health-care professionals as well as the patient.[2]

Pharmacy students should have the opportunity to participate in the physical examination process during many practices of pharmacy courses, both introductory and advanced. To prepare for learning and practicing these skills, it is important to own the proper tools. A stethoscope and sphygmomanometer for use during formal education should be purchased prior to the first course that incorporates physical examination (Fig. 10.1).

**Figure 10.1.** Stethoscope and sphygmomanometer.

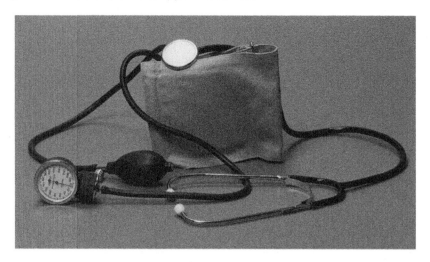

Familiarity with the process of performing physical examination maneuvers and the language used to document physical findings allows for comprehensive planning to be completed during patient encounters and when rounding as a member of the medical team. This chapter introduces basic concepts and provides discussion of relevant aspects of the physical examination that are pertinent to patient-centered care, disease management, and medication therapy management. A summary of the physical examination approach found in this chapter, along with emphasis on key findings related to drug therapy, should be used in conjunction with other resources to strengthen your knowledge and test your skills.

## BASIC PHYSICAL ASSESSMENT TECHNIQUE

The skilled clinician is able to complete systematic, thorough, and accurate physical examinations quickly in a variety of situations. The order of the examination may differ between clinicians, but the systematic approach taken by a single practitioner should remain the same from patient to patient. Develop your own style as you progress through the introductory and advanced-practice experiences always doing the examination in the same order by organ system. During the examination, a practitioner engages five skills. These are communication (listening), inspection, palpation, percussion, and auscultation. It is important to listen to the patient during medical interviews and the physical examination. Inspection refers to observation and looking at the patient or the region of the body being examined and taking note of things such as symmetry, presence or absence of hair, redness (erythema), scars, or lesions of any kind. Palpation involves touching the part of the body being examined taking care to notice any wincing or grimacing on the part of the patient to indicate pain. In addition, the clinician should note any masses that are not obvious by inspection alone. Percussion utilizes a tapping motion with the finger to determine whether a compartment is filled with air, fluid, or solid materials. For example, normal lungs have a tympanic sound to percussion, while a person with pneumonia will have a lung sound that is dull by comparison indicating such things as consolidation or fluid, which is an abnormal finding. Finally, auscultation refers to listening to a part of the body for normal or abnormal sounds with the help of a stethoscope.

Before beginning the actual physical examination, it is necessary to gather specific information by asking questions and listening to the patient. Conducting the medical interview and taking the medical history may help you understand more about the patient than any other component of the physical assessment. During this phase, the pharmacist asks essential questions about the patient's health history. The importance of taking a good medical and medication history should not be underestimated. Sir William Osler, considered the Father of Modern Medicine, once said, "Listen to the patient, he is telling you the diagnosis." Many times patients go to a physician or other health professional because a specific problem is of concern to them. The way the patient identifies the problem becomes their chief complaint and this guides much of the history taking (Table 10.1). The clinician should ask when and where the symptoms first began, qualitative (subjective) and quantitative (objective) factors relating to the complaint, associated symptoms, and any exacerbating or alleviating factors. The interviewer will also want to know if the patient has any history of the same or similar complaints, as well as any prior treatments and tests for this complaint. Included in the complete medical history, regardless of chief complaint, is information about the patient's other medical problems and family history, significant illnesses or surgeries, allergies, medications, habits such as cigarette smoking, caffeine intake, drug and/or alcohol use, as well as a review of organ systems not directly related to the chief complaint. Some patients will be unable to provide an accurate history, young children, patients with dementia, or other memory problems and the seriously injured may require help or input from family or friends to provide the information. If there are no family members or medical records to consult, then being confident in one's physical assessment skills become even more important. Table 10.2 provides sample questions that may aid in obtaining a medical history.

## PRECAUTIONS

Before beginning any examination, members of the health-care team must take the time to observe universal precautions to protect themselves and their patients. Health-care workers should also make sure they are up-to-date on all immunizations as well as undergo yearly tuberculosis screening via purified protein derivative (PPD)

---

**TABLE 10.1.  PATIENT MEDICAL HISTORY**
..........................................................................................................................

The following categories of information should be obtained during a medical history:
The pharmacist/student should meet with the patient to review this information to verify
completeness and accuracy

- *Patient information:* name, date of birth, address, phone number, insurance company, gender, height, weight.

- *Chief complaint:* document this in the patients exact choice of words.

- *Lifestyle, social information:* tobacco, alcohol, caffeine use; impairments; exercise; pregnancy/breastfeeding issues; diet.

- *Doctor information:* determine if the patient is currently under the care of a physician, and if so, obtain a list of all physicians and their phone numbers, whenever possible, to facilitate communication.

- *Allergies:* list drugs, foods, chemicals, others—have the patient describe all symptoms or reaction they experienced when taking the drug, when it occurred, how long it lasted, and the treatment. Identifying all symptoms will help determine if the event was an allergic reaction or whether the patient just did not tolerate a treatment.

- *Over-the-counter (OTC) medications:* have the patient indicate which conditions they occasionally or regularly self-treat with nonprescription (OTC) medications, herbals, vitamins, minerals, or homeopathic remedies. Then, have the patient identify the OTC products used occasionally or regularly, including the category of nutritional/natural products.

- *Medical conditions/diseases:* identify all conditions for which the patient is receiving medical care or may be self-treating.

- *Prescription medications:* the patient should list all prescription medications they are currently using. Patients should be sure to include any medications obtained via mail order, Internet pharmacies, or physician samples.

If appropriate, complete vital signs and other physical assessment parameters as appropriate for setting.

Document all findings in order beginning with the chief complaint. Document the subjective information first, followed by the facts as you are able to determine them.

This is the objective component and includes laboratory findings that are available, and the physical examination findings.

---

placement (and any other screening modalities required by the specific institution). Universal precautions involve the creation of a barrier between the clinician's skin and mucus membranes from potentially infectious materials. Hand washing should take place before and after every patient encounter. Gloves should be worn any time

---

**TABLE 10.2.** SAMPLE QUESTIONS TO BE ASKED OF PATIENTS DURING
A HISTORY

- What brings you here today?
- When did this problem start?
- Describe the symptom. If pain, is it stabbing, burning, sharp, etc?
- Where on your body is this located? Does it move anywhere else?
- Rate your discomfort on a scale from 1 to 10.
- How long during the day does this last? Is there a time that it is worse than others?
- What do you think is the cause of your discomfort?
- Is this problem associated with any other symptoms?
- What makes the symptom worse? What makes it better?

---

there is a chance that the clinician will be in contact with bodily fluids. All bodily fluids should be considered potentially infectious. Masks and gowns may be required during certain procedures, even for observers. Masks may also be required if a patient is under droplet precautions and gowns are required for patients under contact isolation. Precautions must be taken to prevent injury to the health-care worker through needle-stick or other sharps injury. All sharps (including needles, scissors, lancets, and scalpels) should be disposed of immediately following their use into the appropriately marked puncture-resistant containers. Additional information about Universal Precautions may be accessed at the Centers for Disease Control and Prevention web page, http://www.cdc.gov/.

## GETTING STARTED

Good communication is vital to conducting and assembling an accurate medical history and physical examination. All members of the health-care team should clearly identify themselves to patients upon first meeting and determine the language and hearing ability of the patient. When giving directions to the patient, explaining outcomes of testing, or offering other information the clinician should use the primary language of the patient if necessary and possible, avoid the use of medical jargon, and use plain and simple language. Asking the patient to repeat back what they heard is a good way to assess understanding. It is important to be interested, empathetic, and nonjudgmental while approaching the patient's problem.

Many times patients feel some degree of anxiety when being examined. This feeling may be heightened by the presence of additional clinical personnel including students, nurses, and other health-care observers. Remember that the patient may feel exposed and vulnerable; they may not be familiar with the setting, or worried about their diagnosis. Always bear in mind that the patient's rights for privacy and respecting their modesty and comfort is a very important part of building patient rapport. When performing a physical examination, it is crucial to develop a systematic approach for not only completeness, but also to minimize the number of times the patient is asked to change positions.

As a pharmacy student member of the medical team, you should participate in the review of laboratories or diagnostic testing and the physical examination of the patient when possible. If your patient has a heart murmur, listen; an abdominal mass, palpate; a rash, attempt to describe. Actively participating in the physical examination of patients while on rounds and during your practice of pharmacy courses will improve your ability to make good clinical judgments later, and aid in the provision of patient-centered care and medication therapy management.

## General Survey and Vital Signs

Beginning from the time the clinician and the patient meet, there are important observations about the patient that should be made. For example, does the patient appear to be in distress or anxious, or does he or she appear to be well? Does he or she walk with a limp, use an ambulatory assistant device, wear glasses, and appear his or her stated age? Is the patient overweight or cachectic? Take notice of the patient's level of consciousness, affect, and manner of speaking. These observations should be continuous throughout the medical history and physical examination components.

Vital signs should be collected in the beginning of the examination and include height, weight (from which body mass index (BMI) may be calculated), temperature, pulse, respiratory rate, and blood pressure. All values, whether normal or abnormal, should be noted for each patient. Any abnormal values require further investigation and recheck. The BMI is important to determine if the patient falls into guidelines that indicate obesity or other risk factors. To calculate the BMI refer to Table "Calculation of Body Weight, Mass, and Surface Area" (Table 6.2 from Chap. 6). Practice calculating your own BMI and that of your family members. Normal BMI ranges from 18 to 25 (Table 10.3).

Temperature is often considered an optional vital sign in the ambulatory patient. Normal oral temperature values can vary considerably throughout the day with a

| TABLE 10.3. BMI RANGES AND THEIR MEANING | |
| --- | --- |
| What Does BMI No. Measurement Suggest? | Guidelines Established in 1998 by the National Heart Lung and Blood Institute |
| Underweight | BMI < 18.5 |
| Normal | BMI of 18.5 through 24.9 |
| Overweight | BMI of 25.0 through 29.9 |
| Obese | BMI of 30.0 or greater |

| TABLE 10.4. NORMAL TEMPERATURE VALUES | | |
|---|---|---|
| Oral | 35.8°C–37.3°C | 96.4°F–99.1°F |
| Axillary | 36.3°C–37.8°C | 94.9°F–99.6°F |
| Rectal | 36.3°C–37.8°C | 94.9°F–99.6°F |

low of 35.8°C (96.4°F) in the morning and an afternoon high of 37.3°C (99.1°F). Rectal and tympanic membrane temperatures tend on average to be higher than oral temperatures while axillary temperatures are lower. Axillary temperatures are considered the least reliable of the methods and are not preferred. An oral temperature greater than 38°C (100.4°F) is considered fever. Normal temperature values are listed in Table 10.4. Patients with a fever may have tachycardia, due to increased metabolic demands, and it is important for pharmacists to obtain an accurate pulse.

Pulse is measured by pressing the pads of the clinician's index and middle fingers to the patient's radial pulse as shown in Figure 10.2. The clinician should note whether or not the patient's pulse is regular and if the rate seems to be within normal limits. Normal pulse for an adult ranges between 60 and 100 beats per minute. A pulse rate that is faster than 100 beats per minute in an adult is defined as tachycardia, and a pulse that is slower than 60 beats per minute is defined as bradycardia. Whether this is determined to be an irregular pulse depends on numerous patient

**Figure 10.2.** Proper way to take a pulse.

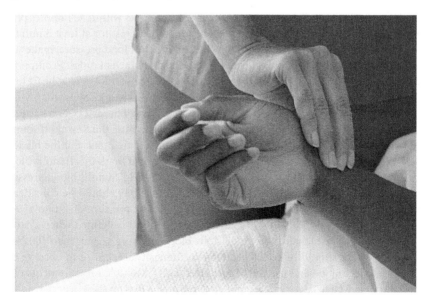

characteristics. Bradycardia may be found in athletes (and is nonpathologic), or may be found in individuals taking β-blockers or people with certain conditions such as hypothyroidism. Tachycardia may be caused by pain, anxiety, or volume depletion.

Other abnormal heart rhythms create a pulse considered irregular. Patients with atrial flutter or certain conduction abnormalities may have regularly irregular pulses while patients with atrial fibrillation will have irregularly irregular pulses. Electrocardiogram (ECG) better assesses rhythm abnormalities and may be a necessary diagnostic test to order after the physical examination revealing an irregular pulse.

When observing a patient's respirations, consider the effort and depth of breathing as well as the rate. It is best to observe subtly the patient's respirations while taking the pulse, as many people will change their natural pattern of breathing if they are aware of being watched. Most normal values fall between 12 and 16 breaths per minute. Respiratory rates less than 12 may be caused by a medication-induced stupor and rates higher than 16 can be caused by anxiety, pain, and pulmonary disease. Various patterns of breathing exist including Cheyne-Stokes (apnea alternating with maximal deep breaths), which may be observed in heart failure patients. Kussmaul breathing is a pattern of deep, rhythmic breathing often seen in diabetic ketoacidosis.

Blood pressure is measured by the use of a sphygmomanometer. It is important to use the appropriate size cuff and proper technique to ensure an accurate reading. The width of the bladder and cuff should be approximately 40% of the upper arm circumference. Care should be taken when attempting to get accurate blood pressure readings of the obese or very thin patient, as getting the wrong size cuff will give an inaccurate reading. The length of the bladder should be about 80% of the upper arm circumference (nearly long enough to encircle the arm). The patient should ideally not have smoked or consumed caffeinated beverages within 30 minutes prior to blood pressure measurement. The patient should be at rest for at least 5 minutes with his or her back and feet supported. When taking the blood pressure, make sure the arm being used is free of clothing and has a viable brachial pulse. Position the arm so that the brachial artery at the point of the antecubital fossa is at heart level (Fig. 10.3). You may have to hold the arm to maintain this critical position while taking the blood pressure. Center the inflatable bladder over the artery, and place the bell of the stethoscope over the brachial artery (this is because the Korotkoff sounds are low pitched). The first sounds heard during the deflating phase of the bladder mark the systolic blood pressure and the last sounds heard mark the diastolic blood pressure. Normal blood pressure is less than 120/80 mm Hg. Systolic blood pressure from 120 to 139 or diastolic blood pressure from 80 to 89 should be considered prehypertension. Stage I hypertension is a systolic blood pressure of 140 to 159 or a diastolic blood pressure 90 to 99. Stage II hypertension is defined when systolic blood pressure greater than 160 or a diastolic blood pressure greater than 100. Any abnormal values should be rechecked later in the visit taking care to observe the appropriate technique and use the proper sized cuff.[3] Multiple measurements over a few visits may be necessary to accurately determine a diagnosis of hypertension as

**Figure 10.3.** Proper way to take a blood pressure.

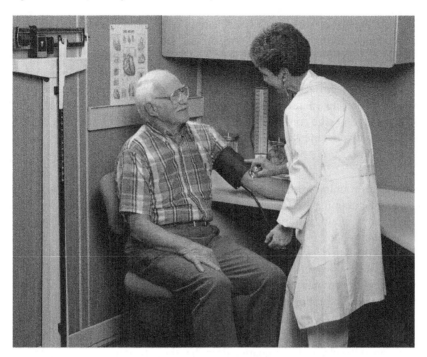

there are several variables, including the white coat syndrome which can raise blood pressure. The white coat syndrome is referred to when patients have anxiety related to seeing a physician and this concomitantly increases their blood pressure giving a false indication that the patient may be hypertensive.

Pain is considered the "fifth vital sign." Pain, as defined by the American Pain Society, is always subjective and is an unpleasant sensory and emotional experience associated with the actual or potential tissue damage or described in terms of such damage. There are various standardized pain assessment tools including the Initial Pain Assessment, the Brief Pain Inventory, and the McGill Questionnaire. In addition, there are pain-rating scales that assist with documenting baseline intensity and improvement with various therapeutic modalities, including pharmacotherapy. Examples of pain rating scales include Visual Analog Scales such as Figure 10.4 or

**Figure 10.4.** Visual analog scale. (From Tintinalli JE, Kelen GD, Stapczynski JS (eds): *Emergency Medicine*. 6th ed. New York: McGraw-Hill; 2004, p. 259.)

|———————————————————————————————|

No
pain

Worst
imaginable pain

numeric scales that ask a patient to select a number that rates the level of their pain with 0 being no pain and 10 being the worse pain they can imagine; the Wong Baker FACES Pain Rating Scale which uses faces with different expressions to demonstrate the level of pain; and descriptor scales that use words such as "no pain, mild pain, moderate pain, and severe pain" for assessment.[4] The clinician shows the patient the scale and asks them to indicate what on the scale indicates the amount of pain they have. These scales can be a helpful way to take a subjective measure (pain) and try to give it a more objective nature. In managing pain in patients, a pharmacist can get a sense of the level of pain control as they follow this number over time. This is also a good measure to document as part of your patient history.

## Review of Systems

The physical examination and its documentation typically follow a particular sequence. The examination begins with general appearance, vital signs, skin, head, ears, eyes, nose, mouth and throat, neck, breasts, heart, lungs, abdomen, genitourinary, rectal, musculoskeletal, vascular, and lymphatic and the neurological evaluation. Table 10.5 describes an abbreviated list of physical examination findings. The remainder of this chapter provides descriptions of pertinent systems mentioned above, reviewing common complaints attributed to each, questions to better elicit a complete history of present illness, and physical examination techniques.

## General Appearance

This section of the physical examination describes the patient from an age and background perspective in addition to how they look and act. Included in this section are age, race, and gender. General appearance may also mention nutritional condition (such as thin or obese), distress (none to severe), mental status (alert, confused, comatose), and a description of general health. An example of the written description: "This is a 45 YOWF NAD" (This patient is a 45-year-old white female who presents in no acute distress) or "This is a 24 YOWDWNBM" (This is a well-developed and well-nourished black male).[5]

## Documentation

The previous description is a standard form of documentation. Physicians and other health-care professionals have used this system of abbreviations, but those who work for accrediting agencies and hospital leaders are asking that abbreviations be limited or discontinued from chart notes to reduce confusion. Follow the standard practice described by your faculty, and preceptors when documenting patient information.

## Skin, Hair, and Nails

Regardless of the area of practice for pharmacists, patients will want to show you their skin and ask, "What is this?" "How can I treat this?" "Is this contagious?" Because of this, pharmacists should feel comfortable completing a basic skin

---

**TABLE 10.5.** STEPS OF THE PHYSICAL EXAMINATION

1. Patient's comfort
   Be certain that the patient is in a relaxed position, properly gowned or draped.

2. The optimal environment
   The examination surface should be at a height appropriate for the examiner. Light sources and curtains should be optimally arranged. Television sets, radios, and other noisy distractions should be eliminated.

3. Vital signs and general inspection
   Evaluate the radial pulse for rate and rhythm. Measure brachial blood pressure. Inspect nails, skin, and hair. Note the general appearance, body habitus, hair distribution, muscle mass, movement coordination, odors, and breathing pattern.

4. Head
   a. Eyes: Examine the conjunctiva, sclera, cornea, and iris of each eye. Test pupils for irregularity, accommodation, and reaction. Evaluate visual fields and visual acuity (cranial nerve II). Assess extraocular movements (cranial nerves III, IV, VI). Test the corneal reflex (cranial nerve V).
   b. Ears: Examine the pinnae and periauricular tissues, Test auditory acuity, perform Weber and Rinne maneuvers (cranial nerve VIII).
   c. Ophthalmo-otoscopy: The ophthalmoscope can now be used after darkening the room to examine the interior of the eye through the pupillary aperture. Particular emphasis should be placed on the retina, optic disc, vessels, and macula lutea. Attention must be given to the media, lens, and cornea. Keeping the room darkened, attach the otoscope head and observe the auditory canals and tympani.
   d. Nose: Connect the nasal speculum to the otoscope and examine the nares, noting the condition of the mucosa, septum and turbinates.
   e. Mouth: Examine the vermilion border, the oral mucosa, the tongue. Identify the salivary duct papillae. Assess the dentition for decay, repair, condition of bite. View the pharynx. Evaluate the function of cranial nerves IX, X, and XII. If appropriate, evaluate sensory divisions of cranial nerves V, VII.
   f. Face: Evaluation of symmetry, smile, frown, and jaw movement will provide information about motor divisions of cranial nerves V and VII.

5. Neck
   Palpate the neck with emphasis on the salivary glands, lymph nodes, and thyroid. Look for tracheal deviation. Identify the carotid arteries and auscultate for bruits. Note jugular venous distention. Reexamine the thyroid from behind the patient. Certain parts of evaluation of this area, jugular venous filling, may warrant review with the patient reclining. Test shoulder strength of the sternocleidomastoid and trapezius muscles (cranial nerves XI and XII).

6. Anterior torso
   With the patient sitting, examine the epitrochlear and axillary nodes. Examine the breasts. Define the PMI and examine the heart, having the patient lean forward if necessary.

*(continued)*

**TABLE 10.5.** STEPS OF THE PHYSICAL EXAMINATION (*Continued*)

7. Posterior torso
   Observe for spinal curvature or chest deformity. Evaluate the vertebral column and the costovertebral areas. Auscultate the posterior and lateral lung fields.

8. Completion of the "sitting" portion of the examination
   Evaluate proximal and distal motor strength, deep tendon reflexes, distal pulses and sensation.

9. With the patient supine

   a. Thorax: Examine the breasts; reexamine the heart, turning the patient to the left lateral decubitus position if appropriate. Auscultate the anterior lung structures.

   b. Abdomen: After inspection, auscultate, listening for bowel sounds and bruits. Next inspect, percuss, and palpate the abdomen, taking special notice of hepatic or splenic enlargements.

   c. Proximal lower extremities: Examine the inguinal, femoral, and popliteal regions for adenopathy and pulses. Evaluate range of motion of hips, knees, and ankles.

10. With the patient standing
    Examine external genitalia of the male. In both male and female, evaluate station and gait.

11. Pelvic and rectal examination
    In females, the pelvic examination should be performed on an examining table provided with stirrups. Rectal examination and occult blood testing should be done simultaneously. In males, the rectal examination is best performed with the patient in the bent forward position.

From Walker HK, Hall WD, Hurst JW (eds): *Clinical Methods: The History, Physical, and Laboratory Examinations*, 3rd edition. Boston, Butterworth, 1990. Used with permission from Elsevier.

---

examination. The skin examination may provide clues to a number of patient disease problems. Dermatologic manifestations may be the first sign of disease that a patient notices. The skin should be assessed during the general survey and the rest of the examination. Note the following characteristics of the skin: color, moisture, temperature, textures, turgor, and lesions, including size and location.

The most common complaints from patients regarding the skin are rashes, lesions, changes in skin color, itching, and changes in hair or nails. It is important to determine a time period associated with the complaint and any changes the patient has noticed. Ask about any other systemic side effects the patient may be experiencing in conjunction with the skin condition.[5–7] Evaluate the patient's medication regimen for any drugs that may cause dermatologic problems. During an infusion of vancomycin, patients may experience flushing and redness with itching, nicknamed redman syndrome. Tetracycline, sulfonamides, diuretics, and the quinolone antibiotics make people more sensitive to the sun, and patients will often present with sunburns. Exposure to the sun while on amiodarone will cause a blue-gray discoloration of the skin.[5] It is important but often forgotten during the examination of a skin disorder to inquire about a travel history, occupational exposure, or any close contacts who may have similar problems.[8] Ascertain what products the patient has already used on the skin because this may have altered the clinical presentation.

When a patient complains of skin color changes, it is important to note whether the change is generalized or local. Generalized color changes include jaundice from liver failure or cyanosis from hypoxia. Localized color changes may indicate cancerous changes or age spots.[8,9]

Patients who complain about hair or nail problems should be evaluated for environmental exposure, especially if the problem is associated with the hands.[8] Hair loss can accompany use of certain neoplastic agents and it is important to reassure the patient that this is to be expected. Hair loss may also occur when patients have anemia and hypothyroidism. Alternatively, patients taking minoxidil or cyclosporin may experience an increase in hair growth. Patients who suffer from hyperthyroidism may complain of very thin, silky hair, a key finding in supporting a hyperthyroidism diagnosis.[5,6] For any skin, hair, or nail complaint, investigate a past medical history to find a link or cause for the problem.

## Head, Ears, Eyes, Nose, and Throat

The examination of the head, ears, eyes, nose, and throat (HEENT) may reveal signs and symptoms of a number of disease states. The examination of the head often involves inspection and palpation. Common terms used to describe findings include normocephalic (normal head), microcephalic (small head), or atraumatic (without trauma).[6] When examining the head, look for patterns in hair growth, nits (eggs of lice) on the scalps, and lumps. Certain diseases can manifest hallmark signs on the head and face. Patients afflicted with Cushing syndrome often present with puffy faces, known as moon-pie facies, because of excess corticosteroid production. Patients with Parkinson disease may present with an expressionless, mask-like face. Patients with hyperthyroidism often have characteristic bulging eyes called exophthalmos.[5,6]

A basic eye examination includes visual fields, ocular movement, and visual acuity. Typically, the eye examination begins with a standard Snellen test or pocket eye card (Fig. 10.5). Visual acuity measures eyesight at an established distance based on population norms. Acuity is expressed as a fraction (20/20). For example, a Snellen result of 20/40 indicates that this patient sees an object at 20 ft that a normal patient would see at 40 ft. The larger the bottom number, the worse the visual acuity.[9] The Snellen eye chart is used to test the patient's ability to see objects in the distance, but does not assess the patient's ability to read close up. As patients age, reading vision often changes requiring correction for objects that are near. Charts are available to assess reading. In addition, the practitioner should perform an external eye examination. External structures of the eye include the lid, eyebrows and lashes, and

**Figure 10.5.** Snellen eye chart.

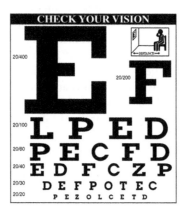

the orbits or eye sockets. Patients may complain of redness, itching, and/or pain in any of the external areas to the eye.[8-10]

The ophthalmoscope helps visualize the internal structures of the eye, most importantly the retina. It is also important to examine the fundus and the blood vessels of the retina. By visualizing the blood vessels, one can determine eye damage secondary to uncontrolled disease. As an example, uncontrolled hypertension can cause papilledema, A-V nicking, and hemorrhages. The ophthalmic examination can also detect forms of retinopathy caused by diseases such as diabetes or hypertension, which becomes present when these diseases remain uncontrolled. It is very important for patients with hypertension or diabetes to have regular eye examinations.[5,8,10]

The most common complaints associated with the eyes are loss of vision, pain, diplopia, tearing, dry eyes, discharge, and redness. If the patient is squinting or tearing, find out if the patient is in pain or experiencing burning in the eyes. If the patient complains about itchy, watery eyes, investigate an allergy history.[8] Note any eye movement that is abnormal. A common sign of anticonvulsant therapy that is associated with toxicity is nystagmus, a fine rhythmic oscillation of the eye, seen especially on extreme movement to the left or right.[7] If the patient is experiencing a loss of vision, ascertain whether it was sudden or gradual. Always determine when the last eye examination was to note if a significant change has occurred.[8]

Examination of the ear also involves external and internal examination. Examine the outer ear for deformities, lumps, and lesions.[8] Tophi deposits along the pinna or auricle (external ear) may be a sign of gout. Check for drainage, pain, and inflammation. If drainage is present, note the color and consistency to assist in diagnosing an infection. Note any hearing aids or devices. Ask questions about earaches, ringing, and dizziness. Ringing in the ears (tinnitus) can be induced by some medications including aspirin. Aminoglycosides and loop diuretics can damage vestibular and auditory function. An ear canal examination, utilizing an otoscope, will visualize the tympanic membrane.

Many common complaints and reasons for visits to a health-care professional include nasal congestion and stuffiness or discharge. Patients who have allergies may present with inflamed nostrils, sinus pain, and postnasal drip. Examine nares (nostrils) to assess patency, color (erythema or pallor), septum, turbinates, and discharge. Note or ask the patient what is the color of mucus from the nose. Thick, purulent mucus typically represents infection.[8] Medications can be the cause of a number of common nasal complaints. Warfarin, which is used to prevent the blood from forming unnecessary clots, can cause epistaxis (nose bleeding) if the patient is prescribed more than needed. Overuse of nasal decongestants can cause a condition known as rhinitis medicamentosus.[5] α-Blockers may cause nasal congestion due to their vasodilatory properties.[7]

Check the mouth for sores, tooth and/or gum inflammation, or nodules. Ask if the patient has complaints of dry mouth, hoarseness, or a change in voice.[8] If the patient has mouth sores, review his list of medications. Many chemotherapeutic agents, such as methotrexate, can cause severe mouth sores called stomatitis. Medications such as phenytoin and cyclosporin can cause gingival hyperplasia (gum swelling).[7] During the examination, have the patient stick out his tongue to examine its symmetry. Look at the area under and around the tongue carefully, as these are common areas for cancerous growth. The first sign of jaundice may be noted underneath the tongue. Note the patient's breath; since an odor can be a clinical clue to certain disease states. Acetone-smelling breath can signal diabetic ketoacidosis, and a fishy smell is associated with chronic renal failure. Patients with an infection of the respiratory tract will often have malodorous breath.[5,8]

Palpate the neck looking for any unusual lumps, masses, or scars. The patient should be in a relaxed position to facilitate feeling lymph nodes and enlargement. Lymph nodes should not be palpable unless enlarged. Assess the position of the trachea and examine the carotid arteries. Note if the patient is complaining of any pain or stiffness during the examination. If the patient complains of sudden stiffness with headache, refer immediately for emergency care. Neck stiffness with headache can signal meningitis, a medical emergency.[5,8,10]

## Respiratory

The respiratory examination begins by inspecting the chest. Notice the patient's posture, as certain diseases that interfere with posture (osteoporosis, scoliosis) can also cause difficulty in breathing. Watch the patient breathe and appreciate the pattern. Is the patient depending on accessory muscles to breathe? Note if breathing is rapid and shallow or slow and irregular. Make note if the patient seems to "favor" one side, called splinting, to protect broken ribs.[6] Patients with chronic obstructive pulmonary disease (COPD) may need to lean forward in order to breathe. They often place both hands upon their knees (tripod position) in order to support respiration.[8] COPD patients may also have clubbed fingers, resulting from years of hypoxia. Patients with COPD may have a thorax that resembles a barrel due to enlarged anterior posterior diameter. Patients referred to as barrel chested have large, round chests that appear very muscular after years of using all of their thorax muscles to breathe.[4,10] After noting any malformations in appearance, palpate the chest. Note if the patient seems tender in any area. Patients may display crepitus, which feels like packing bubbles when a hand is run over the patient's back. Use percussion to determine the lung composition. Dull sounds usually represent fluid-filled compartments, whereas hyperresonant sounds indicate overinflation.[5,6] Listen to detect any abnormal sounds including wheezing, crackles, or stridor. Note if the patient is coughing and whether it is a dry, hacking cough, or a productive "wet" cough. If the patient is coughing up material, record the amount, consistency, and color.[8] Other findings of concern include dyspnea (shortness of breath) and hemoptysis (coughing blood).[9] If either dyspnea or hemoptysis are present, determine when the patient last had a PPD test and their last chest X-ray. As a pharmacist, it is important to ascertain a smoking history and how many, or if any, attempts at smoking cessation have been made by the patient. Make sure to check the patient's medication history to make note of any drugs affecting the respiratory system. For example, narcotics can dramatically slow the respiratory rate in an overdose; angiotensin-converting enzyme inhibitors may cause a persistent, dry cough; β-blockers can exacerbate the bronchoconstriction (narrowed airways) seen in asthma, whereas β-agonists improve shortness of breath during an acute asthma exacerbation.[7]

## Cardiovascular

The cardiovascular examination begins by inspecting the patient to determine the color of skin. Skin can look normal to pale or possibly even blue, denoting lack of oxygen. Next palpate the chest for the point of maximal impulse (PMI), located usually at the fifth intercostal space.[8] Murmurs, thrills, and rubs can also be felt on the skin. Murmurs are heard differently than normal heart sounds, as murmurs are longer. Murmurs are caused by turbulent blood flow and can be the result of septal defects, obstructed vessels, dilated vessels, or incompetent valves. When listening to a murmur, it is important to note the time the murmur occurs in the cardiac cycle, the location the murmur is heard, the "shape" of the murmur, and the quality of the murmur. Murmurs are graded on intensity from I to VI (see Table 10.6).

**TABLE 10.6. HEART MURMURS**

| Grade | Description of Murmur |
|---|---|
| I | Very faint, heard only after listening with stethoscope |
| II | Quiet, heard immediately after placement of stethoscope |
| III | Moderately loud |
| IV | Loud |
| V | Very loud, possible to hear with stethoscope partly away from chest |
| VI | Can be heard without the stethoscope |

Thrills are areas palpated on the skin representing areas of turbulence below. Rubs have a "grating" sound, resulting from inflamed tissue rubbing together. Two types of rubs can occur, pericardial and pulmonary. To differentiate between the two, instruct the patient to hold his breath. The pulmonary rub will become silent while holding one's breath, but the pericardial rub will still be audible.[5,8,9]

Auscultation assists in identifying appropriate heart sounds and determining the quality and importance of abnormal sounds. There are four distinct areas for appreciating the various heart sounds. The first area is over the aortic valve, located in the right second intercostal space, 2 cm from the midsternal line. Next, the tricuspid valve is best heard from the lower left sternal border. The mitral valve is best heard around the cardiac apex. Finally, the pulmonic valve is most appreciated in the area of the left second intercostal space, 2 cm from the midsternal line.[9] When listening to the heart, pay attention to the pitch, volume, and duration of heart sounds. Normal heart sounds, $S_1$ and $S_2$, are typically referred to as "lub-dub." $S_1$ represents the closure of the tricuspid and mitral valves. $S_2$ occurs as the pulmonic and aortic valves close. Two other sounds, $S_3$ and $S_4$, can be heard in normal, healthy people but often represent abnormalities.[5,6] In patients older than 30 years of age, $S_3$ is associated with congestive heart failure (CHF), and $S_4$ can result from a noncompliant left ventricle. Coronary artery disease and hypertension are common causes of a noncompliant ventricle.[6]

If a patient is being assessed for an event of cardiac nature such as a myocardial infarction (heart attack), it is important to not only get objective information including pulse and blood pressure but also obtain a subjective history. Subjective complaints include pain, radiation, and palpitations. Subjectively, patients with CHF may complain of becoming short of breath and requiring more than one pillow to breathe comfortably at night (pillow orthopnea). Patients who are experiencing heart failure may also have systemic signs of disease, manifesting as extremity edema, hepatomegaly, or jugular venous distension.[8,9]

The peripheral vascular examination requires examining the extremities for varicose veins, signs of claudication, or Raynaud phenomena (digits turn blue on cold exposure). Investigate complaints of calf swelling and tenderness for a possible clot preventing blood flow, known as deep vein thrombosis or DVT.

## Breast

Although a pharmacist may never perform a breast examination, it is important to understand the examination since counseling on self-breast examinations and understanding the documentation of the examination relates to information that the pharmacist can provide as part of patient-centered care. Palpation and inspection are the most important skills utilized in performing the breast examination. Practitioners will look for lumps, changes in skin texture and color, and nipple discharge. The most common findings on examination are fibrocystic disease and fibroadenoma. Up to 50% of women have these conditions.[8,9] Inquire when the patient's last mammogram and/or breast examination occurred and note any changes and encourage them to do regular self-examinations and to get a mammogram annually over age 50. Current information has shown that breast self-examinations are not enough for prevention of breast cancer and that mammograms are vital.

## Gastrointestinal

The abdomen is divided into four quadrants to describe the anatomic features (Fig. 10.6). The right upper quadrant (RUQ) contains the liver, gallbladder, pylorus, duodenum, and head of the pancreas; right adrenal gland; upper right kidney; hepatic flexure; a portion of the ascending colon; and a portion of the transverse colon. The left upper quadrant (LUQ) houses the left lobe of the liver, spleen, stomach, the body of the pancreas, the left adrenal gland, the upper left kidney, the splenic flexure, and portions of the transverse and descending colons. The lower quadrants contain kidneys, colon, ovaries, fallopian tubes, ureters, spermatic cords, and the uterus and bladder if enlarged. In addition, the appendix can be found in the right lower quadrant (RLQ).[5,8]

There are also nine anatomically descriptive areas on the abdomen used as a "map" to mark various findings (Fig. 10.6). All four aspects of physical examination are employed during examination of the abdomen. It is important to auscultate the bowel sounds before percussing or palpating the area, as the latter can influence the sound that will be heard.[6] If the patient is complaining of abdominal pain in a particular area, leave that area for last in the physical examination of the abdomen.

**Figure 10.6.** Abdominal quadrants. (From Bates[9] with permission.)

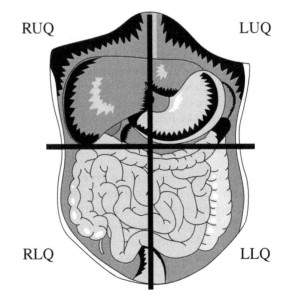

Many symptoms associated with the gastrointestinal system are subjective for the patient and can be assessed by questioning. Start by asking about changes in appetite, nausea, vomiting, or diarrhea. Also, ask if the patient has symptoms of heartburn, bloating, belching, or reflux symptoms. Common concerns for patients include a change in bowel habits or blood in their stool. When blood is present in the stool, attempt to gain insight into the exact symptomatology. When the blood is bright red, it can be a result of hemorrhoids or lower GI tract malignancy. Dark black, bloody stools, referred to as melena, represent bleeding that is occurring higher in the GI tract. Examine all patients for jaundice, abdominal distension, and masses. If jaundice is discovered, ascertain history on drugs of abuse, tattoo history, transfusions, and alcohol consumption, as all can contribute to liver damage.[8] Listen for bowel sounds and the intensity of the sound if present. Bowel sounds should be heard every 5 to 10 seconds as a high-pitched sound. The absence of bowel sounds may represent paralytic ileus, and hyperactive bowel sounds may signal early obstruction. The use of opioid medication can slow bowel sounds considerably and potentially result in obstruction.

## Genitourinary

Like the breast examination, a pharmacist may never perform a genitourinary examination. However, it is important to understand the examination for documentation and counseling purposes. Examination of the genitourinary tract can be an uncomfortable experience for both men and women. It is the examiner's responsibility to remain professional and place the patient at ease to facilitate a thorough examination.

Examining the male genitals involves inspection for abnormalities and palpation for masses and enlargement. Common genitourinary complaints include pain on urination (dysuria), discharge, frequent urination (polyuria), and incontinence.[8] It is important to ask older men about hesitancy, dribbling, and strength of urine stream, as these questions may assist in diagnosing benign prostatic hypertrophy (BPH). In addition, men may be questioned about their testicular self-examination history. Inquire whether the patient has swelling, masses, or pain. Infertility can also affect men, and it is theorized that up to 30% of infertility problems can be linked to the man.[8]

With the evolution of drugs to treat impotence, many men are coming forward to seek help for this condition. Impotence can be described as either erectile or ejaculatory. Causes of impotence can be organic or psychogenic, with the latter accounting for 90% of cases. Diabetes, spinal cord injuries, multiple sclerosis, and direct injury are common organic causes of impotence. Antihypertensive, antidepressant, and antipsychotic medications may cause sexual dysfunction and should be investigated when a patient presents with complaints of this nature.[8]

The examination of a woman's genitourinary system involves both an external and internal examination. The outer examination involves noting normal structures and examining for lesions and discharge. The internal examination employs a speculum to visualize the cervix and internal structure and to perform the Pap smear. Women should have regular gynecologic examinations every 1 to 3 years. It is important to note menstrual history, date of last period, premenstrual symptoms, and quality of menses (heavy versus light, duration, regularity). As a pharmacist, ask about contraception use and satisfaction with this regimen. Ask about any problems with itching, discharge, pain, irregular bleeding, dyspareunia (painful intercourse), and postcoital bleeding. Note any problems the patient has had with fertility and any attempts to correct them.[5,8] Women may also complain of dysuria, polyuria, hematuria, and incontinence. Urinary tract infections are more common in women than men and can be easily treated.[8]

A sexual history is very important in both sexes to assess infection risk and need for testing. Although they may be uncomfortable topics, certain areas must be addressed, including number of partners, sexual activity of partners, activities, protection used, frequency, and any problems that may be occurring.[8]

## Musculoskeletal

Examining the musculoskeletal system involves inspecting for asymmetry, nodules, masses, and any signs of muscle atrophy. When palpating, check for signs of inflammation including warmth, redness, and tenderness. Clinicians will inspect a patient's gait, spine, extremities, neck, and specific joints. For example, rheumatoid arthritis is easily recognized by the deformities on the joints of the hands.[8]

Common complaints attributed to the musculoskeletal system include pain and stiffness, weakness, cramping, back pain, and limited movement. Pharmacists should inquire about methods the patient has used to relieve pain and stiffness, if it helped, and any side effects incurred. Many times, joint difficulties are the result of a previous illness or injury. A good history and physical should contain a thorough investigation of past medical history and evidence of joint- or muscle-damaging incidents.[8]

## Neuropsychiatric Examination

A complete physical examination should include at least a screening neurologic examination and some attention toward mental status and mental health. This includes testing the orientation, cranial nerves, sensation, motor systems, reflexes, coordination, and gait. The screening neurologic examination also requires some special tools. These are a penlight, reflex hammer, a clean safety pin (new for each patient), and a 128 Hz tuning fork. The screening neurologic examination may be more time-consuming than other portions of the physical examination, but it is important as many of the medications used in neurologic or psychiatric disease have side effects that affect this portion of the examination. Some of these side effects may include tremor and other uncontrolled movements, weakness, and ataxia.

Assess mental status by asking for the patient's full name, the (current) location, and the date. If the patient is not oriented to any one of those, it may be important to complete a more in-depth mental status examination, such as the MMSE (mini-mental status examination). At this time, pay special attention to the patient's speech.

Does he or she speak fluently; is naming intact? Look also for very rapid, pressured speech, or very slow speech. Note whether the patient's thoughts follow a logical pattern or if there is looseness of associations. It may be appropriate to take note of the patient's affect, and whether or not it is mood congruent (if the patient appears to feel as they describe themselves). If the patient reports either sadness or loss of interest, it is very important to proceed with more detailed questions pertaining to depression, which are beyond the scope of basic assessment. These include questions about thoughts, intentions, or plans to harm self or others.

Cranial nerves II through XII (including funduscopy) should be assessed. Check for papilledema with the funduscope, and (using the pen light) pupils should be equally round and reactive to light. Also, assess the patient's extraocular movements. Look for symmetry in facial movements and sensation, palatal elevation, tongue movements, and strength of the sternocleidomastoid and trapezius muscles. This examination will often result in several common abbreviations which include PERRLA (pupil equal, round reactive to light and accommodation) and EOMI (extraocular muscles intact).

Sensation is assessed through light touch, pinprick, and vibration. Compare each modality separately comparing side-to-side. If the patient reports a difference, try to have him or her quantify the difference. Motor strength should also be assessed comparing side-to-side, stabilizing one joint at a time. Normal strength is noted as 5/5. Deep tendon reflexes should be evaluated using a reflex hammer. Normal reflexes are documented as 2+. Test coordination by asking the patient to alternate between touching his or her nose and your index finger and by asking the patient to slide his or her heel up and down the shin. Take time to watch the patient walk and take note of the gait, one may also assess tandem gait and the patient's ability to walk on his or her heels and toes.

Pharmacists can utilize the neuropsychiatric examination for therapeutic drug monitoring. Many drugs used in neurologic or psychiatric diseases cause side effects that may only be seen on examination. Some anticonvulsants in elevated concentrations may cause ataxia, falling, confusion, and slurred speech. Lithium may also cause ataxia and slurred speech as well as a fine tremor. Patients on antipsychotics may develop Parkinsonism, which includes symptoms of shuffling gait and pill rolling tremor. Even patients not exhibiting neurologic or psychiatric disease may benefit from a directed neurologic examination for drug therapy monitoring. Patients using inhaled β-agonists may develop a tremor related to medication use, whereas patients taking β-blockers may appear sluggish and tired.[7] Patients requiring thyroid hormones may have changes in deep tendon reflexes depending on whether the hormone levels are low (delayed or slow relaxing reflexes) or elevated (brisk reflexes).

## PUTTING IT ALL TOGETHER

Knowledge and practice of the physical examination by pharmacists is becoming essential to the practice of patient-centered care and medication therapy management. It is befitting for you to become proficient in these skills. Acquiring and sharpening physical assessment skills will lead to improved communication with members of the health-care team, more complete data collection, better assessment and monitoring, and ultimately optimal drug therapy selection and management for the patient.[11] Take every opportunity to practice your skills and ask for feedback on technique. Inquire as to the availability of simulation laboratory tools at your institution, such as a heart sounds generator, for the cardiac examination. Also, inquire about recommended internet sites that highlight heart and lung sounds or videos that demonstrate examination technique. A quick search of the Internet will yield many sites that provide this kind of information. Most importantly, when assessing a patient's drug therapy ask yourself, "What physical examination is relevant to monitor or assess effectiveness and adverse drug events?"

## APPLICATION EXERCISES

1. What are four skills involved in the physical examination?
2. What is the "fifth" vital sign?
3. What are the steps involved in obtaining an accurate blood pressure reading?
4. List medication adverse effects that may be discovered during a neurologic examination.
5. What physical examination parameters may be used to monitor a patient on β-Blocker therapy?
6. What physical examination parameters may be used to monitor a patient on thyroid hormone replacement?
7. What physical examination parameters may be used to monitor a patient on inhaled β-agonists?
8. List techniques to make the patient comfortable during the physical examination.
9. What physical examination skills do you consider "basic skills" for pharmacists? Why?
10. Why are physical assessment skills important for pharmacists?

## ACKNOWLEDGMENT

The authors wish to acknowledge the contributions of Catherine Meier and Rachel H. Bardowell to this chapter.

## REFERENCES

1. Hepler CD, Strand LM. Opportunities and responsibilities in pharmaceutical care. *Am J Hosp Pharm.* 1990;57:533–543.
2. Camara CC, D'Elia RP, Swanson LN. Survey of physical assessment course offerings in American colleges of pharmacy. *Am J Pharm Educ.* 1996;60:343–347.

3. Chobanian AV, Bakris GL, Black HR, et al. National Heart, Lung, and Blood Institute Joint National Committee on Prevention, Detection, Evaluation, and Treatment of High Blood Pressure; National High Blood Pressure Education Program Coordinating Committee. The Seventh Report of the Joint National Committee on Prevention, Detection, Evaluation, and Treatment of High Blood Pressure: The JNC 7 report. *JAMA.* 2003;289:2560–2572.

4. Jarvis C. *Physical Examination and Health Assessment.* 4th ed. St. Louis, MO: Saunders; 2004.

5. Boh LE. *Clinical Clerkship Manual.* Vancouver, WA: Applied Therapeutics; 1993.

6. Longe RL, Calvert JC, Young LY. *Physical Assessment: A Guide for Evaluating Drug Therapy.* Vancouver, VA: Applied Therapeutics; 1994.

7. Lacy CF, Armstrong LL, Lance LL, et al. *Drug Information Handbook.* Hudson, OH: Lexi-Comp; 2000.

8. Swartz MH. *Textbook of Physical Diagnosis: History and Examination.* 3rd ed. Philadelphia, PA: WB Saunders; 1998.

9. Bates B. *A Guide to Physical Examination and History Taking.* 6th ed. Philadelphia, PA: JB Lippicott; 1995.

10. Tietze KJ. *Clinical Skills for Pharmacists.* St Louis, MO: Mosby-Year Book; 1997.

11. Longe RL. Teaching physical assessment to doctor of pharmacy students. *Am J Pharm Educ.* 1995;59:151–155.

CHAPTER

11

# Interpretation of Clinical Laboratory Data

## Karen L. Whalen, Nancy Borja-Hart

**Objectives: Upon completion of the chapter and exercises, the student pharmacist will be able to**

1. Recognize normal ranges for common laboratory values in adults.
2. Identify common causes for abnormal laboratory values.
3. List circumstances that may produce false-negative or false-positive laboratory results.
4. Interpret the clinical significance of abnormal laboratory values.
5. Utilize clinical laboratory data to monitor various disease states.

---

### Patient Encounter

#### Part 1

You are rounding on an internal medicine advanced pharmacy practice experience with the ICU team. When preparing for rounds, note that there was a new admission last night—an Olympic bicyclist who was struck by a car. Begin reviewing the patient's laboratory data in preparation for rounds.

On admission to the hospital last night, patient X had the following CBC:

WBC: 7200 cells/mm$^3$

RBC: $3.7 \times 10^6$ cells/mm$^3$

Hgb: 10 g/dL

Hct: 30%

MCV: 92 μm$^3$/cell

*(continued on next page)*

MCH: 30 pg/cell

MCHC: 35 g/dL

**Discussion Questions—Part 1:**

What do the above abbreviations represent?

Which of the laboratory values are abnormal?

What type of anemia is present?

What is the most likely cause of the anemia in this patient?

In addition to the CBC, what other laboratory tests were most likely ordered for this patient upon admission to the hospital?

What abnormalities (if any) would you expect to see on these laboratory tests?

**Part 2**

Several days later the patient begins to spike fevers. A CBC, chest X-ray, UA, and blood and urine cultures are done to look for possible sources of infection. The CBC and UA results are as follows:

CBC with differential

WBC: 17,900 cells/mm$^3$

WBC differential

-Segs: 65%

-Bands: 10%

-Lymphocytes: 17%

-Monocytes: 5%

-Eosinophils: 2%

-Basophils: 0.5 %

RBC: 4.2 × 10$^6$ cells/mm$^3$

Hgb: 14 g/dL

Hct: 42%

MCV: 90 μm$^3$/cell

MCH: 31 pg/cell

MCHC: 36 g/dL

*(continued on next page)*

Urinalysis

Urine color: straw, cloudy

SG: 1.010

pH: 7.2

Protein: trace

Glucose: negative

Ketones: negative

Blood: trace

Bilirubin: zero

Leukocyte esterase: positive

Nitrites: positive

**Discussion Questions—Part 2:**

What abnormalities are noted in the CBC?

What is a "left shift," and what does it indicate? Is a left shift present?

What abnormalities are noted on the UA?

What is the most likely cause of these abnormalities?

What follow-up actions/treatments will probably be needed as a result of these abnormal laboratory tests?

## INTRODUCTION

This chapter is designed to provide an overview of common laboratory tests used in clinical practice. The most frequently used tests such as complete blood count (CBC), electrolytes and blood chemistries, and urinalysis (UA) are provided first, followed by other clinical and diagnostic tests grouped by disease state or body system.

## CLINICAL PEARLS WHEN INTERPRETING LAB DATA

- Normal values may vary from lab to lab depending on techniques and reagents used.
- Normal values may also vary depending on the patient's age, gender, weight, height, and other factors.

- Laboratory error is a fairly uncommon occurrence; however, it can happen. Potential causes of laboratory error include technical error, improper calculation, inadequate specimen, incorrect sample timing, improper sample preservation, food substances affecting specimen, or medication interference with lab tests.[1]
- If laboratory error is suspected, the test should be repeated.

## Complete Blood Count

The complete blood count (CBC) is an extremely common laboratory test that provides values for hemoglobin (Hgb), hematocrit (Hct), white blood cells (WBCs), red blood cells (RBCs), and red cell indices—mean corpuscular volume (MCV), mean corpuscular hemoglobin (MCH), and mean corpuscular hemoglobin concentration (MCHC).[1,2] In addition, some laboratories may also include platelet count and WBC differential.[3] Sometimes clinicians use shorthand schematics (also known as "Fishbones") like those below to denote the values in the CBC.

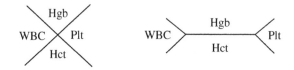

## Hemoglobin (Hgb)

*Normal Range*

| | | |
|---|---|---|
| Male | 14–18 g/dL | SI 8.7–11.2 mmol/L |
| Female | 12–16 g/dL | SI 7.4–9.9 mmol/L |

*Description*

Hgb is the oxygen-carrying compound found in the RBCs.[2–4] Hgb level is a direct indicator of the oxygen-carrying capacity of the blood.[2,3] Adaptation to high altitudes, extreme exercise, and pulmonary conditions may cause variations in Hgb values.[2]

*Clinical Significance*

Increased Hemoglobin

Hgb values may be increased in diseases such as polycythemia vera and chronic obstructive lung disease.[2] Hgb may also be increased in chronic smokers and individuals who engage in regular vigorous exercise or live at high altitudes.

Decreased Hemoglobin

Hgb is decreased in anemia of all types, particularly iron deficiency anemia (IDA).[1] Hgb is also reduced with blood loss, hemolysis, pregnancy, fluid replacement, or increased fluid intake.[1–3]

## Hematocrit (Hct)

*Normal Range*

| Male | 39–49% | SI 0.39–0.49 |
|------|--------|--------------|
| Female | 33–43% | SI 0.33–0.43 |

*Description*

The Hct describes the volume of blood that is occupied by RBCs.[4] It is expressed as a percentage of total blood volume. Another name for Hct is packed cell volume (PCV).[2] As a rule of thumb, the Hct value is generally about three times the value of Hgb.[3,4]

*Clinical Significance*

Increased Hematocrit

Similar to increases in Hgb, increases in Hct are associated with polycythemia vera, chronic obstructive lung disease, and individuals who live at high altitudes.[2,3] Increased Hct may also be seen in cases of dehydration and shock.[1,2]

Decreased Hematocrit

Hct is decreased in all types of anemias, blood loss, hemolysis, pregnancy, cirrhosis, hyperthyroidism, and leukemia.[2,3]

## Red Blood Cell (RBC) Count or Erythrocyte Count

*Normal Range*

| Male | $4.3–5.9 \times 10^6$ cells/mm$^3$ | SI $4.3–5.9 \times 10^{12}$ cells/L |
|------|------------------------------------|-------------------------------------|
| Female | $3.5–5.0 \times 10^6$ cells/mm$^3$ | SI $3.5–5.0 \times 10^{12}$ cells/L |

*Description*

RBCs are produced in the bone marrow.[1] They are released into the systemic circulation and serve to transport oxygen from the lungs to the body tissues.[1,2] After circulating for a life span of approximately 120 days, the RBCs are cleared by the reticuloendothelial system.[1,3] The actual amount of RBCs per unit of blood is the RBC count.[4]

*Clinical Significance*

Increased RBCs

Increased RBC counts (*erythrocytosis*) are associated with polycythemia vera, high altitudes, and strenuous exercise.[2]

Decreased RBCs

RBC counts are decreased in various types of anemias, lymphomas, and leukemia.[2] After puberty females have lower RBCs and Hgb due to menstrual bleeding.[3]

## Mean Corpuscular Volume or Mean Cell Volume (MCV)

*Normal Range*

76–100 μm³/cell          SI 76–100 fL

*Description*

The MCV provides an estimate of the average volume of the erythrocyte. The higher the MCV, the larger the average size of the RBC. Cells with an abnormally large MCV are classified as *macrocytic*.[1,3,4] Conversely, cells with a low MCV are referred to as *microcytic*. *Normocytic* RBCs have an MCV that falls within the normal range.[3,4]

*Clinical Significance*

Increased MCV

An increase in MCV is associated with folate deficiency, $B_{12}$ deficiency, alcoholism, chronic liver disease, hypothyroidism, anorexia, and use of medications such as valproic acid, zidovudine, stavudine, and antimetabolites.[1,3,4]

Decreased MCV

Decreased MCV may result from iron deficiency anemia, hemolytic anemia, lead poisoning, and thalassemia.[1,3]

## Mean Corpuscular Hemoglobin or Mean Cell Hemoglobin (MCH)

*Normal Range*

27–33 pg/cell          SI 27–33 pg/cell

*Description*

The MCH indicates the average weight of Hgb in the RBC.[4] Cells with a low MCH are pale in color and are referred to as *hypochromic*.[1] Cells with an increased MCH are *hyperchromic*, and cells with normal amounts of Hgb are *normochromic*.

*Clinical Significance*

Increased MCH

Elevated MCH may be caused by folate or Vitamin $B_{12}$ deficiency.[4] In individuals with hyperlipidemia MCH may be falsely elevated because of specimen turbidity.[2]

Decreased MCH

Decreased MCH is associated with iron deficiency anemia.[3]

## Mean Corpuscular Hemoglobin Concentration or Mean Cell Hemoglobin Concentration (MCHC)

*Normal Range*

33–37 g/dL              SI 330–370 g/L

*Description*

MCHC is a measure of average Hgb concentration in the RBC.[1]

*Clinical Significance*

Increased MCHC

Increased MCHC is associated with hereditary spherocytosis.[1,2]

Decreased MCHC

MCHC may be decreased in iron deficiency anemia, hemolytic anemia, lead poisoning, and thalassemia.[2–4]

## Reticulocytes

*Normal Range*

0.1–2.4% of RBC          SI 0.001–0.024 RBC

*Description*

Reticulocytes are immature RBCs formed in the bone marrow.[1] An increase in reticulocytes usually indicates an increase in RBC production, but may also be indicative of a decrease in the circulating number of mature erythrocytes.[1,4]

*Clinical Significance*

Increased Reticulocytes

Increased reticulocyte counts (*reticulocytosis*) are associated with hemolytic anemia, hemorrhage, and sickle cell disease.[2,3] Increased reticulocytes are also indicative of response to treatment of anemias secondary to iron, $B_{12}$, or folate deficiency.[1]

Decreased Reticulocytes

Reticulocytes may be decreased as a result of infectious causes, alcoholism, renal disease (from decreased erythropoietin), toxins, untreated iron deficiency anemia, and drug-induced bone marrow suppression.[2]

## White Blood Cell (WBC) or Leukocyte Count

*Normal Range*

3200–11,300 cells/mm$^3$          SI 3.2–11.3 × 10$^9$ cells/L

*Description*

The WBC count represents the total number of WBCs in a given volume of blood. Mature WBCs exist in many forms, including neutrophils, lymphocytes, monocytes, eosinophils, and basophils.[1] A WBC count with differential provides a breakdown of the percentage of each type of WBC.[1,2]

*Clinical Significance*

Increased WBCs

An increase in WBC count is referred to as *leukocytosis*.[2] Leukocytosis may be caused by infection, leukemia, trauma, thyroid storm, and corticosteroid use. Emotion, stress, and seizures may also increase WBC count.[1,2] When WBC count is >50,000 cells/mm$^3$, false elevations in Hgb and MCH can occur.[2]

Decreased WBCs

A decrease in WBC count is referred to as *leukopenia*.[2] Decreased WBCs may be seen in viral infection, aplastic anemia, and in bone marrow depression caused by the use of chemotherapy or anticonvulsants.

## Neutrophils (Polys, Segs, PMNs)

*Normal Range*

| | | |
|---|---|---|
| Segs | 36–73% | SI 0.36–0.73 |
| Bands | 3–5% | SI 0.03–0.05 |

*Description*

Neutrophils are the most common type of WBC. Their primary function is to fight bacterial and fungal infections by phagocytosis of foreign particles.[5] Neutrophils may also be involved in the pathogenesis of some inflammatory disorders, for example, rheumatoid arthritis and inflammatory bowel disease.[1] Bands are immature neutrophils.[3] An increase in bands, often referred to as a "shift to the left" or "left shift," may occur during infection or leukemia.[1,3]

*Clinical Significance*

Increased Neutrophils

An increase in circulating neutrophils is called *neutrophilia*.[2] Neutrophilia is associated with infection, metabolic disorders (eg, diabetic ketoacidosis, DKA), uremia, response to stress, emotional disturbances, burns, acute inflammation, and use of medications such as corticosteroids.[1]

Decreased Neutrophils

A decrease in the number of circulating neutrophils is called *neutropenia*.[2] Neutropenia may result from viral infections (eg, mononucleosis, hepatitis), septicemia, overwhelming infection, and use of chemotherapy agents.[1,2]

Absolute neutrophil count (ANC) is the total number of circulating segs and bands and is calculated from the equation:[1]

$$ANC = WBC \times [(\%segs + \%bands) /100]$$

The risk of infection increases dramatically as the ANC decreases. An ANC less than 500/mm$^3$ is associated with a substantial risk of infection.[2]

## Lymphocytes

*Normal Range*

20–40%          SI 0.20–0.40

*Description*

Lymphocytes are the second most common type of circulating WBC.[1] They are important in the immune response to foreign antigens.[1,5]

*Clinical Significance*

Increased Lymphocytes

An elevated lymphocyte count is called *lymphocytosis*.[2] Lymphocytes may be elevated in hepatitis, mononucleosis, chickenpox, herpes simplex, herpes zoster, and other viral infections.[1,2] Some bacterial infections (eg, syphilis, brucellosis), leukemia, and multiple myeloma are also associated with lymphocytosis.

Decreased Lymphocytes

A decreased lymphocyte count is referred to as *lymphopenia*.[2] Lymphopenia may result from acute infections, burns, trauma, lupus, HIV, and lymphoma.

## Monocytes

*Normal Range*

0–11%

*Description*

Monocytes are synthesized in the bone marrow, released into the circulation, and subsequently migrate into lymph nodes, spleen, liver, lung, and bone marrow.[3,5] In these tissues, monocytes mature into macrophages and serve as scavengers for foreign substances.

*Clinical Significance*

Increased Monocytes

An elevated monocyte count is referred to as *monocytosis*.[1] Monocytosis may be observed in the recovery phase of some infections, subacute bacterial endocarditis (SBE), tuberculosis (TB), syphilis, malaria, leukemia, and lymphoma.[1,2]

Decreased Monocytes

A reduced monocyte count is called *monocytopenia*. Monocytopenia is usually not associated with a specific disease but may be seen with use of bone marrow suppressive agents or severe stress.[2]

## Eosinophils

*Normal Range*

0–8%

*Description*

Eosinophils are phagocytic WBCs that assist in the killing of bacteria and yeast. They reside predominantly in the intestinal mucosa and lungs.[3] They are also involved in allergic reactions and in the immune response to parasites.[1] Eosinophil count must be taken at the same time daily due to diurnal variation.[2]

*Clinical Significance*

Increased Eosinophils

An increased eosinophil count, or *eosinophilia*, is associated with allergic disorders, allergic drug reactions, collagen vascular disease, parasitic infections, immunodeficiency disorders, and some malignancies.[1,3]

Decreased Eosinophils

A decreased eosinophil count is called *eosinopenia*.[2] It is commonly attributed to increases in adrenal steroid production.

## Basophils

*Normal Range*

0–3%          SI < 0.03

*Description*

Basophils are phagocytic WBCs present in small numbers in the circulating blood.[3] They contain heparin, histamine, and leukotrienes and are probably associated with hypersensitivity reactions.[3,5]

*Clinical Significance*

Increased basophils (*basophilia*) may be seen in hypersensitivity reactions to food or medications, certain leukemias, and polycythemia vera.[1-3]

## Platelets

*Normal Range*

150,000–450,000/μL          SI 150–450 × 10⁹/L

*Description*

Platelets are a critical element in blood clot formation. The risk of bleeding is low unless platelets fall below 20,000–50,000/μL.[6]

*Clinical Significance*

Increased Platelets

Increased platelets (*thrombocytosis, thrombocythemia*) may be caused by infection, malignancies, splenectomy, chronic inflammatory disorders (eg, rheumatoid arthritis), polycythemia vera, hemorrhage, iron deficiency anemia, or myeloid metaplasia.[2,6]

Decreased Platelets

Decreased platelet counts (*thrombocytopenia*) may occur in autoimmune disorders such as idiopathic thrombocytopenic purpura (ITP) and also with aplastic anemia, radiation, chemotherapy, space-occupying lesion in the bone marrow, bacterial or viral infections, and use of heparin or valproic acid.[2,5,6]

## URINALYSIS

### Description

Urinalysis (UA) is a useful laboratory test that enables the clinician to identify patients with renal disorders, as well as some nonrenal disorders. Components of the UA are gross appearance, specific gravity (SG), pH, protein, glucose, ketones, blood, bilirubin, leukocyte esterase, and nitrites.[1]

### Appearance and Color

On visual examination, the normal urine color should range from clear to dark yellow.[1,2] Some cloudiness is normal and may be caused by phosphates or urate.[7] The presence of WBCs, RBCs, or bacteria may cause abnormal urine cloudiness. Abnormal urine colors include the following:

- *Red-orange* may be caused by presence of myoglobin (from muscle breakdown from seizures, cocaine, or injuries), Hgb, medications (rifampin, phenazopyridine, phenolphthalein, phenothiazines), or foods (beets, carrots, blackberries).[1,2,7]
- *Blue-green* may result from administration of amitriptyline or methylene blue, or pseudomonal infection.[2,7]
- *Brown-black* may be associated with presence of myoglobin or porphyrins from porphyria or sickle cell crisis, phenol poisoning, or rhubarb ingestion.[2,7]

## Specific Gravity (SG)

*Normal Range*

1.002–1.030

*Description*

SG is an indication of the ability of the kidney to concentrate urine.[7] Unusually low SG would suggest that the kidneys are not able to concentrate urine appropriately.[1]

*Clinical Significance*

Low Specific Gravity

Low SG (*hyposthenuria*) may occur in chronic renal failure or diabetes insipidus.[2,7]

High Specific Gravity

High SG (*hypersthenuria*) may be associated with dehydration, excretion of radiologic contrast media, heart failure (HF), toxemia of pregnancy, or SIADH.[1,2] In addition, increased excretion of glucose or protein greater than 2 g per day may also increase urine SG.[2,7]

## pH

*Normal Range*

4.5–8

*Description*

Normal urine specimens are acidic. The average pH value is approximately 6.[1,2]

*Clinical Significance*

Alkaline urine may be found in certain urinary tract infections (UTIs caused by urea-splitting organisms *Proteus, Pseudomonas*), renal tubular acidosis, and with use of acetazolamide or thiazide diuretics.[1,2,7]

Acidic urine may be caused by metabolic acidosis, pyrexia, or diabetic ketosis.[2]

## Protein

*Normal Range*

0 (< 30 mg/dL) to 1 + (30–100 mg/dL)

*Description*

Trace protein in the urine is a common clinical finding and often has no clinical significance.[7]

*Clinical Significance*

Repeated positive tests or *proteinuria* of greater than 150 mg/dL may be a marker of renal disease.[1,7]

Causes of protein in the urine include diabetic nephropathy, interstitial nephritis, hypertension, fever, exercise, pyelonephritis, multiple myeloma, lupus, and severe HF.[2]

## Glucose and Ketones

*Normal Range*

Glucose negative; ketones negative

*Description*

Glucose begins to spill into urine (*glucosuria*) when serum blood glucose is greater than 180 mg/dL.[8,9]

*Clinical Significance*

Glucose in the urine suggests diabetes mellitus or, in a known diabetic, suggests the need for improved glucose control.[8] Glucose in the urine may also be associated with Cushing's disease, pancreatitis, and use of thiazide diuretics, steroids, or oral contraceptives.

Excess amounts of ketones form when carbohydrate metabolism is altered.[8] DKA, starvation, high protein/low carbohydrate diets, and alcoholism may produce ketones in the urine.[1,8]

## Blood

*Normal Range*

Negative to trace

*Description*

Blood in the urine (*hematuria*) may indicate urinary tract damage.[7]

*Clinical Significance*

Common causes of hematuria are infection, nephrolithiasis, malignancies, and benign prostatic hypertrophy (BPH).[2]

False-positive results for blood in the urine may occur when povidone iodine is used as a cleansing agent before urine specimen collection.[7]

False-negative results may occur in patients taking high doses of vitamin C or ascorbic acid.[7]

## Bilirubin

*Normal Range*

Zero to trace

*Description*

Bilirubin in the urine usually produces a dark yellow or brown color.[2] It appears in the urine before other signs of liver dysfunction appear.

*Clinical Significance*

Bilirubin in the urine may be associated with liver disease (eg, hepatitis), septicemia, or obstructive biliary tract disease.[2,7]

Phenazopyridine or phenothiazines may cause a false-positive result for bilirubin in the urine.[7]

## Leukocyte Esterase

*Normal Range*

Zero to trace

*Description*

Positive leukocyte esterase provides an indication of WBCs in the urine.[7]

*Clinical Significance*

Leukocyte esterase in the urine is associated with infections and/or inflammation of the urinary tract.[2]

## Nitrites

*Normal Range*

Negative

*Description*

Gram-negative bacteria are capable of converting dietary nitrates to nitrites.[7]

*Clinical Significance*

Presence of nitrites in the urine suggests colonization or infection with gram-negative organisms.[2,7]

## ELECTROLYTES AND BLOOD CHEMISTRY

Electrolytes and blood chemistries are usually the first set of labs ordered upon initial patient presentation. Depending on the institution, these labs may be ordered using different acronyms. A basic metabolic panel (BMP) or Chem-7 includes sodium, potassium, chloride, carbon dioxide ($CO_2$), glucose, blood urea nitrogen (BUN), and creatinine.[2] A comprehensive metabolic panel (CMP) includes albumin, alkaline phosphatase (ALP), alanine aminotransferase (ALT), aspartate aminotransferase (AST), total bilirubin, calcium, and $CO_2$, in addition to the components of the BMP. Other examples of biochemical profiles are SMA-6, SMA-12, and Chem

Profile-20.[1] Lab values in the BMP may be denoted using the shorthand diagram ("Fishbone") shown below:

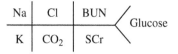

## Sodium (Na⁺)

*Normal Range*

135–147 mEq/L          SI 135–147 mmol/L

*Description*

Sodium is the most prevalent cation in the extracellular fluid.[2] Sodium is important in regulating serum osmolality, fluid balance, and acid-base balance. In addition, sodium also assists in maintaining the electric potential necessary for transmission of nerve impulses.[2]

*Clinical Significance*

Increased Sodium

Increased sodium (*hypernatremia*) may result from increased sodium intake or increased fluid loss.[2,10] Thirst is the primary mechanism to prevent hypernatremia, and, therefore, hypernatremia usually occurs in individuals who are unable to obtain adequate fluid intake. Fluid loss from gastroenteritis, diabetes insipidus, Cushing's disease, hyperaldosteronism, and administration of hypertonic saline solution are causes of hypernatremia.[10]

Decreased Sodium

Decreased sodium (*hyponatremia*) may be caused by a decrease in total body sodium, but is more commonly attributed to excess accumulation of body water (*dilutional hyponatremia*).[10]

Common causes of dilutional hyponatremia include HF, cirrhosis, severe burns, chronic renal failure, and nephrotic syndrome.[2,10] Sodium depletion may also be seen in SIADH, cystic fibrosis, mineralocorticoid deficiency, or fluid replacement with solutions that do not contain sodium.[10]

SIADH may be associated with disease states such as cancer or the use of medications, including chlorpropamide, thiazide diuretics, carbamazepine, and oxcarbazepine.[2]

## Potassium (K⁺)

*Normal Range*

3.5–5 meq/L          SI 3.5–5 mmol/L

*Description*

Potassium is the main intracellular cation.[2] Serum concentrations of potassium are not always an accurate indicator of potassium levels because potassium is an intracellular ion. Potassium plays a key role in many bodily functions, including regulation of nerve excitability, acid-base balance, and muscle function.[2,10] Cardiac function and neuromuscular function can be significantly affected by either an increase or decrease in potassium levels.[2]

*Clinical Significance*

Increased Potassium

Causes of increased potassium (*hyperkalemia*) include metabolic or respiratory acidosis, renal failure, Addison disease, dehydration, and massive cell damage from burns, injuries, and surgery.[2,10] Medications such as ACE inhibitors, angiotensin receptor blockers (ARBs), potassium supplements, potassium-sparing diuretics, and oral contraceptives containing drospirenone are also contributing factors to hyperkalemia.[1,10]

It is important to remember that a high potassium value may be reported if the specimen was hemolyzed when the laboratory test was performed.[2,10]

Decreased Potassium

Causes of decreased potassium (*hypokalemia*) include severe diarrhea and/or vomiting, respiratory alkalosis, hyperaldosteronism, Cushing's disease, alcoholism, and use of amphotericin B or thiazide, loop, or osmotic diuretics.[1,2,10]

If a patient is hypokalemic and potassium supplements have not helped to correct the low potassium, check to see if the magnesium is also low. Decreased potassium is difficult to correct while magnesium remains low.[10]

## Chloride

*Normal Range*

95–105 mEq/L          SI 95–105 mmol/L

*Description*

Chloride is the principal extracellular anion.[2,10] Chloride primarily serves a passive role in the maintenance of fluid balance and acid-base balance. Serum chloride values are useful in identifying fluid or acid-base balance disorders.[10]

*Clinical Significance*

Increased Chloride

Increased chloride (*hyperchloremia*) may be seen in metabolic acidosis, respiratory alkalosis, dehydration, diabetes insipidus, eclampsia, and renal disorders.[1,2,10]

Decreased Chloride

Decreased chloride (*hypochloremia*) may be associated with prolonged vomiting, gastric suctioning, metabolic alkalosis, HF, SIADH, Addison disease, or use of acid suppressants (H2 blockers and proton pump inhibitors (PPIs)).[10]

## Carbon Dioxide ($CO_2$) Content

*Normal Range*

22–28 mEq/L          SI 22–28 mmol/L

*Description*

The majority of $CO_2$ in the plasma is present as bicarbonate ions, and a small percentage is dissolved $CO_2$. The $CO_2$ content is the sum of both bicarbonate ions and dissolved $CO_2$.[1] $CO_2$ and bicarbonate are extremely important in regulating physiologic pH.[1,11] It is important not to confuse the terms $CO_2$ content and $CO_2$ gas (ie, $pCO_2$). $CO_2$ content is composed mostly of bicarbonate ($HCO_3^-$) and is a base. $CO_2$ content is regulated by the kidneys. $CO_2$ gas is acidic and is regulated by the lungs.[2]

*Clinical Significance*

Increased $CO_2$ Content

Increased $CO_2$ is seen in metabolic alkalosis.[1,2] Some common causes of metabolic alkalosis include diuretic therapy, primary aldosteronism, and Bartter syndrome.[2]

Decreased $CO_2$ Content

Decreased $CO_2$ is associated with metabolic acidosis.[1,2] Common causes of metabolic acidosis include DKA, methanol or salicylate toxicity, lactic acidosis, and renal failure.[2]

## Anion Gap

*Normal Range*

3–11 mEq/L          SI 3–11 mmol/L

*Description*

The anion gap is calculated using the following formula:[11]

$$\text{Anion gap} = [Na^+ - (Cl^- + HCO_3^-)]$$

Anion gap is reflective of unmeasured acids.[1] An increase in anion gap suggests an increase in the number of negatively charged weak acids in the plasma.[1,11] Anion gap is useful in evaluating causes of metabolic acidosis.[11]

*Clinical Significance*

Anion gap may be elevated in conditions such as renal failure, lactic acidosis, ketoacidosis, and salicylate, methanol, or ethylene glycol toxicity.[1,11]

## Glucose

*Normal Range*

Fasting          70–99 mg/dL          SI 3.9–5.5 mmol/L

*Description*

Glucose is an important energy source for most cellular functions.[1] Blood glucose regulation is achieved through a complex set of mechanisms that involves insulin, glucagon, cortisol, epinephrine, and other hormones.[2]

*Clinical Significance*

Increased Glucose

The most common cause of increased glucose (*hyperglycemia*) is diabetes mellitus.[1,11,12] A fasting blood sugar greater than 126 mg/dL on two occasions or a random blood sugar greater than 200 mg/dL (along with symptoms of diabetes) is consistent with a diagnosis of diabetes mellitus.[12] Patients are diagnosed with impaired fasting glucose (IFG) if blood glucose levels are 100 to 125 mg/dl when fasting. Impaired glucose tolerance (IGT) is defined as a random glucose level greater than or equal to 140 mg/dl but less than 200 mg/dl.[12] Both IFG and IGT are suggestive of pre-diabetes. Other causes of hyperglycemia include Cushing's disease, sepsis, pancreatitis, shock, trauma, myocardial infarction, and use of corticosteroids or niacin.[13]

Decreased Blood Glucose

Decreased blood glucose (*hypoglycemia*) may result from missing a meal, oral hypoglycemic agents, insulin overdose, or Addison disease.[2,8,14]

## Blood Urea Nitrogen (BUN)

*Normal Range*

6–20 mg/dL          SI 2.1–7.1 mmol/L

*Description*

Urea nitrogen is an end product of protein catabolism.[2] It is produced in the liver, transported in the blood, and cleared by the kidneys. BUN concentration serves as a marker of renal function.[7]

*Clinical Significance*

Increased BUN

Increased BUN (*azotemia*) may be associated with acute or chronic renal failure, HF, gastrointestinal bleeding (gut flora metabolizes blood to ammonia and urea nitrogen), high-protein diet, shock, dehydration, anti-anabolic and nephrotoxic medications.[2,7]

Decreased BUN

Decreased BUN is seen in liver failure because of inability of the liver to synthesize urea, and in disease states such as SIADH and acromegaly.[2,7]

## Creatinine

*Normal Range*

0.6–1.2 mg/dL              SI 53–106 μmol/L

*Description*

Muscle creatine and phosphocreatine break down to form creatinine.[2,7] Creatinine is released into the blood and excreted by glomerular filtration in the kidneys.[1] As long as muscle mass remains fairly constant, creatinine formation remains constant.[7] An increase in serum creatinine in the face of unchanged creatinine formation suggests a diminished ability of the kidneys to filter creatinine.[7] Thus, serum creatinine is used as a tool to identify patients with renal dysfunction.[1,2]

*Clinical Significance*

Increased Creatinine

Increased creatinine is associated with renal dysfunction, dehydration, urinary tract obstruction, vigorous exercise, hyperthyroidism, myasthenia gravis, increased protein intake, and use of nephrotoxic drugs such as cisplatin and amphotericin B.[2,7]

Decreased Creatinine

Serum creatinine may be reduced in patients with cachexia, inactive elderly or comatose patients, and spinal cord injury patients.[7]

BUN/Creatinine Ratio

Calculating the BUN/creatinine ratio may suggest an etiology for renal dysfunction.[7] A BUN/creatinine ratio greater than 20 suggests a prerenal cause such as GI bleeding. A BUN/creatinine ratio between 10 and 20 indicates intrinsic renal disease. [2,7]

Creatinine Clearance (CrCl)

This calculation provides an estimate of the creatinine clearance (CrCl).[7] In addition to assessing kidney function in patients with renal failure, the CrCl can be used to monitor patients on nephrotoxic medications and to assess need for renal dosing adjustments.[7]

The estimated CrCl using the Cockroft and Gault formula is calculated as follows:[7]

$$\text{Estimated CrCl (ml/min)} = \frac{[(140\text{-age}) \times \text{weight in kg}]}{(\text{SCr} \times 72)}$$

The equation must be multiplied by 0.85 if the patient is female. Ideal body weight is used in this equation except if the patient's actual body weight is less than their ideal body weight. In that case, the actual body weight should be used.

## Calcium (Ca⁺⁺)

*Normal Range*

8.5–10.5 mg/dL          SI 2.1–2.6 mmol/L

*Description*

The majority of calcium in the body (98–99%) is found in the skeletal bones and teeth.[2,10] The remainder is found in the blood, muscle, and other tissues. In addition to playing a role in bone mineralization, calcium is important in cardiac and skeletal muscle contraction, blood coagulation, enzyme activity, glandular activity, and transmission of nerve impulses.[10] In the blood, approximately half of the calcium is in the ionized "free" state, and the other half is bound to proteins or complexed with anions. Only calcium in the free state may be utilized in physiologic functions.[10] Calcium levels are regulated by a complex system that involves the skeleton, kidneys, intestines, parathyroid hormone, vitamin D, and serum phosphate.[2,10]

*Clinical Significance*

Increased Calcium

The most common causes of increased calcium (*hypercalcemia*) are malignancies and primary hyperparathyroidism.[2,10] Other causes include Paget's disease, sarcoidosis, vitamin D intoxication, milk alkali syndrome, Addison disease, and use of thiazide diuretics and lithium.

Decreased Calcium

Causes of decreased calcium (*hypocalcemia*) include hypoparathyroidism, vitamin D deficiency, hyperphosphatemia, acute pancreatitis, alkalosis, alcoholism, renal disease, and use of loop diuretics.[2,10]

Pseudohypocalcemia

Approximately one-half of serum calcium circulates bound to plasma proteins such as albumin.[2,10] A decreased albumin concentration may lead to a decreased total serum calcium concentration, and calcium levels may appear falsely low in the presence of low albumin.[2] Serum calcium levels may be corrected for low albumin as follows:

Corrected calcium: Reported serum calcium + 0.8 (4.0 − patient's albumin)

## Inorganic Phosphorus (PO₄)

*Normal Range*

2.5–4.5 mg/dL          SI 0.8–1.45 mmol/L

*Description*

Phosphate is an intracellular anion involved in several critical physiologic functions.[10] Phosphate is necessary for formation of the cellular energy source adenosine triphosphate (ATP) and the synthesis of phospholipids. Phosphate also plays a role in protein, fat, and carbohydrate metabolism, as well as acid-base balance.[2] Phosphate has an inverse relationship with calcium.[10]

*Clinical Significance*

Increased Phosphate

Increased phosphate (*hyperphosphatemia*) can result from renal dysfunction, increased vitamin D intake, increased phosphate intake, hypoparathyroidism, bone malignancy, and use of laxatives.[2]

Decreased Phosphate

Decreased phosphate (*hypophosphatemia*) can be associated with overuse of aluminum- and calcium-containing antacids (these bind phosphorus in the GI tract), alcoholism, malnutrition, hyperparathyroidism, and respiratory alkalosis.[2,10]

## Magnesium (Mg$^{++}$)

*Normal Range*

1.5–2.4 mg/dL                  SI 0.75–1.2 mmol/L

*Description*

Magnesium is a necessary cofactor in physiologic functions utilizing ATP.[2] It is also vital in protein and nucleic acid synthesis, carbohydrate metabolism, and contraction of muscle tissue.[2]

*Clinical Significance*

Increased Magnesium

Increased magnesium (*hypermagnesemia*) may result from renal failure or Addison disease.[2] In addition, the administration of Mg supplements or Mg-containing antacids or laxatives to patients with renal dysfunction may also result in hypermagnesemia.[2,10]

Decreased Magnesium

Reduced magnesium (*hypomagnesemia*) may be associated with diarrhea, renal wasting, vomiting, malabsorption, alcoholism, hyperaldosteronism, chronic pancreatitis, diabetes mellitus, hypercalcemia, and use of loop diuretics, amphotericin B, cisplatin, or PPIs.[2,10]

## Uric Acid

*Normal Range*

| | | |
|---|---|---|
| Male | 3.4–8.5 mg/dL | SI 202–506 μmol/L |
| Females | 2.3–6.6 mg/dL | SI 137–393 μmol/L |

*Description*

Uric acid is the main metabolic end product of the purine bases of DNA.[2,15]

*Clinical Significance*

Increased Uric Acid

Increased uric acid (*hyperuricemia*) may be caused by excessive production of purines or inability of the kidney to excrete urate.[15] Common causes of hyperuricemia are renal dysfunction, metabolic acidosis, tumor lysis syndrome, purine rich diet, and use of furosemide, thiazide diuretics, and niacin.[2,15]

    Hyperuricemia may be associated with the development of gouty arthritis, nephrolithiasis, and gouty tophi.[2]

Decreased Uric Acid

Decreased uric acid levels (*hypouricemia*) are usually of little clinical significance but may occur with a low-protein diet, deficiency of xanthine oxidase, or use of allopurinol, probenecid, or high doses of aspirin or vitamin C.[2,15]

## Osmolality

*Normal Range*

280–303 mOsm/kg       SI 280–303 mmol/kg

*Description*

Plasma osmolality describes the osmotic concentration or number of osmotically active particles in the plasma.[2] It can be used to evaluate water and electrolyte balance. Sodium, glucose, and BUN are the main components that determine serum osmolality.[2] The serum osmolality may be calculated as follows:

$$\text{Serum osmolality} = 1.86\,[\text{Na}^+] + \text{glucose}/18 + \text{BUN}/2.8$$

*Clinical Significance*

Increased Serum Osmolality

Increased serum osmolality (*hyperosmolality*) may occur with dehydration, DKA, and ethanol, methanol, or ethylene glycol toxicity.[2]

Decreased Serum Osmolality

Decreased serum osmolality may be caused by overhydration, hyponatremia, or diabetes insipidus.[2]

## Total Serum Protein

*Normal Range*

6.0–8.5 g/dL      SI 60–85 g/L

*Description*

The total serum protein is the sum of albumin, globulins, and other circulating proteins in the serum.[2] Albumin and globulins are indicators of nutritional status.[2]

*Clinical Significance*

Increased Protein

Increased protein (*hyperproteinemia*) may be associated with collagen vascular diseases (lupus, rheumatoid arthritis, scleroderma), sarcoidosis, multiple myeloma, and dehydration.[2]

Decreased Protein

Decreased serum protein (*hypoproteinemia*) may result from a decreased ability to synthesize protein (liver disease) or an increased protein wasting as seen in renal disease, nephrotic syndrome, and third-degree burns.[2]

## Cholesterol

For a complete discussion of cholesterol, please see the section in cardiac tests.

## CARDIAC TESTS

### Creatine Kinase (CK)

*Normal Range*

The normal range may vary with the assay used.

Total CK

| Male | 38–200 IU/L |
| Female | 26–150 IU/L |

CK-MB

<12 IU/L or <4% of total CK

*Description*

CK is an enzyme that is found primarily in skeletal and cardiac muscle and in smaller fractions in the brain.[13] CK levels may be fractionated into isoenzymes to distinguish CK from muscle (CK-MM), brain (CK-BB), and cardiac tissue (CK-MB). CK-MB is an important marker in the diagnosis of acute myocardial infarction (AMI).[13]

*Clinical Significance*

The CK-MB levels begin to rise 4 to 8 hours after onset of acute myocardial infarction.[2,13] The concentration usually peaks between 12 and 24 hours, and levels return to normal 2 to 3 days after AMI.[2,16] Serial CK-MB tests are useful in the diagnosis of AMI. An elevated CK-MB level or a CK-MB fraction greater than 4% to 5% of total CK is suggestive of AMI.[2,13]

An elevation of total CK may be seen with trauma, surgery, shock, seizures, muscular dystrophy, cerebrovascular accident, polymyositis, dermatomyositis, chronic alcoholism, Reye syndrome, and malignant hyperthermia.[13]

## Troponin

*Normal Range*

| | |
|---|---|
| Troponin I (cTnI) | <1.5 ng/mL (varies with assay) |
| Troponin T (cTnT) | <0.2 ng/mL |

*Description*

Troponin I and T are sensitive markers of cardiac injury.[13,16] Troponin I is found solely in the cardiac muscle, and Troponin T is found in both cardiac and skeletal muscle.[1]

*Clinical Significance*

Troponin levels begin to rise within 4 hours of onset of chest pain.[13] Levels should be drawn on admission and within 8 to 12 hours thereafter. Patients with elevated troponin levels are considered at high risk for a significant cardiac event.[2,13]

Approximately 30% of patients with no elevation in CK-MB may demonstrate elevated troponin and thus be diagnosed with a non-Q-wave myocardial infarction.[1,2]

## Brain Natriuretic Peptide (BNP)

*Normal Range*

<100 pg/ml        SI < 100 ng/L

*Description*

BNP is released from the heart in response to increased workload.[1]

*Clinical Significance*

Patients with HF usually have BNP levels greater than 100 ng/L, and if levels are over 500 ng/L this is indicative of left ventricular dysfunction.[1]

## C-Reactive Protein (CRP)

*Normal Range*

0–1.6 mg/dL        SI 0–16 mg/L

*Description*

CRP is produced in the liver and can aid in the diagnosis of inflammatory conditions such as rheumatoid arthritis or infections. It may also be useful as an indicator of risk for heart disease.[1]

*Clinical Significance*

This test is nonspecific in nature, and a more sensitive test for this parameter is the high sensitivity (hs-CRP).[1] This newer test can identify patients with cardiovascular disease earlier in the disease progression. An hs-CRP level less than 1.0 mg/L indicates low risk for a coronary event, and a value greater than 3.0 mg/L indicates high risk.[1]

## Lactate Dehydrogenase (LD, LDH)

For a complete discussion on LDH, please see the section in gastrointestinal tests.

## LIPOPROTEIN PANEL

## Total Serum Cholesterol

*Blood Levels*[17]

| | | |
|---|---|---|
| Desirable Level | <200 mg/dL | SI <5.17 mmol/L |
| Borderline High | 200–239 mg/dL | SI 5.17–6.19 mmol/L |
| High Cholesterol | ≥ 240 mg/dL | SI >6.20 mmol/L |

*Description*

Cholesterol is an important component of cell membranes and is necessary for the synthesis of many hormones and bile acids.[18] Elevated total serum cholesterol is well known to be associated with an increased risk of developing coronary heart disease (CHD). Total serum cholesterol is a useful screening test to determine CHD risk.[2]

*Clinical Significance*

Adults over 20 years of age should have a baseline fasting lipoprotein profile, and testing should be repeated at least every 4 to 6 years thereafter.[19] Cholesterol levels should be performed after the patient has fasted for at least 9 to 12 hours.[18]

Increased Serum Cholesterol

In cases of elevated cholesterol (*hypercholesterolemia*), the need for diet or drug therapy should be based on the individual components of the lipid profile (LDL, HDL, and triglycerides) and patient-specific factors, such as the presence of diabetes or clinical atherosclerotic cardiovascular disease (ASCVD), which includes CHD, stroke, and peripheral arterial disease. Some causes of hypercholesterolemia include obesity, familial hypercholesterolemia, and cholestasis.[2,18]

Decreased Serum Cholesterol

Decreased cholesterol levels may be seen in malabsorption, malnutrition, hyperthyroidism, chronic anemia, or severe liver disease.[2,18] However, low total serum cholesterol usually indicates good health.

## Low-Density Lipoprotein (LDL)

*Desired Range*[17]

| | |
|---|---|
| Optimal | < 100 mg/dL (2.58 mmol/L) |
| Near optimal/above optimal | 100–129 mg/dL (2.58–3.35 mmol/L) |
| Borderline high | 130–159 mg/dL (3.36–4.13 mmol/L) |
| High | 160–189 mg/dL (4.14–4.90 mmol/L) |
| Very high | ≥ 190 mg/dL (4.91 mmol/L) |

*Description*

Low-density lipoprotein is a major cholesterol transport protein which comprises 60% to 70% of total serum cholesterol. LDL is considered the "bad" cholesterol, and has been linked to atherosclerosis.[2]

*Clinical Significance*

LDL is not normally measured directly due to expense and time required; however, it should be measured in this manner if triglycerides are more than 400 mg/dl.[2,18] When the triglycerides are less than 400 mg/dL, LDL may be calculated using the Friedwald formula as follows[2]:

$$LDL = total\ cholesterol - HDL - (TG/5)$$

LDL levels should be interpreted in conjunction with patient-specific risk factors, such as the presence of clinical ASCVD or diabetes. Patients who fall into one of four specific groups are likely to benefit from LDL-lowering with HMG-CoA reductase inhibitors (statins).[19] The four statin benefit groups include:

- Patients with clinical ASCVD
- Patients with LDL cholesterol ≥ 190 mg/dL
- Patients with type 1 or 2 diabetes between the ages of 40 and 75 years
- Patients 40 to 75 years of age with an estimated 10-year ASCVD risk of ≥ 7.5%

In addition to lipid disorders, elevated LDL may also be associated with diabetes mellitus, diets high in cholesterol and saturated fat, hypothyroidism, and nephrotic syndrome.[2]

## High-Density Lipoprotein (HDL)

*Blood Levels*[17]

| | | |
|---|---|---|
| Low | <40 mg/dL | SI <1.03 mmol/L |
| High | >60 mg/dL | SI >1.55 mmol/L |

*Description*

High-density lipoproteins are responsible for transport of 20% to 30% of serum cholesterol.[2] HDL removes excess cholesterol from peripheral tissues to the liver. It is considered the "good" cholesterol, and elevated HDL levels are associated with a decreased risk for CHD.[2]

*Clinical Significance*

Decreased HDL may be associated with cigarette smoking, poorly controlled diabetes mellitus, lack of exercise, familial hypertriglyceridemia, and use of anabolic/androgenic steroids or β-blockers.[2]

It is estimated that CHD risk increases by 2% to 3% with each 1 mg/dL decrease in HDL.[18] Elevated HDL may be seen with moderate alcohol intake or in patients taking estrogen, oral contraceptives, or niacin.[18]

## Triglycerides

*Blood Levels*[2,17]

| | | |
|---|---|---|
| Normal range | <150 mg/dL | SI <1.7 mmol/L |
| Borderline High | 150–199 mg/dL | SI 1.7–2.26 mmol/L |
| High | 200–499 mg/dL | SI 2.26–5.64 mmol/L |
| Very High | ≥500 mg/dL | SI >5.64 mmol/L |

*Description*

Triglycerides are the main storage form of fatty acids, and they account for greater than 90% of dietary fat intake.[2]

*Clinical Significance*

Triglycerides may be significantly elevated in the nonfasting state and should be measured after a fast of at least 12 to 14 hours.[18] When triglycerides are greater than 2000 mg/dl it may cause xanthomas on the elbows, knees, and buttocks.[18]

In addition to lipid disorders, elevated triglycerides (*hypertriglyceridemia*) may be associated with a nonfasting sample, poorly controlled diabetes mellitus, pancreatitis, nephrotic syndrome, chronic renal failure, alcoholism, gout, and use of oral contraceptives or intravenous lipid infusion.[2,18] Most patients with elevated triglycerides may also have some of the other characteristics of the metabolic syndrome such as abdominal obesity, insulin resistance, hypertension, or low HDL.[17]

Decreased triglycerides may be associated with malnutrition or brain infarction.[2]

## ENDOCRINE TESTS: THYROID FUNCTION

### Thyroid-Stimulating Hormone (TSH)

*Normal Range*

0.3–5 mIU/L          SI 0.3–5 mIU/L

*Description*

TSH is a sensitive screening test used to detect hypothyroidism or hyperthyroidism.[8] An abnormal TSH level should be followed up with further thyroid testing, for example, free thyroxine. TSH is also useful for monitoring therapy for hypothyroidism or hyperthyroidism.[8]

*Clinical Significance*

Elevated TSH

Elevated TSH levels are indicative of hypothyroidism.[2] In patients taking thyroid replacement therapy, an elevated TSH suggests the need for an increase in the dose of thyroid medication. Metoclopramide and other dopamine antagonists may increase TSH.[8,14]

Low TSH

Abnormally low TSH levels (<0.10) are associated with hyperthyroidism. In patients taking thyroid replacement therapy, a decreased TSH indicates the need to reduce the dose of thyroid medication. Medications with dopaminergic activity (eg, dopamine, levodopa, and glucocorticoids) can decrease TSH levels.[2,8,14]

TSH should be monitored 6 to 8 weeks after initiation or a change in therapy. A desirable TSH in the normal range indicates a return to euthyroid state.

### Total Thyroxine (Total $T_4$)

*Normal Range*

4–12 μg/dL          SI 51–154 nmol/L

*Description*

$T_4$ is the predominant circulating thyroid hormone. Total serum thyroxine measures both free thyroxine and thyroxine bound to thyroxine-binding globulin, albumin and prealbumin.[14,20] Only the unbound thyroxine is active. $T_4$ levels are a measure of the functional status of the thyroid gland. $T_4$ may also be used to monitor thyroid therapy. $T_4$ levels may be affected by conditions that increase or decrease the thyroxine-binding proteins.[8]

*Clinical Significance*

Increased $T_4$

$T_4$ can be increased in hyperthyroidism, pregnancy, hepatitis, and with the use of estrogen replacement therapy, oral contraceptives, tamoxifen, and raloxifene.[2,14,20,21]

Decreased $T_4$

Decreased $T_4$ is most commonly seen in hypothyroidism, but may also be associated with renal failure, malnutrition, liver disease, and use of medications that compete for $T_4$ binding sites on $T_4$ binding proteins (eg, salicylates).[2,14] In addition, medications that increase the clearance of $T_4$ (eg, phenytoin, phenobarbital, and carbamazepine) may result in decreased $T_4$.[8,14,20]

# Free Thyroxine (Free $T_4$)

*Normal Range*

0.8–2.7 ng/dL          SI 10–35 pmol/L

*Description*

Because total $T_4$ levels can be affected by conditions that alter the amount of thyroxine binding proteins, free $T_4$ is a more accurate reflection of clinical thyroid status.[2]

*Clinical Significance*

Free $T_4$ is a diagnostic test that may be used to confirm the diagnosis of hypothyroidism (decreased free $T_4$) or hyperthyroidism (increased free $T_4$).[1] Free $T_4$ levels may be increased or decreased by amiodarone and iodides and decreased with lithium.[8]

# Total Triiodothyronine ($T_3$)

*Normal Range*

80–200 ng/dL          SI 1.2–3.1 nmol/L

*Description*

Although $T_3$ is not the predominant circulating thyroid hormone, $T_3$ is three to four times more potent than $T_4$.[1,2,8] The majority of $T_3$ is formed from deiodination of $T_4$

in the kidney and liver. Total $T_3$ measures both bound and unbound $T_3$. $T_3$ is usually used in the diagnosis of hyperthyroidism or $T_3$ toxicosis, but has little utility in the diagnosis of hypothyroidism.[2,8]

*Clinical Significance*

Increased $T_3$

Increased $T_3$ is seen in hyperthyroidism, $T_3$ thyrotoxicosis (Graves' disease), and with high doses of levothyroxine. Pregnancy and use of estrogens or oral contraceptives may also be associated with elevated $T_3$.[2,8]

Decreased $T_3$

Decreased $T_3$ may be associated with hypothyroidism, malnutrition, and anorexia. Corticosteroids and propranolol decrease peripheral conversion of $T_4$ to $T_3$ and may result in reduced $T_3$ levels.[2,8]

## ENDOCRINE TESTS: DIABETES MELLITUS

### Glycosylated Hemoglobin (Hemoglobin A$_{1c}$, HbA$_{1c}$)

*Normal Range*

4–5.6%

*Description*

The $HbA_{1c}$ measures the percentage of Hgb A molecules that are glycosylated (bound to glucose).[22] During the life span of a RBC, glucose binds irreversibly to Hgb in the RBC. As the serum glucose becomes more elevated, more glucose binds to the Hgb. Because the RBC has a life span of approximately 120 days, the $HbA_{1c}$ reflects average blood glucose for the previous 2 to 3 months.[2,22]

*Clinical Significance*

The $HbA_{1c}$ may be used to assess glucose control over the 2 to 3 months preceding the test.

The American Diabetes Association recommends a target $HbA_{1c}$ of less than 7% for most diabetic patients.[23] A $HbA_{1c}$ greater than 7% indicates the need for improved diabetic control through adjustment of diet, exercise, or medication regimen.

The correlation between $HbA_{1c}$ and the estimated average blood glucose can be described by the following formula[23,24]:

$$eAG(mg/dL) = 28.7 \times A1c - 46.7$$

| A1c (%) | Glucose (mg/dL) |
|---------|-----------------|
| 6 | 126 |
| 7 | 154 |
| 8 | 183 |
| 9 | 212 |
| 10 | 240 |
| 11 | 269 |
| 12 | 298 |

It is important to remember that the $HbA_{1c}$ does not provide an indication of the variability in glucose levels, only an estimate of the average. $HbA_{1c}$ may not be a reliable indicator of the average glucose in patients with anemia, hemolysis, or acute blood loss.[22,23]

## ENDOCRINE TESTS: ADRENAL GLAND

### Cortisol

*Normal Range*

| | | |
|---|---|---|
| Morning | 6–25 µg/dL | 165–690 nmol/L |
| Evening | 3–16 µg/dL | 83–441 nmol/L |

*Description*

Cortisol is a hormone produced by the adrenal cortex. It plays a critical role in carbohydrate metabolism and response to stress. Cortisol plasma levels undergo a normal diurnal variation and are highest in the early morning hours.[2,14]

*Clinical Significance*

Increased Cortisol

Increased cortisol levels are associated with Cushing syndrome, Cushing disease, hyperthyroidism, pregnancy, stress, and morbid obesity.[2]

Decreased Cortisol

Decreased cortisol may be secondary to Addison disease, hypothyroidism, or decreased pituitary function.[2]

### Urine Free Cortisol

*Normal Range*

Cortisol level 24 to 108 mcg/24 hours (varies with assay)

*Description*

Urine free cortisol is a screening test for Cushing syndrome. Urine is collected for 24 hours, and cortisol and creatinine levels are measured.[8,14]

*Clinical Significance*

Cortisol levels greater than 200 to 250 mcg/24 hours are highly suggestive of Cushing syndrome.[8,14]

## Overnight Dexamethasone Suppression Test

*Normal Range*

Cortisol < 5 µg/dL at 8:00 AM.

*Description*

In the overnight dexamethasone suppression test, 1 mg of dexamethasone is given at 11 PM, and plasma cortisol levels are drawn at 8:00 AM. In a normal patient, the administration of exogenous steroid (dexamethasone) should suppress the release of cortisol from the adrenal gland. The dexamethasone suppression test is useful in the diagnosis of Cushing syndrome.[2,14]

*Clinical Significance*

A plasma cortisol level >5 µg/dL suggests the diagnosis of Cushing syndrome.[8,14] Further testing may be necessary to determine if the hypercortisolism is due to adrenal gland hyperplasia, an adrenocorticotropic hormone (ACTH)-producing tumor, or a pituitary adenoma (Cushing disease). Elevated cortisol levels may also be seen in patients who are under various types of stress, including acute illness, pregnancy, and major depression. Results should be interpreted with caution in these populations.[2]

## Adrenocorticotropic Hormone (ACTH)

*Normal Range*

<60 pg/mL          SI < 13.2 pmol/L

*Description*

ACTH is a hormone secreted from the anterior pituitary. It controls the release of cortisol from the adrenal gland.[8]

*Clinical Significance*

Increased ACTH

Increased ACTH may be associated with Cushing disease, adrenal hyperplasia, Addison disease, or ectopic ACTH production.[14]

Decreased ACTH

Decreased ACTH may be seen in adrenal malignancy or states of pituitary insufficiency.[14]

## ACTH Stimulation Test (Cosyntropin)

*Description*

The ACTH stimulation test is used to detect adrenal insufficiency. In the ACTH stimulation test, a baseline cortisol level is drawn. Then synthetic ACTH (cosyntropin) is administered, and cortisol and aldosterone levels are collected 30 and 60 minutes postadministration.[8,14]

*Clinical Significance*

Normal

A normal response is a rise in cortisol greater than 10 mcg/dL above baseline or a cortisol level greater than 20 mcg/dL.[2,8,14]

Abnormal

If plasma cortisol remains low and fails to rise greater than 10 μg/dL above baseline, this is indicative of adrenal insufficiency. The aldosterone level will help determine if the adrenal insufficiency is related to failure of the adrenal (primary adrenal insufficiency) or malfunction of the pituitary (secondary adrenal insufficiency).[14]

## GASTROINTESTINAL TESTS

### Alanine Aminotransferase (ALT)

Formerly called serum glutamic pyruvic transaminase (SGPT).

*Normal Range*

0–35 U/L          SI 0–0.58 μkat/L (varies with assay)

*Description*

ALT is an intracellular enzyme present in liver tissue. It is also located in myocardial, muscle, and renal tissue.[1,2,25]

*Clinical Significance*

High serum ALT concentrations are indicative of hepatocellular disease. Elevations greater than three times the upper limit of normal are considered significant. ALT is present in higher concentrations in the liver as compared to other tissues, and is considered a specific marker for liver disease.[1,25]

Increased levels of ALT may occur with hepatitis, alcoholic liver disease, mononucleosis, and cholestasis.[1,14] Elevated ALT may be caused by a number of medications, including HMG-CoA reductase inhibitors, niacin, phenytoin, and valproic acid.[26]

## Aspartate Aminotransferase (AST)

Formerly called serum glutamic oxaloacetic transaminase (SGOT).

*Normal Range*

0–35 U/L          SI 0–0.58 µkat/L (varies with assay)

*Description*

AST is another intracellular aminotransferase found in the liver. It is also present in the heart, kidney, pancreas, lungs, and skeletal muscle.[1,14,25] Injury to these tissues will release AST into the systemic circulation and result in serum AST elevation. Of the two amino-transferase enzymes, ALT is considered a more specific marker of liver disease than AST.[1,25]

*Clinical Significance*

Elevated AST is associated with hepatitis, alcoholic liver disease, cholestasis, peri-carditis, acute myocardial infarction, trauma, HF, mononucleosis, severe burns, renal infarction, pulmonary infarction, and acute pancreatitis.[1,25] In alcoholic liver disease, the ratio of AST to ALT is usually greater than 2:1.[1,25]

Elevations of AST may also be seen with drug toxicity. Acetaminophen, eryth-romycin, levodopa, methyldopa, and tolbutamide may falsely elevate AST by inter-fering with the assay.[25]

## Alkaline Phosphatase (Alk Phos or ALP)

*Normal Range*

30–120 U/L (varies with age and assay)

*Description*

ALPs are a group of isoenzymes located in the bone and liver. Some alkaline phos-phastase is also present in the intestine, kidneys, and the placenta.[1,2,25]

*Clinical Significance*

Elevated concentrations of ALP may be seen in a variety of conditions, including obstructive liver disease, cholestasis, cirrhosis, healing bone fractures, bone growth, Paget's disease, bone metastases, hyperthyroidism, pregnancy, and sepsis.[1,25]

If the source of elevated ALP is unclear, the isoenzyme may be fractionated to discern if the cause is liver, bone, or other. Alternatively, an increased γ-glutamyl transpeptidase (GGT) with an elevated ALP is highly suggestive of a liver source for the increased ALP (see section on GGT).[2,25]

## Ammonia (NH₃)

*Normal Range*

30–70 µg/dL          SI 17–41 µmol/L

*Description*

Ammonia is generated through metabolism of protein by intestinal bacteria. Usually, ammonia is absorbed into the systemic circulation, metabolized by the liver, and the by-product urea is excreted by the kidneys.[2,25] Ammonia concentration is most often used in the diagnosis and monitoring of hepatic encephalopathy.

*Clinical Significance*

Elevated concentrations of ammonia are associated with cirrhosis, other liver diseases, Reye syndrome, GI hemorrhage, total parenteral nutrition, and inherited disorders of the urea cycle.[2,25]

## Bilirubin (Bili)

*Normal Range*

| | | |
|---|---|---|
| Total bili | 0.1–1.0 mg/dL | SI 1.7–17.1 μmol/L |
| Indirect | 0.2–0.7 mg/dL | SI 3.4–12 μmol/L |
| Direct | 0–0.2 mg/dL | SI 0–3.4 μmol/L |

*Description*

Bilirubin is a breakdown product of Hgb. The bilirubin produced from Hgb metabolism is referred to as unconjugated or indirect bilirubin. Unconjugated bilirubin is converted to conjugated or direct bilirubin by the liver through the process of glucuronidation. Conjugated bilirubin is excreted into the bile and subsequently into the intestine. In the intestine, some bilirubin is metabolized to urobilinogen. The majority of urobilinogen is excreted in the feces, and the remainder is reabsorbed and later excreted in the bile or the urine.[1,25]

*Clinical Significance*

Increased levels of indirect bilirubin may result from hemolysis, pernicious anemia, large hematomas, and the inherited disorder Gilbert syndrome.[2] Elevated direct bilirubin may be associated with hepatocellular disease and cholestasis.[25]

Total bilirubin is the sum of the direct and indirect bilirubin. Jaundice is a classic sign of hyperbilirubinemia that usually occurs when total bilirubin exceeds 2 to 4 mg/dL. Other signs of hyperbilirubinemia include scleral icterus and dark urine.[2,25]

## γ-Glutamyl Transpeptidase (GGT, GGTP)

*Normal Range*

| | |
|---|---|
| Male | 0–65 U/L |
| Female | 0–40 U/L |

*Description*

GGT is an enzyme found in the liver, kidney, and pancreas. GGT levels are useful in the diagnosis and monitoring of alcoholic liver disease.[1,25]

*Clinical Significance*

Increased GGT may be seen in alcoholic liver disease, metastatic liver disease, obstructive jaundice, cholelithiasis, and pancreatitis.[1,25]

Enzyme inducers that cause microsomal proliferation such as phenobarbital, rifampin, phenytoin, carbamazepine, and ETOH may also increase GGT levels.[1,2] GGT is considered a sensitive marker of ETOH intake.[1,2]

As mentioned previously, an elevated GGT associated with an increased ALP suggests a hepatic source for the abnormal ALP. Conversely, a normal GGT in the face of an elevated ALP points to a nonhepatic cause of the elevated ALP.

## Lactate Dehydrogenase (LD, LDH)

*Normal Range*

100–210 U/L           (may vary with assay)

*Description*

LDH is an enzyme involved in the interconversion of lactate and pyruvate. It is found in many tissues, including heart, brain, liver, skeletal muscle, kidneys, lungs, and RBCs.[1,2,25] Elevated LDH is not a very specific finding, as it may occur with damage to any of the aforementioned tissues. If LDH is elevated, it may be fractionated into five isoenzymes to better determine the source of the abnormality.[25]

*Clinical Significance*

$LDH_4$ and $LDH_5$ are present in liver tissue, and elevations may be seen in liver disease such as hepatitis and cirrhosis.[1,25] $LDH_1$ and $LDH_2$ may be useful in the diagnosis of myocardial infarction. After an acute MI, levels of LDH begin to rise within 8 to 12 hours, and the ratio of $LDH_1$: $LDH_2$ will be greater than 1 (referred to as a "flip" because levels of $LDH_2$ normally exceed $LDH_1$).[2,13]

Other conditions associated with an increased LDH include hemolysis, trauma, pulmonary infarction, acute renal infarction, malignancy, and myocarditis.[2,14]

## Amylase

*Normal Range*

35–120 units/L (may vary with assay)

*Description*

Amylase is an enzyme that aids in digestion by breaking down complex carbohydrates into simple sugars.[1] The majority of amylase is produced in the pancreas and salivary glands, and lesser amounts are secreted by the fallopian tubes, lungs, thyroid, and tonsils.[25] Serum amylase levels are most often used in the diagnosis of acute pancreatitis. The amylase level begins to rise 2 to 6 hours after the onset of acute pancreatitis.[2,25]

*Clinical Significance*

Increased concentrations of amylase may be seen in acute pancreatitis, exacerbation of chronic pancreatitis, cholecystitis, appendicitis, ectopic pregnancy, mumps, alcoholism, and DKA.[1,2,14,25]

Alcohol abuse and cholecystitis are the two most common causes of pancreatitis in adults.[14] Some medications associated with a risk for pancreatitis include cimetidine, didanosine, estrogens, sulfonamides, tetracycline, valproic acid, DPP-4 inhibitors (eg, sitagliptin, saxagliptin) and GLP-1 agonists (eg, exenatide, liraglutide).[25,27]

## Lipase

*Normal Range*

0–160 U/L (may vary with assay)

*Description*

Lipase is an enzyme that aids in the digestion of fat. It is primarily secreted by the pancreas. Lipase is also useful in the diagnosis of pancreatitis and is considered a more specific marker for pancreatitis than amylase. Like amylase, the lipase level begins to rise within 2 to 6 hours of onset of acute pancreatitis.[1,14,25]

*Clinical Significance*

Elevations of lipase are most often associated with acute pancreatitis.[14] Lipase may also be elevated with cholecystitis, biliary cirrhosis, pancreatic cancer, and small bowel obstruction; however, it is usually to a lesser extent than that seen with acute pancreatitis.[2,14,25]

If lipase is normal and amylase is elevated, this suggests a nonpancreatic origin for the increased amylase.

## Helicobacter pylori IgG

*Normal Value*

Negative

*Description*

*Helicobacter pylori* is a gram-negative rod that is responsible for the majority of cases of peptic ulcer disease. *H. pylori* can be detected in 90% to 100% of patients with duodenal ulcers and 70% to 80% of patients with gastric ulcers. *H. pylori* IgG is a serologic test that detects antibodies to *H. pylori*. A positive test indicates the presence of *H. pylori*.[2,25]

*Clinical Significance*

A positive *H. pylori* IgG in the presence of symptoms is highly suggestive of peptic ulcer disease, and a course of antibiotic therapy is warranted. *H. pylori* IgG may remain positive for many months after treatment of the infection. *H. pylori* has been linked to some types of gastric lymphoma and gastric cancer.[25]

## Hemoccult

*Normal Value*

Negative

*Description*

The Hemoccult test is used to detect the presence of occult blood in the stool.[28]

*Clinical Significance*

A positive Hemoccult test indicates blood loss in the gastrointestinal tract and deserves further work-up.

A false-positive result may be obtained if the patient has consumed red meat, broccoli, turnips, or radishes within 3 days of the test.[28] Aspirin (in doses >325 mg daily), NSAIDs such as ibuprofen, and excess ETOH consumption have also been associated with false positives. False negatives may occur in patients taking high doses of vitamin C or consuming large amounts of citrus fruits or juices.[28]

A Hemoccult test should be performed yearly in all patients more than 50 years of age.

## HEMATOLOGIC TESTS

### Iron

*Normal Range*

| | | |
|---|---|---|
| Male | 80–180 µg/dL | SI 14–32 µmol/L |
| Female | 60–160 µg/dL | SI 11–29 µmol/L |

*Description*

The serum iron measures the concentration of iron bound to the iron transport protein transferrin.[1-3] Under normal circumstances, approximately one-third of transferrin molecules are bound to iron.

*Clinical Significance*

Increased Serum Iron

Increased iron may be associated with excessive iron therapy, frequent transfusions, pernicious anemia, hemolytic anemia, thalassemia, and hemochromatosis (iron overload).[2]

Decreased Serum Iron

Reduced serum iron is most commonly associated with iron deficiency anemia, a microcytic, hypochromic anemia. Causes include poor dietary intake, pregnancy, blood loss associated with menses, peptic ulcer disease, and gastrointestinal bleeding. Other causes of decreased iron are malignancies, anemia of chronic disease, chronic renal disease, and hemodialysis.[2,14]

In iron deficiency anemia, serum iron levels may remain within the lower limit of normal. Thus, serum iron levels are best interpreted along with total iron-binding capacity (TIBC).[3]

## Ferritin

*Normal Range*

| Male   | 15–250 ng/mL | SI 15–250 µg/L |
| Female | 10–150 ng/mL | SI 10–150 µg/L |

*Description*

Ferritin is the storage form of iron. The serum ferritin level provides an accurate reflection of total body iron stores.[2]

*Clinical Significance*

Increased Serum Ferritin

Increased ferritin may result from hemochromatosis. Since ferritin is an acute phase reactant it may also be elevated in patients with malignancies, inflammatory disorders, or infection/fever.[2,3,14]

Decreased Serum Ferritin

Decreased serum ferritin is associated with iron deficiency anemia.[2]

## Total Iron-Binding Capacity (TIBC)

*Normal Range*

250–460 µg/dL          SI 45–82 µmol/L

*Description*

Total iron-binding capacity is an indirect measurement of the iron transport protein transferrin.[3] The test is performed by adding an excess of iron to a plasma sample. Any excess unbound iron is removed from the sample, and the serum iron concentration in the sample is determined. The measured serum iron concentration reflects the TIBC of serum transferrin.

*Clinical Significance*

Increased TIBC

Increased TIBC may be associated with iron deficiency anemia, pregnancy, and oral contraceptive use.[3,14]

Decreased TIBC

Decreased TIBC may be caused by anemia of chronic disease, malignancy, infections, uremia, cirrhosis, hyperthyroidism, and hemochromatosis.[2,3]

## Vitamin B$_{12}$ (Cobalamin)

*Normal Range*

200–900 pg/mL          SI 148–664 pmol/L

*Description*

This test measures serum levels of vitamin B$_{12}$. Vitamin B$_{12}$ is important in DNA synthesis, neurologic function, and hematopoiesis.[3,29] Deficiency of vitamin B$_{12}$ produces a macrocytic anemia. Patients may also present with glossitis, paresthesias, muscle weakness, gastrointestinal symptoms, loss of coordination, tremors, and irritability.

*Clinical Significance*

Decreased vitamin B$_{12}$ may be caused by inadequate dietary intake (rare except for vegan diets), deficiency of intrinsic factor (necessary for absorption of B$_{12}$), or increased requirements.[3,29] Decreased levels of B$_{12}$ are associated with pernicious anemia, gastrectomy, Crohn's disease, small bowel resection, intestinal infections, and use of colchicine or neomycin.[3,14]

## Folate

*Normal Range*

3.0–25 ng/mL          SI 6.8–56.8 nmol/L

*Description*

This test measures serum folate. Like vitamin B$_{12}$, folic acid is a vitamin necessary for synthesis of DNA. Deficiency of folic acid results in megaloblastic anemia.[29]

*Clinical Significance*

Inadequate intake (major cause), decreased absorption, or inability to convert folic acid to the active form tetrahydrofolate may cause decreased folate.[3,29] Folic acid deficiency is associated with alcoholism, poor nutrition, pregnancy, hyper-thyroidism, Crohn's disease, small bowel resection, celiac disease, and the use of medications such as trimethoprim, triamterene, methotrexate, phenytoin, and sulfasalazine.[3,29]

## COAGULATION TESTS

### Prothrombin Time (PT)

*Normal Range*

10–13 seconds (varies with thromboplastin and test method used)

*Description*

The prothrombin test is sensitive to changes in the levels of clotting factors pro-thrombin (factor II), factor VII, and factor X.[30] It is performed by adding thrombo-plastin and calcium to a plasma sample. After addition of these reagents, the time it takes the blood to clot is measured.

*Clinical Significance*

The PT is used to monitor warfarin therapy. Because the PT may vary according to the thromboplastin used to test the sample, the international normalized ratio (INR) is a better monitoring tool.[6,30]

The normal PT in a person not on anticoagulation therapy is 10 to 13 seconds. An increased PT may be seen with anticoagulation therapy, liver disease, vitamin K deficiency, and clotting factor deficiencies.[2,14]

### International Normalized Ratio (INR)

*Desired Range*

Depends on indication for anticoagulation (see below)

*Description*

Because the PT may vary due to the thromboplastin used, the INR is used to stan-dardize the PT.[6,30] The INR adjusts the PT ratio based on the sensitivity of the thromboplastin used to perform the test.

The INR may be calculated as follows:

$$INR = [(Patient\ PT)/(Mean\ Normal\ PT)]^{ISI}$$

ISI is the international sensitivity index rating assigned to a particular thromboplastin.

Desired ranges for the INR are as follows[30,31]:

| INR 2.0–3.0 | Atrial fibrillation |
|---|---|
| | DVT treatment |
| | PE treatment |
| | Prophylaxis of venous thrombosis |
| | Tissue heart valves |
| | Valvular heart disease |
| | Mechanical heart valves (certain types only)* |
| INR 2.5–3.5 | Mechanical heart valves (valves not meeting criteria for INR 2–3)* |
| | |
| *Refer to CHEST guidelines[31] for a thorough discussion of desired INR. | |

*Clinical Significance*

An INR below the desired range indicates suboptimal anticoagulation and a need to increase warfarin dosage. Conversely, an INR above the desired range indicates a need to omit and/or reduce the warfarin dosage. Patients with elevated INRs and/or bleeding may require the administration of vitamin K, fresh frozen plasma, or clotting factors.[30]

To appropriately interpret an INR value and decide on the need for dosage adjustments, patients should be questioned regarding dosage of warfarin, missed doses, dietary intake, alcohol intake, and concomitant medications.

## Activated Partial Thromboplastin Time (aPTT)

*Normal Range*

20–35 seconds (Varies per reagent used; please check at your institution!)

*Description*

The aPTT is sensitive to changes in the intrinsic and common coagulation pathways. It is used to monitor heparin therapy.[2,6] Monitoring of the aPTT is usually not required for patients receiving low molecular weight heparin (LMWH).

*Clinical Significance*

The normal value above represents a control range for patients not on anticoagulation therapy. Patients on heparin therapy will have an elevated aPTT. Much like the PT, the aPTT can vary depending on the reagent (partial thromboplastin) used to test the sample. Therefore, a therapeutic range should be established for each institution based on the partial thromboplastin used at that laboratory.[32] An aPTT below the desired therapeutic range indicates the need to rebolus and/or increase the heparin infusion rate. An aPTT above the desired therapeutic indicates the need to hold and/or reduce the dose of heparin. Patients with clinically significant bleeding may require reversal with protamine sulfate.[32]

## IMMUNOLOGIC TESTS

### Antinuclear Antibodies (ANA Titer)

*Normal Value*
Negative at 1:20 dilution (varies)

*Description*
Antinuclear antibodies (ANA) are antibodies directed against structures in the cell nucleus, for example, nucleic acids.[15] The ANA test is used as a diagnostic tool for autoimmune and connective tissue diseases, particularly systemic lupus erythematosus (SLE).[14,15]

*Clinical Significance*
High titers may be associated with SLE, rheumatoid arthritis, scleroderma, Sjögren syndrome, polymyositis, dermatomyositis, and drug-induced lupus (hydralazine, procainamide).[14,15] False-positive ANA test results may occur in 2% to 5% of healthy patients.

### Rheumatoid Factor (RF)

*Normal Value*
<1:20 or 0–20 IU/mL

*Description*
RF is an immunoglobulin whose activity is directed against IgG. Thus, a positive RF test (titer > 1:20 or level > 20 IU/mL) is indicative of an autoimmune process.[15]

*Clinical Significance*
A positive RF test is most commonly associated with rheumatoid arthritis, but may also be seen with SLE, Sjögren syndrome, scleroderma, malignancy, and infectious diseases such as TB, syphilis, mononucleosis, and endocarditis.[14,15]

### Erythrocyte Sedimentation Rate (ESR)

*Normal Range*

| Male   | 1–15 mm/hr (varies with age) |
|--------|------------------------------|
| Female | 1–20 mm/hr (varies with age) |

*Description*

The erythrocyte sedimentation rate measures the rate of erythrocyte settlement in anticoagulated blood. In the presence of proteins known as acute phase reactants, erythrocytes settle much more quickly. Acute phase reactants are often associated with infectious or inflammatory disorders. Thus, the ESR is a nonspecific diagnostic test that may be used to support a diagnosis or monitor the progress of an inflammatory or infectious process.[14,15]

*Clinical Significance*

The ESR is most valuable in the diagnosis and monitoring of polymyalgia rheumatica and temporal arteritis.[2,14,15] The ESR may also be elevated in bacterial infections such as TB and syphilis, malignancies, rheumatoid arthritis, SLE, scleroderma, and other collagen vascular diseases.

## INFECTIOUS DISEASE DIAGNOSTIC TESTS

### Enzyme Immunoassay (EIA or ELISA) for HIV

*Description*

The ELISA for HIV detects antibodies to HIV. It is a highly sensitive and specific test and is the most commonly used screening test for HIV.[14,33]

*Clinical Significance*

False Positive

False-positive results may occur in patients with lupus, syphilis, lymphoma, liver disease, and renal failure.[14,33] Positive tests should be repeated to assure positive results. Repeatedly positive samples should be confirmed with the Western blot test or immunofluorescence assay.[14,33]

False Negative

False negatives may be seen in early HIV infection and bone marrow transplant.[14]

### Western Blot

*Description*

The Western blot is a confirmatory test used following a positive ELISA result. It detects antibodies to specific proteins of the HIV virus.[14,33]

*Clinical Significance*

Positive Result

A positive result following a positive ELISA test confirms the diagnosis of HIV.

Negative Result

A negative result indicates no HIV antibodies. The ELISA in this case can be considered a false positive.[14]

Indeterminate Result

Indeterminate results may occur if seroconversion is not complete (ie, it is too early in the disease process). Individuals should be retested at a later date.[2,33]

## CD4 T-Cell Count (CD4 Count)

*Normal Range*

$700-1100/mm^3$

*Description*

CD4 cells are a subset of T lymphocytes also known as "helper" cells. CD4 cells play an important role in the immune system and are a good marker of immune status in HIV patients.[34]

*Clinical Significance*

As the CD4 count decreases, the HIV patient is at increased risk of acquiring opportunistic infections. When the absolute CD4 count falls to less than 200, the diagnosis is no longer just HIV but AIDS.[34]

Current guidelines recommend initiation of antiretroviral therapy for all HIV-infected individuals regardless of CD4 count. CD4 count may also be used to assess immunologic response to antiretroviral therapy. With appropriate medication and adherence to treatment the CD4 count may increase.[34]

## HIV Viral Load

*Range of Assay*

HIV–1 RNA          5–1,000,000 copies/mL  (varies with assay)

*Description*

HIV viral load testing measures the amount of HIV virus detectable per milliliter of plasma. Higher viral loads are associated with a poorer prognosis and progression of disease. Viral load should be measured at baseline, 2 to 8 weeks after initiation or change of therapy, and approximately every 3 to 4 months thereafter.[34]

*Clinical Significance*

Desirable viral loads are below the limit of detection; for example, "undetectable" is < 50 copies/mL for the Amplicor assay, and <10 copies/mL for the NucliSens EasyQ HIV-1 assay.[14] Increasing viral loads may indicate viral resistance or nonadherence to therapy. HIV drug resistance testing may be useful in selecting new regimens for patients with virologic failure or suboptimal virologic suppression.[34]

## RPR (Rapid Plasma Reagin)

*Normal Value*

Nonreactive

*Description*

Syphilis is caused by the spirochete *Treponema pallidum.* The RPR is a nontrepone-mal serologic test used to screen for syphilis. It may also be used to assess response to syphilis therapy.[14,33,35]

*Clinical Significance*

A positive RPR titer is suggestive of syphilis and should be followed up with a con-firmatory treponemal test such as the fluorescent treponemal antibody absorbed test (FTA-abs) or the *T. pallidum* particle agglutination (TP-PA).[33,35]

False Positive

False-positive results may occur with other infectious diseases such as measles, chickenpox, malaria, mononucleosis, hepatitis, early HIV infection, and conditions such as pregnancy, lupus, and connective tissue disease.[2,14]

False Negative

False-negative results may be seen early in infection, and in late infection the test may also be nonreactive.

Most patients revert to a nonreactive test following successful treatment. A fourfold decline in the RPR titer after 6 months may also be considered an adequate response to treatment.[35]

## Venereal Disease Research Laboratory Test (VDRL)

*Normal Value*

Nonreactive

*Description*

The VDRL is a nontreponemal serologic test used to screen for syphilis. It may also be used to assess response to syphilis therapy.[33,35]

*Clinical Significance*

A positive VDRL titer is suggestive of syphilis and should be followed up with a confirmatory treponemal test such as the fluorescent treponemal antibody absorbed test (FTA-abs) or the *T. pallidum* particle agglutination (TP-PA).[35]

False Positive

False-positive results may be caused by other infectious diseases such as measles, chickenpox, malaria, mononucleosis, hepatitis, early HIV infection, and other con-ditions such as pregnancy, lupus, and connective tissue disease.[2,33]

**False Negative**

False-negative results may be seen early in infection, and in late infection the test may also be nonreactive.

Most patients revert to a nonreactive test following successful treatment. A fourfold decline in the VDRL titer after 6 months may also be considered an adequate response to treatment.[35]

## HEPATITIS A

### Anti-HAV IgM

*Normal Value*

Negative

*Description*

Hepatitis A IgM antibodies may be detected in the serum 4 to 6 weeks after exposure to hepatitis A and often coincide with the onset of symptoms and jaundice.[2,14,25]

*Clinical Significance*

The presence of anti-HAV IgM indicates acute or recent hepatitis A infection. In most cases, anti-HAV IgM becomes negative within 3 to 6 months after acute hepatitis.[2,14,25]

### Anti-HAV IgG

*Normal Value*

Negative

*Description*

Anti-HAV IgG can be detected 8 to 12 weeks after exposure to hepatitis A.[2,25]

*Clinical Significance*

Presence of anti-HAV IgG indicates previous infection or HAV immunization and immunity to the virus.[2,25]

## HEPATITIS B

### HBsAg (Hepatitis B Surface Antigen)

*Normal Value*

Negative

*Description*

HBsAg is an envelope protein on the surface of the hepatitis B virus. It can be detected in the serum 4 to 12 weeks after infection.[14,25,36]

*Clinical Significance*

A positive test for HBsAg indicates acute hepatitis B. Persistence of HBsAg for 6 months or more after acute infection is indicative of chronic hepatitis B.[2,14]

## Hepatitis B "e" Antigen (HBeAg)

*Normal Value*

Negative

*Description*

HBeAg is used to assess the degree of infectivity of patients with hepatitis B.

*Clinical Significance*

Presence of HBeAg is associated with active viral replication and a high degree of infectivity. HBeAg is usually present for 2 to 6 weeks after acute infection. Persistence of HBeAg is indicative of ongoing viral replication, that is, chronic hepatitis B.[14,25]

## Hepatitis B Core Antibody (Anti-HBc)

*Normal Value*

Negative

*Description*

Anti-HBc IgM and IgG may be detected in the blood a few weeks after the appearance of HBsAg.[2,14]

*Clinical Significance*

Positive anti-HBc IgM is a sensitive marker for acute hepatitis B infection. The presence of anti-HBc IgG indicates past infection with hepatitis B. Anti-HBc IgG antibodies seem to persist for life.[2,14,36]

## Hepatitis B Surface Antibody (Anti-HBs)

*Normal Value*

Negative

*Description*

Anti-HBs is usually detected in the blood 3 to 4 months after infection.[37]

*Clinical Significance*

Presence of anti-HBs indicates recovery and immunity to hepatitis B.

Individuals who have been vaccinated for hepatitis B will test positive for anti-HBs. Anti-HBs concentrations may decline and/or reach undetectable levels several years after vaccination; however, immunity persists for most patients.[37]

## HEPATITIS C

### Hepatitis C Antibody (Anti-HCV)

*Normal Value*

Negative

*Description*

Anti-HCV is used as a screening test for hepatitis C virus.

*Clinical Significance*

Presence of anti-HCV indicates prior exposure to or chronic infection with hepatitis C. Unlike antibodies to hepatitis A and hepatitis B, antibodies to hepatitis C do not confer immunity.[2,25] Antibodies may not be present until 6 to 12 weeks after acute infection.[25]

A positive test for Anti-HCV should be followed by a confirmatory test such as the radioimmunoblot assay (RIBA) or hepatitis C viral load (HCV RNA by PCR).[14]

## QUESTIONS

1. Which of the following would be considered an abnormal laboratory value?
   A. Potassium level—5.9
   B. TSH—5.0 µg/dL
   C. Urine protein—trace
   D. WBC—5600 cell/mm$^3$
2. Which of the following laboratory values is most consistent with the diagnosis of iron deficiency anemia in a female?
   A. Ferritin < 10 ng/mL
   B. Hgb 14 g/dL
   C. MCV 106 µm$^3$/cell
   D. TIBC 350 µg/dL
3. Which of the following laboratory values is most consistent with metabolic acidosis?
   A. Decreased chloride
   B. Elevated anion gap
   C. Increased $CO_2$ content
   D. Blood pH 7.45

4. A patient is taking a three-day course of phenazopyridine. Which of the following laboratory parameters is most likely to be altered by administration of phenazopyridine?

   **A.** Blood glucose

   **B.** Hemoccult test

   **C.** Magnesium

   **D.** Urine appearance and color

5. Which of the following laboratory values would suggest the need for a change in pharmacotherapy to better achieve patient outcomes?

   **A.** An AST of 35 U/L in a patient taking an HMG-CoA reductase inhibitor

   **B.** A fasting glucose of 195 in a patient with diabetes

   **C.** An LDL level of 70 mg/dL in a patient with a history of CHD

   **D.** A uric acid level of 5.0 mg/dL in a patient with a history of gout

## REFERENCES

1. Schwartz CR, Garrison MW. Chapter 2. Interpretation of clinical laboratory tests. In: Alldredge BK, Corelli RL, Ernst ME, Guglielmo BJ, eds. *Koda-Kimble & Young's Applied Therapeutics: The Clinical Use of Drugs*. 10th ed. Baltimore, MD: Lippincott Williams & Wilkins; 2013:16–41.

2. Fischbach FT, Dunning MB, eds. *A Manual of Laboratory and Diagnostic Tests*. 8th ed. Philadelphia, PA: Lippincott Williams & Wilkins; 2009.

3. Hutson PR. Hematology: red and white blood cell tests. In: Lee M, ed. *Basic Skills in Interpreting Laboratory Data*. 4th ed. Bethesda, MD: American Society of Health-System Pharmacists; 2009:339–362.

4. Cook K, Ineck B, Lyons W. Chapter 109. Anemias. In: Talbert RL, DiPiro JT, Matzke GR, Posey LM, Wells BG, Yee GC, eds. *Pharmacotherapy: A Pathophysiologic Approach*. 8th ed. New York, NY: McGraw-Hill; 2011.

5. Rybak MJ, Aeschlimann JR, Laplante KL. Chapter 113. Laboratory Tests to Direct Antimicrobial Pharmacotherapy. In: Talbert RL, DiPiro JT, Matzke GR, Posey LM, Wells BG, Yee GC, eds. *Pharmacotherapy: A Pathophysiologic Approach*. 8th ed. New York, NY: McGraw-Hill; 2011.

6. Allen SM, dela Pena LE. Hematology: blood coagulation tests. In: Lee M, ed. *Basic Skills in Interpreting Laboratory Data*. 4th ed. Bethesda, MD: American Society of Health-System Pharmacists; 2009:363–390.

7. Trombetta DP, Foote EF. The kidneys. In: Lee M, ed. *Basic Skills in Interpreting Laboratory Data*. 4th ed. Bethesda, MD: American Society of Health-System Pharmacists; 2009:161–178.

8. Vivian EM. Endocrine disorders. In: Lee M, ed. *Basic Skills in Interpreting Laboratory Data*. 4th ed. Bethesda, MD: American Society of Health-System Pharmacists; 2009:271–318.

9. Dowling TC. Chapter 50. Clinical Assessment of Kidney Function. In: Talbert RL, DiPiro JT, Matzke GR, Posey LM, Wells BG, Yee GC, eds.

*Pharmacotherapy: A Pathophysiologic Approach.* 8th ed. New York, NY: McGraw-Hill; 2011.

10. Lau A, Chan LN. Electrolytes, other minerals, and trace elements. In: Lee M, ed. *Basic Skills in Interpreting Laboratory Data.* 4th ed. Bethesda, MD: American Society of Health-System Pharmacists; 2009:119–160.

11. Hall TG. Arterial blood gases and acid-base balance. In: Lee M, ed. *Basic Skills in Interpreting Laboratory Data.* 4th ed. Bethesda, MD: American Society of Health-System Pharmacists; 2009:79–190.

12. American Diabetes Association. Diagnosis and classification of diabetes mellitus. *Diabetes Care* 2013;36(Suppl 1):S67–S74.

13. Dahdal WY, Dahdal SY. The heart: laboratory tests and diagnostic procedures. In: Lee M, ed. *Basic Skills in Interpreting Laboratory Data.* 4th ed. Bethesda, MD: American Society of Health-System Pharmacists; 2009:207–234.

14. Bakerman S, Bakerman P, Strausbach P. *ABC's of Interpretive Laboratory Data.* 4th ed. Scottsdale, AZ: Interpretive Laboratory Data; 2002.

15. Schwinghammer TL. Rheumatic diseases. In: Lee M, ed. *Basic Skills in Interpreting Laboratory Data.* 4th ed. Bethesda, MD: American Society of Health-System Pharmacists; 2009:449–474.

16. The Joint European Society of Cardiology/American College of Cardiology Committee. Myocardial infarction redefined—a consensus document of The Joint European Society of Cardiology/American College of Cardiology Committee for the Redefinition of Myocardial Infarction. *European Heart Journal* 2000;21(18):1502–1513.

17. Executive summary of the third report of the National Cholesterol Education Program (NCEP) expert panel on detection, evaluation, and treatment of high blood cholesterol in adults (Adult Treatment Panel III). *JAMA* 2001(19);285:2486–2497.

18. Burkiewicz JS. Lipid Disorders. In: Lee M, ed. *Basic Skills in Interpreting Laboratory Data.* 4th ed. Bethesda, MD: American Society of Health-System Pharmacists; 2009:319–338.

19. Stone NJ, Robinson J, Lichtenstein AH, Bairey Merz CN, Blum CB, Eckel RH, Goldberg AC, Gordon D, Levy D, Lloyd-Jones DM, McBride P, Schwartz JS, Shero ST, Smith SC Jr, Watson K, Wilson PWF. 2013 ACC/AHA guideline on the treatment of blood cholesterol to reduce atherosclerotic cardiovascular risk in adults: a report of the American College of Cardiology/American Heart Association Task Force on Practice Guidelines. *Circulation.* 2013;00:000–000.

20. Dong BJ, Schneider EF. Chapter 52. Thyroid disorders. In: Alldredge BK, Corelli RL, Ernst ME, Guglielmo BJ, eds. *Koda-Kimble & Young's Applied Therapeutics: The Clinical Use of Drugs.* 10th ed. Baltimore, MD: Lippincott Williams & Wilkins; 2013:1186–1222.

21. American Association of Clinical Endocrinologists. Medical guidelines for clinical practice for the evaluation and treatment of hyperthyroidism and hypothyroidism. *Endocr Pract.* 2002;8:457–469.

22. Williams C, Kroon LA. Diabetes mellitus. In: Alldredge BK, Corelli RL, Ernst ME, Guglielmo BJ, eds. *Koda-Kimble & Young's Applied Therapeutics: The Clinical Use of Drugs*. 10th ed. Baltimore, MD: Lippincott Williams & Wilkins; 2013:1223–1300.

23. American Diabetes Association. Standards of medical care in diabetes—2013. *Diabetes Care* 2013;36(Suppl 1):S11–S66.

24. Nathan DM. Kuenen J, Borg R, Zheng H, Schoenfeld D, Heine RJ. Translating the A1C assay into estimated average glucose values. *Diabetes Care*. 2008;31:1–6.

25. Farkas JD, Farkas P. Liver and gastroenterology tests. In: Lee M, ed. *Basic Skills in Interpreting Laboratory Data*. 4th ed. Bethesda, MD: American Society of Health-System Pharmacists; 2009:235–270.

26. Holt CD, Arriola ER. Adverse effects of drugs on the liver. In: Koda-Kimble MA, Young LY, Kradjan WA, Guglielmo BJ, eds. *Applied Therapeutics: The Clinical Use of Drugs*. 8th ed. Baltimore, MD: Lippincott Williams & Wilkins; 2005:30-1–30-29.

27. Byetta [package insert]. Amylin Pharmaceuticals, Inc., San Diego, CA; 2011. Available at http://documents.byetta.com/Byetta_PI.pdf. Accessed March, 2014.

28. Hemoccult [package insert]. Beckman Coulter, Inc., Fullerton, CA; 2005. Available at https://www.beckmancoulter.com/wsrportal/wsr/diagnostics/clinical-products/rapid-diagnostics/hemoccult/index.htm. Accessed March, 2014.

29. O'Bryant CL, Thompson LA. Anemias. In: Alldredge BK, Corelli RL, Ernst ME, Guglielmo BJ, eds. *Koda-Kimble & Young's Applied Therapeutics: The Clinical Use of Drugs*. 10th ed. Baltimore, MD: Lippincott Williams & Wilkins; 2013: 232–251.

30. Ageno W, Gallus AS, Wittkowsky A, Crowther M, Hylek EM, Palareti G. Oral anticoagulation therapy: antithrombotic therapy and prevention of thrombosis, 9th ed: American College of Chest Physicians Evidence-Based Clinical Practice Guidelines. *Chest*. 2012;141(2 suppl):e44S–e88S.

31. Whitlock RP, Sun JC, Fremes SE, Rubens FD, Teoh KH. Antithrombotic and thrombolytic therapy for valvular disease. *CHEST* 2012;141(suppl 2):e576S–e600S.

32. Garcia DA, Baglin TP, Weitz JI, Samama MM. Parenteral anticoagulants: antithrombotic therapy and prevention of thrombosis, 9th ed: American College of Chest Physicians Evidence-Based Clinical Practice Guidelines. *Chest* 2012;141 (2 suppl):e24S–e43S.

33. Erdman SM, Atkinson KM, Rodvold KA. Infectious diseases. In: Lee M, ed. *Basic Skills in Interpreting Laboratory Data*. 4th ed. Bethesda, MD: American Society of Health-System Pharmacists; 2009:391–448.

34. Panel on Antiretroviral Guidelines for Adults and Adolescents. Guidelines for the use of antiretroviral agents in HIV-1-infected adults and adolescents. Department of Health and Human Services. Available at http://aidsinfo.nih.gov/ContentFiles/AdultandAdolescentGL.pdf. Accessed March, 2014.

35. Centers for Disease Control and Prevention. Update to CDC's Sexually transmitted diseases treatment guidelines, 2010: oral cephalosporins no longer a recommended treatment for gonococcal infections. MMWR Morb Mortal Wkly Rep. 2012 Aug 10;61(31):590–594.
36. Holt CD. Chapter 77. Viral hepatitis. In: Alldredge BK, Corelli RL, Ernst ME, Guglielmo BJ, eds. *Koda-Kimble & Young's Applied Therapeutics: The Clinical Use of Drugs.* 10th ed. Baltimore, MD: Lippincott Williams & Wilkins; 2013:1790–1827.
37. Centers for Disease Control and Prevention. A comprehensive immunization strategy to eliminate transmission of hepatitis B virus infection in the United States. *MMWR* 2006;55(No. RR-16):1–25.

CHAPTER

# 12

# Designing Patient Treatment Plans: Pharmacokinetic Foundations

*Sandra B. Earle*

**Objectives: Upon completion of the chapter and exercises, the student pharmacist will be able to**

1. Define components of a dosage regimen (dose rate and dose interval) and predict how they influence concentrations of drug in the plasma. ($C_{ss,avg}$ and $P{:}T$).
2. List the factors influencing the bioavailability of an orally administered drug.
3. List the determinants of volume of distribution and why volume changes may or may not matter.
4. List the determinants of renal clearance and determine how drugs and disease may alter renal clearance and thus alter $C_{ss,avg}$ and/or $P{:}T$ of a given drug cleared by the kidney.
5. List the determinants of hepatic clearance and determine how drugs and disease may alter hepatic clearance and thus alter $C_{ss,avg}$ and/or $P{:}T$ of a given drug cleared by the liver.
6. Given appropriate concentration-time data, calculate $k$, $t_{1/2}$, $C_{max}$, $C_{min}$, and AUC for that drug in that patient.
7. Explain the reasons for drug monitoring and how that will impact the patient's outcome.
8. Discuss the attributes of extended-interval dosing and traditional dosing for aminoglycosides.

---

### Patient Encounter

You are the student pharmacist rounding with the team this month and patient X is not doing as well as the neurology team would like. The neurology resident and medical student come to you to discuss what they might do about pain control and seeing if they can "wake the patient up by reducing his medications." There are really two issues. They have started to reduce the morphine dose in an effort to see if the patient will begin to respond to the team, but so far he

*(continued on next page)*

has not. Alternatively, they are slightly hesitant to reduce the dose because even though the dose of morphine seems to be high enough to keep him from responding to pain, he appears to the team to be agitated. The team is coming to you to see what other drugs on the patient profile may be confounding patient improvement.

As the student pharmacist responsible for working with the team this month, you are expected to participate in solving the problem. First, you must decide what the problem is.

1. What other drugs is the patient being given that may interact?

2. You find there are no pharmacologic or pharmacokinetic drug interactions. What problems are specifically related to the morphine?

3. What do you know about the absorption of morphine across the blood-brain barrier (BBB)? What happens to the $T_{max}$ or AUC?

4. Does trauma cause any change in protein binding or transport, $\alpha_1$-acid glycoprotein, albumin, or P-glycoprotein?

5. What happens to the metabolism of morphine in the brain? What happens to the $T_{\frac{1}{2}}$? Are the active metabolites responsible?

6. Once you have determined the answers to the above questions, what would be your response to the medical student and resident?

Hypothesize several scenarios for the morphine problem above; include not only pharmacologic considerations, but also the pharmacokinetics of absorption, distribution, metabolism, and elimination as possible culprits for the issues at hand.

## INTRODUCTION

The word *pharmacokinetics* strikes fear into the hearts of many students. It should not. The knowledge of pharmacokinetic principles and the ability to apply that knowledge empowers us to do our job well. We are expected to know how to use drugs effectively and safely. To do this we need to understand how drugs affect the body and also how the body affects the drug. Pharmacokinetics is the study of the body's effect on a given drug. Many health-care practitioners have a good understanding of how drugs work, but the pharmacist is the most well educated in pharmacokinetics. Therefore, pharmacists must take on the challenge of mastering these principles and their application.

Bioavailability, distribution, and clearance of a drug are important pharmacokinetic parameters to understand. They are introduced early in the chapter and discussed in more detail later. When a drug is introduced to the body, it first must get to the bloodstream in order to reach the systemic receptors. The fraction of given drug that reaches the systemic circulation is the bioavailability ($F$) of the drug. It will be reported as a percentage or fraction. If a drug's bioavailability is altered, that will affect how much drug is available to work. How the drug distributes in the body is also important to consider. The volume of distribution ($V_d$) of a drug relates the amount of drug in the body to the measured plasma concentration; or, how much volume does there have to be to account for the known amount of drug in the body and the concentration measured. It may help to think of the volume as how much space the drug moves around in, in the body. A large volume of distribution implies a higher amount of tissue binding and slower elimination from the body. Elimination rate constant ($k$) is dependent on the volume of distribution and the clearance of a drug. The elimination rate constant determines how long it takes for the drug to be eliminated from the body. The faster the $k$ the faster the drug leaves the body. Clearance (CL) is often confused with elimination rate or elimination rate constant. Clearance is defined as the volume of blood that can have all the drug removed from it per unit time. Therefore, the units for clearance are volume per time. How fast a drug can be eliminated from the body is dependent on elimination rate constant. The elimination rate constant is dependent upon how efficiently the body can eliminate the drug (CL) and how readily available the drug is to the clearance organ ($V_d$). A drug that has a large volume is not easily available to the clearance organ. Therefore, it will take a longer time for elimination even if the efficiency or clearance of the organ of elimination is large. Bioavailability, volume of distribution, and clearance are the parameters that might be affected by drugs, disease, and other interacting entities. Understanding of these principles enables the pharmacist to predict drug and disease interactions and changes can be made in the individual dosage regimen to accommodate the interaction.

## DOSAGE REGIMEN DESIGN

Pharmacists are often asked to predict and/or react to individual patient outcomes due to pharmacokinetic variations. Practitioners cannot easily affect pharmacokinetic parameters such as bioavailability, distribution, or clearance. The best practice is to alter the dosing regimen that a patient is getting of a particular drug to control the outcome. The dosing regimen is made up of two components: dose rate (DR) and dose interval ($\tau$).

Dose rate (DR) is the amount of drug the individual is receiving per time, so the units will be amount of drug per time. A constant infusion is an easy example. If a patient is getting a 2 mg/min drip of lidocaine, his dose rate is 2 mg/min. If a patient is getting 1 g of cefotaxime every 8 hours, the dose rate is 125 mg/h or

3 g/day. The dose interval ($\tau$) is how often the patient is receiving the drug. The units for dose interval ($\tau$) will be time. In the above example, the cefotaxime dose interval is every 8 hours. These two components work together to determine the dose. Do not confuse dose with dose rate. For the patient getting 1 gram of cefotaxime every 8 hours, if he develops renal impairment the DR would need to be decreased (because the concentrations would increase) and the $\tau$ could be increased (since it is not being cleared as rapidly it could be given less often). This might mean that the dose remains the same. The dose may continue to be 1 gram but it would be given every 12 hours rather than every 8 hours. This would decrease the DR from 3 grams/day to 2 grams/day while keeping the dose constant.

## Average Concentration at Steady State

Commonly, the two factors targeted when trying to maximize efficacy and minimize toxicity are the average concentration at steady state ($C_{ss,avg}$) and the peak-to-trough ratio ($P{:}T$) (Fig. 12.1). Think of steady state as a type of equilibrium. $C_{ss,avg}$ gives a good picture of the overall average concentration seen during a dosing interval at

**Figure 12.1.** Giving the same dose rate with differing results in different peak-to-trough ratios but the same AUC and same $C_{ss,avg}$.

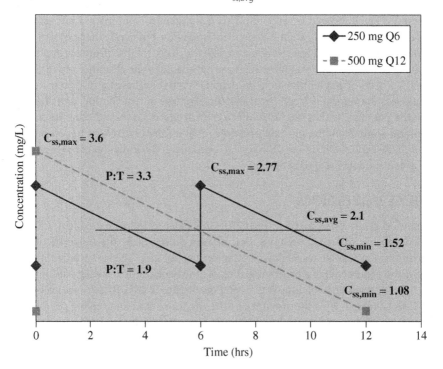

steady state. It is often the parameter that is targeted for maintenance within a given range for a drug. The determinants of $C_{ss,avg}$ are therefore very important. They include bioavailability (F), dose rate (DR), and clearance (CL) (Eq. 12.1).

$$C_{ss,avg} = \frac{F \times DR}{CL} \qquad (12.1)$$

Therefore, if there is a change in CL, F, or DR, there will be an alteration in $C_{ss,avg}$. This may result in possible toxic or subtherapeutic concentrations. The DR could then be either decreased (if toxic) or increased (if subtherapeutic) to accommodate that change. For example, if a patient is on a drug that is cleared by the kidneys and they go into acute renal failure, the clearance (CL) will decrease. The result will be an increase in $C_{ss,avg}$ and possible toxicity. The pharmacist will therefore recommend a decrease in the DR of drug the patient is receiving. The consequence of the decreased DR will be a decrease in the $C_{ss,avg}$. In another case, if a patient were given an additional drug that decreased the bioavailability (F) of a drug the patient was already on, a decrease in $C_{ss,avg}$ would occur possibly causing a loss of efficacy. The pharmacist would respond by suggesting an increase in the DR of the drug the individual was initially taking to increase the $C_{ss,avg}$ and therefore increasing the effectiveness of the drug.

$C_{ss,avg}$ represents total drug, which includes both drug bound to plasma proteins and drug free from plasma proteins. There are proteins (eg, Albumin) present in the blood and plasma that can bind to drugs making them inert. When the laboratory measures drug in a blood or plasma sample it typically measures total drug concentration. This includes both protein bound (inert) and unbound (active) drug. Only unbound drug can interact at the pharmacologic site, so it alone is the active component. To determine the free/unbound concentration at steady state, the fraction unbound must be known (Eq. 12.2).

$$C_{ss,avg,free} = \frac{F \times DR}{CL} \times f_{up} \qquad (12.2)$$

Note that the determinants of $C_{ss,avg}$ and $C_{ss,avg,free}$ are the same other than the addition of the measure of plasma protein binding. ($f_{up}$ is the fraction of drug that is unbound in the plasma.) The $f_{up}$ will range from 0 to 1, which corresponds to none of the drug being free (0 or 0% free) to all of it being free (1 or 100% free).

## Peak-to-Trough Ratio

The peak-to-trough ratio (P:T) is also important in determining a safe, effective dosing regimen. This tells you how much the concentration varies between the highest concentration achieved (peak) and the lowest concentration achieved (trough). The peak concentration is the highest concentration achieved during a dosing interval sometimes called $C_{max}$ or maximum concentration. The trough concentration is the lowest concentrations achieved during the dosing interval sometimes called a $C_{min}$ or minimum concentration. If a drug is not given often enough, it may have an unacceptable $P{:}T$ meaning that there is too much variation between the peak and trough concentrations. For example, if the drug is given once a day rather than three times daily and the dose rate or total daily dose is the same, the peak concentration will be relatively high and the trough concentration relatively low. This could result in toxic peak concentrations and sub-therapeutic trough concentrations (Fig. 12.1). The smaller the pieces that you divide the daily dose into (the smaller the $\tau$), the less variation there will be between the peak and trough concentrations. This may be desirable, but it has to be weighed carefully with the ability of patients to comply with difficult dosing regimens (eg, taking a drug every 4 hours is very difficult for a patient). In addition, it is not always desirable to have a small $P{:}T$. For example, it is advantageous for aminoglycosides to have a large $P{:}T$. High peak concentrations are associated with better bacterial kill, and low trough concentrations may decrease the risk for nephrotoxicity from aminoglycosides. Elimination rate constant ($k$) and dosing interval ($\tau$) determine the $P{:}T$ (Eq. 12.3).

$$P : T = \frac{1}{e^{-k\tau}} \qquad (12.3)$$

The elimination rate constant ($k$) is a fractional rate of drug elimination. The units are inverse time, meaning a fraction per minute or per hour. It is a *dependent* variable meaning that it is determined by clearance (CL) and volume of distribution ($V_d$). Clearance (CL) is not determined by $k$, neither is volume ($V_d$) (Eq. 12.4).

$$k = \frac{CL}{V_d} \qquad (12.4)$$

If there is a change in CL, $V_d$, or dosing interval ($\tau$), there will be a change in $P{:}T$. (Eq. 12.3) This may result in unacceptably high or low peak concentrations and/ or unacceptable trough concentrations. It may be helpful to think about the relationship of elimination rate constant and half-life ($t_{1/2}$). They are inversely proportional (Eq. 12.5). Half-life is the time required for the serum concentration to decrease by 50%. Therefore, the determinants of half-life are also volume of distribution ($V_d$) and clearance (CL) (Eq. 12.6). Half-life is also important in determining time to steady state.

$$t_{1/2} = \frac{0.693}{k} \qquad (12.5)$$

$$t_{1/2} = \frac{0.693 \times V_d}{CL} \qquad (12.6)$$

## Steady State

Recall that steady state is a type of equilibrium. Technically, absolute 100% steady state never occurs, but each half-life cuts the remaining percent needed to reach steady state in half. Consider this illustration from the sport of football. Pretend the penalty for holding in football is half the distance to the goal. If a team were on the opposite goal line and had the whole field to go (100 yards) and benefited from this penalty, the team would gain 50 yards or half the field. If this penalty was called again, there would be only 50 yards remaining so they would gain 25 yards or half of the remaining 50 yards to the goal line. They would now have advanced 75 yards and have only 25 yards to go to the goal line. The third penalty would put the team only 12.5 yards away, etc. If the team continues to get this call over and over they would never reach the goal line. This idea can be applied to achievement of steady state. After 1, 2, 3, 4, and 5 half-lives, 50%, 75%, 87.5%, 93.8%, and 96.9% of steady state, respectively, has been achieved. Thus, it takes 5 half-lives to achieve approximately 97% of steady state. Five half-lives is commonly used as a proxy for steady state. Therefore when dosing a drug with a $t_{1/2}$ of 10 hours, it would take 50 hours or approximately 2 days to achieve steady state.

It is helpful to realize that with dosing every half-life, the peak-to-trough ratio will be 2. Therefore, the peak concentration will be twice the trough concentration. If dosing is more frequent, there will be less variation between the peak and trough concentrations, and if dosing is less frequent, there will be a greater deviation between peak and trough concentrations (Fig. 12.1). Remember the patient taking the drug cleared by the kidneys who suddenly goes into acute renal failure? That individual will have a decrease in CL. This decrease in clearance will result in an increase in the $C_{ss,avg}$ but will also decrease the elimination rate constant ($k$) and decrease the $P{:}T$. This may or may not be clinically acceptable. If this drug were an aminoglycoside, it might be unsatisfactory. To get the peak-to-trough ratio back to what it was before the onset of the acute renal failure, the dosing interval would need to be extended. In this case, the dose rate (DR) would need to decrease to lower the $C_{ss,avg}$, as discussed above. This would happen automatically if the dose interval were increased and the dose kept the same, because there would be less drug per unit time given, thus decreasing the dose rate.

If a decrease in volume of distribution occurred, it would cause an increase in the elimination rate constant ($k$) and a resulting increase in the peak-to-trough ratio. If the dosing regimen is not changed in this scenario, the peak-to-trough ratio will increase, possibly causing peak concentrations that result in toxic side effects or subtherapeutic trough concentrations or both. In this case a decrease in the dosing interval (giving the drug more frequently) would be important to avoid the large peak-to-trough ratio. However, the dose rate should be kept constant because the $C_{ss,avg}$ has not changed (no change in CL or F, Eq. 12.1). In this example, the dose per administration would decrease to maintain the same DR and therefore $C_{ss,avg}$.

In order to determine how to alter the dosage regimen, it is important to understand what factors will alter the bioavailability, volume of distribution, and clearance of drugs.

## Bioavailability

For a drug to work it must be made available to the appropriate receptors in the body. In most cases, this means that it must be made available to the systemic blood flow to enable the drug to get to the appropriate site of action. Bioavailability defines the fraction of given drug that is able to reach the systemic blood flow or made available to the receptors. It will range between 0 and 1. If the bioavailability is zero, 0% or none of the administered drug will reach the systemic circulation. If the bioavailability of a drug is one, then 100% or the entire dose of drug is reaching the circulation. A drug given intravenously will have a bioavailability of 100%. If given via the oral route, the drug would first have to be absorbed from the gut lumen into the gut wall; this is the fraction absorbed ($f_a$). That fraction of drug is then exposed to possible metabolism in the gut wall or expulsion from the gut wall back into the gut lumen (efflux). The fraction that escapes gut metabolism and efflux is symbolized by $f_g$. Finally, the drug that has been absorbed and not metabolized or effluxed ($f_a \times f_g$) would then be transported via the portal vein first to the liver where it may undergo some metabolism. The fraction that is able to avoid metabolism in the liver is called the fraction that escapes the first-pass effect ($f_{fp}$). Therefore, the bioavailable fraction ($F$) would be the fraction able to be absorbed and then avoid metabolism as it passes through the gut wall and liver (Eq. 12.7).

$$F = f_a \times f_g \times f_{fp} \qquad (12.7)$$

### Fraction Absorbed

The bioavailability of a drug is determined by many factors including route of administration, dosage form, physiological status of the patient, and the properties of the drug itself. Following the path of an orally administered drug, the obstacles of getting the drug to the site of action can be identified. First, the drug must be absorbed from the lumen into the gut wall. Most drug absorption in the gut follows the properties of passive diffusion. This means that for a drug to be absorbed, there must be a concentration gradient, and the drug must be in an absorbable form: small enough, relatively lipophilic, and un-ionized. Most absorption occurs in the small intestine because of the great amount of surface area available. Therefore, the rate of absorption is dependent on the drug getting to the site of absorption. Gastric emptying time is often the rate-limiting step in this process. Drug may not have time to be absorbed. This is especially true if there is an increase in gastric motility or if the drug does not have rapid enough dissolution. In this case the drug will be found unchanged in the feces. Another possibility is that the drug may decompose or be adsorbed or complexed in the lumen and thus will be found in the feces in the changed or complexed form (Fig. 12.2).

### Fraction Escaping Gut Metabolism

Once the drug makes it out of the lumen into the gut wall, there are both Phase I and Phase II enzymes in the gut wall that may be able to metabolize a portion of

**Figure 12.2.** Depiction of the trip a drug takes to undergo absorption.

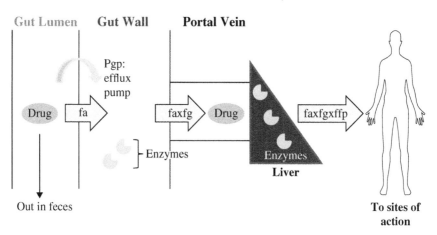

the drug (Fig. 12.2). Cytochrome P450 3A enzymes account for more than 70% of the small intestinal cytochrome enzymes (CYP).[1] There are also drug transport systems that can efflux drug from the gut wall back into the gut lumen. The most studied of these drug efflux systems is p-glycoprotein (P-gp), a member of the ABC cassette family of transporters. P-gp has been found in the cells lining the blood-brain barrier, kidney, adrenal glands, and lungs as well as many other tissues. The cells lining the intestinal tract all exhibit P-gp, with the concentrations increasing as you travel down from the esophagus to the colon.[2] The concentrations of CYP in the cells decrease as you travel down the intestinal tract. Many drugs are substrates, inducers, or inhibitors (Chap. 8) of both the CYP3A family and P-gp. There is some evidence to suggest P-gp may act as a gatekeeper to regulate the exposure of drug to the CYP enzymes in the gut wall.[3] There are examples of drug-drug and drug-food interactions that can now be explained by this mechanism of gut wall efflux and metabolism. Grapefruit juice is an important example of this. Grapefruit juice can inhibit the enzymes in the gut wall and therefore allow more of some drugs to reach the site of action. There is great potential for utilizing inducers and inhibitors of these systems to alter the fraction of drug escaping gut metabolism ($f_g$).

*Fraction Escaping Hepatic First Pass*

Finally, once a drug has been absorbed from the lumen to the gut wall ($f_a$) and escapes metabolism or efflux from the gut wall ($f_g$), it is then taken by the portal vein to the liver. The liver is a major organ responsible for the clearance of drugs by metabolism. It is rich with enzymes for both Phase I and Phase II reactions. Drugs extensively metabolized by hepatic enzymes in the liver, called high-extraction drugs, will have a very low bioavailability if given by a first-pass route.

---

**TABLE 12.1.  EXAMPLES OF DRUGS UNDERGOING A HIGH FIRST-PASS EFFECT**

| | |
|---|---|
| Amitriptyline | Labetalol |
| Chlorpromazine | Lidocaine |
| Cytarabine | Methylphenidate |
| Desipramine | Metoprolol |
| Dihydroergotamine | Morphine |
| Diltiazem | Naloxone |
| Doxepine | Neostigmine |
| Doxorubicin | Nicardipine |
| Encainide | Nicotine |
| Estradiol | Nifedipine |
| 5-FU | Nitroglycerin |
| Hydralazine | Pentoxifylline |
| Imipramine | Propranolol |
| Isoproterenol | Scopolamine |
| Isosorbidedintrate | Testosterone |
| Labetolol | Verapamil |

---

(Table 12.1) These drugs must be administered by a non-first-pass route in order to attain sufficient concentrations of parent drug at the receptor site. An example of this is nitroglycerin; it must be given intravenously, sublingually, or transdermally (Chap. 8) to be effective.

*Enterohepatic Cycling and Biliary Clearance*

A drug may also undergo biliary elimination and/or enterohepatic cycling (See also Chap. 8 for medical terminology). In this case, the drug is absorbed and delivered via the portal vein to the liver; then a portion may be secreted into the bile and stored in the gallbladder. The drug now in the bile will then reenter the intestine. At this point it might be reabsorbed to complete what is called an enterohepatic cycle or it may be excreted in the feces. The drug may also be metabolized in the liver. The new form of the drug is now called a metabolite. The metabolite may also be secreted into the bile so the metabolite can undergo the enterohepatic cycle or be excreted in the feces. The biliary transport of drugs is similar to renal tubular active secretion and can be competitively inhibited. Drugs that have a high biliary clearance have the following characteristics. They are polar, ionized, and have a molecular weight >250 g/mol.

**Figure 12.3.** Area under a concentration time curve.

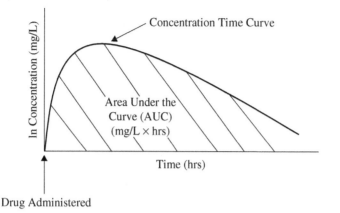

If a drug is enterohepatically cycling, it is continuously being reintroduced to the systemic circulation.

### Measuring Bioavailability

To determine the bioavailability of a drug by a given route of administration, a dose is given intravenously (IV) and by the route being measured. It is given orally (PO) in the example below. Concentrations are drawn periodically to determine a concentration-time curve for each route given. The area under the curve (AUC) for each dose/route combination is measured (Fig. 12.3). The bioavailable fraction will be equal to the quotient of the areas if equivalent doses are given (Eq. 12.8). If inequivalent doses are given, Eq. 12.9 is used to correct for the different doses.

$$F = \frac{AUC_{PO}}{AUC_{IV}} \tag{12.8}$$

$$F = \frac{Dose_{IV} \times AUC_{PO}}{Dose_{PO} \times AUC_{IV}} \tag{12.9}$$

The bioavailability of a drug is important because it is a determinant of the concentration at steady state ($C_{ss,avg}$) (Eq. 12.1). It is also important for determining a loading dose (LD) if the drug is not given intravenously (Eq. 12.10).

$$LD = \frac{C_{target} \times V}{F} \tag{12.10}$$

It is important to recognize all the potential drug-drug, drug-disease, and drug-nutrition interactions that might occur altering the bioavailability of a drug. This may be a problem when changing between products. If there is a change in the dissolution properties, or if the formulation has vehicles that could alter factors involved with $f_a$ or $f_g$, the bioavailability could be altered. This change in bioavailability might alter the $C_{ss,avg}$ and AUC, thus possibly necessitating a change in dose rate. The FDA does require testing to prove that a generic drug has an equivalent bioavailability to the brand name drug.

## Distribution

Once a drug has been made available to the receptors and rest of the body by entering the bloodstream, it distributes, which is the reversible transfer of drug from one place to another. Where a drug distributes is important both therapeutically and from a toxicologic standpoint. The extent of distribution is measured as a volume of distribution.

$$V_c, V_{ss}, V_z$$

There are three different volumes used as pharmacokinetic parameters, each having a different purpose. Initially when a drug is given it will distribute into the blood and highly perfused tissues. This is called the central volume of distribution ($V_c$) and is used to calculate loading doses (Eq. 12.11).

$$V_c = \frac{\text{Loading Dose (LD)}}{\text{Initial Concentration}} \qquad (12.11)$$

The volume of distribution at steady state ($V_{ss}$) represents the volume that the drug occupies when steady state is reached and the drug has been able to come to a distribution equilibrium (Eq. 12.12). It represents physiological spaces that describe the determinants of distribution. It is very difficult to measure because it requires measuring drug concentrations in tissues.

$$V_{ss} = \text{Blood Volume} + \left( \text{Tissue Volume} \times \frac{\text{Unbound fraction in blood}}{\text{Unbound fraction in tissues}} \right) \qquad (12.12)$$

The apparent volume of distribution ($V_z$) is a measurable but calculated volume not a physiologic space. (Eqs. 12.13 and 12.14). It is determined using the elimination rate constant. It is in most cases very similar to the $V_{ss}$. Therefore, the measurable $V_z$ is commonly used to represent the more physiological $V_{ss}$ and call that the volume of distribution ($V_d$).

$$k = \frac{\text{CL}}{V_z} \qquad (12.13)$$

$$t_{\frac{1}{2}} = \frac{0.693 \times V_z}{\text{CL}} \qquad (12.14)$$

The $V_c$ is the smallest volume of distribution, followed by $V_z$, with $V_{ss}$ being the relatively largest volume. When a volume of distribution of a drug $(V_d)$ is referred to, often one is considering the physiological determinants of $V_{ss}$ but measuring the $V_z$.

The volume of distribution can be thought of as the parameter that relates the amount of drug in the body to the measured plasma concentration. Or, how much volume does there have to be to account for the known amount of drug in the body and the concentration measured. The range of volumes of drugs varies widely from 0.04 to >500 L/kg. One may consider it impossible for a drug to have a volume of distribution of 65 L/kg such as amiodarone. How could this be? It is very highly bound to tissues. Consider this analogy.[4] Oil is discovered on an empty lot and the well is drilled. To calculate how much oil there is in the well a known amount of oil-miscible dye is added to the oil in the well and stirred to bring it to equilibrium. A sample of the oil is measured to determine the concentration of dye in the oil so the oil volume can be calculated.

Volume of oil in well (L) = $C_{ss}$ of dye (mg/L) × Known amt of dye added (mg)

By doing this, the oil well is calculated to have a very large volume. However, when the oil is pumped out, there is much less than calculated. What went wrong? There are rocks in the oil well that had bound up much of the dye. If the rocks bound up the dye, then the concentration of dye in the oil was more dilute, appearing as if the volume was much greater than it was when measured. Think of those rocks as tissue binding sites. The larger the volume of distribution, the higher the fraction of drug outside the plasma, which usually means it resides in the tissues bound there.

*Determinants of Distribution*

A volume of distribution will be dependent on the drug's binding to proteins in the blood and tissues, its ability to cross tissue membranes, and the degree to which it partitions into fat. Delivery of the drug by the blood to the tissues is highly dependent on the perfusion rate of the tissue. The rate of tissue uptake is proportional to how well it is perfused. Recall that a drug must be small enough, unbound, un-ionized, and lipophilic (Chap. 8) enough to pass through a tissue membrane.

*Plasma Protein Binding*

Distribution to extravascular tissues can happen only if the drug is not bound to protein in the plasma. Drugs are often bound to proteins in the plasma, most commonly albumin, followed by $\alpha_1$ acid glycoprotein (AAG), lipoproteins, and corticosteroid-binding protein.

The extent of plasma protein binding varies widely among drugs, ranging from less than 0.1% to 100% unbound. Drugs and disease can alter the number of binding sites available, thereby changing the fraction unbound of a drug. Also, there can be competition for available binding sites, resulting in an altered fraction unbound of a drug. The more highly a drug is bound the more likely that a binding interaction

| TABLE 12.2. EXAMPLES OF DRUGS HIGHLY BOUND TO PLASMA PROTEINS | |
| --- | --- |
| Alfentanil | Phenytoin |
| Amiodarone | Propranolol |
| Carbamazepine | Quinidine |
| Ibuprofen | Valproic acid |
| Nifedipine | Verapamil |
| Phenobarbital | Warfarin |

will be significant (Table 12.2). It is important for pharmacists to be able to recognize and anticipate these interactions.[5]

*Binding Proteins*

The two most important binding proteins in the plasma are AAG and albumin. Albumin is the most prevalent binding protein in the plasma. It preferentially binds acidic drugs but has a relatively lower binding affinity than AAG. Disease and drugs that can alter albumin concentrations are listed in Table 12.3. $\alpha_1$ acid glycoprotein (AAG), in contrast, is present in the plasma in low concentrations. But it is an acute-phase reactant and may increase fivefold when in an inflammatory state. Some diseases that increase AAG include those listed in Table 12.3. AAG preferentially binds to basic and neutral compounds. It has a very high affinity for the drugs it binds.

Plasma protein binding interactions are important to anticipate and recognize when a drug is highly protein bound (Table 12.2). When a laboratory measures a drug concentration, it is in most cases a total concentration. This includes both bound and unbound drug in the plasma. Only unbound drug is free to interact

| TABLE 12.3. EXAMPLES OF CONDITIONS THAT ALTER PLASMA PROTEINS | |
| --- | --- |
| **Decrease Binding to Albumin** | **Increase Binding to AAG** |
| Nephrotic syndrome | Crohn's disease |
| Nephritis | Cancer |
| Renal failure | Rheumatoid arthritis |
| Alcoholism | Surgery |
| Hepatic cirrhosis | Acute myocardial infarction |
| Burns | Nephrotic syndrome |
| Pregnancy | Trauma |
| Surgery | |

with the pharmacologic receptors. Therefore, the free concentration is what is important therapeutically. The total concentration will always reflect what is happening with the free concentration as long as there is no change in plasma protein binding. If there is a change in the fraction unbound in the plasma, total concentrations cannot be relied on to give a true reflection of what is happening to the active unbound concentration. This is most important with drugs that are highly bound to plasma proteins, with a $f_{up} \leq 0.25$ (Table 12.2). In this case, a small change in the $f_{up}$ will result in a large-magnitude change in the free concentration.

*Tissue Binding*

Although plasma protein binding is relatively easily measured, tissue binding is very difficult to determine. Tissue binding can be inferred by measuring the plasma protein binding and volume of distribution (Eq. 12.12). Only unbound drug in the plasma ($f_{up}$) can enter and leave the tissue sites. The relationship between the fraction unbound in the plasma and the fraction unbound in the tissues will determine if the drug is predominately in the tissue or predominately in the plasma. If the drug is more highly bound to plasma proteins than to tissue proteins ($f_{up} < f_{ut}$), it will have a relatively small volume. Even a drug with a strong affinity for its plasma protein binding site can be more highly bound in the tissue ($f_{up} > f_{ut}$). In this case, most of the drug will reside in tissue stores, and therefore, it will have a relatively large volume of distribution. Partitioning into fat is also a tissue-binding site and can result in a depot-like effect increasing the volume of distribution and thus the half-life of a drug in a patient with more fat stores.

## Clearance by Hemodialysis

The major factors that determine the ability of hemodialysis (See also Chap. 8 for medical terminology) to remove a drug are how available the drug is to the hemodialysis machine and if it is available for passive diffusion through the membrane. If a drug has a large volume of distribution, the drug is primarily in the tissues and not in the plasma. The drug must be in the plasma to reach the dialysis machine. If a drug has a sufficiently small volume of distribution it can reach the dialysis machine but it also must not be highly protein bound to be dialyzed. If it is highly protein bound, the drug-protein complex is too big to diffuse passively through the dialysis membrane and will not be dialyzed. Size itself can be a limiting factor. If a drug is larger than the molecular weight cut off of the membrane used, it will not be eliminated by hemodialysis. Gwilt and Perrier came up with a quick way to surmise if a drug would be significantly eliminated by hemodialysis[4] (Eq. 12.15). If the resulting number is <20, then the drug would not be significantly removed. If it is >80 a significant portion would be removed. If in-between these numbers, it is difficult to tell.

$$\frac{f_{up} \times 100}{V_d \left( \dfrac{L}{kg} \right)} \qquad (12.15)$$

*Clearance*

Clearance is a measure of the efficiency of drug removal from the body. The two major organs of clearance in the body are the kidneys and the liver. The clearance of a drug by any organ is primarily dependent on the blood flow to that organ ($Q$) and the efficiency of that organ to eliminate the drug (extraction efficiency, $E$). The specific factors are different depending on the organ of clearance. In general, if a compound is not polar enough to be removed by the kidneys, it is metabolized to more polar compound by the liver, making it more likely to be removed by the kidneys. To determine which organ of clearance is predominant, the fraction of parent drug excreted unchanged in the urine ($f_e$) must be determined. For example, if a 100-mg dose of a totally bioavailable drug is given and 80 mg is recovered in the parent form in the urine, the $f_e$ would be 0.8. The remaining 20 mg or 20% of the dose would be cleared by nonrenal routes. These could include the bile, skin, lungs, and/or liver. The determinants of both renal and hepatic clearance are discussed.

*Renal Clearance*

The kidneys rely on three mechanisms to determine renal clearance of drugs. They include glomerular filtration clearance, active secretion, and passive reabsorption. First, drugs are filtered through the glomerulus; then there may be active secretion of the drug from the bloodstream into the proximal tubule (urine); and finally, it can be reabsorbed in the distal tubule by passive diffusion (Fig. 12.4). The determinants of each of these components are discussed below.

*Glomerular Filtration Clearance*

The glomerulus works as a filter. When a drug arrives at the glomerulus via the renal artery, it will either pass through the filter and into the renal tubule or will not. Whether or not a drug will be filtered is dependent on size of the molecule. If a drug has a very large molecular weight, it will not be filtered. In addition, if a drug is bound to a very large protein molecule, it will not be filtered because the protein is too big to be filtered. Recall that a major function of the glomerulus is to keep valuable proteins in the bloodstream and not allow them to be lost via the kidneys. Therefore, if a drug is highly bound to plasma proteins, it will not be filtered. Remember, the clearance of any organ is dependent on the blood flow to the organ and the extraction efficiency of the organ. In this case, the glomerular filtration rate (GFR) is the blood flow, and the extraction efficiency is dictated by the fraction of drug that is free of plasma proteins in the plasma ($f_{up}$). Therefore, GFR and $f_{up}$ determine glomerular filtration clearance ($CL_{gf}$) (Eq. 12.16).

$$CL_{gf} = GFR \times f_{up} \qquad (12.16)$$

**Figure 12.4.** Representation of renal clearance in kidney.

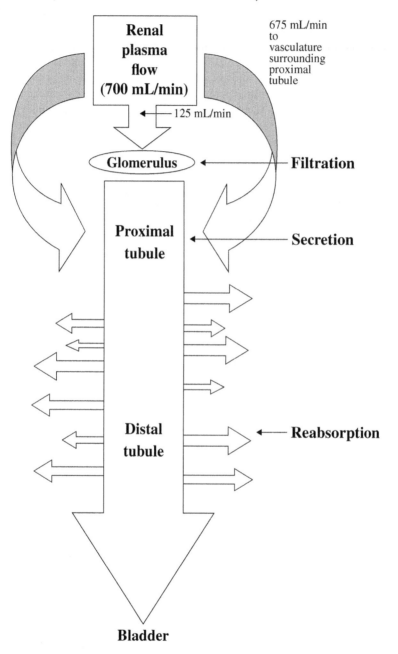

*Active Secretion*

After a drug is filtered into the tubule it will then travel down to the proximal tubule. As the fluid is traveling down the tubule, there is a vast reabsorption of water. Therefore, tubular fluid becomes more concentrated as it is more distal from the glomerulus. Drugs may be actively secreted from the bloodstream back into the renal tubule in the proximal tubule. Because it is an active process, it requires energy and a carrier system. This is a capacity-limited process analogous to hepatic enzymatic metabolism and may be saturated. There are at least two types of carriers known for tubular secretion, one for acids and one for bases. Thus, secreted acids will compete with other secreted acids, and bases will compete with bases for their appropriate carriers. This is an important site for drug-drug interactions. (Recall that biliary clearance is a similar process, with active secretion into the bile containing acid and base carrier systems.) p-glycoprotein may also be an important carrier here.

When two drugs are competing for the same carrier site, the one with the higher affinity for the carrier will be preferentially secreted, leaving the drug with a lesser affinity in the bloodstream. This will result in a decrease in the renal clearance of the drug with a lesser affinity for the carrier, which will produce an increase in $C_{ss,avg}$ and a prolonged half-life. A classic example of this is the probenecid interaction with penicillin. Both of these drugs are competing for the acid secretion carrier sites in the proximal tubule. Probenecid is preferentially secreted because it has a higher affinity for the carrier. Therefore, when probenecid is added to the regimen of a patient taking penicillin, the clearance of penicillin is decreased, resulting in an increased $C_{ss,avg}$ and longer half-life. This is used therapeutically to increase concentrations achieved and allow for less-frequent dosing. Obviously, this type of interaction could result in adversely high concentrations of interacting drugs, so this must be considered when screening for possible drug-drug interactions. Some actively secreted drugs are listed in Table 12.4.

*Tubular Reabsorption*

Tubular reabsorption, a primarily passive process, occurs in the distal tubule. (Lithium is an exception to this, as it is actively reabsorbed in the proximal tubule.) Passive reabsorption is dependent on the principles of a passive diffusion. Therefore, a drug in the tubule must be relatively lipophilic and uncharged to be reabsorbed. Because it is passive, it is not dependent on a carrier system and cannot be saturated. It is, however, dependent on the concentration gradient. Recall that as fluid moves through the tubule there is a vast reabsorption of water, resulting in urine that is more concentrated. (Just think what it would be like if our urine output were equal to that of a normal GFR of 125 mL/min.) Therefore, the concentration of drug in the urine will be higher than that of drug in the bloodstream. The drug will passively diffuse from the distal tubular fluid into the less concentrated bloodstream if it is lipophilic enough and uncharged. This would decrease the renal clearance of the drug. Changing the concentration gradient or the fraction of un-ionized drug alters the fraction of drug reabsorbed. Giving an osmotic diuretic such as mannitol alters the concentration gradient. This drug will decrease water reabsorption and therefore minimize the concentration gradient, resulting

**TABLE 12.4. EXAMPLES OF DRUGS UNDERGOING ACTIVE TUBULAR SECRETION**

| Organic Acids | Organic Bases |
|---|---|
| Cephalosporins | Amantadine |
| Ciprofloxacin | Cimetidine |
| Clavulanate | Didanosine |
| Furosemide | Dopamine |
| Methotrexate | Famciclovir |
| Penicillins | Meperidine |
| Probenecid | Morphine |
| Salicylates | Pseudoephedrine (denantiomer) |
| Sufonamides | Quinine |
| Thiazides | Zalcitabine |
| | Zidovudine |

in less drug being reabsorbed. This would increase renal clearance, decrease $C_{ss,avg}$, and make the half-life shorter. Changing the pH of the tubular fluid alters the ionic character of the drug. For example, a weak acid must be in an acidic environment to be in the primarily un-ionized state. If the pH of the urine is alkalinized, a weak acid will have a smaller fraction of drug in the un-ionized, reabsorbable form, and therefore tubular reabsorption will be decreased. This will result in an increase in renal clearance causing a decreased $C_{ss,avg}$ and a shorter half-life. This is another important area to consider for drug-drug interactions.

*Summary*

When a drug arrives at the glomerulus, it will be filtered. The fraction of drug that will be filtered is dependent on the protein-binding characteristics. The drug then may be actively secreted or passively reabsorbed in the tubule, increasing or decreasing the renal clearance, respectively. The dominant process is determined by comparing the renal clearance to the filtration clearance (Eq. 12.16). If the renal clearance is greater than the filtration clearance, secretion must be the predominant process (Eq. 12.17).

$$CL_R > GFR \times f_{up} \qquad (12.17)$$

Passive reabsorption must be the prevailing process if renal clearance is less than the filtered clearance (Eq. 12.18).

$$CL_R < GFR \times f_{up} \qquad (12.18)$$

Once the predominant process is identified, drug-drug interactions can be more readily anticipated and acted upon.

### Hepatic Clearance

Any organ of clearance is primarily dependent on the blood flow to that organ ($Q$) and the efficiency of that organ in eliminating the drug (extraction efficiency). Hepatic extraction ratio ($E$) is dependent on liver blood flow ($Q$), free intrinsic clearance ($CL_{int}$), and free fraction in the plasma ($f_{up}$). The extraction ratio ($E$) and the fraction that escapes the first pass effect in the liver ($f_{fp}$) are interrelated.

### Fraction Escaping Hepatic First Pass

The fraction that escapes the first-pass effect is that fraction that is not extracted by the liver. For example, if 0.8 or 80% of the drug is extracted or metabolized as it passes through the liver, the extraction ratio ($E$) would be 0.8. In other words, each time that the drug passes through the liver, 80% will be metabolized. This will leave only 0.2 or 20% to escape the first-pass effect and enter the systemic bloodstream. Thus, the same factors that determine the extraction ratio ($E$) will determine the fraction that escapes the first pass effect ($f_{fp}$).

Liver blood flow ($Q$), intrinsic clearance ($CL_{int}$), and free fraction in the plasma ($f_{up}$) are the three factors that determine hepatic CL ($CL_H$), hepatic extraction ratio ($E$), and fraction that escapes the first pass effect ($f_{fp}$).

### Liver Blood Flow

Liver blood flow ($Q$) is the volume of blood entering and exiting the liver per unit time. An average liver blood flow ($Q$) is about 90 L/h or 1.5 L/min, although disease and drugs can alter it. Table 12.5 lists some of these conditions and drugs.

### Intrinsic Clearance

The hepatic free intrinsic clearance ($CL_{int}$) of a drug is the hypothetical measure of the removal of drug by the liver if the drug were not bound to plasma proteins

---

**TABLE 12.5.  EXAMPLES OF DRUGS AND CONDITIONS ALTERING LIVER BLOOD FLOW**

| Decreased Q | Increase Q |
|---|---|
| (any ↓ in Cardiac Output) | (any ↑ in Cardiac Output) |
| Arrhythmias | Food intake (transient) |
| β-Blockers | Positive inotropes |
| Cardiomyopathy | |
| CHF | |
| Hepatic cirrhosis | |
| Shock (transient) | |

and the delivery to the liver were not limited by liver blood flow. It is easiest to think of hepatic intrinsic clearance as enzyme activity. It can be induced and inhibited by drugs that are enzyme inducers and inhibitors. Three factors determine the intrinsic clearance ($CL_{int}$) of a drug: $V_{max}$, $K_m$, and concentration ($C$) (Eq. 12.19).

$$CL_{int} = \frac{V_{max}}{K_m + C} \qquad (12.19)$$

*Michaelis-Menten*

$V_{max}$ is the maximum rate of metabolism. It represents the number of metabolizing enzymes or the capacity of the enzyme system. $K_m$ is the Michaelis constant, which is the concentration at which the rate is half-maximal or $\frac{1}{2}V_{max}$. This is an inverse association constant and gives a measure of the affinity of the drug for the enzyme. The smaller the concentration at which $\frac{1}{2}V_{max}$ is achieved, then the greater is the affinity of the drug for the enzyme. Finally, the concentration of drug is a determinant of intrinsic clearance. For most drugs, the $K_m$ is much greater than the concentrations achieved in the therapeutic range. Mathematically, when there is a sum in the denominator of a fraction and one number is much greater than the other, the smaller number becomes relatively insignificant and can be considered unimportant to the result (Eq. 12.19a).

$$CL_{int} = \frac{V_{max}}{K_m \gg \underset{\searrow 0}{C}} \qquad (12.19a)$$

If this is done, it is apparent that for most drugs in the therapeutic range, the intrinsic clearance ($CL_{int}$) will be dependent on $V_{max}$ and $K_m$ only, not concentration. If the concentrations achieved are not much less than the $K_m$ of a drug, concentration becomes a factor determining intrinsic clearance. This will then become nonlinear hepatic clearance. In other words, the intrinsic clearance ($CL_{int}$), and therefore hepatic clearance ($CL_H$), will be changing as the concentration changes. This is also called concentration-dependent or Michaelis-Menten kinetics. Phenytoin is a typical example of a drug that has a $K_m$ similar to the concentrations achieved therapeutically. Any drug can exhibit nonlinear clearance if enough is given to permit the concentration to approach the $K_m$ of the drug, as in some overdose situations. Some drugs exhibit nonlinear hepatic clearance in the recommended range. Phenytoin is a classic example of this.

*Cytochrome P450 System*

Drugs and disease can alter intrinsic clearance. The hepatic enzymes metabolize drugs by either Phase I or Phase II reactions. Phase I reactions are nonsynthetic and include oxidation and reduction reactions. Synthetic or Phase II reactions include conjugations, acetylation, and transulfuration. Cytochrome P450 (it maximally absorbs light at 450 nm, which is how it got its name) is an important group of enzymes needed to catalyze most of the oxidation and reduction reactions in the liver. CYP450 can be broken down into several families and subfamilies. Some of the substrates of those families are listed in Table 12.6. Substrate means that these are drugs that are dependent on that family of enzymes for metabolism. They would therefore be vulnerable if there were induction or inhibition of that particular CYP450 family. Some of the known enhancers and inhibitors of the families are listed in Tables 12.7 and 12.8. An inducing drug will increase the number of enzymes available for metabolism. Therefore, the $V_{max}$ and therefore Clint for that enzyme system would increase. The time it takes to induce depends on the half-life of the inducing drug and the enzyme turnover rate, which is 1 to 6 days.[6] Induction is dose dependent and reversible. Inhibition, on the other hand, can occur in several ways. The most common is competitive inhibition. Two drugs may be vying for the same enzyme for metabolism. The drug with the strongest affinity would be preferentially metabolized, thus inhibiting the metabolism of the drug with the lesser affinity. This affinity is called the $K_i$. This is analogous to the Michael is constant. The smaller the value of $K_i$, then the stronger the affinity for the enzyme. There can also be noncompetitive inhibition. Time to onset of inhibition is dependent on the enzyme and may be immediate.

Within the families of the CYP there are genetic polymorphisms that have become apparent. Each patient is genetically programmed to have a certain genotype for each family of CYP. This may result in a slower or faster rate of metabolism, depending on the genotype of the patient. Patients with a less common type of slow metabolizing ability for a particular family of CYP enzymes might explain the interpatient variability seen in the pharmacokinetics and adverse events of drugs cleared via these pathways. Drug probes and geneotyping have been studied and are being used clinically.[18] This is not done routinely in patient care in all areas, but is becoming more common as the tests are made available and payers realize the benefits.

*Fraction Unbound in Plasma*

Unbound fraction in plasma is also an important factor in determining the hepatic clearance of a drug. Factors altering the protein binding of a drug are reviewed in the Distribution section of this chapter.

*High Hepatic Extraction Drugs*

Some drugs undergoing hepatic clearance have a very high extraction ratio and therefore undergo a significant first-pass effect. These drugs can be considered independently from those drugs with a low extraction ratio. Drugs with a high extraction ratio have a very strong attraction for the metabolizing enzyme. Therefore, the rate-limiting step for clearance is delivery of the drug to the enzymes or liver blood flow ($Q$). Assuming that liver blood flow is much less than the ability of the liver

**TABLE 12.6. EXAMPLES OF SUBSTRATES OF THE CYP FAMILIES AND P-GLYCOPROTEIN[6,17,19]**

| | | CYP | | | |
|---|---|---|---|---|---|
| **1A2** | | **2C19** | | **2C9** | |
| Acetaminophen | Nortriptyline | Amitriptyline | Nilutamide | Amitriptyline | Losartan |
| Amitriptyline | Olanzapine | Carisoprodol | Omeprazole | Carvedilol | Montelukast |
| Caffeine | Ondansetron | Cilostazol | Pantoprazole | Celecoxib | Naproxen |
| Clomipramine | Propafenone | Citalopram | Pentamidine | Clomipramine | Omeprazole |
| Clopidogrel | Propranolol | Clomipramine | Phenytoin | Desogestrel | Phenytoin |
| Clozapine | Riluzole | Cyclophosphamide | Progesterone | Diazepam | Piroxicam |
| Cyclobenzaprine | Ropinirole | Desipramine | Proguanil | Diclofenac | Rosiglitazone |
| Desipramine | Ropivacaine | Diazepam | Propranolol | Fluoxetine | Sildenafil |
| Diazepam | Tacrine | Esomeprazole | Rabeprazole | Flurbiprofen | Sulfamethoxazole |
| Estradiol | Theophylline | Formoterol | Teniposide | Fluvastatin | Tolbutamide |
| Flutamide | Verapamil | Hexobarbital | Thioridazine | Glimepiride | Torsemide |
| Fluvoxamine | (R)-warfarin | Imipramine | Tolbutamide | Glipizide | Valdecoxib |
| Haloperidol | Zileuton | Indomethacin | Voriconazole | Glyburide | Valsartan |
| Imipramine | | Lansoprazole | (R)-warfarin | Ibuprofen | (S)-warfarin |
| Mexiletine | | Mephobarbital | | Imipramine | Zafirlukast |
| Mirtazapine | | Moclobemide | | Indomethacin | Zileuton |
| Naproxen | | Nelfinavir | | Irbesartan | |

*(continued)*

335

**TABLE 12.6.** EXAMPLES OF SUBSTRATES OF THE CYP FAMILIES AND P-GLYCOPROTEIN[6,17,19] (*Continued*)

| | CYP | | | | |
|---|---|---|---|---|---|
| **2C8** | **2D6** | | | **3A** | |
| Amiodarone | Amitriptyline | Fluoxetine | Perphenazine | Alprazolam | Diltiazem |
| Benzphetamine | Amphetamine | Fluphenazine | Pindolol | Amitriptyline | Donepezil |
| Carbamazepine | Atomoxetine | Fluvoxamine | Propafenone | Amiodarone | Doxorubicin |
| Docetaxel | Bisoprolol | Haloperidol | Propoxyphene | Atorvastatin | Efavirenz |
| Fluvastatin | Carvedilol | Hydrocodone | Propranolol | Budesonide | Ergotamine |
| Isotretinoin | Chlorpromazine | Imipramine | Quetiapine | Buspirone | Erythromycin |
| Paclitaxel | Chlorpropamide | Maprotiline | Risperidone | Carbamazepine | Ethinyl estradiol |
| Phenytoin | Clomipramine | Meperidine | Thioridazine | Chlorpheniramine | Ethosuximide |
| Pioglitazone | Clozapine | Methadone | Timolol | Clarithromycin | Etoposide |
| Repaglinide | Codeine | Methamphetamine | Tramadol | Clindamycin | Fentanyl |
| Retinoic acid | Cyclobenzaprine | Metoprolol | Trazodone | Clomipramine | Fexofenadine |
| Retinol | Desipramine | Mexiletine | Venlafaxine | Clonazepam | Haloperidol |
| Rosiglitazone | Dextromethorphan | Morphine | | Clopidogrel | Hydrocodone |
| Tolbutamide | Donepezil | Nortriptyline | | Cyclobenzaprine | Hydrocortisone |
| Tretinoin | Doxepin | Olanzapine | | Cyclosporine | Imipramine |
| Verapamil | Fenfluramine | Ondansetron | | Dexamethasone | Indinavir |
| Warfarin | Fentanyl | Oxycodone | | Dextromethorphan | Ketoconazole |
| Zopiclone | Flecainide | Paroxetine | | Diazepam | |

## CYP

| 3A | | | | P-GP | |
|---|---|---|---|---|---|
| Lansoprazole | Norethindrone | Salmeterol | Trazodone | Cyclosporine | Saquinavir |
| Loratadine | Omeprazole | Saquinavir | Verapamil | Dexamethasone | Verapamil |
| Losartan | Ondansetron | Sildenafil | Vinblastine | Diltiazem | Vinblastine |
| Lovastatin | Paclitaxel | Simvastatin | Vincristine | Estradiol | Vincristine |
| Methylprednisolone | Pantoprazole | Tacrolimus | (R)-warfarin | Etopside | |
| Miconazole | Prednisone | Tamoxifen | Ziprasidone | Hydrocortisone | |
| Mirtazapine | Progestins | Temazepam | Zolpidem | Nicardipine | |
| Montelukast | Rifampin | Tiagabine | Zonisamide | Paclitaxel | |
| Nifedipine | Ritonavir | Tramadol | | Ritonavir | |

**TABLE 12.7.** EXAMPLES OF ENHANCERS OF THE CYP FAMILIES AND P-GLYCOPROTEIN[6,17,19]

| | | CYP | | |
|---|---|---|---|---|
| 1A2 | 2C19 | 2C8 | 2C9 | 2D6 |
| Carbamazepine | Carbamazepine | Carbamazepine | Aprepitant | Carbamazepine |
| Charbroiled food | Norethindrone | Phenobarbital | Carbamazepine | Ethanol |
| Lansoprazole | Phenobarbital | Rifabutin | Phenobarbital | Phenobarbital |
| Omeprazole | Phenytoin | Rifampicin | Phenytoin | Phenytoin |
| Phenobarbital | Prednisone | Rifampin | Primidone | Primidone |
| Phenytoin | Rifampin | | Rifampin | Rifampin |
| Primidone | | | Rifapentine | Ritonavir |
| Rifampin | | | | St John's wort |
| Ritonavir | | | | |
| Smoking | | | | |
| St John's wort | | | | |

| CYP | | P-GP |
|---|---|---|
| **3A** | | **P-GP** |
| Aminoglutethimide | Nevirapine | Grapefruit juice? |
| Aprepitant | Oxcarbazepine | Flavinoids |
| Carbamazepine | Phenobarbital | Kaaepferol |
| Dexamethasone | Phenytoin | Quercetin |
| Efavirenz | Primidone | |
| Ethosuximide | Rifabutin | |
| Garlic supplements | Rifampin | |
| Glucocorticoids | Rifapentine | |
| Glutethimide | St John's wort | |
| Griseofulvin | | |
| Modafinil | | |
| Nafcillin | | |

**TABLE 12.8.** EXAMPLES OF INHIBITORS OF THE CYP FAMILIES AND P-GLYCOPROTEIN[6,17,19]

| CYP | | | |
|---|---|---|---|
| **1A2** | **2C19** | **2C9** | **2C8** |
| Amiodarone | Citalopram | Amiodarone | Anastrozole |
| Cimetidine | Delavirdine | Chloramphenicol | Gemfibrozil |
| Ciprofloxacin | Efavirenz | Cimetidine | Nicardipine |
| Citalopram | Felbamate | Clopidogrel | Quercetin |
| Clarithromycin | Fluconazole | Cotrimoxazole | Sulfaphenazole |
| Diltiazem | Fluoxetine | Delavirdine | Sulfinpyrazone-trimethoprim |
| Enoxacin | Fluvastatin | Disulfiram | |
| Erythromycin | Fluvoxamine | Efavirenz | |
| Ethinyl estradiol | Indomethacin | Fenofibrate | |
| Fluvoxamine | Isoniazid | Fluconazole | |
| Isoniazid | Ketoconazole | Fluorouracil | |
| Ketoconazole | Letrozole | Fluoxetine | |
| Methoxsalen | Modafinil | Fluvastatin | |
| Mexiletine | Omeprazole | Fluvoxamine | |
| Nalidixic acid | Oxcarbazepine | Gemfibrozil | |
| Norethindrone | Paroxetine | Imatinib | |
| Norfloxacin | Sertraline | Isoniazid | |
| Omeprazole | Telmisartan | Itraconazole | |
| Oral contraceptives | Ticlopidine | Ketoconazole | |
| Paroxetine | Topiramate | Leflunomide | |
| Tacrine | Voriconazole | Lovastatin | |
| Ticlopidine | | Metronidazole | |
| Troleandomycin | | Modafinil | |
| | | Omeprazole | |
| | | Paroxetine | |
| | | Sertraline | |
| | | Sulfonamides | |
| | | Ticlopidine | |
| | | Voriconazole | |
| | | Zafirlukast | |

| 2D6 | CYP — 3A | CYP — P-GP |
|---|---|---|
| Amiodarone | Acitretin | Amiodarone |
| Bupropion | Amiodarone | Clarithromycin |
| Celecoxib | Amprenavir | Cyclosporine |
| Chloroquine | Aprepitant | Diltiazem |
| Chlorpheniramine | Cimetidine | Erythromycin |
| Cimetidine | Ciprofloxacin | Indinavir |
| Citalopram | Clarithromycin | Itraconazole |
| Clomipramine | Cyclosporine | Ketoconazole |
| Cocaine | Danazol | Nelfinavir |
| Desipramine | Delavirdine | Nicardipine |
| Diphenhydramine | Diltiazem | Propafenone |
| Fluoxetine | Efavirenz | Quinidine |
| Fluphenazine | Erythromycin | Ritonavir |
| Halofantrine | Ethinyl Estradiol | Saquinavir |
| Haloperidol | Fluconazole | Tacrolimus |
| Imatinib | Fluoxetine | Tamoxifen |
| Methadone | Fluvoxamine | Verapamil |
| Moclobemide | Gestodene | |
| Norfluoxetine | Grapefruit | |
| Paroxetine | Indinavir | |
| Perphenazine | Imatinib | |
| Propafenone | Isoniazid | |
| Propoxyphene | Itraconazole | |
| Quinacrine | Ketoconazole | |
| Quinidine | Metronidazole | |
| Ranitidine | Methylprednisolone | |
| Ritonavir | Miconazole | |
| Sertraline | Mifepristone | |
| Terbinafine | Nefazodone | |
| Thioridazine | Nelfinavir | |
| | Nicardipine | |
| | Nifedipine | |
| | Norethindrone | |
| | Norfloxacin | |
| | Norfluoxetine | |
| | Oxiconazole | |
| | Prednisone | |
| | Quinine | |
| | Ritonavir | |
| | Roxithromycin | |
| | Saquinavir | |
| | Sertraline | |
| | Synercid | |
| | Troleandomycin | |
| | Verapamil | |
| | Voriconazole | |
| | Zafirlukast | |
| | Zileuton | |

enzyme to metabolize free drug, some mathematical simplifications can be made to establish the important factors determining clearance and bioavailability. The factor determining hepatic clearance becomes hepatic blood flow ($Q$). This makes sense considering that the rate-limiting step is hepatic blood flow. It is very important to realize that for a high-extraction drug only an alteration in liver blood flow will change the hepatic clearance. Therefore, only drug and disease interactions that affect $Q$ will cause a change in $CL_H$ (Eq. 12.20).

$$CL \sim Q \tag{12.20}$$

The factors determining the fraction escaping the first pass effect ($f_{fp}$) can be determined by applying the above assumption. These are high-first-pass drugs, so considering the factors that will affect first pass is important. Changes in Clint or $Q$ can alter the $f_{fp}$ of high extractions drugs (Eq. 12.21). Therefore, changes in P450 ($CL_{int}$) may alter the bioavailability of high extraction drugs.

$$f_{fp} \sim \frac{Q}{CL_{int}} \tag{12.21}$$

These factors are important because predictions about what drugs and/or disease could alter $C_{ss,avg}$ and peak-to-trough interval can be made if the factors influencing these pharmacokinetic parameters are known. These can be contrasted with the factors determining the clearance and first-pass effect of the drugs with a low hepatic extraction.

### Low-Hepatic-Extraction-Ratio Drugs

In contrast to high-extraction drugs, low-extraction drugs have a relatively lessor attraction for the metabolizing enzyme. The rate-limiting step for the clearance of these drugs is the enzyme activity or intrinsic clearance of unbound drug, not delivery of the drug to the liver. Therefore, CL is primarily determined by $CL_{int}$ and $f_{up}$ (Eq. 12.22).

$$CL \sim CL_{int} \times f_{up} \tag{12.22}$$

This is very helpful when one is trying to make predictions about drug and disease interactions. Alterations in $CL_{int}$ would be expected to alter $CL_H$ of these drugs. Therefore, when monitoring drugs that are low extraction, it is very important to be aware if they are P450 substrates. If so, they could be subject to drug interactions involving alterations in the P450 system. Also, plasma protein binding interactions will cause a change in clearance. It is also useful to remember that the first-pass effect is not a factor for these drugs.

### Predictions

Using the above assumptions simplifies determining how drugs and diseases can interact and change the resulting $C_{ss,avg}$ and peak-to-trough ratio. Recall these are the targets for designing a dosage regimen. When either $C_{ss,avg}$ or $P{:}T$ or both of these are altered by a change in $F$, $V_d$, or CL, changes may need to be made in the patient's dosage regimen.

*Low-Extraction Drugs*

A low-extraction drug $C_{ss,avg,tot}$ and $C_{ss,avg,free}$ are determined by the following parameters (Eqs. 12.23 and 12.24).

$$C_{ss,avg,tot} \sim \frac{f_a \times f_g \times DR}{CL_{int} \times f_{up}} \tag{12.23}$$

$$C_{ss,avg,free} \sim \frac{f_a \times f_g \times DR}{CL_{int}} \tag{12.24}$$

A change in $f_a$, $f_g$, $CL_{int}$, or $f_{up}$ would alter the total concentration at steady state. But an alteration in $C_{ss,avg,free}$ would be realized only if there were a change in $f_a$, $f_g$, or $CL_{int}$. A change in binding would not alter the free concentration at steady state but would alter the total concentration at steady state. Because total concentration is what is typically measured, the measured concentration would not reflect accurately what was happening with the active free concentration. In this case, it is important to anticipate this problem and react not to the total measured concentration but to what will be occurring with the free drug. If, for example, a drug that is highly bound to plasma proteins (primarily to albumin) and is a low-extraction drug cleared only by the liver is being given to a patient that is malnourished who has a decrease in albumin, the total concentration at steady state will have decreased. The patient is not experiencing any s signs or symptoms of lack of efficacy or toxicity, but the physician is concerned because the measured concentration has fallen below the recommended range. The physician wants to increase the dose rate to increase the $C_{ss,avg,tot}$. The pharmacist should caution against this considering that a decrease in albumin could have increased the free fraction of the drug. When additional free drug was available to the hepatic enzymes, clearance increases, decreasing the total concentration but there would be no change in the free (active) concentration at steady state. In this case, although the total concentration was decreased because of an increase in clearance, the free concentration was not changed at steady state. The dose rate should remain the same. This is an important reminder that an individual should never be treated based solely on the measured concentration. A free concentration may be ordered to make a better dosage regimen adjustment and clinical judgment may be the best practice.

*High-Extraction Drugs*

Drugs with a high affinity for their metabolizing enzymes are high-extraction drugs. The rate-limiting step to their clearance is liver blood flow ($Q$). Since high-extraction drugs undergo a significant first pass effect, the determinants of $f_{fp}$ become important. Liver blood flow ($Q$) is a determinant of both $f_{fp}$ and CL; they eliminate each other as factors in determining the $C_{ss,avg,tot}$ for a high-extraction drug given orally (Eq. 12.25).

$$C_{ss,avg,tot,PO} \sim \frac{f_a \times f_g \times \dfrac{Q}{CL_{int}} \times DR}{Q} \quad (12.25)$$

Notice that the determinants of $C_{ss,avg,tot}$ for both high-extraction drugs given orally and low extraction drugs are the same. The difference is that $CL_{int} \times f_{up}$ determines clearance for a low-extraction drug but is a factor of $f_{fp}$ for a high extraction drug given orally. These drugs are high-first-pass drugs; therefore, we would expect different factors to determine the $C_{ss,avg}$ for drugs given by a non-first-pass route. If a high extraction drug were given intravenously, the $C_{ss,avg,tot}$ would be dependent on (Eq. 12.26)

$$C_{ss,avg,tot,IV} \sim \frac{DR}{Q} \quad (12.26)$$

Thus, only a change in liver blood flow or dose rate would alter the total concentration of a high-extraction drug given intravenously. The factors determining $C_{ss,avg,free}$ would be (Eq. 12.27):

$$C_{ss,avg,free,IV} \sim \frac{DR}{Q} \times f_{up} \quad (12.27)$$

Therefore, if a high-extraction drug were given intravenously, and there was a displacement of the drug from its protein binding site, there would be an increase in the $C_{ss,avg,free}$ with no change in the $C_{ss,avg,tot}$. This could result in the measured total concentration being within the recommended range but the patient suffering from concentration-related side effects. In this case, the dose rate should be decreased because of the protein binding displacement.

## BASIC CALCULATIONS TO DETERMINE INDIVIDUAL PHARMACOKINETIC VARIABLES

### Characterization of a Concentration-Time Curve

To determine the initial pharmacokinetic parameters of a given drug, the drug will be administered, and the concentrations of drug in the plasma will be measured over time. If a drug is given as a bolus intravenous injection, bioavailability and rate of administration do not have to be considered. When this is done, the maximum concentration ($C_{max}$) will be achieved immediately after the drug is given at time zero. The drug will be distributed and cleared from the body. Because a known amount of drug was introduced into the body, if the $C_{max}$ is measured, the initial volume of distribution $(V_c)$ can be calculated (Eq. 12.27). Note this is a variation on Eq. 12.11.

$$V_c = \frac{\text{Dose (amt)}}{C_{max} \left(\text{amt}/\text{vol}\right)} \qquad (12.27)$$

To determine the rate of elimination from the body ($k$), plasma concentrations will be collected and measured from at least two different points in time after administration. From these two points in time concentrations, the slope of the line describing the elimination of the drug can be determined (Eq. 12.28). See Figure 12.5.

$$k = \frac{\ln C_2 - \ln C_1}{t_2 - t_1} \qquad (12.28)$$

Notice that this is a simple "rise over run" calculation. Memorization is not necessary if you understand that principle. This number will be negative. That is because it is a negative slope or movement from a higher concentration to a lower one with increasing time. The elimination rate constant is used in equations from this point on as an absolute value. The elimination rate constant is important in determining the fraction of drug eliminated per unit time. The units of this constant are accounted for per time (ie, second$^{-1}$ or hour$^{-1}$). Once the elimination rate constant ($k$) is calculated, it is quite easy to determine the half-life of the drug ($t_{\frac{1}{2}}$) (Eq. 12.29).

$$t_{\frac{1}{2}} = \frac{0.693}{k} \qquad (12.29)$$

**Figure 12.5.** A one compartment linear degradation.

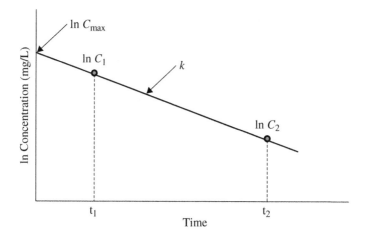

Once the elimination rate constant and one other concentration on the concentration-time curve are known, any concentration at any time point can be determined (Eq. 12.30).

$$C_2 = C_1 \times e^{-k \times t} \qquad (12.30)$$

This is just a rearrangement of the above "rise over run" calculation for $k$ (Eq. 12.28). If the natural log were taken of each side of this equation, the result would be (Eq. 12.31):

$$\ln C_2 = \ln C_1 \times (-k \times t) \qquad (12.31)$$

A simple rearrangement will result in the equation to determine $k$ (Eq. 12.28). The realization that $C_1$ represents the concentration closer to the time of administration and $C_2$ the concentration further from the administration time or time zero is important. For example, if the $C_{max}$ is known, which, as in our above example, occurred at time zero, Eq. 12.32 would look like this:

$$C_2 = C_{max} \times e^{-k \times t_2} \qquad (12.32)$$

Therefore, the concentration at any time after $C_{max}$ has occurred can be determined by inserting the measured $C_{max}$, the calculated $k$, and the time at which you would like to know the concentration. It is helpful to note that the mathematical phrase $e^{-kt}$ represents the fraction remaining at that time $t$. For example, if the $C_{max}$ was 100 mg/L and 10 hours later the concentration was 30 mg/L, then the fraction remaining ($e^{-kt}$) at time 10 hours after administration would be 0.3, or 30% remains 10 hours after administration.

$$C_2 = C_{max} \times e^{-k \times t_2}$$

$$30\ \text{mg/L} = 100\ \text{mg/L} \times e^{-k \times t}$$

$$\therefore e^{-k \times t} = 0.3$$

The log concentration-time curve for a one-compartment model that is linearly cleared is a straight line. It is instructive to think about the equation describing this drug's behavior in terms of a line. Recall, the equation for a line is $y = mx + b$, where $x$ and $y$ are the parameters on the $x$ and $y$ axes, $m$ is the slope of the line, and $b$ the $y$-intercept. Eq. 12.31 is in that form. If the first concentration is the initial concentration ($C_0$ or $C_{max}$) and the second concentration ($C_2$) is any concentration at time "$t$" ($C_t$). The linear equation is:

$$\ln C_2 = \ln C_0 \times (-k \times t) \qquad (12.31)$$

$$\ln C_t = -kx\ t + \ln C_0$$

$$y = mx + b$$

where $y = \ln C_t$, $m = -k$, $x = t$, and $b = \ln C_0$.

Therefore, the $y$ coordinate will be the natural log of the unknown concentration, and the $x$ coordinate will be the time that the unknown concentration occurs. The slope is the elimination rate, and the $y$-intercept the natural log of $C_{max}$. This is a simplified look at a one-compartment model when a drug is given by intravenous bolus.

## Multiple Compartments

The simplistic example above is helpful when trying to grasp the basic concepts of a time-concentration curve and the information that can be gathered. It is important to realize that drugs are rarely given by IV bolus and rarely if ever have instantaneous distribution. Most often drugs distribute into several groups of tissues at different rates. These are called compartments. Most drugs have at least two compartments; many have more. We do most of our calculations based on the assumption that a drug follows one-compartment, linear pharmacokinetics. This is done for the sake of simplicity, in most cases, assuming one compartment does not result in an unacceptable margin of error.

A two-compartment model is often represented schematically as shown in Figure 12.6. In a typical two-compartment model, the first compartment is called the central compartment. It represents the tissues where the drug is presented, and from which the drug is distributed and eliminated. It is physiologically thought of as the blood and highly perfused organs. The second compartment is called the peripheral compartment. This represents the groups of tissue that the drug distributes into more slowly. The drug will also have to move back out of the tissues in the peripheral compartment and return back to the central compartment to be removed. If a concentration-time curve of a two-compartment-model drug were characterized, the line depicting the log concentration versus time would not be straight (Fig. 12.7). There would be an initial steeper decline, representing the distribution of the drug. The second phase of the line would be flatter, depicting the slower elimination of the

**Figure 12.6.** A representation of a two-compartment model.

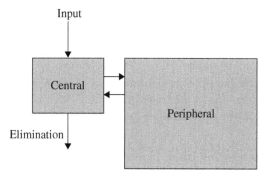

**Figure 12.7.** Concentration-time curve of two-compartment model.

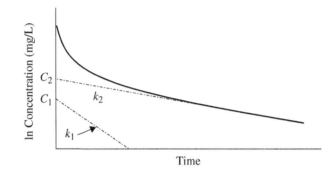

drug. This second phase is called the terminal phase for a two-compartment model. The slope of this terminal phase is what is used to determine $k$ and $t_{\frac{1}{2}}$. The biexponential line that is formed by this data can be analyzed to determine a characterization for both compartments, each having a slope ($k$) and $y$-intercept ($C_0$) to describe them. When the two compartmental lines are added, the equation to describe the concentration at any time can be determined (Eq. 12.33).

$$C_t = C_1 e^{k_1 \times t} + C_2 e^{k_2 \times t} \tag{12.33}$$

As more compartments are added, the describing equations and models become increasingly more complex. Most calculations become very cumbersome with a model that assumes more than two compartments.

### Area Under the Curve

Area under the curve is a model-independent parameter that is a good measure of drug exposure (see Fig. 12.3). The total body clearance can be determined from the dose administered and the area under the time-concentration curve (AUC) (Eq. 12.34).

$$\text{AUC} = \frac{F \times \text{Dose}}{\text{CL}} \tag{12.34}$$

The area under the time-concentration curve can be determined in several ways. The most common is the trapezoidal rule, which is the sum of the areas between each successive concentration-time points (Eq. 12.35). See Figure 12.8.

$$\text{AUC}_{0-\infty} = \frac{C_1 + C_2}{2}\left(t_2 - t_1\right) + \frac{C_2 + C_3}{2}\left(t_3 - t_2\right) + \cdots + \frac{C_n}{k} \tag{12.35}$$

**Figure 12.8.** Trapezoidal Rule for determining the AUC.

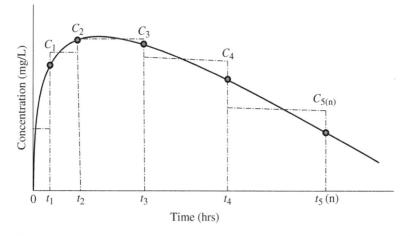

The areas between successive concentrations are treated as rectangles. The height of each rectangle is the average of the two observed points, and the width of the rectangle is the difference between the two time points. The area between the last observed time point and infinity is a triangle that assumes a log-linear decline. It is based upon the quotient of the last time point observed and the elimination rate constant ($K$). The sum of these rectangles and the triangle gives a good estimate of the area under the time-concentration curve. The more measured concentrations the better will be the estimate. The AUC is important for determining clearance but can also be used to determine the average concentration at steady state ($C_{ss,avg}$), and bioavailability (Eqs. 12.34 and 12.36).

$$C_{ss,avg} = \frac{AUC_{0-\tau}}{\tau} \qquad (12.36)$$

## APPLICATION

If a new drug is brought to the market or any drug is analyzed, the first questions about a drug might be physiochemical. Is this a chiral compound? Is it a weak acid or a weak base? How big is it? How lipophilic is it? Is it possibly secreted into bile? Is it highly bound to plasma proteins? If so, which one(s)? What is the volume of distribution?

The next line of questions would address how the drug is cleared. What is its $f_e$? If it were highly cleared by the kidneys, the predominant process, active secretion versus reabsorption, can be determined. If a drug were cleared by the liver, it could be determined if acted like a high or low-extraction drug. If it is cleared by the liver, what enzymes are responsible for the metabolism of the drug? Is it a substrate or known inhibitor or inducer of any of the CYP450 isoenzymes? Are there any active metabolites and, if so, how they are cleared? From this information, possible drug and disease interactions can be anticipated and avoided or adjustments made in the dosage regimen of the drug.

| **TABLE 12.9.** CONDITIONS FAVORING THE USE OF DRUG MONITORING |
| --- |
| **1.** An unpredictable dose-response relationship |
| **2.** A correlation between serum concentrations and efficacy/toxicity |
| **3.** A lack of a clearly observable clinical endpoint (ie, blood pressure reduction) |
| **4.** A narrow toxicity range |
| **5.** Toxicity or lack of efficacy of drug is dangerous |
| **6.** Accurate serum concentration measurement is readily available |
| **7.** Determine effective serum concentration at steady state |
| **8.** Patient infection and correlating change in efficacy of specific drug |
| **9.** Patient adherence in question |

## Drug Monitoring

Many drugs have large effective ranges, meaning there is a large range where the drug is both effective and not toxic. In these cases is not usually necessary to monitor drug concentrations. This does not mean that utilizing and understanding the pharmacokinetic principles learned in the prior discussion cannot be useful to the clinician for these drugs. Table 12.9 lists reasons that drug should have their concentrations monitored. In general, it includes drugs whose efficacy and/or toxicity cannot be measured by any other means.

A few of them are discussed below. The individual parameters of any new or unknown drug can usually be found in the package insert or some other readily available reference.

In general, if a drug is at steady state, it is easy to make needed dose rate adjustments, assuming the drug is cleared linearly and there has been no change in fraction unbound. Recall that the $C_{ss,avg}$ is determined by Eq. 12.1.

$$C_{ss,avg} = \frac{F \times DR}{CL} \qquad (12.1)$$

In most cases it can be assumed that the CL and $F$ are remaining constant. This is assuming linear clearance and no new drugs or diseases introduced that could alter the $F$ or CL. That being the case, the DR and resulting $C_{ss,avg}$ are proportional. Therefore, a proportion can be set up (Eq. 12.37).

$$\text{If } F \text{ and CL remain constant}: C_{ss,avg} \propto DR$$

$$\frac{DR_1}{C_{ss,avg,1}} = \frac{DR_2}{C_{ss,avg,2}} \qquad (12.37)$$

Therefore, if there is a known $C_{ss,avg}$ that results from a certain given DR, a new DR can be easily calculated for the new target $C_{ss,avg}$.

In some cases $C_{ss,avg}$ is not as helpful as peak and trough concentrations. This is the case for aminoglycosides and vancomycin.

## Aminoglycosides and Vancomycin

Most antibiotics have large effective ranges and thus do not warrant drug monitoring. Aminoglycosides and vancomycin are two exceptions. They both have narrow toxicity indices. These are the drugs for which we are very commonly asked to help determine the patient's dosage regimen.

These drugs are cleared exclusively by the kidneys ($f_e$ = 1) and are primarily filtered only. They are not highly protein bound and therefore have a clearance that approximates creatinine clearance. They are not chiral compounds and are not subject to genetic polymorphism. They both exhibit multicompartment pharmacokinetics but are treated as if they had one compartment for dosing purposes.

## Aminoglycosides

The aminoglycosides (AG) have remained very effective for treating gram-negative aerobic infections for more than 50 years. They are commonly used but are known to be potentially nephrotoxic and ototoxic. The most commonly used drugs in this family are gentamicin and tobramycin. Amikacin is reserved for resistant organisms, and others are used only topically because of higher rates of nephrotoxiciy. There are data linking efficacy to the $C_{max}$ of AGs and the $C_{max}$ to the MIC (minimum inhibitory concentration needed to inhibit the growth of the bacteria that you are treating) ratio.[7,8] There are also data linking trough concentrations and length of therapy to nephrotoxicity and ototoxicity. The nephrotoxicity is probably best characterized by correlating it to exposure time to the drug, which would be measured by the AUC. There are data correlating AUC with toxicity.[9,10]

## Traditional Dosing

For many years, a traditional individualized approach was taken to dosing with aminoglycosides (AG). This method, popularized by Sawchuck and Zaske,[7] applied one-compartment pharmacokinetics to determine the patient's individual $k$, $C_{max}$, $C_{min}$, and $V_d$ after measuring two or three serum concentrations within a dosing interval. This method advocated targeting a $C_{max}$ of between 4 and 8 mg/L and a $C_{min}$ of <2 mg/L. The individualized approach targeting these $C_{max}$ and $C_{min}$ has been the mainstay of dosing aminoglycosides until recently, when the pharmacodynamic features of the AGs were considered when thinking about dosing strategies. This approach requires the use of one compartment linear equations rearranged to calculate the Dose (Eqs. 12.38 and 12.39).

$$R_0 = V \times k \times C_{max,tar}\left(\frac{1 - e^{-k\tau}}{1 - e^{-kt_i}}\right) \qquad (12.38)$$

$$\text{Dose} = R_0 \times t_i \qquad (12.39)$$

Utilizing these equations takes practice and expertise. Some clinicians also utilize globalrph.com to do the calculations. It is important before using these equations or utilizing any web assisted tools that the user understands how to use these tools and what assumptions are made when they were developed. These tools can be utilized to start an initial dosage regimen before any concentrations are drawn (empiric dosing) or to adjust the dosing regimen after concentrations are known.

*Extended-Interval Dosing*

Aminoglycosides are concentration-dependent killers of aerobic gram-negative bacteria; the higher the concentration, the greater the ability of the drug to kill bacteria. They are also able to continue to inhibit the growth of bacteria even after the concentration of aminoglycoside (AG) has fallen below the MIC. This is called the post-antibiotic effect (PAE). The PAE allows for an extended dose interval, longer than that predicted based on the MIC of the organism. These two factors taken together make a strong theoretical case for dosing with larger doses less often to enhance efficacy and minimize toxicity. There are several methods published that suggest ways to take advantage of these pharmacodynamic features. The most studied is the Hartford Method.[11] This method has shown to be at least equivalent to traditional methods for both efficacy and toxicities, with a few studies showing a slight advantage to extended-interval dosing for efficacy and nephrotoxicity. A 1998 survey of 249 hospitals nationwide found that approximately 75% report that they are using extended-interval dosing for AG.[12] This approach has been unfortunately named "once-daily dosing." Although using this method does often utilize a q24h schedule, it is not the only dose interval suggested and ought to be increased for those with renal impairment. There are concerns by some practitioners with how these methods are being implemented and whether there is a true advantage to this method.[13]

Empiric regimens and adjustments in the dosage regimen after concentrations are drawn can be done with the nomograms, utilizing equations or globalrph.com. It is important that the person using these tools becomes experienced and knowledgeable before relying on the suggested doses. Always discuss recommendations with the experienced practitioner and supply the data as well as the tool used to create the recommendation for a dose.

*Vancomycin*

Vancomycin is similar to aminoglycosides in that is cleared by the kidneys and the clearance mirrors creatinine clearance. The pharmacokinetic properties differ from the aminoglycosides. Vancomycin has a larger volume of distribution, around 0.7 L/kg, and it is about 50% bound to plasma proteins. The pharmacodynamics of this drug are quite different from those of aminoglycosides. It is not dependent on concentration but more dependent on the time that the microbe is exposed to the antibiotic. In this case, as opposed to the aminoglycosides, it is important to be sure that the concentration of vancomycin does not fall below effective levels. Therefore, a very small peak-to-trough ratio would be preferred when dosing this drug, whereas a large peak-to-trough ratio is the goal in dosing aminoglycosides.

There has been considerable controversy concerning how useful it is to follow the concentrations of this drug.[14-16] Measuring a peak concentration seems to be of little value, but it is important to ensure that the trough concentration does not fall below the concentration necessary to inhibit growth of the organism.

Traditionally, we have assumed a one-compartment model when we calculate individualized pharmacokinetic parameters for patients on vancomycin, but a two- or three-compartment model is probably more accurate. It is hard to justify measuring a peak concentration, but measuring a trough concentration within an hour before administration of the next dose to ensure efficacy is helpful.

One compartment linear equations are utilized to target a given $C_{ss,min}$ (Eqs. 12.39 and 12.40).

$$\text{Dose} = R_0 \times t_i \tag{12.39}$$

$$R_0 = C_{min,ss} \times CL \times \frac{1 - e^{-kt}}{\left(1 - e^{-kt_{inf}}\right) \times \left(e^{-k\left(\tau - t_{inf}\right)}\right)} \tag{12.40}$$

Like aminoglycosides empiric dosage regimens can be calculated using one compartment linear equations or other tools like nomograms or globalrph.com. Adjustments in the dosage regimen after concentrations are drawn can also be done with equations, nomograms, or globalrph.com. It is always important that the person using these is experienced and knowledgeable. Always discuss recommendations with the experienced practitioner and supply the data as well as the tool used to create the recommendation for a dose.

## GLOSSARY

**Bioavailability (F):** Units = none (fraction) The fraction of the administered dose that is available to the systemic circulation. Determined by $f_a$, $f_g$, and $f_{fp}$. It is important in determining the dose rate needed to achieve a certain targeted $C_{ss,avg}$ if given other than by intravenous route.

**Fraction absorbed ($f_a$):** fraction of drug given that is able to be absorbed into the circulation.

**Fraction that escapes gut metabolism ($f_g$):** fraction of drug absorbed that is able to escape metabolism in the gut and escape efflux pumps that are in the gut wall (like P-glycoprotein).

**Fraction that escapes first pass effect ($f_{fp}$):** fraction of drug that escapes metabolism in the liver as the blood passes through the liver before reaching the systemic circulation. $f_{fp}$ is related to the hepatic extraction ratio of a drug (E). $f_{fp} = 1 - E$

**Clearance (CL):** Units = vol/time The volume of serum, plasma or blood that has all of the drug removed per unit of time by the eliminating organ. Total body clearance is the sum of the clearances of all the eliminating organs. It is also the rate of elimination with respect to the given plasma concentration $\left(CL = \frac{k}{c}\right)$. Clearance of any organ is determined by the blood flow to that organ ($Q$) and the extraction efficiency of that organ ($E$). $CL = Q \times E$

**First Order or Linear Elimination:** The rate of elimination is directly proportional to the conentration of drug in the serum. It is independent of concentration.

**Michaelis-Menten or Nonlinear Elimination:** The rate of elimination does not change in proportion to the concentration of drug in the serum. As serum drug concentrations rise the rate of elimination increases less than proportionally. This occurs when there is a capacity limited elimination process. Examples are the hepatic enzymes and the transport sites for renal tubular secretion. When all available or nearly all available receptors are in use, the process reaches a saturation point which results in the rate of elimination becoming fixed.

$$CL = \frac{V_{max}}{K_m + C}$$

**Hepatic Extraction Ratio ($E$):** Units = none fraction of the absobed dose metabolized during each pass through the liver. It is determined by $Q_H$, $CL_{intH}$ and $f_{up}$ and is an important determinant of $CL_H$.

**Dose Regimen (DR):** Units = amt/time The amount of drug administered per time. May be thought of as daily dose. Important in determining the $C_{ss,avg}$. One of the factors that pharmacists can control.

**Dose Interval ($\tau$):** Units = time the frequency of intermittent drug administration. Important in determining the variance between the $C_{ss,max}$ and $C_{min,ss}$ or P:T. One of the factors that pharmacists can control. As a rule of thumb; drugs can be given once every half-life.

**Peak-to-Trough Ratio ($P$:$T$):** Comparison of $C_{max}$ to $C_{min}$. Important for understanding how much variation there is between the $C_{max}$ and $C_{min}$ concentrations within a dosing interval.

**Half-life ($t_{1/2}$):** Units = time Time it takes for one half of the drug to be removed from the body if eliminated by 1st order elimination. Important for determining how often to dose a drug and how long it will take to get to steady state (ss). Determined by total body clearance (CL) and volume of distribution ($V$). Inversily related to elimination rate constant ($k$).

**Elimination rate constant ($k$):** Units = /time The fraction of drug removed in a given time. Determined by measuring the slope of the terminal portion of the slope of the line formed by log serum concentrations vs. time. Important for determining how often to dose a drug and how long it will take to get to steady state. Determined by total body clearance (CL) and volume of distribution ($V$). Inversily realted to half-life ($t_{1/2}$).

**Area Under the Concentration time Curve (AUC):** Units = $\frac{\text{amt} \times \text{time}}{\text{vol}}$ The area measured under the concentration time curve that reults after administration of the drug. It relates patient exposure to a drug better than just a concentration at a point in time. In some cases it may be helpful in determining efficacy and/or toxicity of a given drug. It is determined by the dose given, $F$ if given other than IV and CL.

**Steady state (ss):** The point in therapy when the amount of drug administered exactly replaces the amount of drug removed. SS is never techically achieved, but for clinical purposes 5 $t_{1/2}$ (97% of SS) is considered to be at SS.

    **Maximum Concentration at steady state ($C_{max,ss}$):** Units (amt/vol) The highest concentration achieved after intermittent dosage adminstiration at SS. $C_{max,ss}$ will remain constant from dose to dose. May correlate to possible dose related toxicity problems.

    **Minimum Concentration at steady state ($C_{min,ss}$):** Units (amt/vol) The lowest concentration withing a SS dosing interval. $C_{min,ss}$ will remain constant from dose to dose. May correlate to possible dose related lack of efficiacy.

    **Average Concentration at steady state ($C_{ss,avg}$):** Units (amt/vol) The drug concentration representing the average concentration achieved during a SS dosing interval. It is similar but not determined by the average of the $C_{ss,max}$ and $C_{ss,min}$. It is often the target concentration when determining what dose rate to administer.

**Therapeutic Range (TR):** A statistical range of desirable drug concentrations, for which the *majority* of patients show effective therapeutic response with minimal drug-related side effects. Is *not* an absolute for every patient. Individual patients can have good therapeutic response with "subtherapeutic" drug concentrations or can experience toxicity with "therapeutic" drug concentrations. Therapeutic ranges are indication specific.

**Volume of Distribution ($V$):** Units = volume Where the drug distributes in the body. Important for determining how long the drug stays in the body (determinant of $t_{1/2}$) and whether a drug will be removed by hemodialysis (larger volumes will not be removed significantly). Is primarily determined by binding of the drug to plasma and tissue binding sites as well as lipophilicity.

    **Central Volume of Distribution ($V_c$):** Hypothetical volume into which a drug initally distributes. It includes blood and highly perfused tissues. It is important for determining loading doses.

    **Apparent Volume of Distribution ($V_d$):** Calculated volume that would be necessary to account for all the drug or the concentration of drug in the body. It is calcuated by $V_d = \frac{\text{Dose}}{C}$ or by relating clearance and $kV_d = \frac{\text{CL}}{k}$

    **Volume of Distribution at steady state ($V_{ss}$):** Actual blood and tissue volumes into which the drug distributes. Can estimate the amount of drug in the body. Amount of drug in body = $V_{ss} \times C_{ss,avg}$

## APPLICATION EXERCISES

### Dosage Regimen Design

1. You read the following quote in a paper that you are evaluating: "There was an increase in the elimination rate constant $(K)$; therefore, there was an increase in clearance." Does this make sense or not?
2. Your patient with epilepsy is well controlled on carbamazepine. He then goes to a mail-order pharmacy, which supplies him with a different brand of carbamazepine that is significantly less bioavailable. What would you expect to see? A(n) increase/decrease/no change in clearance, a(n) increase/decrease/ no change in volume, a(n) increase/decrease/no change in $C_{ss,avg}$, and a(n) increase/decrease/no change in half-life.
3. Your patient is well controlled on a drug that is totally cleared by the kidneys. Your patient becomes renally impaired. For this drug, renal impairment decreases the volume of distribution as well as decreasing clearance. Explain how this knowledge will affect your choice of daily dose rate and dose interval.

### Renal Clearance

For the given drugs, identify which of the following may explain an increase in $C_{ss,avg}$ and an increase in half-life. Also, in response to these effects, how would you anticipate needing to alter the patient's dosage regimen?

A. Alkalinzation of the urine
B. Acidification of the urine
C. Giving another weak acid; $f_e = 1$; $CL_r > CL_{gf}$
D. Giving another weak base; $f_e = 1$; $CL_r > CL_{gf}$
E. Giving mannitol, which increases urine flow
F. Giving a drug that displaces the drug from plasma protein binding sites
G. None of the above

1. Drug A: $f_e = 1$; weak acid; $CL_r = 14.4$ mL/min; $f_u = 0.85$
2. Drug B: $f_e = 1$; weak acid; $CL_r = 74$ mL/min; $f_u = 0.04$
3. Drug C: $f_e = 1$; weak base; $CL_r = 19.86$ L/hr; $f_u = 0.85$
4. Drug D: $f_e = 1$; neutral; $CL_r = 4$ L/hr; $f_u = 0.9$
5. Drug E: $f_e = 1$; weak acid; $CL_r = 11$ mL/min; $f_u = 0.85$

### Hepatic Clearance

You will need to refer to the information in Table 12.10 to answer the questions below. The following are physiological factors that influence pharmacokinetic parameters of clearance, volume, and bioavailable fraction:

A. Fraction absorbed $(f_a)$
B. Fraction unbound in the plasma $(f_u)$

**TABLE 12.10. INFORMATION FOR HEPATIC CLEARANCE REVIEW QUESTIONS**

| Drug | $f_e$ | E | $f_u$ | Binding Proteins | Metab CYP Enzymes |
|---|---|---|---|---|---|
| Lidocaine | 0.05 | 0.93 | 0.25 | Alb, AAG | 3A4 |
| Propranolol | 0.05 | 0.7 | 0.1 | Alb, AAG | 3A4, 2D6 |
| Quinidine | 0.18 | 0.05 | 0.25 | Alb, AAG | 3A4 |
| Theophylline | 0.1 | 0.03 | 0.6 | Alb | 1A2 |
| Verapamil | 0.14 | 0.75 | 0.1 | Alb, AAG | 3A4 |
| Warfarin | 0.05 | 0.005 | 0.01 | Alb | 2C9(S) |

**C.** Fraction unbound in the tissue ($f_{ut}$)
**D.** Hepatic enzyme activity ($CL_{int}$)
**E.** Hepatic blood flow ($Q$)
**F.** None of the above

Choose as many of the above as apply for the following questions:

**1.** A change in which of the above would alter phenytoin half-life?
**2.** A change in which of the above would alter the bioavailability of verapamil?
**3.** A change in which of the above would alter the total steady-state concentrations of quinidine, given orally?
**4.** A change in which of the above would alter the free steady-state concentrations of quinidine, given orally?

## Basic Calculations

A patient with epilepsy is successfully treated for seizures with Drug A, 400 mg q12h (8 AM and 8 PM). The usual half-life of the drug is about 12 hours. The patient has been treated for 4 days. The recommended range for your lab for Drug A is 5 to 10 mg/L. Before the patient is discharged, you want to document the serum concentration during a steady-state dosing interval. Four blood samples are drawn:

| Time Postadministration | Serum Concentrations |
|---|---|
| 2 hours | 9.5 mg/L |
| 4 hours | 8.43 mg/L |
| 6 hours | 7.47 mg/L |
| 12 hours | 5.21 mg/L |

1. Plot the serum concentration-time curve
2. What is the concentration at time = 0?
3. Report $k$, $t_{1/2}$, and $C_{ss,min}$. Can you determine $C_{ss,max}$?
4. Report AUC and $C_{ss,avg}$.
5. Determine the concentration at 5 hours

Six months later, the same patient returns to the clinic. He reports "break-through" seizures in the morning and sometimes in the evening. You obtain a blood sample immediately before his next dose. The serum concentration is 2.8 mg/L

What might have caused this?

You measure the following serum concentrations during the dosing interval:

| Time Postadministration | Serum Concentrations |
|---|---|
| 2 hours | 13.2 mg/L |
| 4 hours | 9.68 mg/L |
| 6 hours | 7.10 mg/L |
| 12 hours | 2.80 mg/L |

A. Plot the serum concentration-time curve
B. Report $k$, $t_{1/2}$, and $C_{ss,min}$
C. Report AUC and $C_{ss,avg}$
D. Calculate the concentration at 5 hours
E. What do you think has caused this?

## REFERENCES

1. Watkins PB, Wrighton SA, Schuetz EG, et al. Identification of glucocorticoid-inducible cytochromes P-450 in the intestinal mucosa of rats and man. *J Clin Invest.* 1987;80:1029–1036.
2. Fojo AT, Ueda K, Slamon DJ, et al. Expression of a multidrug-resistance gene in human tumors and tissues. *Proc Natl Acad Sci USA.* 1987;84:265–269.
3. Wacher VJ, Silverman JA, Zhang Y, et al. Role of p-glycoprotein and cytochrome P450 3A in limiting oral absorption of peptides and petidomimetics. *J Pharm Sci.* 1998;87:1322–1330.
4. Gwilt PR. Perrier D. Plasma protein binding and distribution characteristics of drugs as indices of their hemodialyzability. *Clin Pharmacol Ther.* 1978;24:154.
5. MacKichan JJ. Pharmacokinetic consequences of drug displacement from blood and tissue proteins. Clin Pharmacokinet 1984;9(S1):32–41.
6. Kalra BS. Cytochrome P450 enzyme isoforms and their therapeutic implications: An update. *Indian J Med Sci* [serial online] 2007 [cited 2008 Oct 5]; 61:102–16. Available at http://www.indianjmedsci.org/text.asp?2007/61/2/102/30351.

7. Sawchuk RJ, Zaske DE. Pharmacokinetics of dosing regimens which utilize multiple intravenous infusions: gentamicin in burn patients. *J Pharmacokinet Biopharm* 1976;4:183–195.

8. Kashuba ADM, NafzigerAN, Drusano GL, Bertino JS. Optimizing aminoglycoside therapy for nosocomial pneumonia caused by gram-negative bacteria. *Antimicrob Agents Chemother.* 1999; 43:623–629.

9. Rybak MJ, Abate BJ, Kang SL, et al. Prospective evaluation of the effect of an aminoglycoside dosing regimen on rates of observed nephrotoxicity and ototoxicity. *Antimicrob Agents Chemother.* 1999;43:1549–1555.

10. Kirkpartrick CMJ, Buffull SB, Begg EJ. Once daily aminoglycoside therapy: potential ototoxicity. *Antimicrob Agents Chemother.* 1997;879–880.

11. Nicolau DP, Freeman CD, Belliveau PP, et al. *Antimicrob Agents Chemother.* 1995;39:650–655.

12. Chuck SK, Raber SR, Rodvold KA, et al. National survey of extended-interval aminoglycoside dosing. *Clin Infect Dis.* 2000;30:433–439.

13. Brown GH, Bertino JS, Rotschafer JC. Single daily dosing of aminoglycosides—a community standard? *Clin Infect Dis.* 2000;30:440–441.

14. Edwards DJ, Pancorbo S. Routine monitoring of serum vancomycin concentrations: waiting for proof of its value. *Clin Pharm.* 1987;6:652–654.

15. Freeman CD, Quintiliani R, Nightingale CH. Vancomycin therapeutic drug monitoring: is it necessary? *Ann Pharmacother.* 1993;27:594–598.

16. Saunders NJ. Why monitor peak vancomycin concentrations? Lancet 1994;344:1748–1750.

17. Yu DK. The contribution of P-glycoprotein to pharmacokinetic drug-drug interactions. *J Clin Pharmacol.* 1999;39:1203–1212.

18. Streetman DS. Bertino JS, Nafzinger AN. Phenotyping of drug-metbolizing enzymes in adults: a review of in-vivo cytochrome P450 phenotyping probes. *Pharmacogenetics.* 2000;10:187–216.

19. Levien,TL,R.Ph, Baker, DE. *Cytochrome P450 Drug Interactions.* Pharmacist's Letter/Prescriber's Letter. 2003;1–4.

# Topics in Pharmacy Practice

# Drug Information and Drug Literature Evaluation

*Karen L. Kier*

**Objectives: Upon completion of the chapter and exercises, the student pharmacist will be able to**

1. Explain the role that drug information, drug literature evaluation, and professional writing play in establishing a good foundation for a pharmacy professional.
2. Discuss the modified systematic approach to drug information and how it impacts the development of a good search strategy.
3. Specify the differences among primary, secondary, and tertiary literature.
4. Identify essential secondary and tertiary literature used in answering drug information inquiries.
5. Understand the basic concepts of drug literature evaluation and be able to apply them to an article.
6. Recognize and apply key concepts in professional writing.

---

### Patient Encounter

Once the family has been convinced to treat the patient X with antibiotics, they are concerned with the kind of antibiotics that will be used. They have heard that some antibiotics can make a patient lose their hearing and that is the last thing they want. They are also concerned that being on so many antibiotics will make the patient have resistance to their effect and get further or even worse infections.

This is your first day on the ICU ward. What do you need to do first? This family is asking for drug information?

You have reviewed the very specific chart note written in a SOAP format by the student pharmacist who completed the student practice experience last month. You now have an understanding of the family's concern.

*(continued on next page)*

What sources will you use to gather data?

How will you interpret the data to provide them with the information they need, and not too much?

How will you present the data and answer the patient's question: orally, with a slide show, or written information?

Will you provide the information and data to anyone else?

Could the information accessed during the research change the patient's therapeutic plan?

## INTRODUCTION

Drug information is a specialized area of pharmacy focusing on information management. Information management can evolve into many different forms. Drug information can be a verbal answer to a patient's question, or it can involve a detailed monograph presented to the Pharmacy & Therapeutics committee (P&T) in order to decide if a drug will be available through a formulary system. Pharmacists and pharmacy students cannot know every potential or possible question or scenario that might be posed to them during their practice. However, they should be prepared to efficiently and effectively answer questions posed to them from consumers or other health-care professionals. Knowing where to look and how to find the most appropriate information is the basic groundwork for drug information skills. Among the skills of drug information is a knowledge of drug literature evaluation, which allows one to provide a critical analysis of the literature and have a better understanding of the studies done in health and medicine. The goal of this chapter is to provide students with a basic understanding of drug information skills and resources as well as providing the basic tenants of drug literature evaluation. The chapter provides examples of student drug information exercises that could serve as a basic template for written communication.

## DRUG INFORMATION SKILLS

In order to provide an accurate and timely answer to a drug information question, one has to ascertain the nature of the question and has asked all the necessary questions to get to the "ultimate" question. As with many questions, the first question asked is not necessarily the whole picture or representative of the complete question. Many times the first question asked is a lead to open the conversation, and there is more to the question than first appears. Valuable information can be lost when the

| TABLE 13.1. MODIFIED SYSTEMATIC APPROACH | |
|---|---|
| Step I | Secure demographics of requestor |
| Step II | Obtain background information |
| Step III | Determine and categorize the ultimate question |
| Step IV | Develop strategy and conduct search |
| Step V | Perform evaluation, analysis, and synthesis |
| Step VI | Formulate and provide response |
| Step VII | Conduct follow-up and documentation |

pharmacist does not take the time to ask appropriate questions to the requestor. Patients, especially, may not always know the necessary information that is critical for providing a complete and accurate answer. This is why drug information specialists have developed systematic approaches to answering drug information questions. Most specialists today use the modified systematic approach designed by Host and Kirkwood. This approach involves seven steps, which are outlined in Table 13.1.

Looking at each step provides us with a framework for obtaining and answering a drug information request.

## Step I. Secure Demographics of Requestor

Know who is requesting the information because this determines the type of response that is given. A response given to a consumer requesting information would involve much less medical terminology, whereas a response to a health-care professional would involve more technical information including specific medical terminology that would be deemed appropriate. Likewise, it is important to determine the name of the requestor and his or her location (phone, fax, address, e-mail) and affiliation. Some institutions and workplaces have very specific policies and procedures for handling information requests. Always ask for a copy of such policies before answering any questions. For example, some institutions will answer only questions requested by employees, and others may not answer consumer questions. Some pharmacies will not handle consumer questions if the patient does not receive his or her medication from that pharmacy. Often this policy is based on not having available profile information that may be needed to answer questions completely and accurately.

## Step II. Obtain Background Information

Other demographic information that maybe helpful is knowing if the question is patient specific or if the question is one of general knowledge. Most questions are usually a result of a specific patient need rather than purely academic questions that just arise. Patient-specific questions require delving into questions related to the patient. These questions can refer to such things as the patient's age, medication profile, disease state profile, past medication history, family history, social history, current laboratory data, and overall health. The better one understands the conditions, health, and demographics of the patient, the better is one's ability to look at the complete picture and provide an appropriate response. Many drug information centers use a standard response form that guides the collection of this information for each request.

Additional information that may be helpful is where the requestors found the information they already have, including the correct spelling of unfamiliar terms, where they have looked, and how quickly they need to know the information. Many times consumers will read or hear information from television, magazines, friends, or other healthcare professionals. They often do not have the correct spelling of information or even accurate descriptions of the information that they heard. Recent advances in using sources such as the Internet, Lexis-Nexis (a secondary database that contains television transcripts), and Periodicals Index Online (a secondary database with information from both medical and consumer journals and magazines) have provided additional avenues to identifying the questions posed by consumers.

## Step III. Determine and Categorize the Ultimate Question

This step is probably the most critical one in establishing a good search strategy. The first part of this step involves putting the pieces of information together to form the ultimate question. Some interpret the ultimate question as the final iteration of the question. Sometimes the ultimate question is actually more than one distinct question. Once the ultimate question has been determined, the next step is to categorize the question. Many drug information centers have lists of standard categories that they use. A comprehensive list can be found in the textbook called *Drug Information: A Guide for Pharmacists*, 5th edition.[2] Table 13.2 provides some of the most common types. The category is essential to developing the strategy because different references maybe employed for different types or categories of questions. For example, a tablet identification question may require a source such as IDENTIDEX to answer the inquiry, whereas a dosing question may use a standard reference such as *Facts and Comparisons or the Drug Information Handbook*.

## Step IV. Develop Strategy and Conduct Search

Developing an algorithm for searching a question will provide an organized approach to handling the question and assuring that sufficient references and documentation have been acquired to answer the question. A typical algorithm has three essential components, which consist of tertiary, secondary, and primary literature. Primary literature refers to the actual study, case report, or case series. The key to

**TABLE 13.2.** EXAMPLES OF DRUG INFORMATION CATEGORIES

| | |
|---|---|
| Adverse Effects | Identification |
| Availability | Pharmacokinetics |
| Compatibility/Stability | Pharmacology |
| Compounding | Poisoning/Toxicology |
| Dosing and Administration | Pregnancy and Lactation |
| Drug Interaction | Therapeutic Use |
| Herbal | |

this type of literature is that it refers to the actual subjects whether in a clinical trial or as a case report. The primary literature is considered to be the original study or report. In answering drug information requests, the idea is to be able to identify, evaluate, and report on the primary literature whenever possible. Some types of questions do not require a search this extensive. A good example of that type of question would be a tablet identification code or the availability of a drug in the United States. Secondary literature refers to an indexing or abstracting service. Secondary literature is the indexed primary literature. The secondary sources are an excellent tool in obtaining the primary literature. Secondary sources include such very common databases as the IOWA system, International Pharmaceutical Abstracts (IPA), Medline (PubMed), Lexis-Nexis, Google Scholar, Embase, and Reactions. Some secondary sources will provide an abstract of the primary literature, and others will provide a full text version of the article. The key to secondary systems is to become familiar with the best way to search each system and to identify correct key terms. Often the difference between a mediocre search and a good one is the key words used by the researcher. A better understanding of the nature of the question and the related background information will help in determining key search terms. Tertiary literature refers to compilations or reviews of primary literature done by authors who put the actual studies into their own words. Textbooks are a common example of tertiary literature that involves review of material. One problem with tertiary literature is that it is usually at least 2 years out of date by the time it is published, so its timeliness is limited. Another problem is that the reader is dependent on the interpretation and accuracy of the author who did the review, and this interpretation may differ from what others may have considered appropriate. Tertiary literature can also contain misinformation taken out of context or data that were transformed differently from the primary study. Sometimes this results in mistakes in dosing or administration. Some drug information specialists will often refer to a minimum of two tertiary references to find corroborating information. This provides a level of confidence that the information is accurate and consistent. However, this is not always an absolute.

In designing an algorithm, start the research with tertiary literature. Then proceed to secondary sources, which help to identify the necessary primary literature. Knowing what tertiary and secondary references are useful for the question's category facilitates the algorithm design. Table 13.3 provides some common categories with useful tertiary and secondary sources. This table is by no means comprehensive for all references available but is meant to be a basic guide to establishing an algorithm.

### Step V. Perform Evaluation, Analysis, and Synthesis

A good drug information response will demonstrate that the provider took time to evaluate the information, analyze it, and then synthesize it into a good reply. Evaluating the quality of the information is a key. Care should be taken to identify poor data or even controversial data where studies differ on outcomes. Therefore, drug literature evaluation skills become critical to the ability to distinguish good data from poor data. There is no one perfect study, and each study will have some limitations. The professional develops the skills to interpret the merits of a study despite limitations that might be present.

### Step VI. Formulate and Provide Response

Establish an outline that helps formulate a response to the drug information request. As with most professional writing, it is important to have an introduction, body, and conclusion. The introduction should provide a comprehensive but concise review of the disease, drug, or situation proposed in the question. The body of the answer should be a review of the pertinent literature that answers the question. The primary literature should be reviewed and discussed in this section. Any controversy or debate among the studies should be addressed. Studies should be appropriately cited in the reference section. Discussion of study limitations established by either the study authors or by drug literature evaluation is also appropriate within this section. The last section is the conclusion. This section should give a brief synopsis of the information provided and should usually include a professional opinion based on the literature cited.

### Step VII. Conduct Follow-up and Documentation

This step involves checking with the requestor to make sure his or her question has been sufficiently and completely answered. Of vital importance is to document all the steps taken in this process.

### STANDARD REFERENCES

This section provides information on some of the standard references that are used to answer drug information questions. A more extensive review of standard

**TABLE 13.3. COMMON SECONDARY AND TERTIARY REFERENCES BY CATEGORY**

| Category of Inquiry | Tertiary Resources | Secondary Resources |
|---|---|---|
| Adverse Events | AHFS Drug Information, DRUGDEX, Drug Facts and Comparisons, Drug Information Handbook, (Lexi-Comp) | Reactions, IPA, IOWA, MEDLINE |
| Disease State Information | Cecil Textbook of Medicine, Harrison's Principles of Internal Medicine, The Merck Manual Pharmacotherapy | IOWA, MEDLINE, IPA |
| Dosage Guidelines (General) | AHFS Drug Information, DRUGDEX, Drug Facts and Comparisons PDR, Drug Information Handbook, (Lexi-Comp), Pharmacotherapy | IPA, IOWA |
| Dosage Guidelines (Geriatrics) | Geriatric Dosage Handbook (Lexi-Comp), AHFS Drug Information, DRUGDEX, Drug Facts and Comparisons | IPA, IOWA |
| Dosage Guidelines (Pediatrics) | Harriet Lane Handbook, Pediatric Dosage Handbook, AHFS Drug Information, DRUGDEX, Drug Facts and Comparisons, Pediatric Dosing Handbook (Lexi-Comp) | IPA, IOWA, MEDLINE |
| Drug Administration | AHFS Drug Information, DRUGDEX Drug Facts and Comparisons, Drug Information Handbook (Lexi-Comp) | IPA, IOWA |
| Drug Interactions | Drug Interaction Facts, Evaluation of Drug Interactions, DRUGDEX | Reactions, IPA, IOWA |
| Drug Use in Pregnancy and Lactation | Drugs in Pregnancy and Lactation, DRUGDEX, Drug Information Handbook (Lexi-Comp) | Reactions, IOWA, IPA, MEDLINE |
| Herbal and Homeopathic Medications | PDR Herbal, Review of Natural Products, Commission E Monographs | IPA, IOWA, MEDLINE |

(continued)

**TABLE 13.3. COMMON SECONDARY AND TERTIARY REFERENCES BY CATEGORY (Continued)**

| Category of Inquiry | Tertiary Resources | Secondary Resources |
|---|---|---|
| Identification (Domestic) | American Drug Index, IDENTIDEX, DRUGDEX, Handbook of Nonprescription Drugs, USP Dictionary of USAN & International Drug Names | IPA, IOWA, Lexis-Nexis |
| Identification (Foreign) | Index Nominum, Martindale: The Extra Pharmacopeia, USP Dictionary of USAN & International Drug Names, DRUGDEX | IPA, Lexis-Nexis, MEDLINE |
| Identification (Imprint code) | IDENTIDEX, Ident-A-Drug Reference, Clinical Reference Library, Lexi-Comp, www.drugs.com | Lexis-Nexis, www.fda.gov |
| Indications | AHFS Drug Information, DRUGDEX, Facts and Comparisons, Drug Information Handbook (Lexi-Comp) | Lexis-Nexis, www.fda.gov |
| Investigational drugs | USP Dictionary of USAN & International Drug Names, DRUGDEX, Martindale: The Extra Pharmacopeia | IOWA, IPA, MEDLINE, www.clinicaltrials.gov |
| Over-the-counter drugs | Handbook of Nonprescription Drugs, Physicians' Desk Reference for Non-Prescription Drugs, DRUGDEX, POISINDEX | IPA, IOWA, MEDLINE |
| Pharmacokinetics | Applied Pharmacokinetics: Principles of Therapeutic Drug Monitoring, Basic Clinical Pharmacokinetics, AHFS Drug Information, DRUGDEX, Handbook of Clinical Drug Data | IPA, IOWA, MEDLINE |
| Pharmacology | Goodman and Gilman's Pharmacologic Basis of Therapeutics, AHFS Drug Information, DRUGDEX, Facts and Comparisons | IOWA, IPA, MEDLINE, |
| Stability/compatibility | Guide to Parenteral Admixtures, Handbook of Injectable Drugs, AHFS Drug Information, DRUGDEX | IPA, IOWA, MEDLINE |
| Toxicology/poisoning | Clinical Toxicology of Commercial Products, POISINDEX, Poisoning & Toxicology Handbook | Reactions, IPA, IOWA, MEDLINE |

| TABLE 13.4. GENERAL TERTIARY REFERENCES |
| --- |
| Facts and Comparisons eAnswers |
| Drug Information Handbook (LexiiComp) |
| ASHP Drug Information |
| MICROMEDEX (DRUGDEX, IDENTIDEX, POSIONDEX) |

references by categories can be found in the textbook *Drug Information: A Guide for Pharmacists*, 5th edition. Table 13.4 provides some good general tertiary references that can be helpful in answering a wide variety of questions. It is important to note that many of these tertiary references can be found in different formats including hard copy, Web based, CD-ROM based, and PDA based. Table 13.5 outlines some good secondary references that may be available for identifying the primary literature. Table 13.6 provides some guidance to general journals that will often provide good primary literature.

## DRUG LITERATURE EVALUATION

Drug literature evaluation is a key component to providing a good-quality answer to a requestor. Being able to separate good data from poor data is essential.

**TABLE 13.5. COMMON SECONDARY REFERENCES**

| Secondary Source | Brief Description |
| --- | --- |
| IOWA | Index by drug and disease and provides full text articles in PDF format |
| International Pharmaceutical Abstracts (IPA) | Most comprehensive pharmacy database, the best indexing of pharmacy journals from around the world, provides abstracts |
| MEDLINE | Most comprehensive biomedical database that includes medicine, nursing, pharmacy, and veterinary |
| Reactions | Good source for adverse events, drug interactions, problems with herbal therapy, pregnancy and lactation, and toxicology |
| Lexis-Nexis | Provides comprehensive biomedical database, provides TV transcripts |
| Periodicals Online | Provides an index of both medical journals and consumer magazines |

---

**TABLE 13.6.  PRIMARY REFERENCES**

*Annals of Pharmacotherapy*

*Pharmacotherapy*

*American Journal of Health-System Pharmacists*

*Journal of the American Pharmacists Association*

*Journal of the American Medical Association*

*New England Journal of Medicine*

*Annals of Internal Medicine*

---

Knowing the limitations of any study can help in evaluating the usability of its data. Drug information specialists will often use some standard questions to help in this process. Several references provide guides to evaluating the medical and pharmacy literature. A template of 32 questions has been designed by drug information specialists and can be found in some of these references. The questions in Table 13.7 can be used as a template and are adapted with permission from Malone et al.[2] Table 13.8 has some helpful hints for determining the answers to these questions.

---

**TABLE 13.7.  QUESTIONS USED TO GUIDE THE DRUG LITERATURE EVALUATION PROCESS**

1. Is the journal considered reputable? Is the journal appropriate to find an article relating to this particular subject?

2. Do the researchers appear to have the appropriate qualifications for undertaking the study? Was the research performed in an appropriate medical facility?

3. What was the source of financial support for the study?

4. Do the authors give sufficient background information for the study? Did they demonstrate that the study was important and ethical?

5. Are the purpose and the objectives clearly stated and free from bias?

6. Was the study approved by an investigational review board?

7. Does the investigator state the null hypothesis? Is the alternative hypothesis stated?

8. Is the sample size large enough? Is the sample representative of the population?

9. Are the inclusion and exclusion criteria clearly stated, and are they appropriate?

10. Was the study randomized correctly? Even if the study is adequately randomized, are the groups (treatment and control) equivalent?

**TABLE 13.7.** QUESTIONS USED TO GUIDE THE DRUG LITERATURE EVALUATION PROCESS (*Continued*)

11. What is the study design? Is it appropriate?

12. Was the study adequately controlled? Were the controls adequate and appropriate?

13. Was the study adequately blinded?

14. Were appropriate doses and regimens used for the disease state under study?

15. Was the length of the study adequate to observe outcomes?

16. If the study is a crossover study, was the washout period adequate?

17. Were operational definitions given?

18. Were appropriate statistical tests chosen to assess the data? Were the levels of $\alpha$ and $\beta$ error chosen before the data were gathered? Were multiple statistical tests applied until a significant result was achieved?

19. Was patient compliance monitored?

20. If multiple observers were collecting data, did the authors describe how variations in measurements were avoided?

21. Did the authors justify the instrumentation used in the study?

22. Were measurements or assessments of effects made at the appropriate times and frequency?

23. Are the data presented in an appropriate, understandable format?

24. Are standard deviations or confidence intervals shown along with mean values?

25. Are there any problems with type I ($\alpha$) or type II ($\beta$) errors?

26. Are there any potential problems with internal validity or external validity? Internal validity types include history, maturation, instrumentation, selection, morbidity, and mortality.

27. Are adverse reactions reported in sufficient detail?

28. Are the conclusions supported by the data? Is some factor other than the study treatment responsible for the outcomes?

29. Are the results both statistically and clinically significant?

30. Do the authors discuss study limitations in their conclusions?

31. Were appropriate references used? Are references timely and reputable? Have any of the studies been disproven or updated? Do references cited represent a complete background?

32. Would this article change clinical practice or a recommendation that you would give to a patient or healthcare professional?

**TABLE 13.8. HELPFUL HINTS FOR DRUG LITERATURE EVALUATION**

Some helpful hints can also provide some insight to the reader when trying to answer the 32 questions of Table 13.7.

1. A journal is considered reputable if it is peer reviewed.

2. Appropriate qualifications often include some sort of research background or an author on the team who has statistics background. Do the researchers have expertise in the area of study?

3. Often at the end of the article there is information on funding. NIH funding etc. is often considered unbiased. Questions arise if the company marketing the product funds the sponsorship. (This does not necessarily mean it is bad, just a concern.)

4. Sufficient background information would include a good review (timely) of the drug, disease state, or research topic. Was the background concise but comprehensive. Did they indicate why the authors thought this was important or why they needed to know?

5. Purpose is the reason for doing a study, the objectives are how they are going to accomplish the purpose. Very few studies really outline the objectives if they mention the purpose. Some journals now require the authors to state the objective in the abstract.

6. Investigational Review Board (IRB), also known as Institutional Review Board, Human Subjects Committee, etc. They should indicate this over and beyond talking about informed consent.

7. The null hypothesis should be clearly stated as the hypothesis of no difference, with the alternative being the hypothesis of difference. Many times the research question is stated but not in the form of the hypothesis. Ask what you think the null hypothesis would be or should be based on the information given in the article. This formulation of the null hypothesis by the reader will be helpful later to establish type I and type II error as well as trying to obtain information related to external validity.

8. Is the sample large enough, is a good question. The central limit theorem suggests a sample size larger than 30 is necessary to assume normality (normal distribution) and therefore be able to do parametric statistical testing. However, the central limit theorem is not applied here to this question. This question is directed at knowing if the sample is large enough to statistically prove differences between groups or statistically identify trends in the data. It is also directed at knowing if the sample size is large enough to truly represent the overall population being studied. Good research will identify how they arrived at their sample size. This usually involves a calculation that takes into consideration things like type I and type II error (often you will see power used here instead), standard deviation, and the clinical difference to be detected.

9. Inclusion criteria define who is included in the study, and the exclusion criteria define who is eliminated or not included in the study. Exclusion criteria need to make sense and not be so restrictive that they exclude important or good data. Inclusion criteria need to be specific enough that all of the researchers understand who really belongs. Definitions of inclusion criteria are often helpful. For example, the patients must have a fasting blood glucose less than 120 mg/dL.

**TABLE 13.8.  HELPFUL HINTS FOR DRUG LITERATURE EVALUATION (*Continued*)**

10. Did they randomize the study? Really randomize, not just say they did. How did they do it? Random number tables or names pulled from a hat are legitimate ways to do this. Did they provide a table or chart comparing the demographic information between groups? Does it look as though the groups are relatively equal, or are they characteristically (demographically) similar? There are other ways to randomize besides simple random samples. These can be legitimate ways to allocate subjects. Research design textbooks will elaborate on these other methods.

11. What is the study design? Several references including the Malone textbook[2] go into more depth about study designs. Common study designs include the clinical trial (experimental design comparing therapies between groups), cohort studies (long-term studies observing disease patterns related to risk factor exposures), case-control studies (comparison of cases who have a condition with controls without the condition to determine if a risk factor could have caused the differences), intention-to-treat (a type of clinical trial that often controls for subjects dropping out of studies prematurely), and meta-analysis (statistical combination of previous studies' data and determining if the conclusions would be different). Does the type of design they chose make sense? Would a different study design have been better to answer the proposed hypothesis?

12. Did they use controls? Did they compare the controls to the treatment subjects (cases)? Often they will provide a demographics table that allows a comparison of control group to treatment group. Do they look similar? Did they run statistical tests that compare the similarity of the two groups. If they did, $p$-values should be reported; $p$-values less than 0.05 would indicate that the groups are different, whereas a $p$-value greater than 0.05 would show the groups to be similar on that characteristic. The next question would be, did they select the groups appropriately? Where did the controls come from? Is that similar to how they selected the treatment group? Some studies will take a treatment group from the community and then select controls from a hospital group. There could be differences between these two groups just based on their selection and not because of treatments provided. Some studies will actually have more than one control matched to each case. This is actually considered to be a good research technique.

13. Was it single-blinded or double-blinded? Single-blind means either the study subject or the investigator is not aware of the treatment, but not both. Usually in a single-blinded study just the subjects or patients are blinded to the therapy they are receiving. In double-blinded studies both the subjects and the researchers or care providers in the study are blinded to the therapy being given. Usually double-blinded is best!

14. Doses and regimens? Why or why not? What do general tertiary references such as *Facts and Comparisons* say? Also think about pharmacodynamics and pharmacokinetics when considering this question. The authors may have selected appropriate doses and regimens, but did they consider the half-life of the drug and the length of time it takes to get to steady state? Did the authors consider that a drug pharmacodynamically may take some patients 4 to 6 weeks or longer to see clinical benefit?

*(continued)*

**TABLE 13.8.**  HELPFUL HINTS FOR DRUG LITERATURE EVALUATION (*Continued*)

15. If they are talking about adequate treatment with a drug for CHF, and they look at only a 2- to 6-week study, is that really long enough? If they are evaluating only short-term results, that would be fine. If they are looking at long-term outcomes, it needs to be longer, for example, 6 months to a year.

16. Crossover studies mean the same subject gets both treatments, one after the other. Note that the washout period should be at least 5 half-lives of the drug to achieve a plasma level of zero, or the washout needs to be long enough that any pharmacodynamic effects of drug therapy are gone. The drug maybe gone from the plasma but may still have tissue concentrations or have affected receptors for a longer period of time. It is also important in a crossover study that each drug or treatment is started at the beginning of the study and then patients are crossed over to the other drug or treatment. For example, if the study involves 40 patients and they are to get both Drug A and Drug B in the study, this would mean that 20 patients would start the study on Drug A and then be crossed over to Drug B while 20 would start on Drug B and then be crossed over to Drug A. If both drugs are started from the beginning, this helps reduce the chance of error that could have happened because of some other effect that was changing the outcome. For example, CHF usually gets worse with time. If you started all of your CHF patients on an ACE inhibitor and then switched them over to a β-blocker, and then the disease got worse, is that because of the β-blocker, or is that the natural progression of the disease? But if you started half of the group on ACE-I and half on β-blockers and then switched each group to the other treatment, and the CHF got worse on the β-blocker treatment regardless of the timing, one could successfully argue that the β-blocker caused this rather than the disease state itself?

17. Operational definition means definitions of the variables, measurements, etc. When they say subjects have glaucoma, what do they mean by that? When they measure a gentamicin level, how are they doing this, and on what machine? How do they define a gentamicin peak level: is that 1 hour after the infusion or a half-hour? How do they define clinical cure? How do they define an exacerbation of a disease state? Think of these questions as though you were part of the research team receiving this document. Could you adequately perform this study based on the definitions they provide?

18. Some tests you may have to look up in a statistics book. Did they meet the assumptions for a parametric test? How many groups were they comparing on the outcome variable (two, three, etc)? Did they set $\alpha$ (type I) and $\beta$ error (type II) before starting the study? Did they do multiple tests until they found the answer they wanted? Was it a fishing trip—were they just looking for an answer of any type?

19. Did they, and how did they, monitor compliance? Was it a good method?

20. This is important. If there were multiple researchers or multiple sites, how did they coordinate the efforts so that they all did the same thing?

**TABLE 13.8.** HELPFUL HINTS FOR DRUG LITERATURE EVALUATION (*Continued*)

21. Instrumentation is the instrument/gauge they used to measure the variables. This could be an actual instrument such as a blood pressure kit or glucose monitor. This could be an instrument such as a survey or questionnaire. If the research used the Visual Analog Scale for pain, which is a scale from 0 to 10 with 10 being the worst pain, this is an instrument.

22. Did they assess measurements when it was appropriate? If not, what would you or the literature recommend?

23. Format is important. Look at the tables and graphs. Are they easy to read? Do they make sense? Do you know what they measured? Do you know the measurement scale? What are they describing? How many of these are hard to read or make no sense? When you get done looking at it, are you not sure if they were giving you the mean with the standard deviation or standard error of the mean?

24. The study should always give standard deviation and not standard error of the mean, in most cases. Standard error of the mean is only appropriate if more than one sample is being studeed. Confidence intervals are a good alternative when they do not give standard deviations or standard deviations are not appropriate.

25. This is tricky. Did they state a null hypothesis (remember that the null hypothesis is the hypothesis of no difference)? If not, can you infer the null hypothesis? Did they accept or reject the null hypothesis at the end of the study? If they accepted the null hypothesis, it is more likely that they made a type II error. If they rejected the null hypothesis, it is more likely that they made a type I error. Realize that a study is vulnerable to both types of errors.

26. External validity deals with the overall generalizability of the study, whereas internal validity deals with the internal methods used to do the study.

26a. External validity has to do with the generalizability of the study. Can you take the results from the study and generalize them to the rest of the population? The key here is to look at whom they studied (really studied) and what type of conclusions they stated based on the data. For example, if I look at mitral value prolapse (mild and moderate forms) in young men (age 18–40), and I am trying to determine if β-blockers help them with improving exercise tolerance, and my conclusion of the study states that "β-blockers are superior agents in helping improve exercise in mitral value prolapse," there is an external validity problem. From the study, I know that β-blockers are agents that improve exercise tolerance in mild to moderate mitral value prolapse in young men, but I do not know anything about women or serious prolapse problems. You can only make conclusions about what you have studied, and you can only apply your results to your target population. Look for this because it happens often in the medical literature.

26b. Internal validity has to do with the internal structure of the study. This focus is on the materials and methods section of the article. If the internal structure is flawed, then one would question how valid the study would be. For example, some types of internal validity include:

(*continued*)

**TABLE 13.8.** HELPFUL HINTS FOR DRUG LITERATURE EVALUATION (*Continued*)

Instrumentation (mentioned earlier). Is the visual analog scale the best means to measure subjective pain? Is intraocular pressure the best means to measure glaucoma? Is urine output the best means to measure diuretic success in CHF?

History (you may know this as the Hawthorne effect). Did something happen during the study that may have altered the results rather than the intervention or treatment. For example, suppose I established a calcium supplement intervention program for college-age women to improve calcium intake. I designed a good educational program, and I am making the college tour and promoting good calcium intake while in college to prevent later osteoporosis. I then go back and see if the women have changed their behavior and added more calcium to their diets. I have discovered that yes, indeed, they have significantly increased their calcium, and I conclude What a great educational program I have developed! What I did not take into consideration was the Diary Board's latest ad campaign with "Got milk?" In other words, my great program had nothing to do with it, but rather the Milk Board did.

Maturation. This has to do with the subject changing over time. For example, if I gave everyone a copy of the final exam questions as a pretest and then gave the same posttest, I could claim that my superior teaching techniques resulted in an excellent display of knowledge on the final. What is really being displayed is the individual's ability to learn from the pretest. The individual matured. This can happen with disease states as well. For example, a CHF study looking at outcomes must realize that most CHF patients will mature in the disease progression over a 2- to 5-year period of time. Other disease states may improve over time. Some disease states have exacerbations and remissions. How do you know if a drug is preventing exacerbations of multiple sclerosis or if the disease is just in remission as part of its natural course? Did the researchers control for this?

Selection goes back to question 8. How did they select the sample? Was it representative? Did they randomize? Were the controls appropriate?

Experimentation. Did they pick the right study design? Did they pick a cohort study to look at a rare disease when a case-control would have been better? Did they have appropriate treatment groups? Did they have a washout period? Did they cross over treatment groups appropriately?

Attrition refers to dropout rates, morbidity, or even mortality. Did they tell you who dropped out and why? For example, a study will start off with 150 people, but the data are reported on only 132. Where did the rest go, and why?

27. Did they tell you about adverse drug reactions (ADRs)? Was it a good explanation, or did it leave something to be desired? Did they tell you the number of patients who left the study (dropped out) because of ADRs?

28. This is crucial! They can only conclude about what they studied, and a good conclusion will discuss limitations to their study. This is considered good research and not admitting disaster.

**TABLE 13.8.** HELPFUL HINTS FOR DRUG LITERATURE EVALUATION (*Continued*)

29. Statistical significance is usually defined as the *p*-value being less than or equal to α (type I) error rate that was set by the researchers a priori. For example, if the researchers set α at 0.05 and the *p*-value is reported as 0.013, then the results are statistically significant. Clinical significance, however, is not dependent on statistical significance. This is related to one's professional judgment. Do the data suggest a clinical trend but not necessarily have statistical significance?

30. This is also crucial! A thorough discussion of limitations to the study should be included.

31. Were the references timely? Did they have a comprehensive list?

32. This one is up to you to defend! How does this change what you recommend? How good was the study in terms of answering questions 1 through 31? Where the results clinically significant?

## PROFESSIONAL WRITING

Pharmacists and pharmacy students are often required to do professional writing. This may come in different formats, including drug information responses, case presentations, meeting abstracts, research papers, drug monographs, journal clubs, and newsletters.

First steps in professional writing really begin with good preparation. Establish an outline for the paper that is appropriate to the format required for the exercise. Do all the research before establishing the outline. Check to make sure that you have primary literature to support the document when appropriate. Table 13.9 provides some helpful hints for writing.

The following examples are provided as a guide to professional writing. These examples were done by students and represent a good job at the exercise for the information available at the time of the project.

**TABLE 13.9.** HELPFUL WRITING HINTS

- Do not plagiarize any part of the paper (put information into your own words)
- Use proper grammar and spelling (read the paper, do not rely on spell check)
- Keep things concise and to the point (do not stray off on tangents)
- Avoid first person (such words as I and we)
- Avoid abbreviations and acronyms (unless described early in the paper)
- Avoid contractions (can't, couldn't, it's)
- Cite any factual information with appropriate referencing
- Reference throughout the paper starting with the first paper cited (do not put the references in alphabetical order or chronological order)
- Avoid the Internet unless it is specifically appropriate to the document

## Drug Information Professional Writing Examples

### Drug Information Question Response: Renee A. Pothast, Pharm.D., Completed as Part of a Pharm.D. Rotation While a Pharmacy Student at Ohio Northern University

#### Question

Therapy combining an angiotensin-converting enzyme inhibitor with an angiotensin II receptor blocker: is it rational?

#### Introduction

Hypertension and congestive heart failure (CHF) are two cardiovascular conditions common in the American population. In fact, approximately 50 million Americans have hypertension. The incidence increases with age, as one out of every four adults has this condition.[1] Treatment of hypertension is crucial to prevent multiple complications, including coronary heart disease. Control of blood pressure may also decrease the progression of CHF. Medical management of both hypertension and CHF has changed throughout the years. Currently, the effects of the reticular activating system (RAS) have been targeted in designing drug therapy for these conditions.

The RAS is activated in an individual by a variety of states, including sodium restriction and a decline in cardiac output. After the conversion of angiotensinogen to angiotensin I by renin, the angiotensin-converting enzyme (ACE) catalyzes the change of angiotensin I to angiotensin II. It is this peptide hormone, angiotensin II, that mediates the effects of the RAS. Angiotensin receptors can be found in many organs, including the kidneys, heart, blood vessels, brain, and adrenal tissues.[2] Two types of angiotensin II receptor subtypes have been identified. It is believed that activation of the angiotensin II receptor subtype $AT_1$ instigates the effects commonly associated with the RAS. These are an increase in systolic and diastolic blood pressure via systemic vasoconstriction, the release of adrenal aldosterone, and renal sodium reabsorption. Binding to this receptor also mediates cardiac remodeling through hypertrophy and proliferation. On the other hand, the angiotensin II receptor subtype $AT_2$ is now believed to exert opposing effects (vasodilation and antiproliferation), but this must still be fully investigated.[3]

#### The Role of Angiotensin-Converting Enzyme Inhibitors

ACE inhibitors have been found to be very effective when used for hypertension, CHF, and in the post-myocardial infarction (MI) setting. In fact, numerous studies have demonstrated their benefit in these situations, and ACE inhibitors are considered the foundation of combination therapy in CHF patients on the basis of many clinical trials. Enalapril was shown to reduce mortality when used in heart failure patients in the Cooperative North Scandinavian Enalapril Survival Study (CONSENSUS),[4] the Studies of Left Ventricular Dysfunction (SOLVD),[5] and the Veterans Administration Cooperative Vasodilator Heart Failure Trial II (VHeFT II).[6]

The reduction of mortality with ACE inhibitors in post-MI patients has also been demonstrated through clinical trials, including the Survival and Ventricular Enlargement Trial (SAVE)[7] and the Fourth International Study of Infarct Survival (ISIS–4),[8] both of which used captopril. In addition, zofenopril was deemed effective in the Survival of Myocardial Infarction Long-Term Evaluation (SMILE),[9] as was trandolapril in the Trandolapril Cardiac Evaluation (TRACE) study.[10]

The action of ACE inhibitors revolves around the RAS, for they ameliorate some of the effects of angiotensin II by preventing its formation by this pathway. In addition to their effect on the RAS, ACE inhibitors also inhibit the breakdown of bradykinin, enkephalin, and substance P. This most likely contributes to the side effects of cough and angioedema associated with these agents. More recently, the effects on bradykinin are also speculated to contribute to benefits in regard to exercise tolerance encountered by CHF patients on ACE inhibitor therapy.[11] However, this still remains to be fully proven.

Although ACE inhibitors block angiotensin II production by the RAS, long-term suppression of angiotensin II levels are not achieved.[12] One mechanism that is potentially responsible is an increase in angiotensin I levels through the loss of feedback inhibition of renin, overriding the inhibition of ACE.[13] Other mechanisms may be related to alternative pathways of angiotensin II production and activity, including a chymase pathway.[14] Even if the mechanism is not yet clear, it is known that further preventing the detrimental effects of angiotensin II in patients with cardiovascular disease is the goal.

## The Role of Angiotensin II Receptor (AT$_1$) Blockers

The newest class of antihypertensive agents, the angiotensin II receptor blockers (ARBs), also exert their beneficial effects by influence on the RAS and are often compared to ACE inhibitors. Clinical data are being gathered to demonstrate the efficacy of ARBs in patients with heart failure and after an MI. The Evaluation of Losartan in the Elderly Study (ELITE) compared the ARB losartan to the ACE inhibitor captopril in CHF patients. Results actually showed a lower mortality rate in patients taking the ARB compared to the ACE inhibitor.[15] However, these findings were not repeated in ELITE II, which did not find the mortality rates to be significantly different between the two agents.[16] Nevertheless, losartan was found to be better tolerated in both studies.[15,16] Additionally, the Study of Patients Intolerant of Converting Enzyme Inhibitors (SPICE) trial found the ARB candesartan cilexetil to reduce mortality in CHF patients who were unable to tolerate an ACE inhibitor.[17]

ARBs are being assessed for use in post-MI patients in the Optimal Therapy in Myocardial Infarction with the Angiotensin II Antagonist Losartan (OPTIMAAL) trial. This randomized trial, currently in progress, is comparing losartan therapy to captopril in high-risk patients ≥50 years old who have had an acute MI.[18]

ARBs, unlike the ACE inhibitors, exert their effect via binding selectively to the angiotensin II type 1 receptor, $AT_1$. As a result, the hypertensive effects and cardiac remodeling are blocked while angiotensin II is still able to bind to the type 2 receptor, $AT_2$. If binding to the $AT_2$ receptor results in the vasodilation and antiproliferation as currently believed, then there is a theoretical advantage of ARBs over ACE inhibitors. Also, angiotensin II's damaging effects via all pathways are more thoroughly blocked by receptor blocking than by preventing RAS angiotensin II formation as the ACE inhibitors do. Furthermore, the side effect of cough is absent in the ARBs because there is no inhibition of the breakdown of bradykinin.[3,19]

## Rationale of Using an ACE Inhibitor and an ARB in Combination

Because of their different means of preventing angiotensin II from binding to its receptor (either by preventing the formation of angiotensin or direct receptor inhibition), ACE inhibitors and ARBs are being evaluated for combined use. In theory, the benefit stems from complete blockage of the angiotensin II by all pathways, resulting in an additive effect of the two agents and the potential advantage of inhibiting the breakdown of bradykinin.[3] When an ACE inhibitor, an ARB, their combination, or placebo was administered to normotensive male volunteers who were mildly sodium depleted, the ACE inhibitor and ARB combination demonstrated a greater reduction in blood pressure, a major additive effect on renin rise signifying a compensatory mechanism, and no effect on plasma aldosterone levels, most likely because aldosterone is regulated through other pathways than solely the RAS.[20]

## Clinical Studies Validating the Combined Use for Heart Failure

The effects on afterload were studied by Hamroff et al.[21] in 43 patients with severe CHF who were treated with losartan after being maximally treated with an ACE inhibitor. Following evaluation for 1 month in an out-patient facility, patients were started on losartan 25 mg for the first week, followed by an increase to 50 mg thereafter. All other medications and doses remained constant. Blood pressure, heart rate, serum potassium, sodium, blood urea nitrogen, and creatinine were monitored weekly during the 2 weeks of the study. Repeated-measures analysis and a Bonferroni adjusted significance level were used to evaluate the data. Results showed a decline in blood pressure as distinguished by a decline in systolic blood pressure from $122 \pm 18$ mm Hg at baseline to $107 \pm 17$ mm Hg after the 50–mg dose ($p < 0.0001$). There were no significant changes in electrolytes or renal function during treatment duration. Conclusions included that, as indicated by the decline in blood pressure, therapy with an ARB in these patients further reduces afterload. Limitations consist of a small sample size, short treatment duration, lack of a control group, and an insufficient definition of terms.[21]

A double-blind, crossover, placebo-controlled study was conducted by Guazzi et al.[11] in 26 stable CHF patients [New York Heart Association (NYHA) class II to III] with a mean age of 58 years. Following randomization, patients received either placebo + placebo, placebo + enalapril (20 mg/day), placebo + losartan (50 mg/day), or enalapril (20 mg/day) + losartan (50 mg/day), or the same drugs in the reverse order, with all treatment periods lasting 8 weeks. Monitoring was completed by quality-of-life questionnaires, neurohormone evaluations, pulmonary function tests, cardiopulmonary exercise testing, chest x-rays, and left ventricular ejection fraction evaluations. Two patients were excluded from the final analysis because of adverse events (hypotension with the enalapril and losartan combination and cough with enalapril). Results included an increase in exercise oxygen uptake and physical performance when the drugs are used in combination, although improved exercise performance was noted with enalapril only. This is thought to be through action on bradykinin. Also, the inhibitory effect of neurohormones was additive, and combination therapy was safe and well tolerated. Quality of life did not significantly change, although the authors believe this to most likely be because the patients were stabilized in digoxin and diuretic therapy prior to study inclusion. Again, a small sample size is a limitation, as were multiple patient variables with the potential to influence the results and a complicated drug regimen.[11]

The Randomized Evaluation of Strategies for Left Ventricular Dysfunction (RESOLVD) pilot study, conducted by the RESOLVD investigators, compared candesartan, enalapril, and their combination over 43 weeks in this multicenter, double-blind, randomized, parallel, placebo-controlled trial. All patients were in the NYHA functional class II, III, or IV for their CHF. The trial included a run-in of three 1-week phases of enalapril 2.5 mg twice daily + placebo, enalapril 2.5 mg twice daily + candesartan 2 mg daily, and enalapril 2.5 mg twice daily + placebo. Randomization followed, and patients received candesartan alone (4.8 or 16 mg daily), candesartan (4 or 8 mg daily) + enalapril (10 mg twice daily), or enalapril (10 mg twice daily). Endpoints were the change in ejection fraction, the 6-minute walk distance, ventricular volumes, and neurohormone levels. Other measurements made included end-systolic volume (ESV), end-diastolic volume (EDV), and quality of life via the Minnesota Living With Heart Failure questionnaire. Statistical analyses occurred by ANOVA, post-hoc Tukey test, and chi-squared test. There were 899 patients in the run-in phase, and 768 were randomized. Patient characteristics were similar between the groups, although fewer patients in the groups containing candesartan were concomitantly receiving $\beta$-blockers. Although not statistically significant, there was an increase in ejection fraction in the combined group, compared to enalapril or candesartan alone. Both ESV and EDV increased less with combination therapy. Candesartan alone demonstrated the smallest increase in renin levels but the greatest increase in angiotensin II levels. Aldosterone significantly decreased at 17 weeks with combination therapy ($p < 0.01$), but not at 43 weeks. Blood pressure declined the greatest with the combination therapy throughout the study ($p < 0.05$), as did brain natriuretic peptide ($p < 0.01$). Compared to enalapril, potassium decreased with candesartan ($p < 0.05$) and increased with combination therapy ($p < 0.05$). No significant changes in creatinine, 6-minute walk distance, quality of life, mortality, or hospitalization was confirmed. The authors concluded that despite limitations of small number unreliability and not being able to predict net clinical effects because of surrogate outcomes, this pilot study did demonstrate the effectiveness and safety of enalapril and candesartan combination therapy to prevent left ventricular remodeling when compared to either agent given alone.[22]

Baruch et al.[12] carried out a randomized, multicenter, double-blind trial in 83 CHF patients in NYHA functional class II, III, or IV. All patients had to have previous ACE inhibitor therapy and, at baseline, were stratified into low- or high-dose ACE inhibitor therapy based on this previous ACE inhibitor dose. Following a 2-week single-blind placebo phase in which the patient's heart failure and compliance were assessed, patients were randomized to receive 4 weeks of therapy with valsartan 80 mg twice daily, valsartan 160 mg twice daily, or placebo. Hemodynamic monitoring and hormone measurements (plasma norepinephrine, aldosterone, atrial natriuretic peptide, and angiotensin II) were completed on day 0 and day 30. On these days, patients received either 10 mg or 20 mg of lisinopril rather than their usual ACE inhibitor to guarantee sustained ACE inhibition. Statistical analysis included Fisher's exact or Cochran-Mantel-Haenszel test to compare baseline characteristics, ANOVA, ANCOVA, and Student's $t$ test. An overall two-sided significance level was upheld at 0.05 by Bonferroni adjustment. Statistical significance was defined for between-treatment comparisons of valsartan versus placebo at $p < 0.025$ and within-treatment analyses of change from baseline at $p < 0.05$. All patients were male because of the number of Veterans Affairs hospitals included. Immediate effects (day 0) showed valsartan to demonstrate statistical significance over placebo in the reduction in pulmonary capillary wedge pressure (PCWP; $p < 0.025$), right arterial pressure ($p < 0.025$), and systolic blood pressure. No significant change in neurohormone levels was appreciated. When the long-term effect (day 28) was evaluated, the fall in pulmonary artery diastolic pressure ($p = 0.013$) and the systolic blood pressure ($p = 0.013$) were significant in the high-dose valsartan group when compared to placebo. Both valsartan doses caused significant declines in the plasma aldosterone level. The medication was well tolerated, with 89% of patients able to complete the trial. Documented side effects did include hypotension, gastrointestinal disturbances, and dizziness. Also, increases in blood urea nitrogen, serum creatinine, and potassium were noted. The authors made the conclusion that angiotensin II levels do persist despite long-term ACE inhibitor therapy.[12]

A double-blind, randomized, large-scale trial, including 5010 patients and carried out in 300 centers in 16 countries, was recently completed by Cohn et al.[23] This trial, the Valsartan Heart Failure Trial (Val-HeFT), investigated the effect valsartan 160 mg twice daily would have on CHF patients (NYHA functional class II, III, or IV) who were already taking the usual therapies for CHF, including ACE inhibitors, β-blockers, diuretics, and digoxin. Compared to placebo, the valsartan group saw a reduction in all-cause mortality and morbidity by 13.3% ($p = 0.009$) and in hospitalization for CHF by 27.5% ($p < 0.001$). Additionally, therapy with valsartan improved quality of life ($p = 0.005$), NYHA functional class ($p = 0.001$), ejection fraction ($p = 0.001$), and signs and symptoms of heart failure ($p = 0.001$).[23,24]

Swedberg et al.[25] is currently assessing the use of candesartan cilexetil in symptomatic CHF patients in the Candesartan in Heart Failure—Assessment in Mortality and Morbidity (CHARM) trial. This multicenter trial encompasses three parallel, placebo-controlled trials in 6500 patients treated with and without an ACE inhibitor. There is a minimum follow-up period of 2 years, with endpoints including all-cause mortality, effect on MI, hospitalization, and resource utilization.[25]

### Clinical Studies Validating the Combined Use for Post-MI

The feasibility, tolerability, and safety of using captopril and losartan was the aim in a randomized, single-blind pilot study by Pasquale et al.[26] Patients admitted for an anterior acute MI, Killip class I to II, who were successfully reperfused within 4 hours after the onset of symptoms and received the target captopril dose of 75 mg/day 3 days postadmission were included. Randomization occurred, and patients received either placebo or losartan titrated up to 25 mg/day. Captopril 75 mg/day was administered to both groups. Blood pressure, heart rate, and electrocardiogram (ECG) were monitored continuously. Neurohormonal levels were monitored at baseline and on days 3 and 10. A hemodynamic study was also completed on all patients 7 to 10 days after admission. Data were analyzed by two-tailed $t$ test, ANOVA, and chi-squared test. The Bonferroni correction was utilized, and statistical significance was set at $p < 0.05$. A total of 42 patents were included in the results. Only the systolic blood pressure was found to be significantly changed with the ARB and ACE inhibitor combination ($p < 0.001$). Even though the ejection fraction was higher in this group than when captopril was given with placebo, the difference was not significant. No side effects were noted. Because of the small sample size, no significant benefits on remodeling, morbidity, or mortality could be found. Also, the single-blind randomization is not ideal, and results cannot be generalized to all post-MI patients because only those who are low risk, thrombolysed, and reperfused were included. Consistent with the objective of the study, the feasibility and safety of this combination encourages further trials in this area.[26]

Pasquale et al. extended the study to include women and a losartan 50 mg/day-only arm and prolonged it for 90 days, when a second ECG was performed. All other aspects remained identical to the first study except for the objective to verify the efficacy of the combined therapy in the early post-MI setting. The losartan-only group acted as a control to gauge the effects of losartan on angiotensin II levels. Ninety-nine patients were randomized, in addition to 23 patients assigned to the losartan-only group. Data were available for neurohormone and blood pressure assessment from 93 patients. Angiotensin II levels were higher in the losartan-only group on day 10 (this was significantly different from the captopril-only group; $p = 0.006$). Both systolic and diastolic blood pressure was significantly reduced in the captopril + losartan group when compared to the captopril-only group. Patients in the combined group also had a lower ejection fraction than the other two groups, but this did not reach statistical significance. ECG examination at 90 days was completed in 48 patients on captopril only, 47 patients on combined therapy, and 23 patients on losartan only. ESV and ejection fractions were not significantly different between the treatment groups. Nevertheless, there was a statistically significant difference in the ESV within the combination group itself 90 days after treatment ($p = 0.016$). There were six ischemic events observed in the follow-up (one episode of unstable angina in each group, one episode of reinfarction in the captopril-only and combination groups, and one episode of heart failure in the losartan-only group). It may be deduced from this study that combination therapy is safe and beneficial. However, the same limitations as in the first study apply.[27]

Based on results from the previous two studies, Pasquale et al.[28] designed a similar study to further explore the rationale for ACE inhibitor and ARB combined therapy in other post-MI patients. A randomized, double-blind design was used in patients ≥65 years old who were either not receiving thrombolytic treatment or who had received thrombolytic therapy but had unsuccessful reperfusion. Additionally, a coronary angiography 7 to 10 days postadmission had to demonstrate no patency of the infarct-related artery, and captopril 75 mg/day had to be received by day 3 of admission. Among patients excluded were those with heart failure. On day 3, patients were randomized to receive either captopril 75 mg/day + candesartan 4 mg/day initially but later increased to 8 mg/day based on blood pressure, or captopril 75 mg/day + placebo. Monitoring included blood pressure, heart rate, serum creatinine, serum potassium, Holter monitoring, hemodynamic investigations, and an ECG on days 3 and 10. A two-tailed $t$ test, ANOVA, Bonferroni correction, and chi-squared test were all used to analyze the data; $p < 0.05$ was considered significant. Results are based on 71 patients who met the entry criteria and included a statistically significant lower systolic and diastolic blood pressure in the combined group ($p < 0.001$). The combination group showed a higher, but not significantly so, ejection fraction. Follow-up lasted 1 year with a minimum period of observation of 3 months. ESV values after 90 days were significantly lower in the combination group ($p = 0.03$). During the follow-up, there were two episodes of reinfarction and two episodes of unstable angina in the combination group, compared to one episode of reinfarction and four episodes of unstable angina in the captopril-only group. After 10 days of treatment, an increase in serum potassium >5.5 mmol/L and serum creatinine >2.0 mg/L was experienced by four patients in the combination group and by two patients in the captopril-only group. After a reduction of doses, levels declined and patients continued in the relevant treatment groups. No other significant changes were found. It was concluded that the captopril and candesartan combination is beneficial in elderly, post-MI patients as shown by a greater effect on ESV. Limitations are a small sample size causing ungeneraliz-ability and a failure to show possible benefits on morbidity and mortality and a lack of hemodynamic study completion because of age >75 in 28 patients.[28]

Currently, the Valsartan in Acute Myocardial Infarction (VALIANT) trial is under way to assess the use of valsartan alone or in combination with captopril and the effect on mortality in post-MI patients. Random assignments are made in this trial for patients with CHF symptoms or depressed left ventricular ejec-tion fraction. This is the largest clinical trial using an ACE inhibitor and ARB com-bination in post-MI patients, is powered at a 90% level to detect a 15% change in mortality, and is projected to run until 2700 deaths have occurred.[29]

## Conclusion

The RAS plays a considerable role in the detrimental effects of CHF and MI and can be improved by the use of ACE inhibitors and ARBs. Both of these medi-cations have proven to be safe and effective for patients with CHF and in the post-MI setting. It is only recently that their use together has been practiced medically and substantiated by clinical trials. Additional trials are currently being implemented in these settings to further validate this approach.

## References

1. American Heart Association (http://www.americanheart.org/hbp/phys_stats. html) 19 March 2001.

2. Hirsch AT, Pinto YM, Schunkert H, Dzau VJ. Potential role of the tissue renin—angiotensin system in the pathophysiology of congestive heart failure. Am J Cardiol. 1990;66:22D–32D.

3. Carson PE. Rationale for the use of combination angiotensin-converting enzyme inhibitor/angiotensin II receptor blocker therapy in heart failure. Am Heart J. 2000;140(3):361–366.

4. Kjekshus J, Frick H, Swedberg K, Wilhelmsen L. Effects of enalapril on mortality in severe congestive heart failure: results of the Cooperative North Scandinavian Enalapril Survival Study (CONSENSUS). N Engl J Med. 1987;316: 1429–1435.

5. Yusuf S, Pitt B, Davis CE, et al. Effect of enalapril on survival in patients with reduced left ventricular ejection fractions and congestive heart failure. N Engl J Med. 1991;325:293–302.

6. Cohn JN, Johnson G, Ziesche S, et al. A comparison of enalapril with hydrala-zine—isosorbide dinitrate in the treatment of chronic congestive heart failure. N Engl J Med. 1991;325:303–310.

7. Pfeffer MA, Braunwald E, Moye LA, et al. Effect of captopril on mortality and morbidity in patients with left ventricular dysfunction after myocardial infarc-tion. N Engl J Med. 1992;327:669–677.

8. ISIS-4 (Fourth International Study of Infarct Survival) Collaborative Group. ISIS-4: A randomized factorial trial assessing early oral captopril, oral mononitrate,

and intravenous magnesium sulphate in 58,050 patients with suspected acute myocardial infarction. *Lancet.* 1995;345:669–682.

9. Ambrosioni E, Borghi C, Magnani B, for the Survival of Myocardial Infarction Long-Term Evaluation (SMILE) study investigators. The effect of the angiotensin-converting-enzyme inhibitor zofenopril on mortality and morbidity after anterior myocardial infarction. *N Engl J Med.* 1995;332:80–85.

10. Kober L, Torp-Pedersen C, Carlsen JE, et al, for the Trandolapril Cardiac Evaluation (TRACE) study group. A clinical trial of the angiotensin-converting-enzyme inhibitor trandolapril in patients with left ventricular dysfunction after myocardial infarction. *N Engl J Med.* 1995;333:1670–1676.

11. Guazzi M, Palermo P, Pontone G, et al. Synergistic efficacy of enalapril and losartan on exercise performance and oxygen consumption at peak exercise in congestive heart failure. *Am J Cardiol.* 1999;84:1038–1043.

12. Baruch L, Anand I, Cohen IS, et al, for the Vasodilator Heart Failure Trial (VHeFT) study group. Augmented short- and long-term hemodynamic and hormonal effects of an angiotensin receptor blocker added to angiotensin converting enzyme inhibitor therapy in patients with heart failure. *Circulation.* 1999; 99:2658–2664.

13. Schunkert H, Ingelfinger JR, Hirsch AT, et al. Feedback regulation of angiotensin converting enzyme activity and mRNA levels by angiotensin II. *Circ Res.* 1993;72:312–318.

14. Balcells E, Meng QC, Johnson WH, et al. Angiotensin II formation from ACE and chymase in human and animal hearts: methods and species considerations. *Am J Physiol.* 1997;273:H1769–H1774.

15. Pitt B, Segal R, Martinez FA, G, et al. Randomized trial of losartan versus captopril in patients over 65 with heart failure (Evaluation of Losartan in the Elderly Study, ELITE). *Lancet.* 1997;349:747–752.

16. Pitt B, Poole-Wilson PA, Segal R, et al. Effect of losartan compared with captopril on mortality in patients with symptomatic heart failure: randomized trial—the Losartan Heart Failure Survival Study (ELITE II). *Lancet.* 2000;355:1582–1587.

17. Granger CB, Ertl G, Kuch J, et al, for the Study of Patients Intolerant of Converting Enzyme Inhibitors (SPICE) Investigators. Randomized trial of candesartan cilexetil in the treatment of patients with congestive heart failure and a history of intolerance to angiotensin-converting enzyme inhibitors. *Am Heart J.* 2000;139:609–617.

18. Dickstein K, Kjekshus J, for the OPTIMAAL study group. Comparison of the effects of losartan and captopril on mortality in patients after acute myocardial infarction: the OPTIMAAL trial design. *Am J Cardiol.* 1999;83:477–481.

19. Gradman AH. Long-term benefits of angiotensin II blockade: is the consensus changing? *Am J Cardiol.* 1999;84:16S–21S.

20. Azizi M, Chatellier G, Guyene TT, et al. Additive effects of combined angiotensin-converting enzyme inhibition and angiotensin II antagonism on blood pressure and renin release in sodium-depleted normotensives. *Circulation.* 1995;92:825–834.

21. Hamroff G, Blaufarb I, Mancini D, et al. Angiotensin II-receptor blockade further reduces afterload safely in patients maximally treated with angiotensin-converting enzyme inhibitors for heart failure. *J Cardiovasc Pharmacol.* 1997; 30(4):533–536.

22. McKelvie RS, Yusuf S, Pericak D, et al. Comparison of candesartan, enalapril, and their combination in congestive heart failure. *Circulation.* 1999;100: 1056–1064.

23. Cohn JN, Tognoni G, Glazer RD, et al. Rationale and design of the Valsartan Heart Failure Trial: a large multinational trial to assess the effects of valsartan, an angiotensin-receptor blocker, on morbidity and mortality in chronic congestive heart failure [abstract]. *J Card Fail.* 1999;5(2):155–160.

24. Novartis Pharmaceuticals. Novartis issued the following statement in response to the results of the Valsartan Heart Failure Trial (Val-HeFT) announced today at the 73rd Scientific Sessions of the American Heart Association [press release]. Available at http://www.prnewswire.com/news-releases/val-heft-study-to-investigate-benefits-of-diovanr-in-heart-failure-73084397.html

25. Swedberg K, Pfeffer M, Granger C, et al. Candesartan in heart failure-assessment of reduction in mortality and morbidity (CHARM): rationale and design [abstract]. *J Card Fail.* 1999;5(3):276–282.

26. Pasquale PD, Bucca V, Scalzo S, Paterna S. Safety, tolerability, and neurohormonal changes of the combination captopril plus losartan in the early postinfarction period: a pilot study. *Cardiovasc Drugs Ther.* 1998;12:211–216.

27. Pasquale PD, Bucca V, Scalzo S, et al. Does the addition of losartan improve the beneficial effects of ACE inhibitors in patients with anterior myocardial infarction? A pilot study. *Heart.* 1999;81:606–611.

28. Pasquale PD, Cannizzaro S, Giubilato A, et al. Effects of the combination of candesartan plus captopril in elderly patients with anterior myocardial infarction. A pilot study. *Clin Drug Invest.* 2000;19(3):173–182.

29. Pfeffer MA. Enhancing cardiac protection after myocardial infarction: rationale for newer clinical trials of angiotensin receptor blockers. *Am Heart J.* 2000;139:S23–S28.

## NEWSLETTER EXAMPLE: BRIAN E. GULBIS, PHARM.D., PREPARED WHILE A PHARMACY STUDENT AT OHIO NORTHERN UNIVERSITY AS PART OF THE PROFESSION OF PHARMACY COURSEWORK

### Ubiquinone Use in Cardiovascular Disease

Ubiquinone (coenzyme Q-10, CoQ) is a naturally occurring coenzyme found in aerobic organisms. It was given the name ubiquinone because of its universal, or ubiquitous, occurrence in animal tissues. Since its isolation in 1957, CoQ has been studied throughout Japan, Russia, Europe, and the United States.[1] It is found mostly in the inner mitochondrial membrane, especially in the heart, liver, kidney, and pancreas.[2] CoQ plays an important role in the mitochondrial electron transport chain. NADH and succinate dehydrogenases, and other flavoproteins, donate electrons to CoQ, which transfers them to nonheme iron proteins. The oxidation-reduction reactions that CoQ undergoes during electron transport are an essential part of the proton-pumping mechanism that leads to the generation of ATP in the mitochondria.[3] In addition to its role in the electron transport chain, ubiquinone is also an antioxidant and free radical scavenger, and it is believed to possess membrane-stabilizing properties.[2,4]

Since its discovery, coenzyme Q-10 has been used to aid in the treatment of many cardiovascular diseases, such as congestive heart failure (CHF), cardiac arrhythmias, and hypertension. Although it has not been approved for therapeutic use in the United States, ubiquinone is the primary treatment for cardiovascular disease in approximately 12 million Japanese.[1] Grounds for the use of CoQ in cardiovascular therapy were established in the early 1970s by Folkers et al., who found evidence of decreased levels of coenzyme Q-10 in patients with heart disease.[5] Subsequent studies have shown that there is a correlation between cardiovascular disease and low tissue levels of ubiquinone.[6] However, it is not yet known if the lowered CoQ levels are the cause of or a result of the disease states.

In the early 1990s, a multicenter, randomized, double-blind, placebo-controlled clinical trial was performed by Morisco, Trimarco, and Condorelli to study the effects of coenzyme Q-10 on patients with congestive heart failure. Patients were randomly assigned by a computer-generated allocation schedule that matched age, sex, New York Heart Association class, and treatment used for hemodynamic stabilization. A total of 641 patients were enrolled in the study among 33 centers, with 319 patients placed in the coenzyme Q-10 group and 322 patients in the placebo group. During the study, 16 patients died in the CoQ group, and 21 in the placebo group. Twenty-three patients in the CoQ group dropped out of the study, while 18 patients in the control group dropped out. Neither the number of deaths nor the number of patients who dropped out is statistically significant. There were also no statistically significant differences in the age, sex, weight, cardiovascular drug therapy, or noncardiovascular drug therapy of the two groups. The CoQ group was then given 2 mg/kg per day of coenzyme Q-10 in addition to the cardiovascular drug therapy required to reach hemodynamic stabilization. The other group received a placebo in addition to their regular drug therapy. Patients were then examined after 3, 6, and 12 months of the additional therapy. Evaluation of the efficacy of therapy was based on changes in the functional class of patients in the two groups. There was a statistically significant reduction in the class of the patients in the coenzyme Q-10 group. This means there was an overall improvement in functional status of patients in the CoQ group. There were no significant changes in functional class of patients in the placebo group. In addition, physicians and patients were asked to rate the effects of treatment on a scale of 1 to 3. The mean score given by physicians and patients in the placebo group remained unchanged throughout the study. However, there was a continual increase in the mean score given by physicians and patients in the coenzyme Q-10 group. There was also a statistically smaller incidence of cardiovascular complications, including acute pulmonary edema ($p < 0.001$), cardiac asthma ($p < 0.001$), and arrhythmias ($p < 0.05$) in the CoQ group compared to the placebo group. A final observation showed that about 40% of patients in the placebo group required one or more hospitalizations during the follow-up period, whereas only 20% of the patients in the coenzyme Q-10 group required hospitalization ($p < 0.01$).[7]

In a different multicenter study, by Lampertico and Comis, the efficacy and safety of coenzyme Q-10 as supplementary therapy in patients with heart failure were examined. The study took place in Italy, with 378 physicians participating in the trial. Of those 378 physicians, 201 were cardiologists, and 165 were interns. Physicians were asked to choose no more than five of their patients suffering heart failure who had been stabilized on cardiovascular therapy for at least 3 months to participate in the study. In all, 1715 patients were chosen, with 804 being male and 911 female. Coenzyme Q-10 was added to the traditional cardiovascular therapy at a dose of 50 mg per day in 1423 patients, while 192 patients received CoQ as their only therapy. Treatment was given over a 4-week period. In addition to reporting basic patient data, physicians were asked to evaluate a series of subjective and objective symptoms before treatment began, after 15 days, and after 30 days of therapy. Emphasis was placed on adverse events, and the physician was additionally asked to express an opinion on the efficacy of the therapy. The results of the trial showed a statistically significant subjective and objective improvement in the 1423 patients who received CoQ in addition to their conventional medication. Analysis showed an overall reduction in the intensity of symptoms after 2 and 4 weeks of treatment ($p < 0.01$), and statistically significant differences in systolic and diastolic blood pressure and heart rate were found ($p < 0.01$). Also of note, the incidence of clinical improvement in the group of patients who received only coenzyme Q-10 was the same as the group receiving CoQ in addition to their conventional medication. Incidence of adverse effects decreased from 2.2% after 2 weeks to 0.4% at the end of 4 weeks. Physicians' opinion of treatment efficacy was rated as excellent to good for 71.1% of the patients. A limitation of the study is its focus on people of Italian ethnicity.[2]

Although clinical studies provide scientific data to assess the efficacy of coenzyme Q-10 use, most people do not have the results of these studies readily available to them, nor do they have the ability to effectively analyze these results. Therefore, people turn to other resources for product information. Over the past few years, the Internet has become one of the fastest growing sources of information on anything and everything. People use the Internet to find news on world events, the latest sports scores, and information about new products, including natural products. A query of any major search engine for information on ubiquinone will easily yield over 1000 results. A company called Advance Nutrition has a rather extensive site on coenzyme Q-10. The company describes ubiquinone as "a vital catalyst required for the creation of the energy needed to maintain life."[8] Coenzyme Q-10 functions as a proton and electron carrier that "sparks the mitochondrial energy production which runs all vital body functions."[8] The page claims that the use of their coenzyme Q-10 supplement will "Increase energy levels, increase your $VO_2$ reading without exercise, lower high blood pressure, detoxify your body, reduce free radicals dramatically, and aid the function of all living cells..."[8] Other sites make similar claims to those of Advance Nutrition. Another company selling ubiquinone supplements, called Natural Warehouse, alleges that use of their CoQ supplement will result in "energy increase, improvement of heart function, prevention and cure of gum disease, a boost to the immune system, and possible life extension."[9]

There is limited scientific evidence to support some of the claims made by these companies. Several clinical trials have shown that ubiquinone supplements probably improve heart function and aid in the treatment of cardiovascular disease. However, there is not yet any conclusive evidence to support the allegations made by these companies. More studies need to be done, and more data need to be collected and analyzed, before the claims of companies such as Advance Nutrition and Natural Warehouse can be either proved or disproved.

Although no dosage guidelines have been established, the administration of 50–150 mg of coenzyme Q-10 daily is considered to have therapeutic benefits. No major adverse effects have been associated with CoQ use at this dosage level.[2] Rare side effects include nausea, epigastric discomfort, loss of appetite, diarrhea, and skin rash. These adverse events have occurred in fewer than 1% of patients taking coenzyme Q-10 supplements.[1,10]

The results of studies have shown that the use of coenzyme Q-10 supplements appears to be effective in the treatment of cardiovascular diseases such as congestive heart failure, cardiac arrhythmias, and hypertension. The safety of CoQ has been established in studies, and no major side effects have been associated with CoQ use. Based on its safety and apparent efficacy, the use of coenzyme Q-10, in combination with conventional medications, can be recommended for the treatment of cardiovascular disease.

## References

1. Ubiquinone. *Rev Nat Prod.* 1997, August.
2. Lampertico M, Comis S. Italian multicenter study on the efficacy and safety of coenzyme Q10 as adjuvant therapy in heart failure. *Clin Invest.* 1993;71: S129–S133.
3. Marks DB, Marks AD, Smith CM. *Basic Medical Biochemistry: A Clinical Approach.* Baltimore, MD: Williams & Wilkins; 1996:315–316.
4. Ernster L, Dallner G. Biochemical, physiological and medical aspects of ubiquinone function. *Biochim Biophys Acta.* 1995;1271:195–204.

5. Folkers K, Littarru GP, Ho L, Runge TM, Havanonda S, Cooley D. Evidence for a deficiency of coenzyme Q10 in human heart disease. *Int Z Vitaminforsch.* 1970;40(3):380–390.
6. Mortensen SA. Perspectives on therapy of cardiovascular diseases with coenzyme Q10 (ubiquinone). *Clin Invest.* 1993;71:S116–S123.
7. Morisco C, Trimarco B, Condorelli M. Effect of coenzyme Q10 therapy in patients with congestive heart failure: a long-term multicenter randomized study. *Clin Invest.* 1993;71:S134–S136.
8. Advance Nutrition Co. Enzyme Q10. Advance Nutrition. *Infoseek.* Available at http://www.advancenutrition.com/faq.html. Accessed December 28, 1998.
9. Coenzyme Q10. Nutrition Warehouse. *Infoseek.* Available at http://www.nutritionwarehouse.com.au/supplement-blog/bodybuilding-supplements/co-enzyme-q10-%E2%80%93-what-is-it-and-why-do-we-need-it/
10. Anon. Ubidecarenone. DRUGDEX® System. Englewood, CO: MICROMEDEX, Inc., edition expires February 1999.

## JOURNAL CLUB EXAMPLE: DESTA R. BORLAND, PHARM.D., PREPARED WHILE AN OHIO NORTHERN UNIVERSITY PHARMACY STUDENT AS PART OF AN ASSIGNMENT FOR THE CAPSTONE MODULE

### Publication

Abraira C, Colwell JA, Nutall FQ, et al. Veterans Affairs cooperative study on glycemic control and complications in type II diabetes (VA CSDM). Results of the feasibility trial. Veterans Affairs Cooperative Study in Type II Diabetes. Diabetes Care 1995;18(8):1113–1123.

### Objective

The objective of the VA CSDM study was to see if a correlation between the incidence of cardiovascular disease and length and severity of hyperglycemia could be established. The study also looked the possible relationship between glucose levels and macrovascular disease in patients with documented non-insulin-dependent diabetes mellitus (NIDDM). The researchers also wished to assess the need for a long-term trial.

### Background

The Diabetes Control and Complications Trial (DCCT) published in 1993 examined the long-term macrovascular, microvascular, and neurologic complications that occur in patients with insulin-dependent diabetes mellitus (IDDM), including retinopathy, nephropathy, neuropathy, and cardiovascular disease.[1] The results of this study are not generalizable to patients with NIDDM because of the differences between the two disease states. Because the results of the DCCT could not be applied to patients with NIDDM, researchers felt there was a need for a similar study in these patients.

The use of intensive insulin therapy in patients with type II diabetes in considered to be controversial. Some medical personnel believe that insulin use in NIDDM may increase obesity, hypertension, and dyslipidemia. The only study previously done in this area, the University Group Diabetes Program (UGDP), had failed to establish the benefits of insulin therapy in macrovascular disease in patients with NIDDM.

## Methods

The VA CSDM was a multicenter, randomized, prospective feasibility trial conducted in five medical centers over a 2-year period.

## Patients

The trial included 153 men 60 ± 6 years of age who had been diagnosed with type II diabetes an average of 7.8 ± 4 years previous to the start of the study.

## Inclusion Criteria

The patients included in the trial were adult men between the ages of 40 and 69 years of age who required chronic insulin therapy because other medications had shown clinical failure. A $HbA_{1c}$ of >6.55% and a fasting plasma C-peptide of >0.21 pmol/mL were required at initial screening and verified by the coordinating center. Patients were included if they had a history of preexisting retinopathy or previous cardiovascular disease that was not considered severe or incapacitating with no acute attacks in the past 6 months.

## Exclusion Criteria

Patients were excluded if they had a serum creatinine of >141.1 $\mu$mol/L (1.6 mg/dL) or an albuminuria >0.5 g/24 h. Other exclusions were patients with clinically evident autonomic neuropathy, current or previous diabetic gangrene, and those with a serious illness, predicted poor compliance, or a diagnosis of NIDDM >15 years previously.

## Outcome Variables

Patients in the study were monitored by a blinded committee of consultants external to the study itself for variables including new myocardial infarction, congestive heart failure, amputation for ischemic gangrene, stroke, angina, coronary artery disease, angioplasty or bypass graft, claudication, transitory ischemic attacks, ischemic ulcers, or cardiovascular mortality. They were also monitored for episodes of severe, moderate, or mild hypoglycemia with symptoms reviewed to decide which category each case fell into. $HbA_{1c}$ and lipid profiles including HDL, LDL, and triglycerides were measured at each quarterly visit and determined by a central lab that had no knowledge of the treatment groups. Fasting plasma C-peptide was measured at entry and after the 2 years had been completed and was determined by a central lab. Also, at each visit, any current or incurrent cases of angina pectoris, smoking, coronary heart disease, transient ischemic attacks, and dyslipidemia were noted. If the patient was being treated for hypertension, the current therapy was documented along with the blood pressure and absence or presence of a foot ulcer, and clinical neuropathy. A central lab, on each 6-month visit determined a urinary albumin excretion level.

An independent Data Monitoring Board periodically evaluated the central laboratories involved in the study. All laboratory accreditations, proficiency-testing programs, and intraassay and interassay coefficients of variation were reviewed to establish that the laboratory was performing properly.

### Procedures

Initially, 289 patients were screened for possible inclusion into the study, with only 153 enrolled. Each hospital involved received a standardized operations manual on how to proceed with educating the patients on the dietary plan that should be followed throughout the 2 years that the study would take place. The dietary plan was reinforced at each 3-month ambulatory visit. The health professionals involved were instructed to treat all of the patient's other disease states, such as dyslipidemia, obesity, hypertension, and smoking, according to the American Diabetes Association (ADA) guidelines.

Patients were randomized into either the standard treatment group, which would be treated with one injection of insulin per day and two injections if absolutely necessary, not to exceed two, or the intensively treated group, which was broken into four stepped treatment phases.

Patients in the standard treatment therapy group maintained the same dosing regimen of one injection per day unless they were experiencing diabetic symptoms or reached the $HbA_{1c}$ "alert" level of 12.9% whether or not symptoms were present at the time of testing. These patients were monitored by ambulatory visits every 3 months. At each visit the patients underwent urinary glucose testing, ketonuria testing, and blood glucose testing.

Phase I patients were treated with one bedtime dose of either an intermediate- or long-acting insulin. Phase II patients were given both an evening dose and a daytime dose of glipizide. Phase III patients were administered two injections of insulin daily. Phase IV were dosed multiple insulin injections daily. All patients in the intense treatment group did home blood glucose tests twice daily and once a week at 3 AM. Patients were stepped through the various phases if they were not meeting their designated target $HbA_{1c}$ level of as close to the normal range as possible (5.1 ± 1%) and a fasting blood glucose of 4.44–6.38 mmol/L (80–115 mg/ dL). Patients in this therapy group were also monitored at ambulatory visits at 3-month intervals, and the same tests were performed as with patients in the standard treatment group. These patients also received a monthly visit and weekly phone call for the purpose of monitoring the current doses and making changes in the treatment where necessary. The cardiovascular events and other outcome variables listed above were also monitored at each of the 3-month ambulatory visits.

As previously mentioned, all of the laboratory tests were completed at accredited, centrally located labs. The researchers also split 10% of the specimens and sent half of those specimens to another blinded lab to assess accuracy of the central labs participating.

## Statistical Methods

The independent variables of time and treatment were analyzed using a series of chi-squared tests and repeated-measures analysis of variance (ANOVA). Discrete variables and continuous variables were also analyzed using the chi-squared test. All baseline comparisons of the two treatment groups were analyzed using the Student's $t$ test. No $p$-value or $\alpha$ value was mentioned in the article. The Cox regression analysis was used to determine the relationship between new cardiovascular events and previous cardiovascular disease.[2]

## Results/Conclusions

Of the 153 patients involved in the study, 98.6% kept each of their scheduled quarterly visits, and only 4% of those in the intensively treated group were indicated as failing to adhere to the protocol. The average time in the study was 27 months with a range of 18–35 months. Four patients in the intense treatment group failed to complete the study. One left voluntarily at 7 months, one moved without a forwarding address, one fell into an irreversible coma related to a case of septicemia, and one left after being diagnosed with psychotic depression. Results from these four patients, up until their dismissal from the trial, were calculated into the final data. Ninety-six percent of patients in the standard treatment group and 71% of the patients in the intense treatment group were able to follow their treatment protocol throughout the study without interruption.

In the intensively treated group, 85% were in either phase I or phase II, and 15% were in phase III or phase IV at the 1-year marker. By the end of the study most of the patients were receiving two or more daily insulin injections. None of the patients in the standard therapy group were moved to intensified therapy for more than a short period of time. The average insulin dose of patients in the standard treatment group was 23% lower than in the intense treatment group.

Patients in the intense therapy group had fasting glucose levels close to normal range starting at about the 3-month mark and maintained those levels throughout the study. Patients in the standard therapy group were not as close to the normal range, with an average difference between the two groups of 5.46 mmol/L (98.3 mg/dL). The intense therapy group patients were also able to maintain lower $HbA_{1c}$ levels than the patients in the standard therapy group throughout the 2 years of the study. The average difference in $HbA_{1c}$ levels between the two groups was 2.7% starting after the 6-month marker. A small decrease in $HbA_{1c}$ was seen with the addition of glipizide, but the majority of the decrease was seen with the bedtime dose of intermediate- or long-acting insulin. No real change was seen with the twice-daily insulin injections.

At the onset of the study there was no statistical difference in body mass index, patients on therapy for hypertension, hypercholesterolemia, smokers, or those with previous cardiovascular events between the two treatment groups. Throughout the study, there was no statistical difference in body mass index between the two groups. By the end of the 2-year study both groups had experienced a fall in serum triglyceride concentrations with no statistical difference. The fall in LDL levels was also considered not significant for either group. There was a slight increase in patients who required hypercholesterolemia therapy but with no statistical difference. The average blood pressure of the participants did not change throughout. Forty patients experienced 61 new cardiovascular events, but the relationship to each treatment group was not reported. A later article, "Cardiovascular Events and Correlates in the Veterans Affairs Feasibility Trial,"[2] was published in 1997. Sixteen patients (20%) in the standard treatment group and 24 (32%) patients in the intense treatment group experienced new cardiovascular events, but no statistical difference was found in the overall cardiovascular mortality.[2] Five participants in the intensively treated group and two participants in the standard treatment group reported hypoglycemic events. The researchers determined that there was no statistical difference in hypoglycemic events between the two treatment groups.

The major concern of weight gain in NIDDM patients on intense insulin therapy was not seen in this study. It was also determined that patients with type II diabetes could have well-controlled glucose levels without the use of excessively large doses of insulin. A bedtime dose of an intermediate-acting insulin in combination with a daytime glipizide or by itself may be most beneficial in regulating glucose levels. Researchers were also able to establish that "improved glycemic control could be accomplished without differences in adverse events associated with insulin therapy."

Both treatment regimens were considered safe and effective in treating the patients involved. No patients presented with a hyperosmolar state and ketoacidosis throughout the 2-year study. And in the standard treatment group only six patients ever reached the alert $HbA_{1c}$ level of >12.9%.

## Reader's Results/Conclusions

The primary objective of the study was met by the large number of cardiovascular events, proving that a further study with a much larger sample size should be conducted to better monitor the effects of insulin therapy on new cardiovascular events and macrovascular disease in patients with diagnosed type II diabetes.

The study also showed that it might be possible to treat NIDDM patients with chronic insulin therapy without risk of increasing obesity, hypertension, or dyslipidemia, meaning patients could achieve improved glycemic control without increased risk of adverse events.

The article was written in an understandable fashion and an adequate length. The study was funded by various organizations including many drug manufactures and the DVA Medical Research Service, allowing for lack of bias. The study was approved by an Investigational Review Board and used appropriate references.

Although the article was published in a rather reputable journal and was approved by the institutional review board at each of the participating hospitals, many limitations were evident. The study lacks generalizibility because all of the patients involved were men from within a narrow age range and did not include patients with a >15-year history of NIDDM. The sample size was also relatively small, but because the study was only assessing the need for a larger study, this may have been appropriate. The researchers failed to mention how the patients were randomized into the two treatment groups or how their compliance was monitored throughout the study. The article failed to discuss many aspects of the statistical methods used, including power and values. The new cardiovascular events of 40 patients were never discussed except to say that they would be mentioned in a later article.

This article should be used as a starting point for further research to be done in the future. By the time this article was published, a proposal for a long-term trial of 1463 patients had already been established to better assess the use of chronic insulin therapy in NIDDM patients.

## References

1. The Diabetes Control and Complications Trial. The effect of intensive treatment of diabetes on the development and progression of long-term complications in insulin-dependent diabetes mellitus. *N Engl J Med.* 1993;329(14):977–984.
2. Abraira C, Colwell J, Nutall F, et al. Cardiovascular events and correlates in the Veterans Affairs Diabetes Feasibility Trial. *Arch Intern Med.* 1997;157:181–190.

## EXAMPLE OF A DRUG MONOGRAPH: SPARFLOXACIN (ZAGAM®) COMPARISON TO CIPROFLOXACIN (CIPRO®) BY KAREN L. KIER, DRUG INFORMATION CENTER, OHIO NORTHERN UNIVERSITY

### Background

Sparfloxacin is a new once-daily fluoroquinolone antibiotic by Rhone-Poulenc Rorer that was approved by the FDA on December 19, 1996. This fluoroquinolone has demonstrated activity against a broad spectrum of organisms including gram-positive, gram-negative, and anaerobic bacteria. Sparfloxacin is highly active *in vitro* against many penicillin-resistant strains of gram-positive pathogens as well as drug-resistant strains of *Haemophilus influenzae* and *Moraxella catarrhalis*. It may offer an advantage over other fluoroquinolones by its improved gram-positive cocci coverage and its activity against some anaerobes.[1,12]

## What It Is

Sparfloxacin is a difluorinated quinolone antibiotic that is structurally related to ciprofloxacin.[1]

## What It Does

Bactericidal activity by inhibition of the enzyme DNA gyrase, which is necessary for the synthesis of DNA by bacteria.

## Clinical Trials

An *in vitro* study of activity to human infection isolates showed that sparfloxacin has good activity against anaerobes such as *Peptostreptococci*, *Clostridium perfingens*, *Clostridium difficile*, and *Fusobacterium*. Sparfloxacin had significantly better activity against *Bacteroides fragilis* than ciprofloxacin, lomefloxacin, and ofloxacin but was not superior to piperacillin/tazobactam, cefoxitin, imipenem, clindamycin, or metronidazole. This *in vitro* activity may prove to be beneficial in patients with mixed infections that can include anaerobes such as soft tissue infections in patients with diabetes. The limitations of this study included *in vitro* testing, which does not always correlate to *in vivo* response, and the small number of cultures that were performed.[1]

A multicenter, double-blinded, randomized trial comparing sparfloxacin to doxycycline for nongonococal urethritis looked at 725 men. Sparfloxacin was given in a dosing regimen of a 200-mg loading dose on day 1 followed by 100 mg each day for 2 days, and a second group received 100 mg per day for 6 days. This was compared to doxycycline 200 mg once per day for 7 days. For chlamydial infections, rates of relapse or reinfection were similar for both drugs. In addition, the researchers found that 3 days and 7 days of sparfloxacin were also equal in efficacy. Cultures were taken at each office visit by doing an endo-urethral swab to confirm presence of bacteria. Success of therapy was determined by clinical symptoms and bacteriologic response of the urethral smear. For ureaplasmal urethritis or urethritis of unknown etiology, sparfloxacin had a lower relapse/reinfection rate than doxycycline.[4] A limitation of this study is that the results can be applied only to treating men and not to women. In addition, this study was a multicenter trial that did not control for laboratory or observer differences. This study had limitations in the application of statistical tests. The study used only frequency and descriptive data and did not perform any tests to determine statistically significant results.

A double-blinded, multicenter trial that treated 382 patients for acute purulent sinusitis used sparfloxacin 200 mg once per day for 5 days with a 400-mg loading dose on the first day compared to cefuroxime axetil 250 mg two times per day for 8 days. Patients were classified as success or failure based on clinical symptoms as well as bacterial cultures and radiologic exams. Three hundred seventy-four patients were evaluated in the final results. The success rates as defined by the authors was 82.6% with sparfloxacin and 83.2% with cefuroxime axetil. The most common cultured organisms were H. influenzae and S. pneumoniae. The success rate as well as the side-effect profile were similar between the two drugs.[5] The study limitations included some patients lost to follow-up and not evaluated for the study as well as multiple observers collecting data without mentioning how this variation was to be controlled for by the different researchers. The cultures were analyzed all at one location, which was an appropriate measure to improve internal validity. Another limitation was that not all patients had bacterial cultures or radiologic exams performed. Therefore, success or failure was defined differently for some patients.

A double-blinded, multicenter, randomized trial evaluated 733 patients for acute exacerbation of chronic obstructive pulmonary disease (COPD). The study compared sparfloxacin 100 mg every day with a 200-mg loading dose to amoxicillin 500 mg/clavulanic acid 125 mg three times per day for 7 to 14 days. Patients were evaluated if their $FEV_1$/FVC ratio was less than 70% and stable. The primary endpoint was improvement in dyspnea and reduction in sputum purulence and volume. Success rates for both treatment groups were equivalent. Sparfloxacin improved dyspnea in 87.4% of patients compared to 88.8% amoxicillin/clavulanic acid. In terms of bacteriologic eradication, sparfloxacin appeared to be superior to amoxicillin/clavulanic acid for Haemophilus influenzae and Moraxella catarrhalis.[6] The study limitations included lack of culture eradication, and not all types of COPD patients were included.

In a prospective, placebo-controlled double-blind study, sparfloxacin 200 mg once daily with a 400-mg loading dose was compared with amoxicillin 1 g three times a day in combination with ofloxacin 200 mg twice a day. This comparison was done in 211 patients admitted to the hospital for community-acquired pneumonia. The efficacy rate was found to be similar between the two groups, with sparfloxacin having a 91.9% rate of success compared to the combination, which showed a lower rate of 81.5%. The adverse effect profile was also found to be similar between the two study drugs.[7] Study limitations included a multicenter trial that did not control for multiple observers. In addition, statistical analysis was limited to frequency data, and statistical significance was not performed. The efficacy rate was considered to be similar via frequency data, but there is a 10% difference in clinical response. This difference could be enough to prove statistical as well as clinical significance.

### Comparative Studies

A double-blinded, randomized clinical trial involving 686 patients compared ciprofloxacin to sparfloxacin in complicated urinary tract infections (UTI). This was a multicenter study comparing sparfloxacin 200-mg loading dose followed by

100 mg every day with ciprofloxacin 500 mg twice daily for 10–14 days. Complicated UTI was defined as pyruria and bacteriuria. Evaluations were performed at four different time points during the study. The clinical efficacy of the two products was equivalent at the end of treatment, with sparfloxacin having a clinical cure rate of 87.5% compared to ciprofloxacin's cure rate of 85%. Bacteriologic cure was 72.6% in the sparfloxacin group and 81.4% in the ciprofloxacin group. The side-effect profile was similar in the two groups. However, it was noted that in terms of bacteriologic efficacy ciprofloxacin was superior to sparfloxacin because of persistent pathogens of the Enterobacteriaceae species other than *E. coli*.[2] Study limitations included the lack of statistical tests to make comparisons to show statistical significance.

A multicenter, double-blinded, randomized clinical trial compared the efficacy of sparfloxacin with ciprofloxacin in acute gonorrhea. The study compared single oral doses of sparfloxacin 200 mg versus ciprofloxacin 250 mg in 238 men with the diagnosis of *Neisseria gonorrhoeae*. The two drugs were found to be equally effective in the treatment of gonorrhea in men. The primary eradication rate was 99% in the sparfloxacin group and 98% in the ciprofloxacin group. The side effects were similar for both treatment groups.[13] The study was only in the acute environment and does not provide long-term results. The incidence of resistance was not studied. Another limitation was that some patients were lost to follow-up and were dropped from the study analysis.

## Recommendation

Ciprofloxacin and sparfloxacin have good gram-negative coverage for most serious infections. The clinical trials support similar rates of eradication and efficacy. The concerns with sparfloxacin are with the drug interactions and the adverse effect of a prolonged QT interval. Because sparfloxacin has these potential problems, the Pharmacy Department recommends to the P&T committee that ciprofloxacin remain as the fluoroquinolone of choice for the institution.

## References

1. Nord CE. *In vitro* activity of quinolones and other antimicrobial agents against anaerobic bacteria. *Clin Infect Dis.* 1996;23(Suppl 1):s15–s18.
2. Naber KG, Di Silverio F, Geddes A, et al. Comparative efficacy of sparfloxacin versus ciprofloxacin in the treatment of complicated urinary tract infection. *J Antimicrob Chemother.* 1996;37(Suppl A):135–144.
3. Rubinstein E. Safety profile of sparfloxacin in the treatment of respiratory tract infections. *J Antimicrob Chemother.* 1996;37(Suppl A):145–160.
4. Phillips I, Dimian, C, Barlow D, et al. A comparative study of two different regimens of sparfloxacin versus doxycycline in the treatment of non-gonococcal urethritis in men. *J Antimicrob Chemother.* 1996;37(Suppl A):123–134.
5. Gehanno P, Berche P, et al. Sparfloxacin versus cefuroxime axetil in the treatment of acute purulent sinusitis. *J Antimicrob Chemother.* 1996;37(Suppl A): 93–104.

6. Allegra L, Konietzko N, Leophonte P, et al. Comparative safety and efficacy of sparfloxacin in the treatment of acute exacerbations of chronic obstructive pulmonary disease: a double-blind, randomized, parallel, multicentre study. *J Antimicrob Chemother.* 1996;37(Suppl A):93–104.

7. Portier H, May T, Proust A, et al. Comparative efficacy of sparfloxacin in comparison with amoxycillin plus ofloxacin in the treatment of community-acquired pneumonia. *J Antimicrob Chemother.* 1996;37(Suppl A):83–91.

8. Huston KA. Achilles tendinitis and tendon rupture due to fluoroquinolone antibiotics. *N Engl J Med.* 1994;331:748.

9. Johnson JH, Cooper MA, Andrews JM, et al. Pharmacokinetics and inflammatory fluid penetration of sparfloxacin. *Antimicrob Agents Chemother.* 1992;36: 2444–2446.

10. Ritz M, Lose H, Fabbender M, et al. Multiple-dose pharmacokinetics of sparfloxacin and its influence on fecal flora. *Antimicrob Agents Chemother.* 1994;38: 455–459.

11. Takagi K, Yamaki K, Nadai M, et al. Effect of a new quinolone, sparfloxacin, on the pharmacokinetics of theophylline in asthmatic patients. *Antimicrob Agents Chemother.* 1991;35:1137–1141.

12. FDC Pink Sheet. January 6, 1997, 16–17.

13. Moi H, Morel P, Gianotti B, et al. Comparative efficacy and safety of single oral doses of sparfloxacin versus ciprofloxacin in the treatment of acute gonococcal urethritis in men. *J Antimicrob Chemother.* 1996;37(Suppl A):115–122.

14. Anderson PO, Knoben JE. *Handbook of Clinical Drug Data.* 8th ed. Stamford, CT: Appleton & Lange; 1997.

15. Goa KL, Bryson HM, Markham A. Sparfloxacin. *Drugs.* 1997;53(4):700–725.

## EXAMPLE OF PHARMACY & THERAPEUTICS COMMITTEE MONOGRAPH: APRIL M. BAYS, PHARM.D. STUDENT, OHIO NORTHERN UNIVERSITY, AS PART OF A PATIENT CARE ASSESSMENT MODULE ASSIGNMENT: CARVEDILOL (COREG®, SMITHKLINE BEECHAM)

### Pharmacology

Carvedilol is a nonselective $\beta$-adrenergic blocking agent with $\alpha_1$-adrenergic blocking activity and no sympathomimetic activity.[1,2] The $\beta$-adrenoreceptor blocking activity is present in the S(−) enantiomer, and the $\alpha$-adrenergic blocking activity is present in both R(+) and S(−) enantiomers at equal potency.[3] The exact mechanism of the antihypertensive effect produced by the $\beta$-adrenergic blockade is not known, but it may involve suppression of renin production. The $\beta$-adrenergic blocking activity of carvedilol decreases cardiac output, exercise- and/or isoproterenol-induced tachycardia, and reflex orthostatic tachycardia. The $\alpha_1$-adrenergic blocking activity of carvedilol blunts the pressor effect of phenylephrine, causes vasodilation, and reduces peripheral vascular resistance.

Because of the $\alpha_1$-receptor-blocking activity of carvedilol, blood pressure is lowered more in the standing than the supine position.[2]

The mechanisms by which carvedilol slows the progression of heart failure are not known. Possible mechanisms include up-regulation of the $\beta$-adrenergic receptors in the heart, modulation of postreceptor inhibitory G proteins, an effect on left ventricular remodeling, and an improvement in baroreceptor function, which normally can inhibit excess sympathetic outflow.[4]

Carvedilol is rapidly and extensively absorbed following oral administration, with a bioavailability of 25% to 35%, as a result of a significant degree of first-pass metabolism.[1,3] Taking carvedilol with food delays its absorption an additional 1 to 2 hours but does not appear to affect the extent of bioavailability.[3] The volume of distribution at steady-state concentration is approximately 115 L, indicating extensive protein binding (98%), primarily to albumin. Peak plasma concentrations are reached in 1 to 2 hours.[2,5] The drug is extensively metabolized in the liver and primarily excreted by the feces. Small amounts (less than 1%) of unchanged carvedilol are excreted in the urine.[5] The elimination half-life is 7 to 10 hours.[1,5] The primary P450 enzymes responsible for the metabolism of carvedilol are CYP2D6 and CYP2C8.

### Indications for Use

Carvedilol is indicated for congestive heart failure and hypertension. In essential hypertension, carvedilol is indicated either alone or in combination with other antihypertensive agents such as thiazide diuretics. Carvedilol, in the treatment of congestive heart failure, is indicated for use in conjunction with digitalis, diuretics, and/or angiotensin-converting enzyme (ACE) inhibitors. It is used to slow the progression of disease as evidenced by cardiovascular death, cardiovascular hospitalization, or the need to adjust other heart failure medications. Carvedilol may be used in patients who are unable to tolerate an ACE inhibitor or in patients who are not receiving digitalis, hydralazine, or nitrate therapy.[1,3,5] Unlabeled uses for carvedilol include angina pectoris and idiopathic cardiomyopathy.

### Review of Congestive Heart Failure

Congestive heart failure results when the heart cannot pump blood at a rate comparable to the requirements of metabolizing tissues or can do so only from an elevated filling pressure. As a result, the heart cannot produce enough blood circulation to maintain the body in its normal state. The term "congestive" refers to fluid buildup that occurs with the disease. With less blood leaving your heart, blood returning to your heart gets backed up. As back pressure builds, fluid from your blood can collect in your vital organs, including your lungs and liver. Fluid can also seep into surrounding tissues, causing swelling.[6,7]

Heart attacks, congenital heart disease, heart muscle damage caused by alcohol or viruses, high blood pressure, heart valve abnormalities, and abnormal heart rhythms are the major causes of congestive heart failure. Signs of congestive heart failure include reduced ability to exercise, fatigue, breathing problems, and swelling of the legs.[7,8] The amount of impairment from congestive heart failure ranges from none after appropriate compensation by drugs to the patient being totally bedridden and incapable of normal functioning.[9]

In some cases, congestive heart failure can be corrected by treating an underlying cause, but many times the problem cannot be eliminated. Then, the goal of treatment is to prevent further damage to your heart and help it pump as efficiently as possible. This is usually done through ACE inhibitors, diuretics, digoxin, and β-blockers.

## Efficacy

The relatively recent discovery that β-blockers may be used in the treatment of congestive heart failure has lead to many case studies examining the effectiveness of carvedilol. In a double-blinded study by the Australia/New Zealand Heart Failure Research Collaborative Group, 415 patients with chronic stable heart failure were randomly assigned treatment of carvedilol or matching placebo. The primary study outcomes were changes in left-ventricular ejection fraction and treadmill exercise duration. A sample size of 200–225 patients per group was estimated to provide more than 80% power at a statistical significance of 0.05 to detect an absolute change in left ventricular ejection fraction of 2% or more between the groups and a change in treadmill exercise duration of 1 minute or more between groups.

The patients were recruited to the trial from 20 hospitals in Australia and New Zealand. Patients included in the study were those with chronic stable heart failure caused by ischemic heart disease, a left-ventricular ejection fraction of less than 45%, and current New York Heart Association (NYHA) functional class II or III or previous NYHA class II-IV. The mean age of the participants at entry to the study was 67 years, and 80% were men. Principal outcome analysis was by intention to treat. At baseline, 6 months, and 12 months, measurements of left-ventricular ejection fraction and treadmill exercise duration were taken. A double-blinded follow-up continued for an average of 19 months, during which all deaths, hospital admissions, and episodes of worsening heart failure were documented. Results from the study indicate an increase in left ventricular ejection fraction from 28.4% at baseline to 33.5% at 12 months among the patients assigned carvedilol. The placebo group showed little change. However, there was no significant difference between the carvedilol and placebo groups in tread-mill exercise duration at 12 months.

The Australia/New Zealand Heart Failure Research Collaborative Group concluded that in patients with chronic stable heart failure caused by ischemic heart disease, the effects of carvedilol on left ventricular function were maintained for at least 1 year from the start of treatment, with no apparent loss of the initial short-term improvement. The increase in left ventricular ejection fraction suggests a sustained improvement in intrinsic myocardial function. Whether there are benefits of β-blocker therapy for these outcomes in other subgroups of patients with heart failure remains uncertain. There have, however, been some reports of benefits in studies of patients with ideopathic cardiomyopathy and in other trials among patients with more severe heart failure.[10]

There are possible concerns with this study. First, the sample size of patients per group was estimated to provide 80% power. Power is the positive spin indicating that when you say the groups are equal, they are in reality equal. A power of 90% tends to be an acceptable standard for most studies. Therefore, the placebo and carvedilol groups may not be as equal as they seem. Additionally, as a result of dropouts and death during the course of the study, the final number of subjects was smaller than the original sample size calculations. This may increase the possibility of a false-negative result. Last, the increase in left-ventricular ejection fraction may not be clinically significant even though it is statistically significant because of the condition of the patient and the response of the patient to the drug.

In a study determining the long-term efficacy of carvedilol in patients with severe chronic heart failure, Krum and colleagues[11] hypothesized that carvedilol produces clinical and hemodynamic improvements in patients who have severe heart failure despite treatment with angiotensin-converting enzyme inhibitors. Patients with chronic heart failure who remained symptomatic were eligible for the study. Heart failure was defined as the presence of dypsnea or fatigue at rest or on exertion for more than 2 months in association with a left ventricular ejection fraction less than or equal to 0.35 as assessed by radionuclide ventriculography. The cause of heart failure was related to numerous different types of cardiac dysfunction. Fifty-six patients with severe chronic heart failure were enrolled in the double-blinded, placebo-controlled study of carvedilol. The 56 patients consisted of 45 men and 11 women (25 to 79 years old). Forty-nine of the 56 patients were randomly assigned to a long-term therapy of carvedilol (33 patients) or placebo (16 patients) while backround therapy remained constant. Patients treated with carvedilol showed an improvement in symptom scores and functional class, whereas these variables did not change in the patients receiving placebo. These clinical benefits were accompanied by an increase in the distance traveled during a 6-minute walk in the carvedilol group. Carvedilol was also associated with a significant improvement in cardiac performance. Patients being treated with carvedilol showed a significant increase in stroke volume index and left-ventricular ejection fraction. Although there was a rise in stroke volume index, the cardiac index did not increase with carvedilol because the heart rate decreased considerably during long treatment with the drug. Last, the plasma epinephrine decreased with the use of carvedilol when compared to the placebo.

For each of the variables being studied, $p < 0.05$, indicating that there was a difference between carvedilol and placebo. In conclusion, this study demonstrated that the β-blockade of carvedilol produces clinical and hemodynamic benefits in patients with severe chronic heart failure in those who can tolerate low doses of the drug. The addition of carvedilol to conventional therapy led to an improvement in symptoms, functional capacity, and submaximal exercise tolerance. This study also demonstrates that carvedilol may be useful in the management of advanced heart failure, regardless of the cause of cardiac dysfunction. The low number of patients enrolled in this study may not have been large enough to detect a statistically significant difference between the treatments. Also, treatment effects may be overestimated with such a small population. Last, the clinical and hemodynamic improvements from carvedilol may not be clinically significant. The improvements may be so insignificant that less expensive treatment options could be used without harming the patient.[11]

## Safety

Carvedilol is generally well tolerated at doses up to 50 mg daily. It is contraindicated in patients with NYHA class IV decompensated cardiac failure requiring intravenous inotropic therapy, bronchial asthma or related bronchospastic conditions, second- or third-degree AV block, sick sinus syndrome (unless a permanent pacemaker is in place), cardiogenic shock, and severe brachycardia. The use of carvedilol in patients with clinically manifest hepatic impairment is not recommended. Also, carvedilol is contraindicated in patients with hypersensitivity to the drug.[2,5]

Mild hepatocellular injury confirmed by carvedilol challenge after the discontinuation of treatment has occurred in a few patients, but no deaths from liver failure have been reported. Also, hepatic injury has been reversible. In controlled studies of hypertensive patients, the incidence of liver function abnormalities reported as adverse experiences was 1.1% (13 of 1142) in patients receiving carvedilol and 0.9% (4 of 462) in those receiving placebo. In patients receiving carvedilol with abnormal liver function tests, the drug should be discontinued. Additionally, it should not be given to patients with preexisting liver disease. Carvedilol should also be used cautiously in those with peripheral vascular disease, diabetes, hypoglycemia, thyrotoxicosis, and those undergoing anesthesia and/or major surgery.[4,5]

Most adverse effects reported were of mild to moderate severity. In clinical trials comparing carvedilol monotherapy with placebo, 4.9% of patients treated with less than 50 mg of carvedilol and 5.2% of patients taking placebo discontinued use because of adverse effects. Discontinuation of therapy because of postural hypotension was more common among patients treated with carvedilol (1% versus zero). The overall incidence of adverse effects increased with increasing doses of carvedilol. For individual adverse events this could only be distinguished for dizziness, which increased in frequency from 2% to 5% as the total daily dose increased from 6.25 mg to 50 mg.[3,9] Coreg has been evaluated for safety in congestive heart failure in more than 1900 patients worldwide, of whom 1300 participated in United States clinical trials. Approximately 54% of the total treated population received carvedilol for at least 6 months, and 20%

received carvedilol for at least 12 months. The most common side effect among patients was dizziness (32% of the total U.S. treated population). Other common side effects of the U.S. treated population, listed in order of most severe to least severe, are fatigue, upper respiratory tract infection, chest pain, hyperglycemia, diarrhea, bradycardia, hypotension, nausea, and edema. The incidence of adverse reactions does not differ between patients with heart failure who are 65 years of age and older and those who are younger.

Carvedilol has the potential to interact with a number of medications. Because of carvedilol's extensive oxidative liver metabolism, its pharmacokinetics can be profoundly affected by certain drugs that significantly induce or inhibit oxidation. Carvedilol interacts with rifampin, cimetidine, other inhibitors of cytochrome P450 2D6 isoenzyme, digoxin, calcium channel blockers, antidiabetic medications, clonidine, and cyclosporin. Rifampin, an inducer of hepatic metabolism, can reduce plasma concentrations of carvedilol by 70% when carvedilol is coadministered. In contrast, cimetidine may increase plasma concentrations by 30% in patients receiving carvedilol. Other inhibitors of cytochrome P450 2D6 isoenzyme, such as fluoxetine, paroxetine, propafenone, and quinidine, could expect to increase plasma concentrations in patients receiving carvedilol. The concentration of digoxin is increased by 15% when it is used in combination with carvedilol. As a result, digoxin levels should be closely monitored when a combination of these drugs is used. The combination of carvedilol and calcium channel blockers has resulted in rare conduction disturbances. Carvedilol may mask signs and symptoms of hypoglycemia. Clonidine potentiates the blood pressure and heart rate—lowering effects of β-blockers such as carvedilol. When clonidine is used in combination therapy with carvedilol, carvedilol should always be discontinued first. Last, carvedilol increases cyclosporin concentrations.[3,5,8]

When it is taken with food, the rate of absorption is slowed, but the extent of the bioavailability is not affected. Taking with food minimizes the risk of orthostatic hypotension. No food/drug interactions have been noted.

Studies of carvedilol have shown it to have no carcinogenic effect or mutagenicity, and the no-observed-effect dose level for impairment of fertility was 60 mg/kg/day in adult rats. Carvedilol is in pregnancy category C. There are no adequate and well-controlled studies in pregnant women. Carvedilol should be used during pregnancy only if the potential benefit justifies the potential risk to the fetus. It is not known whether this drug is excreted in human milk. Safety and efficacy in patients younger than 18 years of age have not been established. There were no notable differences in efficacy or the incidence of adverse events between elderly and younger patients.[3,5]

Patient monitoring includes blood pressure determinations, blood glucose concentrations, electrocardiogram determinations, heart rate determinations, hepatic function determinations, and renal function determinations.[1] Weight gain of 0.91 to 1.36 kg above their usual "dry" weight should be reported for possible edema. Additionally, at the first sign of liver dysfunction, perform laboratory testing. If the patient has laboratory evidence of liver injury or jaundice, stop therapy and do not restart.[8]

## Dose

In congestive heart failure, an initial oral dose of 3.125 mg twice daily is recommended, and if tolerated, the dose may be doubled every 2 weeks up to a maximum dose of 25 to 50 mg twice daily.[1,3,4] Four strengths of carvedilol are available for use: 3.125 mg, 6.25 mg, 12.5 mg, and 25 mg. Tablets are the only available dosage form. Carvedilol should be taken with food to slow the rate of absorption and reduce the risk of postural hypotension.[4] Dosing must be adjusted to meet the individual requirements of each patient on the basis of clinical response. When carvedilol is discontinued, its dosage should be tapered over a 1- to 2-week period, especially in patients with ischemic heart disease. Only small amounts of carvedilol are excreted unchanged in the urine (less than 1% of the dose), and dosing adjustments are not required in patients with renal insufficiency.

Dosage adjustments are not required in chronic hemodialysis patients. However, dose reductions are suggested in patients with hepatic insufficiency. One study by Neugebauer et al. suggests that carvedilol therapy be initiated with approximately 20% of the normal dose in patients with liver cirrhosis. The manufacturer states that carvedilol should not be administered to patients with liver cirrhosis.[1] If the patient's pulse rate drops below 55 beats per minute, the dosage of carvedilol should be reduced. It may also be necessary to adjust the dosages of the patient's other heart failure medications when carvedilol is introduced. At each dosage increase, the patient should be observed for 1 hour for signs of dizziness or lightheadedness. The maximum recommended dosage of carvedilol is 25 mg twice daily in patients weighing less than 85 kg and 50 mg twice daily in patients weighing 85 kg or more.[8]

## Cost

The cost for a 1-month supply of carvedilol is $93 average wholesale price. The price per day for carvedilol is $3 average wholesale price.[12] Because carvedilol is the only $\beta$-adrenergic blocking agent with $\alpha_1$-adrenergic blocking activity currently on the market, it is not possible to perform a cost-benefit analysis of carvedilol with any one individual drug having the same pharmacological effect. Carvedilol, however, can be compared by evaluating the conventional method of therapy for congestive heart failure plus carvedilol with the conventional method of therapy alone. The conventional method of therapy includes digoxin, diuretics, and angiotensin-converting enzyme inhibitors.

In a study by Delea et al.,[13] the cost effectiveness of carvedilol for the treatment of congestive heart failure was examined. The conventional therapy consisted of digoxin, furosemide, and enalapril. They examined the conventional method plus carvedilol versus the conventional method alone and found that the cost-effectiveness of carvedilol for congestive heart failure compares favorably to that of other generally accepted medical interventions, even under the assumptions regarding the duration of therapeutic benefit.[13]

## Recommendation

Carvedilol appears to be a useful agent in the management of congestive heart failure. Studies have shown that it has a significant impact on the left ventricular ejection fraction, although its benefit in exercise duration remains questionable. Carvedilol is generally well tolerated, and adverse effects appear to be relatively mild to moderate, with dizziness reported as the most common side effect. An unfavorable aspect of carvedilol is its potential to interact negatively with various other medications such as rifampin, cimetidine, inhibitors of cytochrome P450 2D6 isoenzyme, digoxin, calcium channel blockers, antidiabetic medications, clonidine, and cyclosporin. Carvedilol is available only in tablet forms, and dosing ranges from 3.125 mg to 50 mg twice daily.

When one is measuring cost with therapy, patient morbidity must be heavily considered. At a cost of $3 per day average wholesale price (in addition to the conventional therapy), the progression of congestive heart failure can be delayed, resulting in a potentially longer life for the patient.

Considering this information, carvedilol does appear to be a very useful addition to the standard conventional therapy (digoxin, diuretics, and ACE inhibitors) used in the treatment of congestive heart failure and should be available on formulary.

## References

1. USPDI Vol I. *Drug Information for the Health Care Professional.* Englewood, CO: MICROMEDEX, 1999.
2. McEnvoy GK. *American Hospital Formulary Service.* Bethesda: American Society of Health-System Pharmacists, 2000.
3. Kastrup E. *Drug Facts and Comparisons.* St. Louis: Facts and Comparisons, 2000.
4. Frishman W. *Carvedilol. Drug Ther.* 1998;339:1759–1765.
5. Walsh P. *Physicians' Desk Reference.* Montvale, NJ: Medical Economics Company, 2000.
6. Hardman JG, Limbird LE, Molinoff PB, Ruddon RW, Gilman AG, eds. *Goodman and Gilman's the Pharmacological Basis of Therapeutics,* 9th ed. New York: McGraw-Hill, 1996.
7. Senni M, Redfield M. Congestive heart failure in elderly patients. *Mayo Clin Proc.* 1997;72:453–460.
8. Vanderhoff B, Ruppel H, Amsterdam P. Carvedilol: The new role of beta blockers in congestive heart failure. *Am Fam Physician.* 1998;58:1627–1633, 1641–1642.
9. Fisher L, Moye L. Carvedilol and the Food and Drug Administration approval process: an introduction. *Contr Clin Trials.* 1999;20:1–15.

10. Australia/New Zealand Heart Failure Research Collaborative Group. Random-
    ized, placebo-controlled trial of carvedilol in patients with congestive heart
    failure due to ischaemic heart disease. *Lancet.* 1997;349:375–380.
11. Krum H, Sackner-Bernstein J, Goldsmith R. Double-blind, placebo-controlled
    study of the long-term efficacy of carvedilol in patients with severe chronic
    heart failure. *Circulation.* 1995;92:1499–1506.
12. Cardinale V. *Redbook,* 103rd ed. Montvale: Medical Economics Company, 1999.
13. Delea T, Vera-Llonch M, Richner R. Cost effectiveness of carvedilol for heart
    failure. *Am J Cardiol.* 1999;83:890–896.

## SUMMARY

The skills of drug information, drug literature evaluation, and professional communication are essential components of professional pharmacy practice. Information is always a guiding principle in sustaining the professional's knowledge while
opening the door for a better-educated patient. One cannot be expected to have all
of the answers stored away in one's brain, but one should be able to use one's skills
to find the answer.

## APPLICATION EXERCISES

1. What are the seven steps of the modified systematic approach to drug
   information?
2. What does it mean to get to the "ultimate" question, and why is the category of
   the question so vital to a good response?
3. What is the difference among primary, secondary, and tertiary literature?
4. What are examples of internal and external validity?
5. What does it mean when an article states that the results were statistically
   significant?
6. Name five rules for professional writing.

## REFERENCES

1. Host TR, Kirkwood CF. Computer-assisted instruction for responding to drug
   information requests. Paper presented at the 22nd Annual ASHP Midyear Clinical Meeting, December 1997, Atlanta.
2. Malone P, Kier KL, Malone M, Stanovich J. *Drug Information: A Guide for
   Pharmacists.* 5th ed. New York: McGraw-Hill; 2014.

# Community/Ambulatory Care

*Maria Maniscalco-Feichtl, Karen L. Whalen*

**Objectives: Upon completion of the chapter and exercises, the student pharmacist will be able to**

1. Compare and contrast various types of community pharmacy and ambulatory care practice settings.
2. Outline the basic management issues (eg, workflow, staff, and business aspects) of community pharmacy practice.
3. List key steps in the medication order fulfillment process.
4. Define the term medication therapy management services (MTM) and list core elements of MTM.
5. Discuss opportunities for provision of MTM and advanced patient care services in the community and ambulatory care setting.
6. Discuss the impact of technology on present and future community practice issues.

---

### Patient Encounter

A 54-year-old female presents to the pharmacy counter with a new prescription. You recognize her from pictures in the newspaper as the mother of the Olympic cyclist who was severely injured. She hands you the following prescription:

JOHN TAYLOR, M.D.
1234 MIDWAY AVENUE
ANYTOWN, USA 34567

---

Name: *Nelly Nervous*            Date: *9/15/14*
*Lorazepam 0.5 mg #60*
*One tab bid prn anxiety*
Refill: *X 2*                    *J Taylor MD*

---

*(continued on next page)*

When entering the prescription data, you note her current Rx profile as follows:

| Medication | Directions | Qty | Last Refill | Refills Remaining |
|---|---|---|---|---|
| Glyburide 5-mg tab | One po bid AC | 60 | 9/01/14 | 3 |
| Levothyroxine 112-mcg tab | One tab po daily | 30 | 8/25/14 | 2 |
| Lisinopril 10-mg tab | One tab po daily | 30 | 9/01/14 | 3 |
| Metformin 500-mg tab | One po bid with food | 60 | 8/25/14 | 2 |
| Simvastatin 10-mg tab | One tab po qhs | 30 | 6/26/14 | 5 |

For the purpose of this exercise, assume today's date is 9/15/14.

### Discussion questions for introductory pharmacy practice:

- What information should be verified with the patient or caregiver before filling the prescription for lorazepam?
- Is the prescription missing any necessary information?
- Are you familiar with all of the abbreviations used on the prescription and in the prescription profile?
- Describe the steps you would take in completing the medication order fulfillment process.
- What auxiliary labels would most likely be placed on the bottle of lorazepam?
- What open-ended questions should be asked when counseling the patient on the new prescription?
- List at least four counseling points that should be provided to the patient when she picks up her new prescription for lorazepam.

### Discussion questions for advanced pharmacy practice:

- Are you able to answer all of the questions directed at the IPPE (introductory pharmacy practice experience) student?

- Are you concerned about any potential drug interactions with the lorazepam and her current prescription profile? If so, how would you address these issues?
- Based on the current prescription profile, what adherence issues may need to be addressed? How would you address these issues with the patient?

When picking up the prescription, the patient asks you for a recommendation for an over-the-counter (OTC) product that will help her get some sleep.

- What questions should be asked of the patient when performing an OTC consult?
- What concerns do you have about recommending an OTC sleep product for this patient?

Two-and-a-half weeks after picking up the initial prescription for lorazepam, the patient presents to your counter for a refill. When you process the prescription, the computer comes up with the following DUR alert: "Refill too early."

- What questions should you ask the patient prior to making a decision on whether it is appropriate to dispense the prescription?
- What alternatives do we have to offer the patient at this point?

The patient begins to cry at the counter, and sobs that, "The lorazepam is the only thing that has helped me with the stress of coping with my son's injury!" List an empathic response you would provide to the patient. Describe your approach in addressing her request for an early refill, indicating possible overuse of lorazepam.

Shortly after the patient leaves the pharmacy, another patient comes up to the counter and says, "Wow! She was really upset! What's wrong with her? Is she the one whose son was hurt in that biking accident? What's his status? Will he be OK?" How would you respond to this curious patient?

## COMMUNITY AND AMBULATORY CARE: AN OVERVIEW

This chapter provides an introduction to pharmacy practice in the ambulatory patient setting. Two models for types of practice include the community pharmacy and a general ambulatory care clinic for patients with chronic and nonemergent acute conditions. Colleges of pharmacy in the United States may offer introductory pharmacy practice experiences (as discussed in Chap. 1) in either setting. During these experiences, student pharmacists have the opportunity to learn and practice basic skills, and to advance knowledge and skills in preparation for advanced courses in practice. The chapter provides an introduction to community pharmacy and ambulatory care practice settings.

## COMMUNITY PHARMACY PRACTICE: PHARMACY BUSINESS ISSUES

### Introduction

Historically, community pharmacy was synonymous with independent pharmacy. The pharmacist was the chemist, and to patients he was someone who would share counsel, and gain the confidence of all his patrons. Often, the pharmacist was the first stop on the healthcare circuit, with his opinion sought after on how to treat anything from a sore throat to an ingrown toenail.

Community pharmacies now encompass everything from chain drug stores (Boots, CVS, Rite Aid, Walgreens, Pharmasave) to the mass merchandiser pharmacies (Target and Walmart), the supermarket pharmacies (Tops, Stop & Shop, Loblaws, Sobeys), the remaining single-owner independent pharmacies, mail-order pharmacies, and Internet pharmacies. Each type of organization has a unique environment in which professionals dispense medications and work with patients, yet there are many similarities in practices. Each type of organization is briefly reviewed from the perspective of US pharmacy practice to provide students with background information, which may aid in preparation for community pharmacy practice courses.

### Types of Pharmacies

#### Chain

Traditional chain pharmacy describes an operation with multiple locations, similar physical designs, one primary management/leadership team, and a varied mix of merchandise to offer their customers. Chains can be as small as three stores or as large as 7000 stores. Examples of some of the larger chains include Walgreens, CVS, Rite Aid, Boots, and Watson's.

#### Mass Merchant

Mass merchants are retail outlets whose primary goal is generating conventional retail sales, not pharmacy business. Mass merchants have entered into the pharmacy market, primarily to attract new types of customers to their stores and grow the sales of their established products. Most have entered this market with the pharmacy department being a loss leader, meaning they are willing to lose money in the prescription department. Losses are more than offset by sales in other departments. Examples of these types of organizations include Walmart and Target.

#### Supermarket

Supermarkets are another retail outlet whose primary goal is to generate sales of their customary product lines, mainly groceries and related items. Like mass merchants, the prescription department primarily serves as a loss leader. Examples of supermarket organizations that are in the pharmacy business include Kroger, Tops, Stop & Shop, Giant, Vons and Publix Supermarkets.

*Independent Pharmacy*

Independent pharmacies are the long-established type of pharmacy with a single store or two and one or two owners, whose primary product line is the prescription department. Many independent pharmacists have added durable medical equipment (DME), compounding, or other specialty services to their product line.

*Mail-Order Pharmacy*

Many of the larger chain pharmacies and pharmacy benefits managers (PBMs) have developed a mail-order division in order to maximize efficiency, address the insurance companies and third party payers' demands for less costly prescription processing, and to meet customer needs.

*Internet*

Entrepreneurial professionals and business persons have developed systems to obtain the necessary information for processing and dispensing prescriptions using Internet technology. A prescription may be mailed to the Internet pharmacy, transmitted via fax or other electronic means from the prescriber's office, or transferred via phone call from a community pharmacy. The prescription is processed and mailed to the patient. State boards of pharmacy have had to adjust to this type of transaction, and update legislation regarding regulation of online pharmacies. The National Association of Boards of Pharmacy (NABP) has developed a seal of approval program for Internet pharmacies known as the Verified Internet Pharmacy Practice Sites (VIPPS), identifying the sites with proper processes and procedures.

## Pharmacy Employees

In addition to the pharmacist, the staff members play a vital role in the everyday workflow. It is important for you to have a clear understanding and appreciation of the individuals with whom you will be working, what they do, and how they contribute to the success of the business. Some of the employees include the pharmacy technician, cashier, general manager, other management, and support staff. Depending on the size and type of store, there may be various specialists in departments such as greeting cards, gifts, health and beauty aids (HBA), OTC medications, DME, cosmetics, photo, food/groceries, natural products, vitamins and minerals, the information area, and diagnostic/home testing products.

The staff with whom you will spend most of your time works in the pharmacy department. The pharmacist is the licensed professional responsible for the safe, effective, and accurate processing and dispensing of prescriptions. Requirements for licensure vary by state, but one common law in every state is that the *pharmacist* must verify the final prescription product before it is given to the patient. Pharmacists may hold many titles and have additional responsibilities, such as pharmacy manager, store or department manager, or general manager. Pharmacy managers are often responsible for deciding how much inventory to hold, serving as contact persons for third-party payers (especially auditors), training staff on new technologies, addressing customer service issues, and maintaining pharmacy workflow.[4]

Support personnel in the pharmacy may have many job titles and responsibilities. Job titles for other individuals who may work in the pharmacy department are the pharmacy technician and the pharmacy clerk. The role of the pharmacy technician is to support the pharmacist with order fulfillment, manage all tasks not requiring a pharmacist's direct participation or judgment (eg, third-party reconciliation, general inventory management, etc.), and free time for the pharmacist to perform professional responsibilities. Some pharmacy technicians may specialize in the area of processing insurance claims. In some states, the technician must successfully complete a certification examination and maintain continuing education credits in order to work in a pharmacy. The pharmacy clerk manages certain tasks in the store, such as conducting sales transactions, responding to questions about general merchandise, and directing the customers to the correct department. Clerks usually work the cash register in the pharmacy and may assist with accepting new prescriptions, triaging customer inquiries, and helping to answer general questions.

## Pharmacy Department Setup

It is imperative to recognize the impact of "workflow" in regard to managing a pharmacy. Workflow describes the overall process from prescription intake to counseling the patient (Fig. 14.1). Efficiency and productivity are tied into how well the workflow

**Figure 14.1.** Workflow.

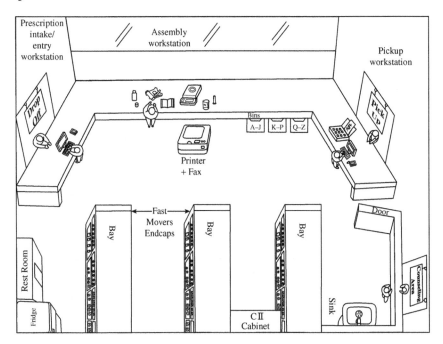

in the pharmacy is maintained. Typically, this task becomes the responsibility of the pharmacy manager. Workflow incorporates the entire pharmacy staff and is a series of multiple workstations involved in efficiently processing a prescription from beginning to end.

## Workstations Overview

The *prescription intake workstation* (also known as the "drop-off window") is where patients present their prescriptions for filling. Prescriptions are reviewed for completeness, and patients are informed about wait times and other possible products and services that may complement the care of the specific condition for which the prescription is being filled.

The *prescription entry workstation* is where information is entered into the computer system, and profiles are maintained and updated. This is usually located in close proximity to the intake station, and it is possible that the same person may work in both areas. Computer software systems in use by pharmacies often require the prescription to be scanned into a database at this station. Scanning the prescription into the database facilitates easy retrieval of the original prescription for reviewing purposes. Scanning the prescription also enables pharmacists, who are working from a facility in another location (central fill), to complete the order fulfillment process and send a packaged prescription to the respective store via courier.

Once prescriptions are ready for filling, they are classified as "waiting" (the patient will wait for their prescription), "later or returning" (the patient will return for pickup at a later time), or "delivery" (if that service is available). Each pharmacy will have a method of prioritizing prescriptions to minimize wait times and maximize the use of pharmacy personnel. Prescriptions for patients who are waiting require immediate entry into the computer system. Once prescriptions have been entered, they must be filled in the proper order based on priority.

The *assembly workstation* is where all the parts of the prescription come together to be assembled: the written prescription, patient medication container with label, stock bottle of medication, patient information leaflet, medication guide and any adherence aids (such as dosing spoon, medication calendar, etc.). The assembly area is the space on the pharmacy counter where medications are packaged and prepared for checking by the pharmacist. It is very important to keep everything organized so that prescriptions are not misfiled. Equipment and resources that may be used in this area include counting devices, calculator, computer, textbooks, prescription containers, auxiliary labels, and a distilled water dispenser.

The *pickup workstation* (often referred to as the "pickup window") is where prescriptions that have been filled and are ready for patient pickup are stored in the pharmacy. Prescriptions are usually kept in baskets or bins and are arranged in alphabetical order according to the patient's last name. This area is where prescriptions are dispensed to the patient and patient counseling takes place, so there should be a designated area where the pharmacist can have a confidential conversation with the patient.

The *medication storage system* usually consists of shelving units called "bays." These are typically horseshoe-shaped units with adjustable shelves to accommodate different bottle sizes. Bays are typically located directly behind the pharmacy counter, and the medications may be arranged in a variety of ways. One commonly used system has medications arranged alphabetically by brand name, with the generic equivalent alongside the brand-name container. Occasionally, the pharmacist may choose to arrange the medications by manufacturer. Since it is difficult to train staff to learn brand and generic names and there are multiple similar products, the use of straight alphabetizing is the preferred method for many pharmacists. A good number of pharmacies also have an area referred to as a "fast mover" section. This section contains medications that are most often dispensed by that pharmacy, and is usually located directly above the filling counter or on the end caps of the bays. This method of singling out fast-mover products is designed to save pharmacy employees time in retrieving medications. Some liquid, suppositories, and injectable medications require refrigeration. A full-sized or compact refrigerator is typically kept in the dispensing area. Prescriptions that have been filled with medications requiring refrigeration will be kept cool until dispensed. A note should be placed with the patient's paperwork indicating that the medication is located in the refrigerator.

## Medication Order Fulfillment (The Packaging Process)

Knapp et al defined the order fulfillment process as "bottling and preparation of the medication to be dispensed," and also stated that "Oversight and quality control of order fulfillment systems are professional functions of pharmacists that cannot be delegated."[12] Medication dispensing involves much more than counting by fives with a spatula and putting pills in a bottle. The dispensing process (*dispensing* indicates the medication has been packaged and is ready to be reviewed by the pharmacist) incorporates many important steps, each offering an opportunity to identify a potential or actual drug-related problem (see Table 14.1).

*Step One: Obtain the Prescription*

The initial step in this process is to acquire the prescription. This may be in person or via telephone, facsimile machine, e-mail, or the Internet. The person receiving the prescription should verify that all information on the prescription is legible and review the prescription for omissions (see Table 14.2). If any part of the prescription is not legible, make the necessary phone calls to verify information and clarify any discrepancies before processing and dispensing. It is critical to review prescriptions

**TABLE 14.1. CATEGORIES OF DRUG-RELATED PROBLEMS**

1. Nonadherence
2. Unnecessary medication
3. Need for additional medication
4. Ineffective medication
5. Dosage too low
6. Dosage too high
7. Adverse drug event
8. Drug-Drug interaction

**TABLE 14.2. INFORMATION TO VERIFY ON THE PRESCRIPTION**

1. Prescriber's name and address
2. Patient name and address
3. Other patient information, where necessary (age, date of birth, weight— esp. important for dispensing to children, etc.)
4. Drug indication, verifying the indication for the medication reduces the risk of medication errors
5. Date of issuance of the prescription
6. Drug name/strength/dosage form
7. Total quantity of medication to dispense
8. Instructions/directions for the medication (SIG), such as amount or units per dose, frequency, route of administration
9. Number of refills
10. DAW (dispense as written) line: indicates whether a generic medication may or may not be dispensed; requirements are state-specific; there may be a check box or additional prescriber signature on the blank to address this issue
11. Prescriber signature and address
12. Prescriber US Drug Enforcement Administration (DEA) number for controlled substance prescriptions (often a required piece of data for filing insurance claims for payment)
13. Length of therapy, this information is useful when reviewing a profile, monitoring for drug-related problems, and counseling patients

for completeness and to use the prescription as a starting point for identifying potential or actual drug-related problems.

Prescriptions telephoned into the pharmacy must be transcribed to written form immediately. Pharmacists, or in some states, licensed/registered pharmacy interns, are authorized to receive phoned-in prescriptions. Some states allow doctor's staff persons to leave phone-in prescriptions on a voicemail system, which are then transcribed to written form by the pharmacist. Interpretation of voicemail messages requires the pharmacist to be able to understand clearly what the prescriber is stating, as well as the prescriber indicating all of the necessary information needed to fulfill the prescription order. It is important to distinguish between physicians and their agents/representatives when prescriptions are called into the pharmacy. These agents/representatives (who could be clerks, administrative assistants, or nurses) may not be as familiar with medical terminology and word pronunciation. All prescription information called in from the doctor's office should be repeated back to the caller to verify all facts.

### Practice Pearl

Often student pharmacists feel rushed or nervous when speaking on the phone and forget to repeat information back to the prescriber. It takes a concentrated effort to make it a habit to repeat back information. It is worth your effort. If you practice in a State that permits interns to take phone-in prescriptions, repeat back the instructions to the prescriber at every phone-in opportunity. Developing this skill early on in your career will increase your professional communication confidence, as well as decrease the potential for a medication error.

Transmission of prescriptions via electronic mail (e-mail), directly through the computer via software, and by facsimile (fax) machine will continue to grow in popularity. With each process comes a new set of potential opportunities and problems. Regardless of how the prescription gets to the pharmacy, the information in Table 14.2 must be reviewed and verified.

The next step is to gather all patient information necessary for dispensing and counseling. Determine who is presenting the prescription: is it the patient, a family member, a caregiver, or another individual? Knowing this information will determine the validity of any information, how the counseling session will move forward, and what other calls might be necessary to address concerns and issues. It is also important to determine if the patient will wait for the prescription, return, or want it delivered or mailed.

## MANAGING THE CLINICAL MESSAGES/DUR MESSAGES/COMPUTER CHECKS

Almost every pharmacy dispensing computer system, and most third parties, incorporate programs designed to alert the pharmacist and support staff about various types of issues. These are commonly referred to as drug utilization review (DUR) alerts or messages. DUR alerts may include drug-drug or drug-disease interactions, allergies, and early or late refills. These alerts are designed to bring to the pharmacist's attention potentially risky situations, should the medication in question be dispensed. It is imperative that someone in a position to render judgment on these issues (ie, pharmacist, student pharmacist with preceptor supervision) reviews each message, takes the appropriate steps, and documents interventions. The goals when taking action on these alerts are to increase patient safety, improve patient care, and decrease liability. Please refer to Table 14.3 for examples of a DUR and pharmacist interventions.

## Technology

New software technology that permits scanning of the prescription into a database has changed the traditional workflow concept of medication order fulfillment. After the pharmacist or technician at the store level scans in the prescription, a central fill pharmacist and/or technician can take over the process. Please see section titled "Step Three: Pharmacist Final Check."

*Step Two: Order Fulfillment*

Once the initial interaction with the patient and/or caregiver has taken place, it is time for the behind-the-counter processes to begin. A patient profile is created or updated in the computer system and the prescription information is entered. The insurance/payment method is verified and any DUR alerts are addressed. The system updates files and prints a label and patient information leaflet. The stock package is retrieved from the shelf, and the prescription is filled, ensuring the dosage, dosage form, and other aspects of the medicine are appropriate for the patient.

*Drug Delivery System—Prescription Compounding*

Determining if the prescribed drug is being administered via an appropriate dosage form is based upon the pharmacist/student pharmacist assessment of the drug and the individual needs of the patient. You should evaluate patient characteristics that may influence the selection of a drug delivery system. Solid (capsules, tablets), liquid (solutions, suspensions, syrups), and topical (creams, lotions, ointments, gels, patches, inhalants) dosage forms are available. Determining the appropriate dosage form will facilitate the patient experiencing positive therapeutic response.

Prescription compounding offers the pharmacist an opportunity to develop a patient-specific product to meet a unique need. A multitude of resources are available to provide training and support for pharmacists interested in becoming

**TABLE 14.3.** DESCRIPTION OF THE PROCESS FOR MANAGING A DUR
MESSAGE/ALERT

Examples of a DUR (drug utilization review):

**Scenario #1.** *Patient presents for a refill on a medication to manage her diabetes (eg, Glyburide)*
*2 weeks early.*

The computer system and/or billing the patient's insurance and/or the pharmacist
review of the patient profile may determine the patient is requesting an early refill on
her prescription. This should prompt the pharmacist/intern to consult with the patient.
One common reason for the early refill is the prescriber tells the patient over the phone
to change directions for use (in this case, an increase in number of tablets used per day)
resulting in the patient running out of the medicine before the scheduled refill. This was
communicated verbally from the doctor to the patient, with no communication to the
pharmacy.

**Pharmacist intervention:** Initiated communication with the patient, verified the information
with the doctor's office, obtained a new prescription with the new SIG, and updated
records. Note: the opposite situation can occur too. A decrease in prescribed dose or
frequency of administration is ordered by the physician, but not communicated to the
pharmacy, resulting in a late refill. It is important to consult with the patient in either
scenario prior to consulting with the prescriber.

**Outcome:** The pharmacist/student should recognize the value of consulting with the
patient, even with respect to a day's supply issue, when evaluating a DUR message.

**Scenario #2.** *Computer software DUR message indicates a major interaction between two drugs on the*
*patient profile.*

Pharmacy computer software programs will often alert the pharmacist to potential
drug interactions via the DUR system. For example, a patient who receives a prescription
for Bactrim DS and is presently taking warfarin will generate a "red flag alert" for
the pharmacist to evaluate the patient profile and initiate efforts to prevent a drug-
related problem.

**Pharmacist intervention:** Initiated communication with the patient to inform of interaction,
initiated consultation with the prescriber and requested an antibiotic suitable for the
patient's condition that did not cause an interaction with the patient's warfarin, obtained
a new prescription and/or documented prescriber's directions for using Bactrim DS
concomitantly with warfarin, communicated discussion with prescriber to the patient,
and updated patient's pharmacy profile.

**Outcome:** The pharmacist/intern should recognize the value of preventing a serious
drug-related problem and also the value of documenting communication with the
patient and provider to facilitate access of information for pharmacy staff and/or
patient request.

compounding specialists. Patient groups such as those taking difficult-to-find medicines, individuals with swallowing problems, children who desire more tasteful flavors, and hospice patients with administration challenges all have special needs that can be met by compounding pharmacists. You are encouraged to participate in these types of services whenever possible, understanding it is essential to follow policy and procedure and to comply with legal regulations.

*Brand and Generic Drugs*

In the United States, each medication approved by the Food and Drug Administration (FDA) has a brand (or trade) name and a generic name. The generic name is the official, chemical name for the product's active ingredient. A brand-name product will usually become available as a generic product once the patent on the brand-name product has expired. In the United States new drug patents expire 17 years from the time the drug is discovered, not from the time the drug is commercially available. Generic drugs are almost always less expensive than the brand-name product, which is an opportunity for pharmacists to offer medications at a reduced cost.

Patients may raise questions about the quality of generic medications, and pharmacists and students must be ready to address and alleviate patient concerns. The FDA approves generic products, and the generic products must meet the same stringent requirements as brand-name products. In some clinical circumstances, brand-name products are preferred over generic products, for example, medications with a narrow range between subtherapeutic, therapeutic, and toxic levels. Examples include Lanoxin (digoxin), Synthroid (levothyroxine), and Coumadin (warfarin). These medications are commonly referred to as narrow-therapeutic-index drugs. A good resource to determine the therapeutic equivalence of approved drug products is the *Orange Book*, a publication updated regularly by the US Department of Health and Human Services (HHS).[23]

Another issue affecting whether or not a generic medication is dispensed is the type of insurance the patient has and the requirements of the specific plan. Some insurance companies mandate dispensing of generics, while others incentivize the use of generics based on lower out-of-pocket costs (co-pays) for the patient. In addition, some state laws require that the pharmacist offer generic products to patients when generics are available. The pharmacist/student pharmacist must address all pertinent issues related to generic medications, so patients receive the greatest benefit from the prescribed medication.

*Auxiliary Label*

During order fulfillment the appropriate auxiliary labels need to be placed on the prescription vial. These are usually applied in a conspicuous place without interfering with information on the prescription label. Auxiliary labels provide additional patient information and instructions for medication use. Examples are listed in Table 14.4.

**TABLE 14.4.** INFORMATION SUPPLIED BY AUXILIARY LABELS

1. How and when to take the drug

2. What to avoid when taking the medication (such as foods, other medications)

3. If the product is a new generic drug for the same medication dispensed previously

4. Possible adverse effects

5. The expiration date, especially if it is a reconstituted medication

6. How to store the medicine

*National Drug Code Number*

Once the prescription is completely assembled, all work should be rechecked by comparing the information on the label with the written prescription and the stock bottle. The best verification for ensuring that the correct product is in the prescription container is through the use of the National Drug Code (NDC) number. The NDC number is assigned by the manufacturer for each specific product. The NDC code has 11 numbers, and provides the following three pieces of information about each product: manufacturer (first five digits), drug name, strength, dosage form (next four digits), and package size (last two digits). An important part of checking prescriptions and verifying drugs prescribed for patients is matching the NDC number on the stock bottle with the product number printed on the label. NDC numbers are also used for billing prescriptions through third parties and insurance companies.

*Step Three: Pharmacist Final Check*

The final check of the prescription must be conducted by the pharmacist. Once it is ready for dispensing, the prescription, the patient information leaflet, and any other necessary information for the patient are placed in a bag. If filling more than one prescription for a patient, the correct information must be kept with the respective prescription. If filling prescriptions for more than one family member, the prescriptions for each family member should be placed in a separate dispensing bag. Putting prescriptions for more than one patient in the same bag increases liability and the chances of mistakenly dispensing a prescription to the wrong individual. Also, when filling prescriptions for someone with a common name, it is important to double check that you are dispensing medication for the correct patient. Pharmacy staff should verify the patient's date of birth and address prior to dispensing the product to prevent a medication error.

Patient adherence with prescribed therapy is important for patients to achieve positive health outcomes. The term "adherence" is selected for this chapter, as it reflects a more participatory action on the part of the patient. Many adherence devices are available to assist patients with taking their medications. Table 14.5 lists the most frequently used devices. Each device should be selected based on specific benefits and patient needs.

---

**TABLE 14.5.** COMMONLY RECOMMENDED ADHERENCE DEVICES

1. Pill boxes

2. Dosing spoons for pediatric use

3. Droppers for small doses of liquids

4. Dial-a-dose containers

5. Medication calendars

6. Beeping devices

7. Telephone call reminders

8. Internet/e-mail reminders

---

## TELEPHARMACY AND TELEHEALTH—UPCOMING CHANGES IN MEDICATION ORDER FULFILLMENT PRACTICE

Telepharmacy may be defined as "the use of electronic information and communication technologies to provide and support health care when distance separates the participants."[1,25]

As social media continues to shape how we interact with one another, the practice of telepharmacy/telehealth will evolve to accommodate these changes. An example of telepharmacy practice is the use of pharmacists and support staff working at a central fill location (not at the store where the prescription was dropped off) to perform prescription entry and/or assembly functions. The intent of using a central order fulfillment process (central fill) is to decrease the amount of time needed to prepare a medication for dispensing, and to reduce the need for additional pharmacy personnel at the store level. In the United States, some state regulations permit the central fill pharmacist to review the prescription and send a label to the store-level printer for the technician to complete the packaging process. The pharmacist at the store level then performs the final verification. Another traditional chain pharmacy has the central fill pharmacist and technician team perform all aspects of medication order fulfillment (packaging, following up with physician for prescription order clarification, etc.) and mail the packaged medication to the store within a defined period of time (eg, 24 hours). In this case, the main responsibility of the store-level pharmacist is to counsel the patient at pickup. In regards to counseling, pharmacists are performing medication reviews telephonically and/or via a webcam.[24]

### Workflow Issues: Quality-Related Events and Continuous Quality Improvement

Training staff to be proficient at each workstation is essential to dispense medications in a timely manner. The pharmacist is ultimately in charge of determining who works at each station, assuring the employee is competent at following the rules of that station, and recognizing when a staff member needs extra training and/or feedback to do the job well. Medication errors are more likely to occur in an environment where the responsibilities at each workstation are not recognized or followed by the staff. In the United States, many state boards of pharmacy have enacted legislation to promote effective management of workflow. The legislation encourages pharmacists to document quality-related events (QREs) as part of a continuous quality improvement (CQI) process to determine workflow issues (not enough staff, technology failure, etc.).[8] A QRE may be defined as the inappropriate dispensing or administration of a prescribed medication product. CQI may be defined as a system of standards or procedures to identify and evaluate QREs to improve patient care.[8] The goal for all staff reporting QREs is to review the workflow issues and determine what part of the process might be compromising patient safety. This is meant to be a nonpunitive process and, therefore, names of persons involved are not listed in the report. Only the incident is documented. For example, if a prescription is dispensed with the wrong directions on the label, the QRE may indicate that the error occurred at the prescription intake station on a day when the electricity was lost for 5 minutes. During the electrical outage, information typed into the computer was lost, and the Rx label was printed incorrectly. A positive outcome of documenting this QRE is the store owner may install generator back-up to prevent future electrical shortages from interfering with order entry. Ideally, QRE reports should be reviewed quarterly, so changes may be implemented in a timely manner. You ought to work closely with the pharmacy staff during the dispensing process in order to learn the workflow, understand the role of each staff member in the process, and recognize areas of concern (eg, a technician calls out sick leaving the pharmacy short-staffed, etc.) which may lead to a potential medication error. Finally, you should be able to document QREs, especially drug-related events, via the policy and procedures of that pharmacy.

## Financial Data in Community Pharmacy Practice

An important aspect of community practice is the financial structure of the business. Although most of your activities are focused on patient care, an understanding of the finances will assist in making sense of many of the organizational decisions, such as staff and resource allocation, product mix, and program development. The balance sheet has two sides: income and expenses. Income into the pharmacy is primarily generated through three sources: sales of prescription medications, sales of nonprescription products, and other income (which varies considerably among organizations). Examples of income gathering services provided by the pharmacist are performing MTM, administration of immunization and/or disease screening.[6]

On the expense/cost side of the ledger, there are many items for which a company has to pay out monies, including costs of goods sold (both prescription and OTC products), interest on loans/line of credit, and the general operating expenses associated with most businesses (including human resources, marketing and advertising, rent and leases, and professional services).

Net operating income or loss before taxes is calculated by totaling sales and income, then subtracting all expenses. Often there is a fine line between making a profit and taking a loss. This is why many managers of community pharmacies are constantly looking to expand sales in their nonprescription departments which offer more margin dollars and greater chances for improved profits.

## Getting Paid for Medication Order Fulfillment

### Third-Party Issues

Third-party prescriptions are paid for by a provider or payer. There are three parties involved in the payment of these prescriptions: the patient, the pharmacist, and the payer. Payers may be private insurance companies, government programs, or any other organization paying for prescriptions. Third-party payers are responsible for payment for an increasing number of prescriptions, and they have had a significant effect on profits and the role of the pharmacist. A key concern with third-party prescriptions is the amount of payment received by the pharmacy. With third-party prescriptions, patients pay a premium for a prescription card obtained through their medical insurance program. The card entitles them to obtain prescriptions from an approved pharmacy under a shared-payment structure. The insurance company pays for part of the prescription cost, while the patient pays either a deductible or co-pay. Often, the total reimbursement is insufficient to make a profit just from prescription sales.

### Prescription Costs—Pharmacy Operations Issues

Community pharmacies are usually reimbursed a percentage of Average Wholesale Price (AWP) as an estimate of the drug cost, plus a dispensing fee for pharmacy services. The difference between the actual acquisition cost of the medication and the drug cost estimate typically offsets operational costs. The Medicare Part D prescription benefit, as well as legislators considering changing the use of AWP as a basis for pharmacy reimbursement has threatened the ability of the pharmacy manager to offset operational costs.

The average percentage of total revenues generated from the prescription department for the different types of pharmacies varies significantly. The number ranges from approximately 6% for the mass merchandisers, to 10% for the supermarkets, 50% for the average large chain, and around 90% for the typical independent pharmacy. What does this mean? The independent pharmacy is at the greatest risk from decreasing reimbursement rates for prescriptions, whereas the other types of organizations have many more options for sales and revenue generation. Independent pharmacy owners report feeling pressured to accept lower reimbursement for their services because they have limited power to leverage when negotiating contract terms with insurers.[3]

## Customer Conveniences

In addition to the dispensing and counseling processes, a number of other issues may have a profound effect on the pharmacist-patient relationship. For lack of a better term, these will be called "customer conveniences." They are listed below:

*Drive-Through Pharmacies*

Drive-through pharmacies are a convenience for patients, especially parents with sick children who do not want to take the child out of the car to get a prescription filled. Drive-through pharmacies are also a convenience for elderly or disabled who may have difficulty getting in and out of the car. However, the lack of face-to-face contact with the patient has the potential to jeopardize optimal health outcomes and affects the pharmacist's ability to address patient concerns.

*Extended Hours*

Many of the larger chain and mass merchandiser pharmacies have extended pharmacy hours to try to meet the needs of our time-conscious society. This can be an opportunity for pharmacists to interact with patients at times when the pharmacy may not be quite as busy.

*Prescription Delivery*

Prescription delivery is a specialty service offered to patients who cannot come to the pharmacy. For refills, where the patient has at least a general understanding of the medication, delivery service can be beneficial in improving adherence. However, for a new prescription, prescription delivery eliminates face-to-face contact with the pharmacist, again reducing the opportunity for a pharmacist to counsel on medication use.

*Drug Kiosks and Other New Technology*

Prescription pickup kiosks are freestanding machines that hold filled prescriptions until customers are ready to pick them up. Kiosks work similar to ATM machines, where customers enter a pin number to retrieve their prescription. In August 2005, a mass merchandiser pharmacy installed a prescription kiosk in a New York store in Penn Station.[11]

The states of Missouri and Hawaii have automated prescription kiosk systems where the pharmacy must maintain a video and audio system to provide effective oral communication between pharmacist and patient. In addition, the kiosk must allow the patient to print written information.[15]

Hospital systems are looking at dispensing medications, including over the counter drugs, via kiosks.[19]

The impact of patients using prescription drug kiosks and bypassing pharmacist face-to-face contact is unknown; however, in the near future, pharmacists should actively approach the concept of counseling patients via mHealth technologies such as their personal computer, web TV, or personal digital devices. Your pharmacy curriculum may include (or soon include) coursework to integrate telehealth technology in pharmacy practice patient care activities.[21,25]

## Third Class of Drugs

The FDA has given consideration to creating a third class of drugs in the United States. The Consumer Healthcare Products association defines a third class of drugs as being available only through a pharmacist.[22] Creating a third class or a transitional class of drugs would require an act of Congress. FDA has repeatedly rejected supporting the creation of the third class based on it causing decreased patient access to meds. A 2007 survey determined 68% of 1000 survey respondents in the United States strongly to somewhat supported the creation of a third class of drugs.[2] With that in mind, certain types of insulin, emergency contraception, products containing pseudoephedrine, and cough medication containing schedule 5 narcotic, all must be kept behind the counter. This is conceptually equivalent to a third class.[13,20] While a pharmacy clerk may sell these items, this is an excellent opportunity for the community pharmacist to counsel a patient.[14]

## COMMUNITY PHARMACY PRACTICE: PATIENT-CARE ISSUES

### Patient Confidentiality

Patient confidentiality is necessary in all aspects of community pharmacy practice. Laws vary from state to state, but all states consider the issue of confidentiality a high priority. Many organizations are transitioning from paper to electronic medical records. Healthcare administrators, legislators, and lobbying groups will be focused on limiting access to electronic data to individuals with proper credentials. Levels of security and individuals with access to specific types of data will be specifically outlined within each organization. It is very important for pharmacists to support the position of their need to access patient information so they can advance their practices, improve patient care, collect outcomes data, and document their value to third-party payers.

Confidentiality in community pharmacy practice during day-to-day operations is a constant challenge. Confidentiality can be unknowingly/accidentally violated in many situations, so it is critical for everyone in the pharmacy to be aware of these situations and to act appropriately. Some examples where confidentiality might be jeopardized are described in Table 14.6. The US Department of Health and Human Services (HHS) established a set of standards for the protection of health information as required by the Health Insurance Portability and Accountability Act of 1996 (HIPAA).[9] The goal of HIPAA is to assure an individual's health information is properly protected, while allowing the transfer of health information necessary for provision of quality health care. You may have already signed a confidentiality

**TABLE 14.6. SITUATIONS IN THE COMMUNITY PHARMACY WITH POTENTIAL FOR BREACH OF CONFIDENTIALITY**

1. **Telephone communications.** When taking a telephoned prescription, calling for a prescription transfer, providing a transfer to another pharmacy, repeating the information for verification purposes, or listening to a voicemail recording, it would be very easy to repeat the patient name and medication loud enough for a customer or patient to overhear the information. Be cognizant of your proximity to the lay population and adjust your tone of voice to avoid inadvertently causing a HIPAA violation.

2. **Patient counseling.** When counseling a patient on his or her medication, it would be easy to share information loud enough for someone to overhear what was being discussed. Chain pharmacies are constantly redesigning their pharmacy department to take this issue into consideration. Management of already established workspaces can reorganize the workflow to increase the pharmacist's opportunity to speak with customers in an area that addresses the confidentiality needs.

3. **Refill request at the intake window.** Some patients will present to the pharmacy for refills of their prescription, yet not remember which medication they need. Asking permission of the patient to read the names of the medications out loud prior to engaging in the activity is one possible solution.

4. **Position of the prescription pickup bins.** If the bins are too close to the register, patients might be able to read the names printed on the prescription bag.

5. **Provision of pharmacy records.** Patients are eligible for a copy of their prescription records as per the Health Insurance Portability and Accountability Act of 1996 (HIPAA). Remember to follow the store policy and procedure to prepare and deliver this information, which usually requires the requesting patient to sign a release form. Only provide the information to the requesting patient and/or approved caretaker, for example, the parent of a child.

agreement on the first day of your practice experience indicating you will follow the policies and procedures regarding confidentiality at your site.

## Prescription Costs

Prescription medications are a vital part of prevention and/or treatment of a medical illness. Prescription drug costs in the United States were approximately $234 billion in 2008, approximately six times the $40.3 billion spent in 1990.[10] Prescription drug prices as measured by the Consumer Price Index increased 3.4% in 2009, 2.5% in 2008, 1.4% in 2007, and 4.3% in 2006. The average annual growth in prescription drug prices from 2000 to 2009 was 3.6 percent, compared to 4.1% for all medical care.[21] Industry data show that retail prescription prices[12] rose from an average price of $38.43 in 1998 to $71.69 in 2008. In 2008, the average brand name prescription price was $137.90, almost 4 times the average generic price of $35.22.[10] Rising costs have raised concerns about the affordability of prescription medications, and patients often exhibit frustration by directing accusations at the pharmacy staff. It is not necessarily the pharmacist or the pharmacy that is responsible for rising prices. Three main factors are directly involved in the increasing cost of prescription medication:

1. **Utilization**—From 1999 to 2009, the number of prescriptions increased 39% (from 2.8 billion to 3.9 billion), compared to a US population growth of 9%. The number of prescriptions dispensed in the US in 2009 increased 2.1% (from 3.8 billion to 3.9 billion), a larger growth rate than the 1.0% increase in 2008 over 2007.[10] Medications are often the least expensive and preferred option for treating disease. As the population ages, more prescriptions will be written and dispensed for the ailments and conditions of this age group.
2. **Availability of new medications/drug advertising**—Although the development of new molecular entities (drugs) is critical to progress in patient care, the cost of bringing a new drug to market continues to rise. Manufacturer research and development (R&D) spending was about $65 billion developing new medicines and vaccines in 2009, an increase of about $1.5 billion over 2008.[10] Manufacturer spending on advertising was over 1.5 times as much in 2009 ($10.9 billion) as in 1999 ($6.6 billion).[10]
3. **Development of formularies**—Private employers, local, state and federal government, and insurers create formularies (a list of medications deemed cost-effective as per respective insuring company), or simply shift the total cost (eg, nonformulary product) to the individual.

## Communication Skills

Development of verbal, nonverbal, and written communication skills is a challenging, yet necessary exercise for you. Communications with patients, physicians and their staff, insurance companies, and others will be vital to your success in the community pharmacy practice environment, and ultimately, your effectiveness in taking care of patients. This section is designed to emphasize a few of the basic aspects of communication skills in the community pharmacy setting. (Communication skills are covered further, with practice exercises in Chap. 4 of this text.)

One of the most important aspects of prescription dispensing is the interaction with the patient. In the United States, the rules of Omnibus Budget and Reconciliation Act of 1990 (commonly referred to as OBRA-90) mandate certain professional responsibilities of the pharmacist when dispensing prescriptions for Medicaid (government third-party payer) patients. These responsibilities include:

1. OBRA-90 mandates that patients who utilize the United States Medicaid program receive an offer from the pharmacist to be counseled on their medications.
2. This legislation also requires that pharmacists maintain patient profiles for Medicaid patients that include information such as a list of disease states, medications, allergies, and adverse events.

**3.** The pharmacist must also perform a prospective drug utilization review of the entire patient profile prior to dispensing a prescription.

The goal of the OBRA-90 requirements is to help reduce the incidence of drug-related problems such as medication-related adverse effects, duplication of therapy, and poor adherence, to prevent negative patient outcomes. Many states have expanded these responsibilities to include all patients, so outcomes and costs can be improved in the entire population of medication users. It is important to understand the state-specific patient counseling requirements applicable for the practice site where you are based.

Written communications are necessary at times to share or to request information. Preparing written materials using the fourth to sixth grade reading level increases the likelihood that most patients will be able to comprehend the document. Try to avoid the use of scientific terminology, as it may confuse or upset patients.

Verbal communications can take place either over the telephone or in person. When answering the phone, be sure to identify yourself. Be sure to familiarize yourself with the verbal communication processes used by your preceptor and staff members at that practice site. Recognize that you will consistently have to triage calls, distinguishing those that you can answer from those that must be referred to staff in the pharmacy or other departments. Ask for examples of when to transfer a call, information to obtain when receiving a refill request, and if there are any specific medications that will require additional effort from the patient such as the patient has to be the individual to sign for it at time of pickup.

Pharmacist-to-patient dialogue is usually prompted through the need for individual counseling or the need to obtain information. Prior to counseling an individual be sure to clarify who will actually be picking up the prescription, as the conversation will take on a different tone if it is someone else. During the counseling session, ask open-ended questions, such as the ones listed in Table 14.7. The information gathered from the open-ended questions will assist you and the pharmacist in knowing the specifics needed to complete the counseling process.

The last step in the counseling process is to assess patient understanding of the information you have communicated. During this assessment the pharmacist/student has the patient repeat the information that was just shared, in order to substantiate patient understanding. A key prompt to ask the patient is "Just to make sure that I did not forget to tell you anything important, please describe how you are going to use the medicine."

## Meeting OBRA-90 Counseling Requirement

A brief overview of a new or refill prescription consult fulfills the OBRA-90 counseling requirement. Community pharmacists while counseling a patient on a new or refilled medication may use the opportunity to refer that patient for an MTM consult. See the section "Medication Therapy Management Services" for detailed information.

TABLE 14.7. PATIENT ASSESSMENT: KEY OPEN-ENDED QUESTIONS TO ASK DURING A COUNSELING SESSION

1. What did the doctor tell you this medication is for?
   a. What problem or symptom is it supposed to help?
   b. What is it supposed to do?
2. How did your doctor tell you to take this medication?
   a. How often did your doctor say to take it?
   b. How much were you instructed to take?
   c. How long were you instructed to take this medication?
   d. What did your doctor say to do when you miss a dose?
   e. How should you store this medication?
3. What did your doctor tell you to expect from the medication?
   a. What good effects are you supposed to expect?
   b. How will you know if the medication is working?
   c. What bad effects did your doctor tell you to watch for?
   d. What should you do if a bad reaction occurs?
   e. What precautions are you to take while on this medication?
   f. How will you know if it is not working?
   g. What are you to do if the medication does not work?

## OTC Medications—the Patient Consultation

One of the unique aspects of community pharmacy practice is the opportunity to counsel patients on the use of over-the-counter (OTC) medications. A medication with OTC status in the United States has been determined by the FDA as "generally recognized as safe and effective." The key areas of focus for the pharmacist/student pharmacist should include cough/cold, allergy, pain/analgesia, GI (antacids, laxatives), dietary aids, vitamins, minerals, supplements, and herbs, products for the skin, self-testing/diagnostics, and feminine hygiene. Other areas include first aid, eye/ear, foot care, oral care, home health care, and baby needs.

The primary goal of the OTC consult is to assist the patient in determining the best approach to a particular situation. The consult may have one or more of the following four outcomes: recommend a product for the individual, refer the individual to the physician, recommend a product and refer the individual to a physician, or provide health education without recommending a product at this time. Individuals with certain disease states require special attention, as their concurrent conditions have a significant impact on OTC recommendations. Special populations include neonates/infants/pediatrics, breastfeeding mothers, pregnant women, elderly patients, some disabled patients, patients with HIV, mental health disorders, or diabetes. Consumers should be made aware of the many risks and benefits of OTC product selection.[7] Utilization of effective questioning techniques, active listening, and assessment of nonverbal cues by the pharmacist often results in an educated and satisfied patient.

OTC medications have pharmacologic, pharmacokinetic, and toxicological properties, in addition to precautions, interactions, and contraindications that must be taken into consideration in discussions with patients. When counseling about OTC medications, it is important to consider these medications as an important part of the patient's overall medication regimen, and to assess for potential interactions or effects on other medications. You should pay special attention to opportunities to become involved as either an observer or an active participant in OTC consults. If you feel the need to follow-up with the individual to assess his or her response to the medication, ensure that this will take place by documenting the interaction in the profile and making a note to contact at a later date. An example of a question and answer session with an individual about an OTC product is included below.

## Example of an OTC Consultation

*Situation:* You are in the pharmacy and notice a woman in the cough/cold section. You approach her, introduce yourself, and ask "How may I help you today?" (Remember to ask open-ended questions.) She replies that she is looking for a product for her daughter. You obtain the following information to help you determine your course of action:

| Student/Pharmacist Questions | Mother's Response |
| --- | --- |
| Who is the patient? | My daughter |
| What are her symptoms? | She has a low-grade fever (100°F–101°F), and a cough |
| How long has she had these symptoms? | Started this morning |
| How old is she? | 7 years old |
| What is her weight? | Approximately 54 lbs |
| What are her allergies/reactions? | Penicillin—she had a rash and hives |
| What are her medical conditions? | History of ear infections between ages 2 and 5; none in past year |
| Have you called your doctor about this yet? | Not yet |
| Do you have access to medical care? | Yes, we have a pediatrician |
| What medications is your daughter taking? | None |
| Did you give her any medicine for the fever this morning? | No |
| Are there other children in the house? | Yes, a 3-year-old and a 9-month-old; both are feeling well so far |

Based on the discussion, the pharmacist may have done the following:

1. Recommended a fever reducing medication formulated for a 7-year-old child.
2. Confirmed the dosage by double checking the child's weight.
3. Educated the mother that the fever temperature should decrease within half hour to hour after administering the medication. Reinforce the importance of always reading the directions and not administering more than prescribed on the label.
4. Educated the mother that if the fever persists more than 24 hours, she should talk to her pediatrician.
5. Educated the mother that she should *not* give this fever-reducing formulation to her 3-year-old or infant child, as the formulation strength is not appropriate.
6. Provided her with the pharmacy phone number and suggested that she should call should she have further questions.

Certainly, there will be situations where this much depth is not necessary. However, you should always be prepared to enter into an OTC consult with this systematic approach in mind.

## Pharmacist Administration of Immunizations

In addition to MTM programs, community pharmacists are also expanding patient-care services into the area of immunizations. All states in the United States currently have legislation permitting pharmacists to administer vaccines. In some states, pharmacist immunization practices are limited to influenza, and/or must be performed under a collaborative agreement with a physician provider.

Other states allow pharmacists to immunize patients for pneumonia, hepatitis, shingles, and tetanus as well as perform immunizations for pediatric patients. The authority to immunize is a major milestone for community pharmacist practitioners. Administration of immunizations and education on vaccine-preventable illnesses is an excellent opportunity for pharmacists to act as health educators and public health advocates for the local community.

## Medication Therapy Management Services

The integration of pharmacist-provided patient care with traditional medication order fulfillment activities has been the goal for many innovative pharmacists (Fig. 14.2).

Pharmacists are considered easily accessible and approachable healthcare providers and are known to give brief, pertinent advice on medication use. Due to the fact more people are taking medication on a daily basis and especially the elderly, who are taking multiple medications per day, the Center for Medicare and Medicaid services (CMS) mandated that plans administering federal pharmacy benefits have to include medication therapy management services (MTM).[17] MTM is the opportunity for pharmacists to provide cognitive care in addition to dispensing medication to their patients.

**Figure 14.2.** Medication use process.

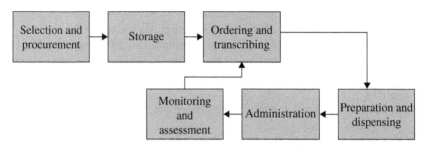

Eleven national pharmacy organizations developed a consensus definition of MTM in July 2004 (see Table 14.8).[16] With the consensus in place, the American Pharmacists Association and the National Association of Chain Drug Stores Foundation developed a model framework for implementation of effective MTM entitled *Medication Therapy Management in Community Pharmacy Practice: Core Elements of an MTM Service Version 2.0.* The goal of the framework is to provide continuity of care for the patient and/or their caregiver by using the five core elements of MTM: medication therapy review (MTR), personal medication list (PML), medication-related action plan (MAP), intervention and/or referral, and documentation and follow-up (see Table 14.8 for definition of MTM Core Elements).[16] The key steps for implementing a successful MTM program include developing and/or updating all relevant policies and procedures, assessing work flow in the pharmacy to decide how MTM will fit into the existing processes, identifying equipment and resource needs, developing a clinical database, assessing the financials, designing a marketing and advertising plan, implementing the program, monitoring progress, and executing a strategy for CQI.

It is important to note the range of MTM. A pharmacist may choose to provide a simple MTM consult by educating a patient on the use of a medical device. On the other hand, pharmacists may also perform a comprehensive assessment of medication use (review of drug profile for drug-drug, drug-disease, drug-diet interactions, appropriate use of medication, appropriate monitoring and management of adverse events) or targeted disease state management (eg, diabetes). In the case of a targeted MTM consult, a pharmacist may provide a very intricate disease state management (DSM) program, with detailed processes outlined to help patients manage the many complexities of a disease such as diabetes. Pharmacists may also perform point-of-care  monitoring for health conditions such as dyslipidemia and osteoporosis.

In 2009, most community pharmacists were engaged in the simple provision of MTM, such as teaching patients how to use metered-dose inhalers or blood glucose meters. Future MTM services will likely include pharmacists assessing and utilizing

---

**TABLE 14.8.** DEFINITION AND FIVE CORE ELEMENTS OF MEDICATION THERAPY MANAGEMENT SERVICES[16]

| | |
|---|---|
| *Definition* | "Medication therapy management is a distinct service or group of services that optimize therapeutic outcomes for individual patients. Medication therapy management services are independent of, but can occur in conjunction with, the provision of a medication product and encompass a broad range of professional activities and responsibilities within the licensed pharmacist's, or other qualified health-care provider's scope of practice." (see Reference for complete definition) |

**FIVE CORE ELEMENTS OF MTM**

| | |
|---|---|
| **1. *Medication Therapy Review (MTR)*** | It is a systematic process of collecting patient-specific information, assessing medication therapies to identify medication-related problems, developing a prioritized list of medication-related problems, and creating a plan to resolve them. |
| **2. *Personal Medication List (PML)*** | It is a comprehensive record of the patient's medications (prescription and nonprescription medications, herbal products, and other dietary supplements). |
| **3. *Medication-Related Action Plan (MAP)*** | It is a patient-centric document containing a list of actions for the patient to use in tracking progress for self-management. |
| **4. *Intervention and/or Referral*** | The pharmacist provides consultative services and intervenes to address medication-related problems; when necessary, the pharmacist refers the patient to a physician or other health-care professional. |
| **5. *Documentation and Followup*** | Interventions are documented, and a follow-up visit is scheduled based on the patient's medication-related needs or the need for continuity of care when transitioning through the healthcare system. |

---

pharmacogenomics to optimize a patient therapy regimen. The next step for these pharmacists is to attain continuing education in their respective areas of interest and consider specialty certification in these areas. Ideally, community pharmacists will join the ranks of their ambulatory care colleagues in developing collaborations with prescribers to provide comprehensive disease state management.

Pharmacists who are apprehensive to engage in MTM may benefit from taking a certification course (offered by many state and national organizations) in MTM or in specific disease state management. Such courses offer the education a pharmacist needs to provide targeted care. At present, the most common programs in the community pharmacy setting are diabetes, hypertension, dyslipidemia, and asthma. Some community pharmacies where you will be placed for an experiential education course may have disease state management programs in place; however, these programs may be in various conditions of development, and may vary in the types and extent of services they provide. One common goal for all MTM programs is to improve patient outcomes.

In order to provide MTM, the pharmacist needs to protect a block of time in the work week away from order fulfillment. For the pharmacy business to sustain such a change, the integration of MTM must incorporate strategies to generate revenues.

Being paid for MTM is a challenging task. In 2007, the American Medical Association approved the following current procedural terminology (CPT) codes for payment of MTM (see Table 14.9 for code definitions).[5] CPT codes for provision of medication management is a major milestone for the pharmacy profession.

Finally, to market the value of patient-care interventions, pharmacists need to take the initiative to develop MTM programs, document their value, and then present data to the decision makers within payer organizations to assist in contracting for payment. In the future, pharmacists who only engage in medication order fulfillment are at risk of being replaced by advancements in automation and technology. As a student pharmacist, you will graduate with the clinical knowledge and aptitude to act as an agent of change and move the practice of community pharmacy into the future—a future including the provision of MTM.

**TABLE 14.9.** CURRENT PROCEDURAL TERMINOLOGY CODES FOR MEDICATION THERAPY MANAGEMENT SERVICES[5]

| CPT Code | Definition |
| --- | --- |
| 99605 | Medication therapy management service(s) provided by a pharmacist, individual, face-to-face with patient, initial 15 minutes, with assessment, and intervention if provided; initial 15 minutes, new patient |
| 99606 | Initial 15 minutes, established patient |
| 99607 | Each additional 15 minutes (To be listed separately in addition to code for the primary service; eg, 99605 or 99606) |

## How to Conduct a Medication Therapy Management Interview

The medication therapy management interview is a goal-directed communication. The purpose is for one person to obtain information from another. The degree of success of the interview is a measure of the effectiveness of communication between the pharmacist/student pharmacist and the individual. The goals in conducting a medication therapy management interview should include the following:

1. Obtain information from the patient to establish a more comprehensive database than what exists in the pharmacy computer.
2. Establish a pharmacist-patient relationship by explaining the benefits of MTM.
3. Incorporate MTM Core Elements (see Table 14.8).
4. Observe the patient's behavior for trends that may affect outcomes.

The following is a description of the content of a comprehensive medication therapy interview:

Each interview must be tailored in emphasis and content to satisfy the needs of the particular patient. In the community setting, a great majority of medication interviews will take place "blind"; that is, the only information the pharmacist will have in advance is the individual profile and whatever he or she knows about the patient from previous visits and discussions. If any additional information is available before the medication interview, it should be reviewed and used to augment the interview process. Pharmacist's access to an individual's electronic medical record (and, therefore, essential data such as laboratory results) may dramatically affect his or her ability to provide optimal direct patient-care services.

In most cases, you will be supervised by a pharmacist during the interview process, especially your first couple of interviews. The level of your participation will vary based on experience and the particular situation. Before an interview is attempted, you should become familiar with as much of the individual's social, medical, and medication information as possible. Introduce yourself and explain your purpose. It is important to seek approval to conduct the interview. Attempt to conduct the interview in a comfortable area with a limited number of outside distractions. Establish professional rapport and keep social conversation to a minimum. It is important to get to the point of the interview, and the individual should feel as though he or she has your complete attention and interest. Allow the individual to speak without interruptions unless the person begins to digress. Verbal and nonverbal cues may be used to keep the patient on track without significant interruption.

Begin the interview with a general question about the patient; then obtain the necessary demographic information. Review the specific information obtained about medications, such as indication, dosing schedules, duration of therapy, and reasons for discontinuing. Remember to include information about both prescription and over-the-counter medications. Special care should be taken when interacting with women to ensure issues such as medication effects in pregnancy and lactation are addressed (if appropriate). Ask if he or she has ever had an adverse effect to a medication and obtain as many details about the event as possible. Close the interview with a summary of the information obtained. This allows the interviewer to check information for accuracy, and it may remind the patient or caregiver of other significant information that may have been overlooked. A statement that you may contact the individual later to ask for more details leaves this option open in case you have forgotten something.

The student/pharmacist may obtain information from individuals in various ways. The comprehensive patient medication history interview is one method to accomplish this goal. However, the person may be unwilling to spend the necessary time with the student/pharmacist. Each individual should be assessed and a determination made regarding the optimal method of obtaining additional information.

## MTM Patient Empowerment—Pharmacist as a Health Educator

The community pharmacist is an accessible health-care provider in a prime position to act as a health educator and a facilitator of patient empowerment. Individual empowerment refers to the concept that providing pertinent health-related information enables the patient to make his or her own informed health-care decisions. Patient empowerment is the key to achieving optimal medication therapy outcomes. Pharmacists may empower the individual by working together to identify the patient's healthcare barriers and designing strategies to overcome them. The use of motivational interviewing and other empowerment techniques may be needed to facilitate these interactions. The key to educating individuals is the act of engaging the patient and tailoring information to their lifestyle—not just telling them what to do. For example, you can tell an individual with asthma who is severely allergic to pollen to never go outside during pollen season. This is impractical and useless. Instead, educate the individual to keep her mouth covered with the cup of her hand or a small scarf in order to minimize the exposure to the pollen. An example related to medication use is to engage the patient in adherence strategies by asking the individual *what time she prefers* to use her controller inhaler and linking the medication use to her daily routine (eg, before breakfast and at bedtime). Ask her to *show* you how she uses the inhaler, and recommend any pertinent changes in technique, as compared to just stating "Use this inhaler twice a day."

## AMBULATORY CARE PHARMACY: PRACTICE ISSUES

### Introduction to Ambulatory Care Practice

In recent years, health care in the United States has been shifting toward an increased emphasis on health promotion, disease prevention, and management of chronic illness in the outpatient setting. With this transition, pharmacy skills in the ambulatory care environment are of increasing importance. Topics covered in other chapters of this textbook, such as drug information (Chap. 13), physical assessment (Chap. 10), and communication skills (Chap. 4) are important for successful performance in the ambulatory care setting.

## Practice Site

Ambulatory care pharmacy is an exciting and diverse area of pharmacy. Pharmacists specializing in ambulatory care may practice in an academic medical center, a community pharmacy, a private physician's office, or another type of practice with an outpatient focus (treatment of chronic and acute nonemergent illnesses). Ambulatory care pharmacists may treat patients with a wide range of chronic conditions such as diabetes, hypertension, asthma, and heart failure, or they may focus on a specialized patient population, such as patients with HIV or specific neurologic disorders. Please see Table 14.10 for a list of potential types of ambulatory care practice sites and common disease states encountered in the ambulatory practice setting.

## Level of Practice

Ambulatory care pharmacists may participate in any number of activities related to patient care, including performing targeted disease state management (MTM), counseling patients on new prescriptions, utilizing techniques to enhance adherence, reporting and tracking adverse drug reactions, administering immunizations,

**TABLE 14.10. TYPES OF AMBULATORY CARE PRACTICE SITES AND DISEASE STATES COMMONLY ENCOUNTERED IN THE AMBULATORY SETTING**

| Practice Sites | Disease States | |
|---|---|---|
| Academic medical center | Asthma | Heart failure |
| Community pharmacy | Atrial fibrillation | Hepatitis |
| Hospital-based clinics | BPH | HIV |
|    Primary care clinics | Chronic kidney disease | Hypertension |
|    Specialty clinics | COPD | Low back pain |
| Indian Health Service | Depression | Osteoarthritis |
| Managed care facilities | Diabetes | Osteoporosis |
| Physician group practice | Dyslipidemia | Peptic ulcer disease |
| Public Health Department | GERD | STDs |
| Rural health clinic | Gout | Thyroid disorders |
| Veteran's Affairs Medical Center | Headaches | Tobacco abuse |

and participating in formulary decision-making processes. In some circumstances, the ambulatory pharmacist may have an advanced scope of practice which includes prescribing privileges for particular medications, the ability to order laboratory tests to monitor therapeutic outcomes, and the authority to adjust medications on the basis of physical examination data and laboratory tests. Examples of these types of practice settings include certain clinical pharmacy specialists practicing in Veterans Affairs hospitals and pharmacists practicing under the Clinical Pharmacist Practitioner (CPP) designation in North Carolina.[18] Regardless of the level of practice at your ambulatory care experiential site, it is important to remember that many of these individuals have been coming to the site long before you were here, and they will continue to be patients here long after you have left this experiential site. Therefore, it is critical that you make every effort to provide optimal care, show concern for their well-being, and help promote continuity of care at every visit. All patient care activities should be conducted under the supervision of your preceptor or a designated licensed pharmacist.

## Source of Patient Referrals

Patients may be referred to the ambulatory care pharmacist through a variety of methods. For ambulatory practice sites within an academic medical center, Veterans' Affairs Healthcare System, or other hospital-affiliated setting, patient referrals usually come from physicians or other healthcare professionals working within that system. Referrals may be made in the form of a traditional consult request, a telephone call, or an electronic order. In some sites (eg, some Veterans' Affairs hospitals) no referral is necessary. In these cases, all individuals receiving a new prescription are required to meet with the pharmacist assigned to that particular clinic area. The pharmacist reviews the patient profile, checks for appropriateness of medication and dosage, and counsels on the new prescription prior to the prescription being filled. The pharmacist may also address formulary issues during this visit. For ambulatory practice sites in the community, individuals may be referred from local physicians, other healthcare professionals, other individuals, or they may self-refer. Pharmacists who are trying to establish ambulatory services in the community pharmacy setting may need to spend a significant amount of time marketing services, developing relationships, and building the trust of local physicians in order to generate referrals. It is important that you understand the referral process for your ambulatory care experiential site.

## Reimbursement for Services

Reimbursement for services has been a challenge faced by many ambulatory care pharmacists over the last several years. With the reluctance of many insurance companies to recognize pharmacists as patient-care providers, ambulatory care pharmacists often have to request that individuals pay directly for services. Many pharmacists have been billing for services "incident to" a physician visit, or to have reduced or waived fees for patients receiving ambulatory services. With the introduction of National Provider Identifiers (NPIs) for health-care providers (including pharmacists) and the development of CPT codes for MTM, reimbursement for ambulatory care services is becoming a reality. A full discussion of reimbursement issues is beyond the scope of this text; however, you should ask your preceptor about mechanisms for reimbursement of ambulatory pharmacy services at your experiential site.

## EXPERIENTIAL EDUCATION COURSES: MANAGING ACTIVITIES AT THE SITE

Up to this point the information in this chapter has been devoted primarily to describing the major who's, what's, where's, when's, and why's of community pharmacy and ambulatory care practice. The remainder of the chapter is devoted to describing specific activities in which you will most likely participate during the community and ambulatory care experiential courses. You will have day-to-day responsibilities, some longer term projects, and many core skills to develop and objectives to meet. Learning objectives for each introductory pharmacy practice and advanced practice course will be outlined in your College of Pharmacy syllabus.

When you begin your course, it is possible you will be exposed to many new aspects of pharmacy practice. The preceptor should conduct an orientation to the site and activities, which will set the stage for a successful experience for both of you. See Table 14.11 for a proposed outline of orientation topics. The list is only a guide and should be customized based on your year of education and the site of your particular practice experience. Coursework in the community and ambulatory care setting is an opportunity for you, the student pharmacist, to be an agent of change and to use your

---

**TABLE 14.11.** PROPOSED OUTLINE FOR COMMUNITY/AMBULATORY CARE PHARMACY EXPERIENTIAL ORIENTATION

1. Philosophy and purpose
2. The pharmacy organization and site description
3. Dress code, parking, other logistical issues
4. Confidentiality of information, communications
5. Attendance
6. Tour of facilities
7. Computer systems to access the pharmacy dispensing system, patient data, and drug information data
8. Student's expectations and goals
9. Preceptor's expectations and goals
10. Conference and meeting schedule
11. Overview of assignments
12. Student evaluation and grading process

motivation, communication skills, disease state knowledge, and imagination to engage in promoting the pharmacist as a health educator and expert of medication management.

You will work with different types of preceptors during your community pharmacy practice and ambulatory care experiential courses. The types of preceptors seen in these settings include shared faculty, full-time academic faculty, and full-time pharmacy employees. Shared faculty members generally have responsibilities to both the university and the practice site. Each type of preceptor will have a different scope of responsibilities with regard to student education and work in the pharmacy/practice site.

## Patient Care Activities

The majority of your time during the experiential course should be devoted to patient care activities. For the introductory community pharmacy practice experience these activities may be limited mainly to the medication order fulfillment process. For advanced pharmacy practice experiences, examples of patient care activities in which you may participate include medication history interviews, patient counseling, OTC consults, provision of MTM, or targeted disease state management in an ambulatory setting. All of these activities should be performed under the supervision of a licensed pharmacist. In addition to patient care activities, you may have a number of other learning opportunities, as described below.

## Drug Information Assignments

During your experiential courses in the community or ambulatory setting, numerous opportunities to answer drug information questions will be identified. Questions will be asked by patients, other health-care professionals, and also the preceptor. It is important to identify the actual question. Attempt to keep the topic narrow enough so that a brief review is possible—work with the preceptor to define the appropriate focus. Do not get involved in answering very general questions such as "Can you tell me about steroids and what they do?" All statements of fact must be referenced. All references used to answer a question, regardless of the perceived significance, must be documented. This will be used for documenting all information related to the question and the response provided. Answers to these requests must be approved by the preceptor or another licensed pharmacist. Please see Chapter 13 for detailed information on the provision of drug information.

## Case Presentations

During an experiential education course, you may be required to complete at least one formal case presentation. Many structures are used for presenting cases, but one common approach is to focus on a drug-related problem. Each preceptor may have different expectations for the format and content of the case presentation, so be sure to obtain that information from your preceptor. There are other examples of these in Chapters 4 and 6 of this book.

The following are suggested guidelines to be used in the preparation of the case presentation:

1. Focus on a patient-specific drug-related problem.
2. Include relevant information useful for patient education, counseling, and outcomes assessment.
3. Include issues such as general health education, if they are important to the case.
4. Prepare a handout and make copies for all attendees. The handout should include all pertinent information about the patient, therapeutic and clinical data, and the plan for problem resolution. In addition, a list of references should be included. Use the template form provided to you by your preceptor. If a template is not available, ask your preceptor for an example of how to document this information.
5. Stay within the specified time parameters for the case presentation (eg, 30 minutes, including time for questions).
6. Prepare the presentation in the desired format. Some preceptors may expect PowerPoint presentations, so be sure to clarify this with your preceptor.

## Journal Club Presentation

In addition to the case presentation, you may also be expected to present a journal club article. In most cases, the journal club article (Chap. 13) will be a clinical trial that is relevant to medications being used in your current setting. For example, if you are doing an ambulatory care experiential course, where you see many patients with diabetes, an appropriate journal club article might be a comparison of two types of combination therapies for Type 2 diabetes. Usually it is up to the student to select an article, but sometimes the article is assigned. Critique of the article should include a brief overview of the article, with an in-depth analysis of the methods, statistics, results, and conclusions. You should look for potential sources of bias, possible confounding factors, and examine the appropriateness of the statistical tests. You should be prepared to make a statement as to the clinical significance of the article in your particular practice setting. Please see Figure 14.3 for a flow chart to guide your evaluation of statistical and clinical significance.

## Other Activities

### Community Outreach

The pharmacist is a respected and involved member of his or her community. As a part of the community or ambulatory experiential course, you may be expected to participate in at least one community service activity. The definition of community is quite flexible and will vary depending on location. For example, if the site where you are completing the course is located in a small town or neighborhood with an elementary, junior high, or high school nearby, you may be asked to provide educational talks to students. If the site is located near a high-rise apartment complex with

**Figure 14.3.** Determining statistical significance, clinical difference and clinical meaningfulness.

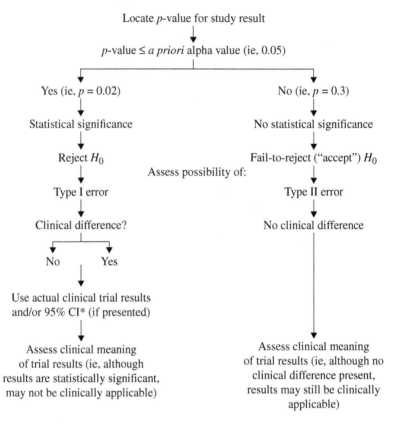

*95% Confidence interval.

Kendrach M, Freeman MK, Wensel TM, Hughes PJ. Literature evaluation I: Controlled clinical trial evaluation. In: KL Kier, PM Malone, JE Stanovich, eds, Drug Information: A Guide for Pharmacists. 4th ed.; 2012, Chapter 4. Available at http://www.accesspharmacy.com/content.aspx?aID=55671079 (subscription required). Accessed March, 2014. (From Kendrach M... Used with permission.)

a large elderly population, you may be asked to create and provide an educational program specifically requested, such as an overview of osteoporosis, for the residents. The particular activity is typically assigned by the preceptor, and any activities must be reviewed and approved by the preceptor in advance. Remember that, above all, you are a representative of the pharmacy organization and your respective college/ university whenever you are in the community or practicing as a student pharmacist. You may have to get the approval of your college/university for participation in certain community outreach projects, so be certain to check on this *prior to* initiation of any projects.

*Professional Organizations*

Many professional organizations serve the needs of community and ambulatory pharmacy. The National Association of Chain Drug Stores, American Pharmacists Association (APhA), National Community Pharmacists Association (NCPA), and the American College of Clinical Pharmacy (ACCP), along with local, state, and other national organizations, offer many programs and services to support community and ambulatory pharmacists. Each organization has their own ideas about the profession and their approach toward business and patient-care aspects, but all are valuable. These organizations are active politically and affect policy decisions that influence pharmacy practice and the business of pharmacy. You are encouraged to learn more about these organizations. Many have student chapters you may want to consider joining for professional and personal growth. Take the opportunity to ask your preceptor about membership in these organizations, and the impact it has had on their career.

Many community pharmacists belong to a local health-based organization (eg, American Lung Association, American Cancer Association, etc.) and volunteer their time to serve as a board member, committee member, or as a liaison. Not only does this benefit the organization, it benefits the pharmacy profession. The impact of pharmacists on public health is demonstrated as more pharmacists engage in community outreach efforts. In addition, the pharmacist benefits by utilizing their skills outside of the traditional setting. During your experiential courses, you may be asked to accompany your preceptor to a health-based organizational meeting or event. Take advantage of this opportunity to learn about ways pharmacists can get involved in their community outside of the pharmacy.

## Student Performance

Evaluating your performance during this type of course is an extremely challenging process. Make sure to review the course objectives and evaluation standards with your preceptor at the beginning of the course, so that you will not have any surprises when it comes time for your evaluation. Many of the course activities offer specific experiences that align with at least one of the primary learning objectives outlined in your course syllabus. Student performance is measured against meeting the objectives. Weighting factors (value) may be assigned to each objective. Objectives with a greater weight suggest that your efforts should be focused on these areas during the course. Each preceptor/site in conjunction with the college or school of pharmacy faculty will determine the best process for measuring and evaluating your performance, and it is important for you to communicate concerns about the grading process early in the course to the preceptor or to the faculty member at the school as appropriate.

## SUMMARY AND CONCLUSION

Tremendous opportunities exist for student pharmacists in community and ambulatory care pharmacy practice. In this chapter we have reviewed the different types of pharmacies and ambulatory settings where you may work while completing an experiential education practice course. We have provided an overview of practice issues, staffing issues, and business issues related to community and ambulatory practice. All of these items are components of the foundation you need to build to practice as a pharmacist. A student in this environment will be exposed to each of these issues and activities, some to a greater degree and in more depth than others. You will also participate in assignments that will build knowledge and skills necessary for you to become an effective pharmacy practitioner. Take advantage of every opportunity to learn as much as possible, especially activities involving direct patient care, because this is the future of pharmacy. If you embrace the many opportunities and challenge yourself, you will achieve a wealth of knowledge and experience in community and ambulatory pharmacy practice.

## REFERENCES

1. Angaran D. Telemedicine and telepharmacy: current status and future implications. *AJHP Official Journal of The American Society of Health-System Pharmacists* [serial online]. 1999;56(14):1405–1426, July 15. Available at Ipswich, MA: MEDLINE. Accessed March, 2014.
2. Behind the Counter Omnibus Survey Results and Analysis. Available at http://www.ncpafoundation.org/downloads/btc_surveyanalysis.pdf. Accessed March, 2014.
3. Brown T. Economic impact and variation in costs to provide community pharmacy services. Available at http://www.ncpafoundation.org/downloads/economicimpact_report.pdf. Accessed March, 2014.
4. Carroll NV. *Financial Management for Pharmacists: A Decision-Making Approach.* Philadelphia, PA: Lea & Febiger; 1991.
5. CPT Codes. Pharmacist services technical advisory committee. Available at http://www.pstac.org/services/mtms-codes.html. Accessed March, 2014.
6. Doucette WR, McDonough RP, Mormann MM, et al. Three-year financial analysis of pharmacy services at an independent community pharmacy. *J Am Pharm Assoc.* 2003;52(2):181–187. doi: 10.1331/JAPhA.2012.11207.
7. Droege M, Maniscalco M, Daniel KL, Baldwin J. Comparing consumers' risk perceptions of prescription and over-the-counter medications. *J Pharm Tech.* 2007;23:142–147.

8. Florida Department of Health. Statute 64B16 Board of Pharmacy; 64B16-27.300 Standards of Practice—continuous quality improvement program. Available at https://www.flrules.org/gateway/ruleNo.asp?id=64B16-27.300. Accessed March, 2014.

9. The Health Insurance Portability and Accountability Act of 1996 (HIPAA). Available at http://www.hhs.gov/ocr/privacy/. Accessed February 2, 2013.

10. Kaiser prescription drug trends fact sheet—May 2010 update. Available at http://www.kff.org/rxdrugs/upload/3057-08.pdf. Accessed March, 2014.

11. Kmart begins offering pharmacy kiosks. Available at http://www.selfserviceworld.com/article/169722/Kmart-begins-offering-pharmacy-kiosks. Accessed March, 2014.

12. Knapp DA. Professionally determined need for pharmacy services in 2020. *Am J Pharm Educ.* 2002;66:421–429.

13. Legal requirements for the sale and purchase of drug products Containing Pseudoephedrine, Ephedrine, and Phenylpropanolamine. Available at http://www.fda.gov/Drugs/DrugSafety/InformationbyDrugClass/ucm072423.htm. Accessed March, 2014.

14. Levy S. Has the time come for a third class of drugs? Available at http://drugtopics.modernmedicine.com/news/has-time-come-third-class-drugs. Accessed March, 2014.

15. Lichtman SS, Youdelman M. Analysis of state pharmacy laws: impact of pharmacy laws on the provision of language services. February 2010. Available at http://www.aacp.org/resources/education/documents/pharmacylawbooklet%20final.pdf. Accessed March, 2014.

16. Medication therapy management in pharmacy practice: core elements of an MTM service model (version 2.0). *J Am Pharm Assoc: JAPhA* [serial online]. May 2008;48(3):341–353. Available at MEDLINE, Ipswich, MA. Accessed March, 2014.

17. Medication Therapy Management. Available at http://www.cms.gov/Medicare/Prescription-Drug-Coverage/PrescriptionDrugCovContra/MTM.html. Accessed March, 2014.

18. North Carolina Board of Pharmacy Clinical Pharmacist Practitioners. Available at http://www.ncbop.org/pharmacists_cpp.htm. Accessed March, 2014.

19. Pharmacy kiosks now dispensing OTC drugs. Available at http://www.selfserviceworld.com/article/183467/Pharmacy-kiosks-now-dispensing-OTC-drugs. Accessed March, 2014.

20. Plan B. Available at http://www.planbonestep.com/. Accessed March, 2014.

21. Provost M, Perri M, Galen R. Teaching telemonitoring and the use of high tech tools for disease management in pharmacy practice. *AACP Annual Meeting* [serial online]. 2003;104(JUL):NIL, January 1. Available at International Pharmaceutical Abstracts, Ipswich, MA. Accessed March, 2014.

22. Third Class of Drugs. Available at http://www.chpa.org/05_27_03_ThirdClass.aspx. Accessed March, 2014.

**23.** U.S. Department of Health and Human Services, Public Health Service, Food and Drug Administration, Center for Drug Evaluation and Research, Office of Information Technology, Division of Data Management and Services. *Electronic Orange Book* [electronic resource]: *Approved Drug Products with Therapeutic Equivalence Evaluations.* Available at http://www.accessdata. fda.gov/scripts/cder/ob/default.cfm. Accessed March, 2014.

**24.** Webcams connect pharmacists to immobile Minn. Seniors by Elizabeth Stawicki, Minnesota Public Radio January 31, 2013 Available at http://www. mprnews.org/story/2013/01/31/health/webcam-connects-pharmacists-to-immobile-seniors. March, 2014.

**25.** What is telepharmacy? Telehealth Resource Centers, part of U.S. Department of Health and Human Services' Health Resources and Services Administration (HRSA) Office for the Advancement of Telehealth,Office of Rural Health Policy. Available from: http://www.telehealthresourcecenter. org/toolbox-module/online-prescribing-and-telepharmacy. Accessed March, 2014.

## PATIENT CASES

### Note to Students

The information provided in the following cases is quite similar to what you might find on review of a typical patient profile in the community or ambulatory practice setting. You should treat the information as if these are real patients and you are now in charge of their care. When evaluating the cases, you may find that not all necessary data are present. If you feel that additional information is necessary in order to make decisions about the medication regimens provided, you should be prepared to elicit this information from your preceptor in the setting of a "role-playing" exercise. Your preceptor will play the role of the patient, while you play the role of the pharmacist. You must also, in some cases, approach your preceptor as "the patient's physician" to get further information. Formulate questions that you might theoretically ask the patient, or physician in order to obtain the information that you feel is lacking.

After reviewing the cases, you should be able to use the methods described in chapters from the textbook to assess each patient problem (ie, SOAPE, FARM). You may identify additional patient problems (need for counseling regarding smoking cessation, inhaler technique, medication compliance, weight loss, etc.).

### Note to Preceptors

We have chosen to omit some information from the following cases in order to challenge the student and to have them practice communication skills to gather additional information. When the student feels that additional information is necessary, engage him or her in a "role-playing" exercise (with the student playing the role of the pharmacist and the preceptor playing the role of patient, physician, or nurse). Remind the student to use open-ended questions, and to communicate at a level suitable for the type of interaction (ie, patient vs. physician interview).

Laboratory tests and medication profiles are provided in table format for each case. Refer to Chapter 11 for additional information on laboratory tests. For each case, the student should try to use the information provided to develop a rationale for medication changes and an appropriate therapeutic plan. For the ambulatory cases, abbreviated progress notes are available, but the student should try to formulate a plan *before* looking ahead to the notes.

## COMMUNITY PHARMACY CASES

### COMMUNITY CASE 1

A 28-year-old WF presents to the pharmacy counter with the following prescription:

RALPH ST. JOHN, M.D.
678 DAIRY ROAD
SMALLVILLE, USA 84326

---

Name: *Kate Stuffie*     Date: *10/1/14*
*Amoxil 875 mg #20*
*One tab po bid for infection*
Refill: *0*                              *R St. John, MD*

---

When entering the prescription data, you note the patient's current Rx profile as follows:

| Medication | Directions | Qty | Last Refill | Refills Left |
|---|---|---|---|---|
| Allegra-D 12 hour tabs | One tab po bid for allergies | 60 | 9/12/14 | 1 |
| Fluticasone nasal spray | 2 sprays each nostril daily | 1 | 9/12/14 | 3 |
| Yaz tablets | One tab po daily | 28 | 9/25/14 | 8 |

For the purpose of this exercise, assume today's date is 10/01/14.

*(continued on next page)*

## DISCUSSION QUESTIONS

- Are you familiar with all of the abbreviations used on the prescription and in the prescription profile?
- What are the indications for the medications included in the current Rx profile?
- Is the new prescription missing any necessary information?
- What information should be verified before filling the prescription for amoxicillin?
- Are you concerned about any potential drug interactions with amoxicillin and her current prescription profile? If so, how would you address these issues?
- Describe the steps you would take in completing the medication order fulfillment process.
- What auxiliary labels would most likely be placed on the bottle of amoxicillin?
- What open-ended questions should be asked when counseling the patient on the new prescription?
- List at least four counseling points that should be provided to the patient when picking up her new prescription for amoxicillin.

## COMMUNITY CASE 2

A teenage girl walks up to the pharmacy counter and asks if she can speak to you in private. She tells you in confidence that she needs the "morning-after" pill Plan B One-Step. She is tearful and appears to be quite upset.

## DISCUSSION QUESTIONS

- List an empathic response you would provide to the patient. How would you handle the upset patient?
- After calming the patient, what questions should you ask the patient prior to deciding if Plan B One-Step is appropriate in this case?
- To whom can Plan B One-Step be sold over-the-counter?
- What counseling points should be provided to patients receiving Plan B One-Step?
- What ethical issues might pharmacists face when dispensing emergency contraceptive products?

## AMBULATORY CARE CASES

The following cases contain information similar to what you will find in an ambulatory care setting. You should treat the information as if these are real patients and you are now in charge of their care. They have been assigned to see you, the pharmacist. You may ask your preceptor questions to get a better patient history, as not all of the information you need may be found in the chart. You should be prepared to present your patient education materials to your preceptor as if he or she is the patient. You will then proceed to complete a SOAPE note and a patient case presentation for your preceptor.

### AMBULATORY PATIENT CASE 1

| | | | |
|---|---|---|---|
| **Patient Name:** Oliver, Ellen | | **Date:** 9/15/14 | |
| **Ht:** 5'4 "  **Gender:** F | **Wt:** 175 lb | **Age:** 60 | **Race:** Black |
| **Allergies:** NKDA | **MD:** Dr. W. Davis | | **Insurance:** |

| CC/HPI: "I'm here to get the results of my blood work." EO is a 60-year-old BF presenting to the clinic for f/u of laboratory results. She was started on pravastatin for her dyslipidemia at the last visit on 8/1. |
|---|

| | |
|---|---|
| **PMH:** Type 2 DM, hyperlipidemia, allergic rhinitis, GERD, HTN | **PSH:** None |
| **FH:** Father ↓ 62, MI  Mother ↓ 88, CVA | **SHx:** Denies tobacco and ETOH |

| Home Meds: | Problem List: |
|---|---|
| **1. Lisinopril** 10 mg po daily | 1. Type 2 DM |
| **2. HCTZ** 25 mg po daily | 2. Dyslipidemia |
| **3. Glipizide XL** 10 mg po QAM | 3. HTN |
| **4. Metformin** 500 mg po bid | 4. GERD |
| **5. Pravastatin** 40 mg po hs | 5. Allergic rhinits |
| **6. Cetirizine** 10 mg po hs | |
| **7. Ranitidine** 150 mg po bid prn | |

**ROS/PE**

| |
|---|
| **GEN:** 60-year-old BF in NAD |
| **HEENT:** Denies vision changes; PERRLA |
| **NECK:** Supple, no JVD |
| **CV:** Denies CP, chest tightness, palpitations; RRR, no M/R/G |
| **LUNGS:** CTA bilaterally |
| **ABD:** Denies N/V/D and abd pain; abdomen S/NT |
| **EXT:** Denies cramping, tingling, numbness in hands, legs, and feet; feet clean and dry, no cuts or lesions; dorsalis pedis 2+ bilat |
| **NEURO:** Grossly intact |

**Vitals and Labs:** EO

| Date | 8/01/14 | 9/15/14 |
|---|---|---|
| BP | 130/80 | 122/78 |
| HR | 76 | 80 |
| RR | 14 | 14 |
| Temp | 98.6 | 97.8 |
| Glucose | 251 | 194 |
| SCr | 1.0 | |
| HbA1c | | 8.4 |
| PT/INR | | |
| Tot Prot | 8.1 | |
| Alb | 4.3 | |
| ALT | 35 | |
| AST | 30 | |
| Alk Phos | 84 | |
| LDH | | |

| Tot Bili | 0.6 | |
|---|---|---|
| TC | 238 | 206 |
| HDL | 37 | 39 |
| LDL | 145 | 115 |
| TG | 280 | 260 |
| TSH | 1.2 | |
| Spot Urine for Albumin | <30 | |

**Progress Note**

1. Type 2 DM—uncontrolled; A1c above goal of <7% on glipizide XL 10 mg QAM and metformin 500 mg twice daily. Recommend increasing metformin to 1000 mg twice daily. SCr WNL for continuation of metformin. Patient needs education on disease, complications, diet, exercise, and home monitoring of blood glucose.
2. Dyslipidemia – Based on the ACC/AHA cholesterol guidelines, this patient with Type 2 DM and a 10-year risk of ASCVD >7.5% is a candidate for high-intensity statin therapy. Recommend switching to more potent statin such as atorvastatin 40 mg daily or rosuvastatin 20 mg daily.
3. HTN—controlled. BP at goal of <140/80 mmHg on lisinopril and HCTZ.

## AMBULATORY PATIENT CASE 2

| | |
|---|---|
| **Patient Name:** Huff, Pam | **Date:** 9/05/14 |

| | | | |
|---|---|---|---|
| **Ht:** 5'5"  **Gender:** F | **Wt:** 288.5 lb | **Age:** 48 | **Race:** White |

| | | |
|---|---|---|
| **Allergies:** Sulfur | **MD:** McIntyre | **Insurance:** |

**CC/HPI:** PH is a 48-year-old WF who presents to the clinic for f/u of asthma exacerbation (secondary to a URI), which required hospitalization. She reports that she is still having symptoms and needs to use her albuterol several times a day.

| **PMH:** Asthma, Type 2 DM, HTN, diabetic peripheral neuropathy, lower back pain 2° OA, hyperlipidemia, URI, bronchitis, nephrolithiasis, anxiety, hypothyroid, HF with reduced EF (EF 30%) | **PSH:** C-section, kidney stones |
|---|---|

| **FH:** Sister: viral meningitis<br>　　Father: HTN, stroke<br>　　Mother: Type 2 DM | **SHx:** (+) tobacco—1 ppd<br>　　No ETOH |
|---|---|
| **Home Meds:**<br>　1. Insulin glargine 35 units SC HS<br>　2. Insulin lispro 10 units tid AC<br>　3. Albuterol MDI 2 puffs tid<br>　4. Albuterol via nebulizer prn<br>　5. Ramipril 5 mg po daily<br>　6. Furosemide 40 mg po daily<br>　7. KCl 20 meq po qd<br>　8. Carisoprodol 350 mg po bid<br>　9. Rosuvastatin 20 mg po daily<br>　　(new Rx two weeks ago)<br>　10. Hydrocodone/APAP 1 tab po<br>　　Q8H prn | **Problem List:**<br>　1. Otitis media<br>　2. Asthma<br>　3. Heart failure with reduced EF<br>　4. Type 2 DM<br>　5. HTN<br>　6. Diabetic peripheral neuropathy<br>　7. Lower back pain<br>　8. Vasomotor symptoms/amenor-<br>　　rhea X 3 mos<br>　9. Hyperlipidemia<br>　10. Tobacco dependency |

## ROS/PE

| |
|---|
| **GEN:** 48-year-old WF slightly anxious, but in NAD |
| **HEENT:** Left TM slightly bulging w/mod. injection/erythema; nares patent w/o discharge; mild pharyngeal erythema; no syncope, dizziness; + coughing, allergic rhinitis; + vision changes recently |
| **NECK:** Nonswollen, nontender, no JVD |
| **CV:** Tachycardia w/o murmur, regular rhythm |
| **LUNGS:** + faint expiratory wheezes bilaterally; + SOB w/exertion, + orthopnea (3–4 pillows) |
| **ABD:** Obese, + BS X 4, soft and nontender; no N/V/D and abd pain, + constipation |
| **GU:** Amenorrhea X 3 mos, + hot flashes |
| **EXT:** 2+ pitting edema bilaterally in LE, +1/4 pulses bilaterally in LE, DTR intact; + tingling/numbness in LE |
| **NEURO:** Grossly intact |

Vitals and Labs: PH

| Date | 8/22/14 | 8/29/14 | 9/05/14 |
|---|---|---|---|
| BP | 136/84 | 140/90 | 138/86 |
| HR | 88 | 80 | 100 |
| RR | 24 | 20 | 18 |
| Temp | | | 99.3 |
| Glucose | 135 | 115 | 124 |
| SCr | 0.7 | | |
| K | 4.3 | | |
| HbA1c | 7.1 | | |
| Alb | 4.0 | | |
| Tot Prot | 8.2 | | |
| ALT | 45 | | |
| AST | 40 | | |
| Alk Phos | 80 | | |
| LDH | | | |
| Tot Bili | 0.6 | | |
| TC | 221 | | |
| HDL | 32 | | |
| LDL | 119 | | |
| TG | 352 | | |
| TSH | 0.653 | | |
| Spot Urine for Albumin | <30 | | |

### Progress Note

1. OM of left ear—begin amoxicillin 500 mg po tid 10 days per provider
2. Asthma—uncontrolled as evidenced by frequent use of albuterol. Pt may benefit from addition of inhaled corticosteroid to help reduce the frequency of symptoms and exacerbations. Pt strongly advised on the need for smoking cessation to help with asthma control.
3. HFrEF—symptomatic. May require temporary increase in furosemide for relief of symptoms. Will discuss with provider. When pt is stable would consider addition of a selective beta-blocker with careful titration and monitoring of both HF and asthma symptoms. Pt may benefit from optimization of ramipril dose.
4. Type 2 DM—controlled as evidenced by glucose and $HbA_{1c}$.
5. Hot flashes + amenorrhea × 3 months—may be candidate for hormone replacement. Encouraged patient to implement lifestyle modifications for now.
6. Hyperlipidemia—recently started rosuvastatin. Recommend reassess lipids in 3 months.

## AMBULATORY PATIENT CASE 3

| | | | |
|---|---|---|---|
| **Patient. Name:** Poulec, Jada | | **Date:** 6/26/14 | |
| **Ht:** 5'2"          **Wt:** 183.5 lb<br>**Gender:** F | | **Age:** 61 | **Race:** White |
| **Allergies:** Sulfa          **MD:** Dr. B. Clot | | **Insurance:** | |
| **CC/HPI:** JP, a 61-year-old WF, presents to clinic for routine PT/INR check. She states that she had unexplained bruising on the right leg a couple of weeks ago that resolved w/o treatment. | | | |
| **PMH:** Atrial fibrillation (12/08)<br>       CABG (12/07)<br>       Hyperlipidemia<br>       Hypertension | | **PSH:** Hysterectomy (1994) | |
| **FH:** Father ↑ 81, CAD<br>       Mother ↓, unknown cause | | **SHx:** (−) tobacco, ETOH, illicit drugs | |

| Home Meds: | Problem List: |
|---|---|
| 1. Warfarin 5 mg po daily except 2.5 mg Tuesday and Thursday<br>2. Digoxin 0.25 mg po daily<br>3. Atorvastatin 20 mg po daily<br>4. Furosemide 40 mg po daily<br>5. KCL 10 meq po qd<br>6. Losartan 50 mg po daily<br>7. Metoprolol 50 mg po twice daily<br>8. Cetirizine 10 mg po daily prn | 1. Chronic anticoagulation |

## ROS/PE

| |
|---|
| **GEN:** WDWN WF |
| **HEENT:** Denies any changes in vision |
| **NECK:** Supple |
| **CV:** Denies CP, chest tightness, palpitations; RRR, no M/R/G click |
| **LUNGS:** Denies SOB, orthopnea; CTA bilaterally |
| **ABD:** Denies N/V/D/C and abd pain |
| **GU:** Denies blood in urine or stool, denies nocturia |
| **EXT:** Denies unusual bruising or bleeding besides bruising on the right leg a few weeks ago, no C/C/E |
| **NEURO:** Grossly intact |

**VITALS AND LABS:** JP

| Date | 2/16/14 | 3/6/14 | 4/26/14 | 5/24/14 | 6/26/14 |
|---|---|---|---|---|---|
| BP | 138/88 | 126/84 | 130/80 | 132/82 | 128/84 |
| HR | 64 | 68 | 62 | 64 | 66 |
| RR | 16 | 14 | 12 | 14 | 16 |
| Temp | | | | | |
| Glucose | 96 | 95 | 95 | 98 | 98 |
| SCr | 1.0 | | 1.1 | | 1.0 |
| HbA1c | | | | | |
| INR | 2.9 | 3.1 | 2.8 | 3.0 | 1.9 |
| Alb | 4.3 | | | | |
| Tot Prot | 7.1 | | | | |
| ALT | 40 | | | | |
| AST | 35 | | | | |
| Alk Phos | 90 | | | | |
| LDH | | | | | |
| Tot Bili | 0.8 | | | | |
| TC | | 216 | | | 208 |
| HDL | | 80 | | | 81 |
| LDL | | 109 | | | 96 |
| TG | | 135 | | | 155 |
| TSH | | | | | |

**Progress Note**

1. Anticoagulation—PT/INR is on the low end of the therapeutic range. Goal INR 2–3. Patient has been therapeutic on current warfarin regimen for past 4 months. Patient states that she has not missed any doses, but did eat a lot of "greens" at a family picnic over the weekend. She also states that she has been eating leftover "greens" all week. Recommend continue current dose. Counsel on consistency in vitamin K intake in diet. RTC 2 weeks for repeat INR.

CHAPTER

# Institutional Pharmacy Practice

*Stephanie D. Garrett, Antonia Zapantis*

**Objectives: Upon completion of the chapter and exercises, the student pharmacist will be able to**

1. Describe the various departments and personnel that you may encounter in an institutional setting.
2. Outline differences between the various drug distribution systems available in institutional settings.
3. List the special needs of acutely ill patients in terms of dispensing oral and intravenous medications that a pharmacist needs to manage.
4. Describe the role of government and accreditation bodies in terms of quality initiatives within institutional settings.
5. State the role of a student during rounds.
6. Identify potential medication regimen assessment activities to assist in patient monitoring.

## Patient Encounter

You have been assigned to the ICU satellite for the day. A nurse approaches you with the following order for Patient X and asks for your help:

**General Hospital**

☐
STAT
(Place X in box if STAT)   **PHYSICIAN ORDER**
ALLERGIES & DESCRIPTION

*Patient X*
*Nurse ICU-5*

| DATE AND TIME | DO NOT USE THIS SHEET UNLESS A RED NO. SHOWS ➡ | ① |
|---|---|---|

9/4   *Transfer from nurse ICU to MICU*
*Resume Nurse ICU meds*
*CM and Crm clidtine Stool*
*BC x2 Stat*
*Hydrocortisone 70mg Q6*
*DC Rocephin*
*Start VANCO 1 Gm IV Q? - Pharmacy to dose*
*Zosyn 4.5gm IV Q8*
*Levophed Gtt Stat @ 1.0 mcg titrate per protocol*
*Albumin 5% now*                        *BP 7 90*

When you pull up patient X in the computer and quickly review his chart, you obtain the following additional information:

Ht: 5'10"

Wt: 70 kg

Allergies: PCN

SCr: 1.3 (baseline: 0.7, 3 days ago: 1)

Vitals: T 101°F, BP 82/56, P 109, R 25

*(continued on next page)*

**Discussion for Introductory Pharmacy Practice Experience (IPPE) Students:**

After receiving the order, what would you do first?

A. Start crying.

B. Put the order aside until your preceptor comes back from lunch.

C. Go home. Your 8-hour shift is over.

D. None of the above.

The choices above may seem funny, but this order requires immediate attention by a licensed pharmacist.

Consider the following issues related to the order above:

• Legibility.

• Do not use abbreviations.

• Transfer orders.

• Missing information.

• Appropriateness of doses.

• Do you know what all of the abbreviations stand for?

• What issues with these orders might have been avoided in a computerized physician order entry (CPOE) environment?

• Do you know what these drugs are and what they are used for? Where would you go to find out?

**Discussion for Advanced Pharmacy Practice Experience (APPE) Students:**

Consider the following issues related to the order above:

• Can you answer all of the questions listed above that are geared toward an IPPE student?

• Is this patient's renal function normal? Why or why not?

• How would you empirically dose vancomycin for this patient? Would you recommend vancomycin levels?

• What is the role of corticosteroids in sepsis?

• What additional information do you need before dispensing the Zosyn?

*(continued on next page)*

- Would this patient be appropriate for prolonged infusion of Zosyn? What is prolonged infusion? If appropriate, what would regimen be?
- What coverage will this antibiotic regimen provide?
- Levophed
  - What is missing from the order?
  - What is the dose?
  - What concentration would you make the drip?
  - What rate should you tell the nurse to set on the pump?
  - What monitoring parameters will you assess?
    - Efficacy
    - Toxicity
- What additional information do you need from the physician or nurse?
- Albumin
  - What is the dose?
  - How should the order be written?
  - Is the order appropriate?
  - How fast should it be infused?
  - What monitoring parameters will you assess?
  - Do you need any more information before you send the albumin to the ICU?
  - Do you need to document anything before you dispense the albumin?
  - Is this a relatively expensive or inexpensive therapy?
  - Is this therapy appropriate if the patient is a Jehovah's Witness?

## GENERAL HOSPITAL OVERVIEW

### Introduction

Welcome to the world of hospitals and health-systems pharmacy! There are over 5700 registered hospitals nationwide with almost 1 million staffed beds accounting for over $773 billion of health care expenses.[1] Hospitals can range from local general hospitals that care for patients with a variety of medical conditions to specialized ones that focus on specific conditions, such as mental illness, pediatrics, or geriatrics. They can range from small critical access institutions with limited services to large hospitals with hundreds of beds offering a variety of services. Critical access hospitals are typically located in rural areas, while urban hospitals tend to be bigger to meet the demands of the city.[2] Though most hospitals treat patients acutely with an average length of stay (LOS) of 4.8 days,[3] there are some long-term care facilities where the LOS can exceed 30 days. These facilities are generally run the same way, though they may have regulatory differences from traditional hospitals. Lastly, ownership and control further differentiate hospitals one from another. There are government hospitals, which include all levels of government and include VA hospitals, military hospitals, public university run hospitals, and county hospitals. Then there are nongovernment hospitals and these are further broken down into *for profit* (eg, Health Care of America—HCA) and *not-for-profit* (St. Luke's Medical Center).[2] The provision of inpatient services (acute and chronic care) and outpatient services (acute and chronic care) within the same organization is collectively called a health-system and pharmacists within these systems are known as health-system pharmacists. These systems may consist of multiple hospitals, clinics, and community pharmacies, but generally run under the auspices of one organization with one overall governing body.

Once you get inside the hospital, many different people are doing their part to provide patient care. Table 15.1 includes some of the departments you may be exposed to during your experiential education courses. You will also interact with persons from the various medical specialties listed in Table 15.2. One thing that is important to learn is the hierarchy of the medical team, which is depicted in Figure 15.1. This teaching team essentially functions as a real-world classroom by offering an

**TABLE 15.1. TYPICAL HOSPITAL DEPARTMENTS**

Pharmacy

Nursing

Administration

Medical records

Radiology

Clinical laboratories

Housekeeping

Business office

Respiratory therapy

Purchasing

Central service

Social service

Information services

Case management

**TABLE 15.2.** TYPICAL MEDICAL SERVICES

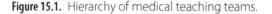

Internal medicine/hospitalist

Surgery

Obstetrics-gynecology

Pediatrics

Anesthesiology

Radiology

Psychiatry

Family practice

**Figure 15.1.** Hierarchy of medical teaching teams.

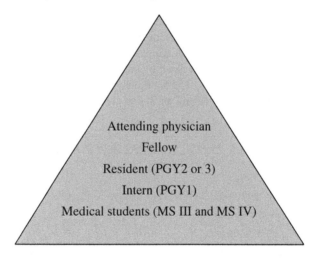

opportunity to apply medical theory and evidence-based medicine to actual patients.[4] Changes in this medical team will be occurring.

## The Department of Pharmacy

You will probably be spending the most time in the department of pharmacy. Depending on the size of the hospital, the size of the pharmacy department may range from a few people to many. Every department is different, but some of the personnel you may encounter are listed in Table 15.3.

The goal of every pharmacy department is to get the right medication to the patient as efficiently as possible. The way each pharmacy department is

TABLE 15.3. TYPICAL PERSONNEL WITHIN A HOSPITAL
DEPARTMENT OF PHARMACY

Chief of pharmacy

Director of pharmacy

Assistant director(s)

Operation manager(s)

Clinical manager(s)

Financial manager

Clinical coordinator(s)

Technician supervisor(s)

Automated dispensing Cabinet (ADC) supervisor

Purchaser

Informatics pharmacist(s)

Clinical pharmacist(s)

Staff pharmacist(s)

Pharmacy resident(s)

Pharmacy intern(s)

Technician(s)

approaching this process is presently being evaluated. The Pharmacy Practice Model Initiative (PPMI) comes from the American Society of Health-System Pharmacists (ASHP) and the ASHP Foundation outlining the efficient use of pharmacists as direct health care providers (HCPs) while advancing the health and wellbeing of patients by developing and supporting a futuristic practice model. The core of this initiative is inference of passion, commitment, and pro-activeness among hospital and health-system pharmacy practice leaders and ultimately putting the patient in the center of health-care as it relates to pharmacy. The five objectives that look to expand the role of a pharmacist in patient care are (1) creating a framework ensuring the provision of safe, effective, efficient, accountable, and evidence-based care; (2) determining pharmacy services to be provided in a consistent manner; (3) identifying emerging technologies supporting patient care, (4) developing a template supporting the optimal utilization and deployment of pharmacy resources, and (5) identifying specific actions pharmacy leaders needed to implement practice model change implementing change.[5]

The system for drug distribution depends on the size and needs of the hospital. Smaller hospitals may not provide pharmacy services 24 hours per day.[6] Regardless, pharmacist review of physician orders is generally required prior to medication administration. This provides the perfect opportunity for pharmacists to intervene in a patient-centered manner when therapeutic regimens are not optimized or when dosage errors, drug-drug interactions, and other contraindications exist. The two circumstances where administration of medications prior to prospective pharmacist review is permitted are when a physician controls the ordering, preparation, and administration of the medication, that is, sedating a patient for intubation, or in urgent situations where the wait time for this prospective review would actually cause patient harm.[7]

## Drug Distribution

Pharmacy departments either have centralized drug distribution (60%) or decentralized drug distribution (40%). Centralized systems include traditional manual systems and fixed robotic systems (ie, robot or carousel) utilizing bar-code technology automating the dispensing process (eg, cartfill). Decentralized systems include medications dispensed directly to the HCP administering the medication via automated dispensing cabinets (ADCs), satellite pharmacies, or floorstock systems. Regardless of the system used, unit-dose dispensing is preferable, where the medication is in a form ready to administer to the patient with appropriate labeling of mediation name, quantity, strength, expiration date, lot number, and name and place of business of the manufacturer, packer, or distributor.[8,9] There could also be combinations of these systems depending on the need of the hospitals and the level of technology implementation. Figure 15.2 illustrates the steps needed for medications to reach the patient once prescribers order them.

Traditionally, hospitals used floorstock systems, though currently it is less common. In the floorstock system, the majority of medications are stored on the nursing unit, with the exception of rarely used or expensive medications. The nurse is responsible for all aspects of medication preparation and administration regardless of dosage form. The floorstock system accomplishes the goal of getting the medication to the patient but leaves room for errors to occur, since certain checks and balances are missing.[8]

The cart-fill system resembles the way prescriptions are filled in an outpatient setting. The first dose may be sent directly from the main pharmacy, a decentralized satellite pharmacy, or an ADC.[6] The remaining patient's medication are filled and sent from the main pharmacy. The day supply may vary by hospital protocol, but is most commonly between 3 and 5 days' supply. The process can be manual or automated by a robot. Robotic dispensing can increase medication fill accuracy by greater than 90%, reduce inventory costs by 30% and reduce technician and pharmacist operation labor by 58% and 58% to 61%, respectively, freeing pharmacists' time to participate in more patient care activities.[10,11] When the medication supply runs out, the nurse requests more medication from the pharmacy. The ADC ensures that medications are secured until the physician order has been reviewed and verified by the pharmacist. Other advantages of the system are reduced time spent by nursing personnel inventorying controlled substances, more efficient and timely resupply of medications on the patient care unit, increased medication security and controlled substance accountability, quick access to first doses

**Figure 15.2.** Drug distribution.

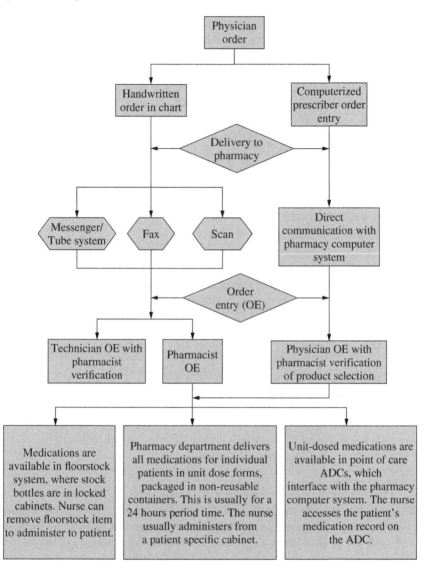

for stat medication orders, and increase efficiency for drug administration billing. Technicians fill the ADC. When inventory is low in the individual ADC or a medication is ordered that is not stored in the ADC, a report is printed in the pharmacy with a refill or a medication load list. When stock medications are pulled in the pharmacy, a pharmacist checks them prior to the loading of medications into the ADC. Some systems also utilize a bar-coding restocking verification system to add another level of safety. Bar-code scanners in the pharmacy ensure that the correct item is removed from the pharmacy stock. Bar-coded labels are generated concurrently. When medications are delivered to the patient care unit, another bar-code scanner double checks that the correct medication is added to the correct location within the ADC.[12]

There are many things to consider when making recommendations to your health-care team regarding the medication therapy of your mutual patient, including the appropriate dosage form of the medication.

## How to Pick the Right Dosage Form

You might think oral medications should be easy. Actually, depending on the patient's situation a "simple per oral" medication may require you to dispense a different dosage form. Review the following three scenarios and decide what dosage form you would dispense for each scenario. Note that each patient has an order for the same medication.

---

**Scenario One**

45-yo female patient with chest pain and indigestion rule out myocardial infarction

Order              Famotidine 20 mg po Q12h

**Scenario Two**

68-yo male patient status post CVA with a recent PEG placement

Order              Famotidine 20 mg po Q12h

**Scenario Three**

7-yo female patient with rhabdomyosarcoma (31 lb)

Order              Famotidine 0.5 mg/kg po Q12h

---

All three patients are getting the same medication, but the common 20-mg tablet may not be the most appropriate dosage form for each patient. In **Scenario One,** the 20-mg tablet would be appropriate, but that same tablet (depending on the size) could get stuck in the feeding tube of the patient from **Scenario Two.** Feeding tubes are placed for a variety of reasons and include nasogastric intubation, orogastric intubation, nasoenteric intubation, gastrostomy, and jejunostomy. Gastrostomy tubes can be placed by laparotomy or percutaneous endoscopy gastrostomy (PEG). You may need to send the nurse famotidine suspension or instruct her to crush the tablet and flush the feeding tube with 15 to 30 mL of water before and after administration of the crushed tablet.[13] Things get a little more complicated with controlled release medications, which typically cannot be crushed. For a complete list of medications that should not be crushed, refer to The Institute for Safe Medication

Practices (ISMP) web site.[14] **Scenario Three** is similar to Scenario Two, but pediatric patients are unique because their dosing is not standardized. This is the reason why a standard 10-mg or 20-mg tablet may not be appropriate for pediatric patients. In addition, pediatric patients may not be able to swallow tablets; therefore, liquids may be more appropriate. The correct dosage for **Scenario Three** is 7 mg; therefore, it would be appropriate to send the nurse an oral syringe with 7 mg of the suspension.

*Continuous Infusions*

So what is the difference between an IV "P" & IV "piggyback"? One of the most confusing concepts is the different methods of intravenous administration of medications: Continuous infusion, IV push, IV piggyback. Continuous infusions are often the primary infusion line and can be used for the administration of vasopressors, total parenteral nutrition (TPN), or replacement fluids. The rate of a continuous infusion is usually expressed in volume per unit of time (mL/h). An example of a continuous infusion label is depicted in Figure 15.3 (adapted from ISMP guidelines—labels).[15]

*Intermittent Doses—Push*

IV push doses are intermittent doses (Q12h, Q8h, etc.) that do not need to be diluted and can be "pushed" relatively quickly. Examples of medications that can be "pushed" are famotidine, ondansetron, metoclopramide, and various antibiotics. Typically, authorized personnel with a high level of training are needed to administer these medications. These medications require a minimum dilution to prevent complications including phlebitis, which is an inflammation of the intimal lining of a blood vessel. It is progressive in nature. Drugs with risk of phlebitis include diazepam, phenytoin, diazoxide, furosemide, cyclophosphamide, and nitrogen mustard.[16] An example of an IV push label is depicted in Figure 15.4 (adapted from ISMP guidelines—labels). [15]

**Figure 15.3.** Continuous infusion label example.

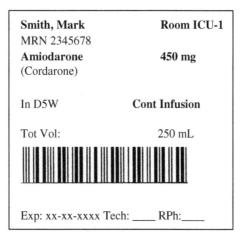

| Smith, Mark | Room ICU-1 |
|---|---|
| MRN 2345678 | |
| **Amiodarone** | **450 mg** |
| (Cordarone) | |
| | |
| In D5W | **Cont Infusion** |
| | |
| Tot Vol: | 250 mL |

Exp: xx-xx-xxxx Tech: _____ RPh:_____

**Figure 15.4.** Push label example.

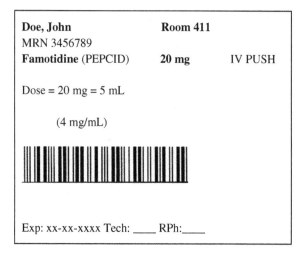

Doe, John                          **Room 411**
MRN 3456789
**Famotidine** (PEPCID)      **20 mg**          IV PUSH

Dose = 20 mg = 5 mL

(4 mg/mL)

Exp: xx-xx-xxxx Tech: ____ RPh:____

*Intermittent Doses—Piggyback*

IV piggyback doses are intermittent doses of medications (Q12h, Q8h, etc.) that need to be diluted or infused slowly. These do not need a high level of monitoring like IV push medications, because it is less likely that complications like phlebitis would occur because the IV solution is more dilute. Examples of medications that can be dosed via piggyback are various antibiotics and concentrated electrolytes (ie, potassium chloride). An example of an IV piggyback label is depicted in Figure 15.5 (adapted from Institute for Safe Medication Practices guidelines—labels).[15]

**Figure 15.5.** Piggyback label example.

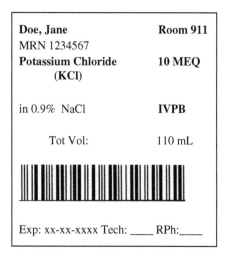

Doe, Jane                          **Room 911**
MRN 1234567
**Potassium Chloride**       **10 MEQ**
     **(KCl)**

in 0.9% NaCl                  **IVPB**

Tot Vol:                       110 mL

Exp: xx-xx-xxxx Tech: ____ RPh:____

## Medication Administration

Medication dispensing can account for 11% of medication errors and administration can account for 38% of medication errors.[12] Use of bar coding medication administration (BCMA) has the potential to decrease these errors dramatically by specifically improving patient identification, verifying medication administration (ie, 5 *rights*: right patient, right drug, right dose, right route, right time) and specimen handling, and ultimately update the medical record electronically.[17]

Additionally, in terms of intravenous medications, smart pumps may be implemented in health-care systems to improve safety. Smart pump technology employs software that can alert users to potential errors within infusion pumps used to administer intravenous medications. The software allows medication libraries to be stored within the pump and aides in providing medication dosing guidelines and clinical advisories, as well as establishing dose and concentration limits.[18] Like all technologies discussed thus far, cost remains an obstacle for full implementation.

## The Medical Chart

The medical chart is divided into various sections. There may be many variations depending on the hospital. Additionally, many hospitals may be documenting all or some of this information electronically, known as the "electronic medical record (EMR)" or "electronic health record (EHR)". Table 15.4 provides a basic list of the sections and their corresponding contents.

### TABLE 15.4.  THE MEDICAL CHART

| Section | Contents | Contents |
|---|---|---|
| Face sheet | Patient medical record number | Unique numerical assignment for each patient; stays the same for each hospital/hospital district |
| | Financial/admission number | Unique numerical assignment for each patient encounter |
| | Patient demographics | Includes information like name, admitting/attending physician, admitting diagnosis, medical service, age, birth date, sex, SSN, address, phone number, next of kin and contact info, religion, insurance, employer information |

*(continued)*

**TABLE 15.4.** THE MEDICAL CHART (*Continued*)

| Section | Contents | Comments |
|---|---|---|
| History and physical (H&P) | Patient demographics | |
| | Chief complaint (CC) | |
| | History of present illness (HxPI) | |
| | Past medical history (PMH) | |
| | Surgical history (SxH) | |
| | Home medications | |
| | Allergies | |
| | Social history (SH) | |
| | Family history (FH) | |
| | Review of systems (ROS) | |
| | Physical examination (PE) | |
| | Impression/assessment | |
| | Plan | |
| Consultations | Cardiology | Same format as H&P |
| | Nephrology | Specialty physicians may be consulted for difficult cases |
| | Infectious diseases | |
| | Neurology | |
| | Psychiatry | |
| | Hematology | |
| | Oncology | |
| Physician orders | Documentation of all orders | Usually in reverse chronological order |
| | Medications | |
| | Treatments | |
| | Tests | |
| Progress notes | Attending physicians | Daily history of what's going on with the patient |
| | Consulting physicians | |
| | Consulting services | |
| | Pharmacokinetic consult service notes | |
| | Case management notes | |
| | Respiratory therapy notes | |
| | Dietary notes | |

**TABLE 15.4.** THE MEDICAL CHART (*Continued*)

| Section | Contents | Contents |
|---|---|---|
| Laboratory | Reporting of laboratory values drawn by date and time | Typically has reference ranges can have summaries (all CBC results for hospital stay) Can have interpretations for uncommon laboratory results |
| Nursing notes | Admission assessment<br><br>Initial height and weight, allergies<br><br>Daily flow sheets<br><br>Documentation of physical assessments and laboratories<br><br>Documentation of vital signs<br><br>IV access documentation<br><br>Intake and outputs documentation<br><br>Weight<br><br>Graphical representation of vitals for trending purposes | Frequency of vital sign assessment determined by level of care patient is receiving |
| Medication administration records (MARs) | Daily documentation of meds administered to patient<br><br>Time medications administered<br><br>Site of injections<br><br>Reasons for not administering<br><br>Reasons for administering prn medications<br><br>Pain scores<br><br>Fingerstick blood glucose levels<br><br>MAR checks | MAR check is when a hospital personnel checks the MAR against the physician orders to verify no orders are missed during order entry |
| Cardiology | ECG strips<br><br>12-lead ECG reports<br><br>Echocardiogram results | |

(*continued*)

**TABLE 15.4.** THE MEDICAL CHART (*Continued*)

| Section | Contents | Contents |
|---|---|---|
| Radiology | X-ray results | |
| | Ultrasounds | |
| | CT scans | |
| | MRI results | |
| | Mammograms | |
| | Nuclear medicine scans | |
| Surgical procedures | Documentation of surgical procedures | |
| Respiratory therapy record | Documentation of respiratory therapy procedures | |
| | Documentation of respiratory medication administration | |
| | Ventilator settings | |
| Documentation of blood products received | Packed red blood cells (PRBC) | |
| | Fresh frozen plasma (FFP) | |
| | Platelets | |
| | Miscellaneous | |
| Legal documents | End of life instructions | |
| | Do not resuscitate (DNR) | |
| | Do not intubate (DNI) | |
| | Living will | |
| Miscellaneous | Emergency medical transport (EMT) records | |
| | Discharge notes from previous hospital stays | |

## Accreditation

Patients, payers and government agencies expect health-care organizations to complete self-assessments and be externally peer-reviewed to accurately assess their level of performance in relation to established standards and to implement ways to continuously improve. This process is commonly known as accreditation, and it provides a report card for the public. In terms of health-care organizations in the United States, there are various accrediting bodies available to this external assessment.[19]

---

**TABLE 15.5.** THE REASONS ORGANIZATIONS SEEK ACCREDITATION

- Enhance the community's confidence in the care provided
- Provide a report card for the public
- Supply a marketing tool in this time of competitive health-care marketplace (failure to meet standards can severely affect an organization's prestige)
- Represent state-of-the-art performance improvement strategies that focus on quality health care while providing safe patient care
- May fulfill all or part of state licensing requirements
- Required by most residency programs (medical, pharmacy, nursing)
- Boost recruitment of qualified personnel
- Encourage staff development
- Acknowledged by some third-party payers for reimbursement of services
- Provides deeming authority for Medicare and in some states Medicaid certification without undergoing separate government inspection
- Lessen liability insurance costs
- Provide outline for favorable organizational structure

---

The Joint Commission (TJC, formerly referred to as JCAHO), and its international branch Joint Commission International (JCI), is an independent not-for-profit organization that provides uniform recognized standards for institutions developed by experts in various health-care fields. TJC accredits over 20,000 (greater than 90%) health-care organizations and programs in the United States through implementation of these standards. This recognition is a symbol of safety and quality reflecting an institution's commitment to optimal achievable care. The reasons organizations seek accreditation are listed in Table 15.5.[20,21] A leading Joint Commission theme is safety, which was emphasized by the implementation of the National Patient Safety Goals in 2003. The initial aim for the development of the goals was to promote specific improvements in patient safety, while realizing that errors were the result of system-wide failures, therefore safety must be a system-wide approach. There are different goals for various types of organizations, however for hospitals, there are 15 goals with 6 underlying themes. Since their inception, the goals are generally updated annually. For a full list of the 2013 National Patient Safety Goals refer to Table 15.6.[22] Additionally, various standards have been developed with the input of HCPs, subject matter experts, consumers, government agencies and employers. Within these standards, various other safety requirements have been incorporated. One such standard you may be exposed to is IM.02.02.01 limiting the use of

| TABLE 15.6. 2013 NATIONAL PATIENT SAFETY GOALS | |
|---|---|
| **Number Goals and Subgoals** | |
| Goal 1 | Identify patients correctly |
| | Use at least two patient identifiers when providing care, treatment, or services |
| | Make sure that the correct patient gets the correct blood type during a blood transfusion |
| Goal 2 | Improve staff communication |
| | Get important test results to the right staff person on time. |
| Goal 3 | Use medicines safely |
| | Before a procedure, label medicines that are not labeled. For example, medicines in syringes, cups, and basins. Do this in the area where medicines and supplies are set up. |
| | Take extra care with patients who take medicines to thin their blood. |
| Goal 7 | Prevent infection |
| | Use the hand cleaning guidelines from the Centers for Disease Control and Prevention or the World Health Organization. Set goals for improving hand cleaning. Use the goals to improve hand cleaning. |
| | Use proven guidelines to prevent infections that are difficult to treat. |
| | Use proven guidelines to prevent infection of the blood from central lines. |
| Goal 15 | Identify patient safety risks |
| | Find out which patients are most likely to try to commit suicide. |
| Universal Protocol 1 | Prevent mistakes in surgery |
| | Make sure that the correct surgery is done on the correct patient and at the correct place on the patient's body. |
| | Mark the correct place on the patient's body where the surgery is to be done. |
| | Pause before the surgery to make sure that a mistake is not being made. |

Prohibited (Do Not Use Abbreviations). Please refer to Table 15.7 for the full list of Prohibited Abbreviations.[23]

Assessment of core measures integrates outcomes into the accreditation process by permitting rigorous comparison of the actual core measure results across hospitals. Specifically, the public can compare core measurement activity from one

**TABLE 15.7.** THE JOINT COMMISSION "DO NOT USE" LIST

| Abbreviation | Potential Problem | Use Instead |
|---|---|---|
| "u" | Mistaken for zero, 4, or cc | Write out |
| "IU" | Mistaken for IV or 10 | Write out |
| "qd" or "qod" | Mistaken for each other or qid | Write out |
| Trailing zero/lack of leading zero | Decimal point missed | Write "x" mg or "0.x" mg |
| MS, $MSO_4$, and $MgSO_4$ | Mistaken for each other | Write out |

institution to another to see how they compare. There are over 14 performance measures evaluated based on therapeutic outcomes, including Surgical Care Improvement Project (SCIP), Venous Thromboembolism (VTE), Pneumonia Measures (PN), Acute Myocardial Infarction (AMI), Heart Failure (HF), Perinatal Care (PC), and Stroke (STK). TJC Oryx Core Measures are continually updated to reflect current practices and evidence based medicine. [24]

Other accreditation bodies, available for hospital assessment are Healthcare Facilities Accreditation Program (HFAP) and Det Norske Vertas (DNV). HFAP accredits all types of health-care organizations. Successful accreditation is based on the facility's ability to correct deficiencies encouraging discovery of these deficiencies during the survey process. DNV utilizes the ISO process, which is known in non-medical industries as a quality-management system with heavy emphasis on leadership and accountability. Quality-management systems within health-care or-ganizations are better prepared to reduce costs, manage work flow, and improve health outcomes. TJC, HFAP, and DNV are all approved accreditation programs by CMS as a requirement for CMS reimbursement. [21]

## Hospital Quality Initiatives

Publicly and privately owned health-care purchasers are continually looking for ways to increase quality by limiting overuse, misuse and waste of health care. This should ultimately increase the value of health care. These undertakings are collec-tively called value-based purchasing (VBP). [25] In order to "move Medicare from a passive payer of claims to a prudent purchaser of healthcare services," the Centers for Medicare and Medicaid Services (CMS) adopted VBP strategies as mandated by the 2010 Affordable Care Act, incentivizing hospitals to meet or improve on performance standards. [26] Measures included are listed in Table 15.8. Patients are ultimately the winners since consumers will have data available to compare hospital performance (www.hospitalcompare.hhs.gov).

**TABLE 15.8.** HOSPITAL QUALITY INITIATIVES

| Types | Quality Measures |
|---|---|
| Hospital Care Quality Information from the Consumer Perspective Survey Elements | 1. Communication with doctors |
| | 2. Communication with nurses |
| | 3. Responsiveness of hospital staff |
| | 4. Pain management |
| | 5. Communication about medicines |
| | 6. Discharge information |
| | 7. Cleanliness of the hospital environment |
| | 8. Quietness of the hospital environment |
| Clinical Process of Care Measures | 1. Fibrinolytic Therapy Received Within 30 Minutes of Hospital Arrival of Acute Myocardial Infarction |
| | 2. Primary PCI Received Within 90 Minutes of Hospital Arrival of Acute Myocardial Infarction |
| | 3. Discharge Instructions for Patients Admitted with Heart Failure |
| | 4. Blood Cultures Performed in the ED Prior to Initial Antibiotic Received in Hospital for Community Acquired Pneumonia (CAP) |
| | 5. Appropriate Initial Antibiotic Selection for CAP in Immunocompetent Patient |
| | 6. Prophylactic Antibiotic Received Within One Hour Prior to Surgical Incision |
| | 7. Appropriate Prophylactic Antibiotic Selection for Surgical Patients |
| | 8. Prophylactic Antibiotics Discontinued Within 24 Hours After Surgery End Time |
| | 9. Cardiac Surgery Patients with Controlled 6 AM Postoperative Serum Glucose |
| | 10. Surgery Patients with Recommended Venous Thromboembolism Prophylaxis Ordered |
| | 11. Surgery Patients Who Received Appropriate Venous Thromboembolism Prophylaxis within 24 Hours |
| | 12. Surgery Patients on a Beta Blocker Prior to Arrival Who Received a Beta Blocker During the Perioperative Period |

**TABLE 15.8.** HOSPITAL QUALITY INITIATIVES (*Continued*)

| Types | Quality Measures |
|---|---|
| 30-day mortality claims-based measures | 1. Acute Myocardial Infarction (AMI) 30-day Mortality Rate |
| | 2. Heart Failure (HF) 30-day Mortality Rate |
| | 3. Pneumonia (PN) 30-Day Mortality Rate |
| Hospital Acquired Condition Measures | 1. Foreign Object Retained After Surgery |
| | 2. Air Embolism |
| | 3. Blood Incompatibility |
| | 4. Pressure Ulcer Stages III & IV |
| | 5. Falls and Trauma |
| | 6. Vascular Catheter-Associated Infections |
| | 7. Catheter-Associated Urinary Tract Infection (UTI) |
| | 8. Manifestations of Poor Glycemic Control |
| AHRQ Patient Safety Indicators (PSIs), Inpatient Quality Indicators (IQIs), and Composite Measures | 1. Complication/patient safety for selected indicators (composite) |
| | 2. Mortality for selected medical conditions (composite) |

## Pharmacy and Therapeutics Committee

The Pharmacy and Therapeutics (P&T) Committee is a multidisciplinary committee charged with ensuring safe medication use in an institution or health system. Committee members vary from institution to institution, but generally consist of physicians, pharmacists, nurses, administrators, other allied HCPs, and representatives from ambulatory care and clinical laboratories. A physician is typically the chair of the committee and the physician members should encompass all disciplines in the institution. A pharmacy representative typically acts as the secretary. Hospital bylaws give the committee the authority to make decisions regarding medication use. Recommendations from the P&T Committee go to various executive committees for final institutional approval. This process varies slightly depending on institution. In addition, TJC stipulates within its standards that the policies regarding medication use of an institution is determined in a multidisciplinary approach. Committee functions include developing and maintaining the drug formulary system, policy development, acting in an advisory capacity for medication-related issues, and providing quality assurance activities and educational programs as needed.[27] Table 15.9 provides a sample P&T Committee agenda.

| TABLE 15.9. SAMPLE AGENDA OF P&T COMMITTEE MEETING | |
| --- | --- |
| **Agenda Item** | **Comments** |
| Previous minutes | Previous meetings minutes are approved by committee members. |
| Formulary review | Drug Formulary System: An ongoing process whereby a health-care organization, through its physicians, pharmacists, and other health-care professionals, establishes policies on the use of drug products and therapies, and identifies drug products and therapies that are the most medically appropriate (including ethical, legal, social, philosophical, quality-of-life, and safety factors) and cost-effective to best serve the health interests of a given patient population. |
| | Drug Formulary: A continually updated list of medications and related information for use in the organization, representing the clinical judgment of physicians, pharmacists, and other experts in the diagnosis and/or treatment of disease and promotion of health. |
| Policy establishment | Regarding anything pertaining to medications within the hospital system, including administration, procurement, storage, etc. |
| Subcommittee reports | Examples include anti-infective and medication safety. |
| Quality assurance activities | Medication error reports. |
| | Adverse drug reaction reports. |
| | Antibiotic utilization review. |
| | Drug usage review. |
| Adjournment | Recommendations go to various executive committees for final institutional approval. |
| | Process varies slightly depending on institution. |

# EDUCATIONAL EXPERIENCES IN AN INSTITUTIONAL SETTING

## Introduction

*Introductory Pharmacy Practice Experiences*

A student pharmacist will be exposed to a variety of people, job responsibilities, and areas in the institutional pharmacy. The information may be overwhelming, but take advantage of the opportunities. Your preceptor and other personnel will be a wealth of knowledge. Remember that learning how to fill physician's orders and interacting with other HCPs appropriately are the two major goals of most introductory pharmacy practice hospital experiences.

### Advanced Pharmacy Practice Experiences

What you learned in your institution introductory pharmacy practice experiences (IPPEs) will lay a foundation for the knowledge and skills needed to begin your advanced pharmacy practice experiences (APPEs). The old adage of "it doesn't matter how great the medication is if it doesn't get to the patient" is very true. Generally, APPE preceptors expect student pharmacists to practice as if they are responsible since you are typically a few short months away from joining the pharmacy profession as a licensed practitioner. This is simultaneously a great responsibility and a great opportunity. Table 15.10 lists selected activities in which students are expected to participate in during APPEs.[28]

### Team Participation

Rounding may be a primary activity during certain institutional experiences. The format of rounds will differ greatly from institution to institution. Even within one institution, medical services or attending physicians may conduct rounds differently. Table 15.11 defines some of the terms associated with rounds. Chapter 5 includes a detailed discussion of appropriate team interactions which you are urged to read and review.

The goal of rounds is to facilitate communication between parties caring for a particular patient. Attending rounds with physicians and other HCP can help you gain insight into why certain treatment decisions are being made. Rounding also

---

**TABLE 15.10. SELECTED ACTIVITIES IN WHICH STUDENTS ON ADVANCED PHARMACY PRACTICE EXPERIENCES SHOULD PARTICIPATE**

- Practicing as a member of an interprofessional team
- Identifying, evaluating, and communicating to the patient and other health-care professionals the appropriateness of the patient's specific pharmacotherapeutic agents, dosing regimens, dosage forms, routes of administration, and delivery systems
- Identifying and reporting medication errors and adverse drug reactions
- Managing the drug regimen through monitoring and assessing patient information
- Providing pharmacist-delivered patient care to a diverse patient population
- Providing patient education to a diverse patient population
- Educating the public and health-care professionals regarding medical conditions, wellness, dietary supplements, durable medical equipment, and medical and drug devices
- Retrieving, evaluating, managing, and using clinical and scientific publications in the decision-making process
- Accessing, evaluating, and applying information to promote optimal health care ensuring continuity of pharmaceutical care among health-care settings

## TABLE 15.11.  ROUNDS AND ASSOCIATED TERMS

- Rounds ("rounds will start at 9 AM on the 6th floor")

  The act of seeing patients

- Walking rounds

  Medical team moves from bedside to bedside to discuss patient cases

  Physical assessment and interaction with the patient may or may not occur

- Sitting rounds

  Patients are discussed while sitting in a conference room or at the nursing station

  The patient chart (or EMR) may or may not be available for review during rounds

  Patients may or may not be physically seen by the entire team after sitting rounds

- Prerounds ("please have your prerounding done before we meet at 8 AM")

  Preparation time before rounds

  Members of the medical team round individually on their assigned patients in order to be prepared for formal rounds with the preceptor or attending physician

  The student pharmacist should consider speaking to each of his/her assigned patients daily during prerounds to assess medication-related issues (ie, tolerability, adverse effects, symptom improvement)

- Grand rounds

  Typically refers to a multidisciplinary teaching conference involving a patient case

affords the student pharmacist an opportunity to make recommendations regarding drug selection, monitoring, and other aspects of pharmacotherapy as depicted in Figure 15.6. Rounds can also occur in nonteaching hospitals without medical students and residents. You may be asked to attend rounds with nurses, respiratory therapists, or pharmacists. In some instances, you and your preceptor (or another pharmacist or student) might round alone allowing for more time and detail to be focused on pharmacotherapy discussions. Some pharmacists might conduct their own rounds in the afternoon in order to prepare for multidisciplinary rounds the following morning.

The role of the student pharmacist on rounds will be specific to each institution. You should discuss the following questions in detail with your preceptor. Are you expected to observe or actively participate? If you believe that something in the medication regimen should be addressed by the team, who should you mention it to and when? Should you proactively bring primary literature to rounds or prepare short educational presentations? What should you do if you cannot answer a question? These are all topics that you and your preceptor should discuss before your first day of rounds. As a student training in an institution, you will also be involved in supporting the clinical and administrative initiatives of the department of pharmacy. Hospitals often have many clinical initiatives underway

**Figure 15.6.** Pharmacy's role on the medical teaching teams.

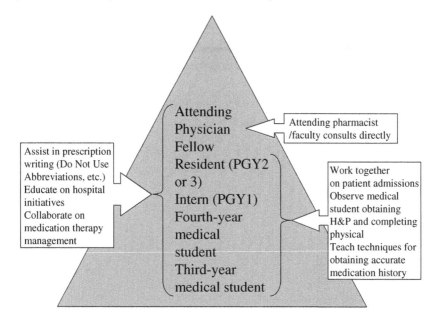

at any given time depending on the priorities of the department. Some of the most common clinical initiatives in hospitals today are listed in Table 15.12. Pharmacy initiatives (and the relative importance of them) will differ from hospital to hospital, but some are mandated by regulatory agencies like TJC. Some of the goals of pharmacy initiatives include maintaining the formulary, reducing unnecessary medication use, reducing cost, optimizing therapy, and improving patient safety.

Site-specific pharmacy initiatives should be reviewed with you during your orientation. As you follow patients and work with the team, you should verify that these initiatives are being met. Your preceptor may print reports for patients on your team who require screening or intervention to meet a particular initiative. For example, you may receive a report of all patients on your team who have an active order for warfarin. It might be your responsibility to conduct patient education or to recommend appropriate warfarin dose adjustments based on the daily international normalized ratios (INRs) of these patients. You may be required to document discharge counseling for all of your patients being discharged on more than five medications.

### "Following" and "Monitoring" Patients

APPEs enable student pharmacists to begin "practicing" pharmacy while still being closely supervised by licensed pharmacists. During your clinical experiences (internal medicine, cardiology, infectious diseases, transplantation, oncology, pediatrics, etc.) you may be assigned certain patients to monitor throughout the hospital admission. The number and complexity of the assigned patients will differ depending on the

## TABLE 15.12. HOSPITAL PHARMACY INITIATIVES

IV to po conversions

Renal dosing conversion

Therapeutic interchanges or formulary interchanges

Anticoagulation monitoring and counseling

Antibiotic streamlining, surveillance, and/or stewardship

Pharmacy consult services (dosing and/or monitoring)

- TPN
- Vancomycin and aminoglycosides
- Phenytoin
- Erythropoietin
- Others

Discharge counseling

Medication counseling

Medication reconciliation

Screening for "do-not-use" abbreviations

The Joint Commission Oryx Core Measure adherence

HCAHPS

structure at the site and your ability. When you are asked to "monitor" a particular patient, it is generally expected that you will have fully assessed the patient's medication regimen for drug-related problems. Monitoring drug therapy and medication safety is the core of what we do as pharmacists. Techniques for monitoring drug therapy have been discussed in detail in Chapter 6. During each APPE, your skills at monitoring drug therapy (even very complicated medication regimens) will improve with practice. On your first APPE it might take an hour or more to obtain all of the necessary information from the medical record and then an additional hour or more to fully assess the regimen and create your own assessment and plan. Do not get discouraged! This is time well spent. Each patient experience will improve your skills. You will want to assess many things in each medication regimen. Table 15.13 groups some of the assessment activities into difficulty level. Strive to complete all of these assessment activities on each and every individual.

Individuals admitted to the hospital often have a complicated medical history. During the inpatient admission, some individuals may be receiving 10 or more medications. Many of the medications will be protocol driven. In other words, individuals admitted to a certain unit or with a certain diagnosis could be required to have certain medications on their profile for "as needed" use. Table 15.14 lists some of the common protocol medications for patients admitted with chest pain.

---

**TABLE 15.13. MEDICATION REGIMEN ASSESSMENT ACTIVITIES (GROUPED BY PRECEPTOR-PERCEIVED DIFFICULTY LEVEL)**

Low-level assessment

Medications are dosed correctly

Medication regimen has been screened for drug interactions

Patient allergies/intolerances have been noted and addressed

Patient's pregnancy and lactation status has been noted and addressed

Mid-level assessment

All medication doses have been adjusted for patient-specific factors (renal and/or hepatic insufficiency)

Indications and contraindications for all medications have been assessed

All institution-specific initiatives have been addressed (IV to po, therapeutic interchange, etc.)

PRN medication use has been assessed

High-level assessment

Medication regimens adhere to evidence-based practice guidelines

Culture and sensitivity results have been assessed and antibiotic regimen has been adjusted accordingly

Appropriate monitoring has been conducted to assess efficacy and safety of all medications

---

**TABLE 15.14. EXAMPLE OF PRN PROTOCOL FOR PATIENTS ADMITTED TO THE CHEST PAIN UNIT**

Nitroglycerin 0.4 mg sublingual tablet prn chest pain

Nitroglycerin drip, start as needed for chest pain not relieved by nitroglycerin sublingual tablets

Morphine 2 mg IV Q15 minutes for pain not relieved by nitroglycerin

Acetaminophen 650 mg po Q6h for temperature >100°F

---

Protocol-driven medications, like those listed above are often difficult for students to discuss and assess. For instance, if your patient has an active order for the protocol medications listed in Table 15.14, you should state that during your presentation of the patient. It will be more important, however, to discuss which of these prn medications your patient has actually received. The individual whose chest pain is relieved by one sublingual nitroglycerin tablet is very different from the individual receiving a nitroglycerin drip and morphine every 15 minutes without relief of the pain. Your preceptor will want to be certain that you understand the distinction. It is generally expected that an advanced student should be able to prioritize the patients that he/she has been assigned to follow or monitor.

*Prioritization*

What if you were asked to prioritize the following three patients based solely on their medication lists? Which patient would you focus on first? Discuss these scenarios with your preceptor to make sure you are managing your time wisely.

| Scenario One—Patient 1 |
| --- |
| Aspirin enteric coated 81 mg po daily |
| Digoxin 0.25 mg po daily |
| Enoxaparin 70 mg SubQ 12h |
| Diltiazem-0.9% NaCl (1 mg/mL) titrate to keep HR<110 |
| Dextrose 5%–0.45% NaCl IV 75 mL/h |
| Sliding Scale Regular Insulin |
| Note: 0–60 = D50W 1 amp and recheck in 1 hour |
| 61–150 = 0 units |
| 151–200 = 2 units |
| 201–250 = 4 units |
| 251–300 = 6 units |
| 301–350 = 8 units |
| 351–400 = 10 units |
| > 400 = 10 units and call MD |

| Scenario Two—Patient 2 |
| --- |
| Aspirin enteric coated 162 mg po chew now |
| Albuterol/Ipratropium1 unit inhaled Q8h and prn for SOB |
| Furosemide 40 mg IV now |
| Morphine sulfate 4 mg IVP now |
| Budesonide 2 puffs inhaled bid (home dose) |

| Scenario Three—Patient 3 |
| --- |
| Acetylcysteine 9800 mg po mixed in cola now, then 4900 mg po Q4h × 17 doses |
| Lisinopril 10 mg po daily |
| Fluoxetine 20 mg po daily |

What if you were asked to prioritize the following three patients by their chief complaint? Which patient would you focus on first? Discuss with your preceptor how they would prioritize these cases.

| |
|---|
| **Scenario One—Patient 1** |
| 45-yo male patient with chest pain radiating down the left arm |
| **Scenario Two—Patient 2** |
| 68-yo male patient with a history of alcoholism and severe pain in the upper middle left part of the abdomen that worsens after eating |
| **Scenario Three—Patient 3** |
| 27-yo female patient who is 27 weeks pregnant with dysuria |

### Working With Students from Other Pharmacy Schools

You may be scheduled to complete introductory or advanced experiences at a site with students from several different pharmacy schools. How should you approach this scenario? Hopefully you will use it as an opportunity to assess your individual strengths and weaknesses, but more importantly you should use this as an opportunity to work together toward a common goal with one of your future colleagues.

### How Will You Stand Out?

Each year a large number of student pharmacists graduate from colleges with the entry level Doctor of Pharmacy degree. Some of these new practitioners will go on to complete residencies, fellowships, and graduate programs. Many will become board certified or obtain other specialized training. How will you stand out and obtain the job you want? One way is to make the most of your APPEs. This will probably be the only time in your life when your only job is to learn! You should make the most of it! Your APPEs will vary in difficulty and required time commitment. How will you spend your free time? You might choose to get involved with extra pharmacy-related projects. Motivated and enthusiastic students tend to seek out additional projects that will broaden their knowledge base, increase their exposure, and/or make them more marketable to potential employers. It might not be possible for you to complete all of the APPEs that you would like. Maybe you had hoped to gain experience in nutrition support, but that particular experience did not fit into your schedule or the preceptor was unavailable. You might ask your institutional preceptor if you could work on a TPN service as an extra project. If you make a request like this, you should be prepared to complete the project on your own time (summer, nights, weekends, or during a break). You should not expect the project to substitute for any of the required aspects of the experience. Table 15.15 lists ideas for extra projects that you might consider. Many of the projects listed in this table might look impressive on

---

**TABLE 15.15.** EXTRA "PROJECTS" FOR THE MOTIVATED STUDENT PHARMACIST

Clinical projects

   Becoming certified in advanced cardiac life support (ACLS)

   Conducting a medication use evaluation (MUE)

   Preparing and presenting an in-service for pharmacy or other staff

   Developing a new policy or procedure

   Shadowing pharmacists or other HCPs with unique practices

Research-related projects

   Designing and conducting a research project

   Collecting data for an ongoing research project

   Working with a preceptor on a grant application

   Presenting a poster at a professional meeting

   Participating in the manuscript development process

Administrative and academic-related projects

   Developing training manuals or tutorials

   Facilitating a laboratory or teaching a class

   Writing a newsletter article

   Writing a review article for publication

   Writing a drug monograph (and presenting it at a Pharmacy and Therapeutics Committee meeting)

---

a student's curriculum vitae, but the point is for you to obtain the experiences and exposure that will make you a better practitioner. You will probably also impress your preceptors with your initiative!

## CONCLUSION

There are many opportunities for learning in an institutional setting. This chapter described areas of institutions and practices that are common. As a student pharmacist, you should integrate the knowledge of laws, accreditation, and various practices into your core skills and knowledge. It is important to know who works in institutions and how the pharmacist interacts with these individuals. It is also important to understand the different kinds of responsibilities the pharmacist must manage including but not limited to medication safety, patient counseling, HCP education, and interaction with professionals. Knowledge of accreditation standards and hospital committees will benefit you during your experiences. As a student pharmacist, you should interact with medical students, nursing students, and other student pharmacists from other colleges. These may be the same individuals you will work with during your professional career. These student interactions are a great way to increase your professional network and knowledge. Take advantage of experiential education to build your core skills and knowledge of practice.

## APPLICATION EXERCISES

1. In which section of the medical chart would you find the "chief complaint" and "past medical history"?
   A. History and physical
   B. Laboratory
   C. Medication administration records
   D. Radiology
2. List some of the personnel in a typical hospital department of pharmacy.
3. Authorized personnel with a higher level of training are typically needed to administer which of the following?
   A. Oral medications
   B. Continuous IV infusions
   C. Intermittent IV push medications
   D. Intermittent IV piggyback medications
4. List several reasons that hospitals seek accreditation by The Joint Commission.
5. Which of the following is a National Patient Safety Goal?
   A. Improve the effectiveness of communication among caregivers.
   B. Accurately and completely reconcile medications across the continuum of care.
   C. Improve the safety of using medications.
   D. All of the above.
6. What is wrong with the order "warfarin 4.0 mg po daily"?
   A. "Daily" should be abbreviated "QD."
   B. Warfarin should always be ordered by brand name.
   C. Trailing zeros should never be used.
   D. Nothing. The order is correct as written.
7. Which committee is charged with ensuring safe medication use in an institution or health system?
   A. The Anti-Infective Monitoring Committee
   B. The Medical Executive Committee
   C. The Joint Commission (TJC)
   D. The Pharmacy and Therapeutics Committee (P&T)
8. Which of the following accurately describes the hierarchy of the medical teaching team?
   A. Intern → medical student → attending physician → fellow
   B. Medical student → resident → fellow → attending physician
   C. Resident → fellow → intern → attending physician
   D. Medical student → resident → attending physician → fellow

9. Which of the following hospital initiatives might you become involved with during your IPPE and/or APPE courses?
   A. Medication reconciliation
   B. Intravenous to oral conversion
   C. Antibiotic stewardship
   D. All of the above
10. Discuss several things you could do to stand out in a positive way during your APPEs.

## REFERENCES

1. American Hospital Association. Fast facts on US hospitals. 2013. Available at http://www.aha.org/research/rc/stat-studies/fast-facts.shtml. Accessed March, 2014.
2. Snook I. Today's hospital. In: Snook I, ed. *Hospitals: What They Are and How They Work*. 2nd ed. Philadelphia, PA: Jones & Bartlett; 2003:9–11.
3. United States Department of Health & Human Services, Centers for Disease Control & Prevention, National Center for Health Statistics. National hospital discharge survey data documentation 2010. 2012(March). Available at ftp://ftp.cdc.gov/pub/Health_Statistics/NCHS/Dataset_Documentation/NHDS/NHDS_2010_Documentation.pdf. Accessed March, 2014.
4. Snook I. Organization. In: Snook I, ed. *Hospitals: What They Are and How They Work*. 2nd ed. Philadelphia, PA: Jones & Bartlett; 2003:17–24.
5. American Society of Health-System Pharmacist. ASHP pharmacy practice model initiative. 2013. Available at http://www.ashpmedia.org/ppmi/index.html. Accessed March, 2014.
6. Otto C, McCloskey. Hospitals. In: McCarthy R, Schafermeyer K, eds. *Introduction to Health Care Delivery*. 4th ed. Sandbury, MA: Jones & Bartlett; 2004: 167–190.
7. The Joint Commission. Hospital accreditation standards. Oakbrook Terrace, IL; 2012:MM 4.10. Available at http://www.jointcommission.org/standards_information/edition.aspx (Login required).
8. Murray MD, Shojania KG. Unit-dose distribution systems. In: *Making Health Care Safer: A Critical Analysis of Patient Safety Practice*. Rockville, MD: Agency for Healthcare Research and Quality; 2001:101–110. Available at http://www.ahrq.gov/clinic/ptsafety/. Accessed March, 2014.
9. United States Food and Drug Administration. CPG Sec 430.100 unit dose labeling for solid and liquid oral dosage forms. Compliance Policy Guides. 1984. Available at http://www.fda.gov/ICECI/ComplianceManuals/CompliancePolicyGuidanceManual/ucm074377.htm. Accessed March, 2014.
10. Shack J, Tulloch S. Integrated pharmacy automation systems lead to increases in patient safety and significant the reductions in medication inventory costs [Shore Memorial Hospital] (Case Study). Fairport, NY; 2008. Available at

http://www.mckesson.com/static_files/McKesson.com/MPT/Documents/ MAIFiles/CaseStudy_Shore_Memorial_Hospital.pdf . Accessed March, 2014.

11. McKesson Automation. Evergreen Hospital Medical Center nursing, pharmacy benefit from ROBOT-Rx: http://singularityhub.com/2012/06/03/meet-robot-rx-the-robot-pharmacist-doling-out-350-million-doses-per-year/. Accessed March, 2014.

12. Murray MD. Automated medication dispensing devices. In: *Making Health Care Safer: A Critical Analysis of Patient Safety Practice*. Rockville, MD: Agency for Healthcare Research and Quality; 2001:111–117. Available at http://www.ahrq .gov/clinic/ptsafety/. Accessed March, 2014.

13. Timby B, Smith N. Caring for clients with disorders of upper gastrointestinal tract. In: Timby B, Smith N, eds. *Introductory Medical-Surgical Nursing*. 9th ed. Philadelphia, PA: Lippincott Wilkinson & Wilkins; 2007:821–846.

14. Mitchell JF. Oral dosage forms that should not be crushed. Institute of Safe Medication Practices. 2012:1–15. Available at http://www.ismp.org/tools/ donotcrush.pdf. Accessed March, 2014.

15. Institute of Safe Medication Practices. Label formats finalized versions. Institute of Safe Medication Practices. 2013. Available at http://www.ismp.org/Tools/ guidelines/labelFormats/default.asp. Accessed March, 2014.

16. Vitale C, Domenici Belisle C, Fanikos J. Chapter 17: Sterile Products. In: Shargel L, Mutnick A, Souney P, Swanson L, eds. *Comprehensive Pharmacy Review for NAPLEX*. 8e. Baltimore, MD: Lippincott Williams & Wilkins; 2013. www. lwwhealthlibrary.com. Accessed March 24, 2014.

17. Wald H, Shojania KG. Prevention of misidentifications. In: *Making Health Care Safer: A Critical Analysis of Patient Safety Practice*. Agency for Healthcare Research and Quality; 2001:487–500. Available at http://www.ahrq.gov/clinic/ ptsafety/. Accessed March, 2014.

18. Institute of Safe Medication Practices. Proceedings from the ISMP summit on the use of smart infusion pumps: Guidelines for safe implementation and use. 2009:1–19. Available at http://www.ismp.org/tools/guidelines/smartpumps/ default.asp. Accessed March, 2014.

19. Groene O. Implementing health promotion in hospitals: Manual and self-assessment forms. 2010. Available at http://www.euro.who.int/__data/assets/ pdf_file/0009/99819/E88584.pdf. Accessed March, 2014.

20. The Joint Commission. About The Joint Commission. 2013. Available at http:// www.jointcommission.org/about_us/about_the_joint_commission_main.aspx. Accessed March, 2014.

21. DerGurahian J. DNV setting new standard. *Modern Healthcare*. 2008:2–4. Available at http://www.nxtbook.com/ygsreprints/ygs/modh-1-25337720/ index.php?startid=2#/2. Accessed March, 2014.

22. The Joint Commission. 2013 Hospital National Patient Safety Goals. 2013. Available at http://www.jointcommission.org/standards_information/npsgs. aspx. Accessed March, 2014.

23. The Joint Commission. Facts about the official "Do Not Use" list of abbrevia-
    tions. 2013. Available at http://www.jointcommission.org/facts_about_the_
    official_/. Accessed March, 2014.

24. The Joint Commission. Core measure sets. 2013. Available at http://www
    .jointcommission.org/core_measure_sets.aspx. Accessed March, 2014.

25. Scanlon DP, Chernew M, Doty HE. Introduction. In: *Evaluating the Impact of
    Value-Based Purchasing: A Guide for Purchasers*. Rockville: Agency for Health-
    care Research and Quality; 2002. Available at http://www.ahrq.gov/qual/
    valuebased/. Accessed March, 2014.

26. Centers for Medicare and Medicaid Services. CMS issues final rule for first year
    of hospital value-based purchasing program. Baltimore, MA; 2011. Available at
    http://www.cms.gov/apps/media/press/factsheet.asp?Counter=3947. Accessed
    March, 2014.

27. Tyler LS, Millares M, Wilson AL, Valentino A, Cole SW, Com- P. ASHP state-
    ment on the Pharmacy and Therapeutics Committee and the formulary sys-
    tem. American Journal of Health-System Pharmacy. 2008;65(24):2384–2386.
    doi:10.2146/ajhp080413.

28. Accreditation Council of Pharmacy Education. Accreditation standards and
    guidelines for the professional program in pharmacy leading to the doctor
    of pharmacy degree. Chicago, IL; 2011:1–97. Available at https://www.acpe-
    accredit.org/pharmacists/standards.asp. Accessed March, 2014.

## APPLICATION EXERCISE ANSWERS

1. In which section of the medical chart would you find the "chief complaint" and
   "past medical history?"
   History and physical

2. List some of the personnel in a typical hospital department of pharmacy.
   See Table 15.3.

3. Authorized personnel with a higher level of training are typically needed to
   administer which of the following?
   Intermittent IV push medications

4. List several reasons that hospitals seek accreditation by The Joint Commission.
   See Table 15.5.

5. Which of the following is a National Patient Safety Goal for 2009?
   Improve the effectiveness of communication among caregivers. Accurately
   and completely reconcile medications across the continuum of care.
   Improve the safety of using medications.

6. What is wrong with the following order "warfarin 4.0 mg po daily?"
   Trailing zeros should never be used.

7. Which committee is charged with ensuring safe medication use in an institution
   or health system?
   The Pharmacy and Therapeutics Committee (P&T)

8. Which of the following accurately describes the hierarchy of the medical teaching team?

    Medical student → resident → fellow → attending physician

9. Which of the following hospital initiatives might you become involved with during your pharmacy practice experience courses?

    Medication reconciliation

    IV to po conversions

    Antibiotic stewardship

10. Discuss several things you could do to stand out in a positive way during your APPEs.

    See Table 15.15.

## HOSPITAL PATIENT CASE 1

| | |
|---|---|
| **Patient Name:** Ewen, Mark | **Admission Date:** 7/16/13 |
| **Gender:** M    **Race:** White | **Weight:** 197 lb    **Height:** 6'1" |
| **Allergies:** NKDA | |

**Chief Complaint:** "I'm having chest pain"

**HPI:**
ME is a 51-yo wm who presents to the ER complaining of stabbing chest pain with radiation to the left arm that woke him from sleep this morning. The pain has been constant since this morning and is rated an 8 of 10. He also complains of chest pressure, diaphoresis, and some shortness of breath. There has been no change in the pain (or associated symptoms) with activity or position.

| **PMH:** | **PSH:** |
|---|---|
| MI and stent placement (11/04) | Stent placement (11/99 in Canada, no |
| DVT and PE (11/04) | records available) |
| CAD (? duration) | Multiple skin grafts to lower extremities |
| Hyperlipidemia (? duration) | |
| Lower extremity PVD | |
| (diagnosed 1985) | |

| **Family History:** | **Social History:** |
|---|---|
| Mother deceased at | (−) tobacco |
| age 50, MVA | (−) illicit drug use |
| Father deceased at age 72, HF | Occasional ETOH |

| **Home Medications:** | **ROS/PE:** | |
|---|---|---|
| Lopressor 50 mg po bid | General: | WDWN wm with chest pain |
| Coumadin 5 mg po daily | Vitals: | BP: 111/76 HR: 82 |
| Aspirin 325 mg po daily | | RR: 20 T: 98.4 |
| Questran 1 packet daily | HEENT: | no abnormalities |
| Darvocet N100 prn | Neck: | (−) JVD |
| Nitrostat SL prn chest pain | CV: | (+) CP, constant; (+) pain on |
| | | chest wall with palpation |
| | Lungs: | (+) SOB; clear to ausculta- |
| | | tion bilaterally |
| | ABD: | (+) BS; (−) tenderness or |
| | | rebound |
| | GU: | deferred |
| | EXT: | multiple healed skin grafts |
| | | on lower extremities; stage |
| | | 2-3 stasis ulcer on LLE |
| | | (2cm diameter); vascular |
| | | insufficiency |
| | Neuro: | AAA × 3 |

## Laboratory Results

| Date: | 7/16 Admission | | 7/17 | | | | 7/18 | | 7/19 |
|---|---|---|---|---|---|---|---|---|---|
| Time: | 1800 | 2400 | 0600 | 1200 | 1800 | 2400 | 0600 | 1800 | 0600 |
| BP | 142/83 | 115/75 | 116/75 | 110/76 | 112/77 | 115/76 | 110/75 | 115/77 | 112/78 |
| HR | 82 | 73 | 54 | 60 | 64 | 70 | 70 | 72 | 75 |
| RR | 20 | 19 | 20 | 19 | 19 | 20 | 19 | 20 | 20 |
| $T_{max}$ | 98.4 | 98.6 | 98.2 | 98.4 | 98.5 | 98.6 | 98.4 | 98.6 | 98.5 |
| Na | 141 | | 139 | | | | 140 | | |
| K | 4.2 | | 4.2 | | | | 4.3 | | |
| Cl | 108 | | 106 | | | | 105 | | |
| $CO_2$ | 27 | | 26 | | | | 26 | | |
| BUN | 7 | | 12 | | | | 10 | | |
| SCr | 0.9 | | 1.0 | | | | 1.0 | | |
| Glucose | 101 | | 84 | | | | 95 | | |
| WBC | 5.85 | | 4.91 | | | | | | |
| Hgb | 15.7 | | 14.9 | | | | | | |
| Hct | 45.7 | | 44 | | | | | | |
| Platelets | 302 | | 293 | | | | | | |
| MCV | 96.1 | | 96 | | | | | | |
| MCHC | 33 | | 34 | | | | | | |
| RDW | 12.2 | | 11.9 | | | | | | |
| CK | 76 | 74 | 58 | | | | | | |
| CKMB | 0 | 0 | 0 | | | | | | |
| Troponin I | <0.3 | <0.3 | <0.3 | | | | | | |
| PT | 11.8 | | | | | | | | |
| INR | 1.4 | | | | | | | | |
| PTT | 27.8 | | | | | | | | |
| TC | | | 509 | | | | | | |
| TG | | | 841 | | | | | | |
| HDL | | | 39 | | | | | | |
| LDL | | | — | | | | | | |

## Hospital Medication Summary

| Start Date | Medication Dose/Route/Frequency | D/C Date |
|---|---|---|
| 7/16 | Metoprolol 50 mg po Q12h | 7/17 |
| 7/16 | Famotidine 20 mg IV Q12h | 7/17 |
| 7/16 | Aspirin 81 mg chew and swallow STAT × 1 | 7/16 |
| 7/16 | Enoxaparin 90 mg/0.9 mL SubQ Q12h | 7/17 |
| 7/17 | NTG Patch 0.2 mg/h apply one patch daily | 7/19 |
| 7/17 | Enteric coated aspirin 325 mg po daily | 7/19 |
| 7/17 | Famotidine 20 mg po Q12h | 7/19 |
| 7/17 | Metoprolol 50 mg po daily | 7/19 |
| 7/16 | NTG 0.4 mg tab SL Q5 minutes × 3 prn chest pain | 7/19 |
| 7/16 | NTG in D5W 50 mg/250 mL IV prn—titrate to relief of chest pain | 7/17 |
| 7/16 | Morphine 2 mg/0.5 mL IV Q4 prn chest pain | 7/17 |
| 7/17 | Alprazolam 0.25 mg po Q8h prn anxiety | 7/18 |

## Hospital Patient Case 2

| | |
|---|---|
| **Patient Name:** Vaughan, Susan | **Admission Date:** 9/15/13 |

| | | | |
|---|---|---|---|
| **Gender:** F | **Race:** African American | **Weight:** 150 lb | **Height:** 5'8" |

**Allergies:** NKDA

**Chief Complaint:** "My legs have been swelling up"

**HPI:**
SV is a 78-yo AAF who presents to the emergency room with swollen and tender legs for 3 days. She states that the swelling and some tenderness started in the morning several days ago. She states that she has tried to elevate her legs and stay off her feet, but the pain and swelling are getting worse.

| **PMH:** | **PSH:** |
|---|---|
| GERD<br>Chronic iron deficiency anemia<br>PE (11/03) | Greenfield filter placement (11/03) |

| Family History: | Social History: |
|---|---|
| Mother deceased; age 85; heart attack | (−) tobacco |
| | (−) ETOH |
| Father deceased; age unknown; cancer | (−) illict drugs |

| Home Medications: | ROS/PE: | |
|---|---|---|
| Acetaminophen prn | General: | WDWN AAF in NAD |
| Multivitamin po daily | Vitals: | BP: 126/65, HR: 70 |
| Pepcid 20 mg po daily | | RR: 24, T: 97 |
| (Pepcid prescribed daily, but patient "takes it when she needs it") | HEENT: | No abnormalities |
| | CV: | RRR; borderline bradycardia |
| | Lungs: | clear to auscultation bilaterally |
| | ABD: | (+) BS × 4 |
| | GU: | deferred |
| | EXT: | bilateral pain and tenderness with touch; (+) Homan sign; decreased strength and ROM; (+) edema with R > L; good pulses |
| | Neuro: | AAA × 3 |

## LABORATORY RESULTS

| Date: | 9/15 Admission | | | 9/16 | 9/17 | 9/18 | 9/19 |
|---|---|---|---|---|---|---|---|
| Time: | 1200 | 1800 | 2400 | 0600 | 0600 | 0600 | 0600 |
| BP | 126/65 | | | 120/57 | 135/74 | 111/57 | 105/62 |
| HR | 70 | | | 66 | 80 | 75 | 73 |
| RR | 24 | | | 20 | 20 | 20 | 18 |
| $T_{max}$ | 97 | | | 99.2 | 98.5 | 98.6 | 98 |
| Na | 139 | | | 140 | 139 | | |
| K | 3.9 | | | 3.9 | 3.9 | | |
| Cl | 100 | | | 102 | 101 | | |
| $CO_2$ | 28 | | | 29 | 29 | | |
| BUN | 10 | | | 9 | 9 | | |

| | | | | | | | |
|---|---|---|---|---|---|---|---|
| SCr | 0.8 | | | 0.9 | 0.9 | | |
| Glucose | 111 | | | 99 | 105 | | |
| WBC | 7.6 | | | 6.5 | | | |
| Hgb | 12.3 | | | 11.3 | | | |
| Hct | 36.8 | | | 36.1 | | | |
| Platelets | 200 | | | 211 | | | |
| MCV | 31.3 | | | 35 | | | |
| RDW | 45 | | | 44 | | | |
| PMN | 65.7 | | | 68 | | | |
| PT | 12.1 | 12.3 | 13.3 | 13.3 | 15.3 | 17 | 17.5 |
| INR | 1.07 | 1.2 | 1.29 | 1.29 | 1.7 | 2.09 | 2.48 |
| PTT | 25.8 | 30.2 | 57.4 | 59.9 | 61.2 | 65.5 | 68 |

## HOSPITAL MEDICATION SUMMARY

| Start Date | Medication Dose/Route/Frequency | D/C Date |
|---|---|---|
| 9/15 | Heparin 250,000 units/250 mL D5W titrate per heparin protocol | |
| 9/15 | Ferrous sulfate 325 mg po tid with meals | |
| 9/15 | Multivitamin tablet po daily | |
| 9/15 | Famotidine 20 mg po bid | |
| 9/16 | Warfarin 7.5 mg po × 1 today | 9/16 |
| 9/17 | Warfarin 5 mg po × 1 today | 9/17 |
| 9/18 | Warfarin 5 mg po × 1 today | 9/18 |
| 9/19 | Warfarin 5 mg po × 1 today | 9/19 |
| 9/15 | Docusate sodium 100 mg po prn constipation | |
| 9/15 | Acetaminophen 500 mg po Q4-6h prn pain or headache | |
| 9/15 | Propoxyphene 100 mg/acetaminophen 650 mg take 1–2 tablets po Q4h for pain not relieved by acetaminophen | |

## HOSPITAL PATIENT CASE 3

| | |
|---|---|
| **Patient Name:** Jones, Nathan | **Admission Date:** 1/27/13 |
| **Gender:** M    **Race:** Hispanic | **Weight:** 174 lb      **Height:** 5'9" |
| **Allergies:** Aspirin, codeine | |

**Chief Complaint:** "I threw up blood"

**HPI:**
NJ is a 57-yo Hispanic male with a LeVeen shunt and reported history of liver disease, who presents to the ER complaining of hematemesis (×1, 2 hours before arrival) and melena (× 2 the day before arrival). Patient denies other complaints; specifically he states he has no abdominal pain, no fever, and no chest pain. Upon arrival in the ER, the patient experienced emesis again with blood clots and bright red blood (witnessed by ER staff).

| **PMH:** | **PSH:** |
|---|---|
| Umbilical hernia | LeVeen shunt placement 5/04 |
| History of "liver disease" | |

| **Family History:** | **Social History:** |
|---|---|
| Mother deceased at age 57, rectal cancer | (+) ETOH approx. 8 beers/week |
| Father deceased at age 80, "old age" | (+) tobacco (20 pack years) |
| | (−) illicit drug use |

**Home Medications:**
Not currently taking any medications
History of taking potassium and a "water pill"

**ROS/PE:**

| | |
|---|---|
| General: | WDWN Hispanic male |
| Vitals: | BP: 96/67 HR: 96 RR: 32 T: 99.4 |
| HEENT: | no abnormalities |
| Neck: | (−) JVD; (−) goiter |
| CV: | tenderness with palpation on chest wall |
| Lungs: | clear to auscultation bilaterally |
| ABD: | (+) BS; mild distention; (+) ascites |
| GU: | (−) gross blood; occult blood (+) |
| EXT: | Bilateral 1+ edema |
| Neuro: | AAA × 3 |

## LABORATORY RESULTS

| Date: | 1/27 Admission | 1/28 | | | 1/29 | 1/30 | 1/31 |
|---|---|---|---|---|---|---|---|
| Time: | 2400 | 0600 | 1200 | 2400 | 0600 | 0600 | 0600 |
| BP | 96/57 | 136/79 | | | 129/76 | 137/82 | 154/89 |
| HR | 96 | 95 | | | 111 | 72 | 80 |
| RR | 32 | 18 | | | 32 | 20 | 21 |
| $T_{max}$ | 99.4 | 99.3 | | | 102.5 | 101 | 102.5 |
| Na | 140 | 142 | | | 144 | 143 | 137 |
| K | 4.2 | 3.5 | | 3.1 | 3.8 | 3.4 | 3.7 |
| Cl | 109 | 122 | | | 116 | 116 | 113 |
| $CO_2$ | 25 | 20 | | | 24 | 24 | 23 |
| BUN | 27 | 25 | | | 26 | 19 | 13 |
| SCr | 0.7 | 0.5 | | | 0.7 | 0.6 | 0.6 |
| Glucose | 124 | 166 | | | 119 | 134 | 114 |
| WBC | 8.77 | 4.78 | 5.01 | 5.89 | 6.06 | 3.11 | 5.53 |
| Hgb | 9.9 | 7.3 | 6.2 | 10.8 | 12.3 | 10.9 | 10.1 |
| Hct | 29.7 | 21.2 | 17.8 | 31.7 | 36.3 | 32.5 | 29.6 |
| Platelets | 91 | 40 | 43 | 43 | 38 | 28 | 42 |
| MCV | 101.4 | 96 | 93.2 | 93.2 | 93.3 | 91.9 | 94.8 |
| RDW | 56.7 | 55.4 | 54.3 | 54.6 | 56.1 | 55.9 | 56 |
| PMN | 72 | 84.8 | 85 | 84.6 | 85.5 | 85.6 | 84.1 |
| AST | | 40 | | | 52 | | |
| ALT | | 39 | | | 39 | | |
| Alk Phos | | 53 | | | 63 | | |
| Bilirubin | | 1 | | | 1.7 | | |
| Albumin | | 1.2 | | | 2.1 | | |
| Ammonia | | 16 | | | 56 | 37 | 18 |
| Mg | | | 0.7 | 1.8 | | | 1.6 |
| Ca | 8.9 | 5.6 | | | 7.4 | | 7.4 |
| PT | 16 | 19.3 | | | 15.3 | | |
| INR | 1.72 | 2.49 | | | 1.58 | | |
| PTT | 30.9 | 41.7 | | | 30.4 | | |

## HOSPITAL MEDICATION SUMMARY

| Start Date | Medication Dose/Route/Frequency | D/C Date |
|---|---|---|
| 1/27 | Pantoprazole 40 mg IV Q12h | 1/30 |
| 1/27 | Multivitamin IV daily (added to first liter of IVF daily) | 1/30 |
| 1/27 | Thiamine 100 mg IV daily (added to first liter of IVF daily) | 1/30 |
| 1/27 | Folate 1 mg IV daily (added to first liter of IVF daily) | 1/30 |
| 1/27 | NS at 150 mL/h | 1/29 |
| 1/28 | Vitamin K 10 mg SubQ daily × 3 days | 1/30 |
| 1/28 | Magnesium sulfate 2 g in 400 mL NS over 2 hours × 1 | 1/28 |
| 1/29 | Cefotaxime 1 gm IV Q6h | |
| 1/29 | Lactulose 30 mL po bid | |
| 1/29 | Spironolactone 50 mg po bid | |
| 1/29 | NS at 75 mL/h | |
| 1/30 | Pantoprazole 40 mg po daily | |
| 1/30 | Multivitamin po daily | |
| 1/30 | Thiamine 100 mg po daily | |
| 1/30 | Folate 1 mg po daily | |
| 1/27 | Lorazepam 0.5 mg IV Q4-6h prn anxiety or agitation | |
| 1/27 | Acetaminophen 650 mg PR Q6h prn pain/fever | |
| 1/27 | Promethazine 25 mg IV Q4-6h prn nausea | |
| 1/27 | Furosemide 20 mg IV prn (after each transfusion) | |

## HOSPITAL PATIENT CASE 4

| | |
|---|---|
| **Patient Name:** Lewis, Jack | **Admission Date:** 7/14/13 |
| **Gender:** M   **Race:** White | **Weight:** 250 lb      **Height:** 5'10" |
| **Allergies:** NKDA | |
| **Chief Complaint:** "I can't stop coughing" | |

**HPI:**
JL is a 34-yo wm who presents to the ER complaining of a cough with some brown-tinged sputum and right upper quadrant pain 7 days. He also complains of subjective fever, chills, and decreased appetite for about 1 week. He has been short of breath, but denies dyspnea on exertion. JL had one episode of hemoptysis the evening prior to admission.

| **PMH:** | **PSH:** |
|---|---|
| Asthma since childhood | Arthroscopic knee surgery (1993) |
| Hyperlipidemia × 2 years | |

| **Family History:** | **Social History:** |
|---|---|
| Mother alive, no known medical problems | (−) ETOH |
| Father alive with arthritis and HTN | (+) tobacco (1 pack per week) |
| | (−) illicit drug use |
| | Occupational exposure to bleach |

| **Home Medications:** | **ROS/PE:** | |
|---|---|---|
| Albuterol inhaler prn | General: | Obese wm with cough |
| Zocor 20 mg po daily: | Vitals: | BP: 136/78 HR: 109 RR: 18, T: 100.6 |
| | HEENT: | no swollen lymph nodes or glands; nares patent |
| | CV | (−) CP; tachycardic (NSR) |
| | Lungs: | decreased breath sounds at right base; dullness to percussion at right base; (+) egophany; bilateral ronchi; no wheezes noted |
| | ABD: | (+) BS; nontender |
| | GU: | deferred |
| | EXT: | good capillary refill; muscle strength 5/5 in all extremities; no rashes or lesions noted |
| | Neuro: | AAA × 3 |

## LABORATORY RESULTS

| Date: | 7/14 Admission | 7/15 | | | 7/16 | 7/17 |
|---|---|---|---|---|---|---|
| Time: | 2200 | 0600 | 1200 | 2400 | 0600 | 0600 |
| BP | 136/78 | 129/82 | 130/81 | | 129/78 | 133/80 |
| HR | 109 | 108 | 110 | | 105 | 101 |
| RR | 18 | 20 | 19 | | 19 | 19 |
| $T_{max}$ | 100.6 | 101 | 100.8 | | 99.5 | 99.2 |
| Na | 137 | 137 | | | 142 | 143 |
| K | 3.2 | 4.5 | | | 4.0 | 4.1 |
| Cl | 94 | 103 | | | 102 | 104 |
| $CO_2$ | 28 | 26 | | | 28 | 28 |
| BUN | 10 | 7 | | | 7 | 6 |
| SCr | 0.9 | 0.8 | | | 0.8 | 0.8 |
| Glucose | 110 | 88 | | | 90 | 92 |
| WBC | 19.8 | 13.9 | | | 12.8 | 12.1 |
| Hgb | 15 | 13 | | | 13.1 | 13 |
| Hct | 42.6 | 40 | | | 40 | 41 |
| Platelets | 199 | 201 | | | 213 | 308 |
| MCV | 90 | 91 | | | 89 | 90 |
| RDW | 45 | 42 | | | 42 | 44 |
| PMN | 89 | 82 | | | 76 | 68.7 |
| Lymphs | 6.1 | 9.2 | | | 10.4 | 13.1 |
| Bands | 3 | 2 | | | 3 | 2 |
| AST | 30 | | | | | |
| ALT | 22 | | | | | |
| Alk Phos | 98 | | | | | |
| Bilirubin | 1.1 | | | | | |
| Albumin | 4.2 | | | | | |
| Mg | | 2.3 | | | | |

## HOSPITAL MEDICATION SUMMARY

| Start Date | Medication Dose/Route/Frequency | D/C Date |
|---|---|---|
| 7/14 | D5 1/2 NS + KCl 40 mEq/L at 125 mL/h | 7/15 |
| 7/14 | Ceftriaxone 1 g IV Q12h | 7/16 |
| 7/14 | Clarithromycin 500 mg po bid | |
| 7/14 | Simvastatin 20 mg po daily | |
| 7/15 | D5 1/2 NS + KCl 20 mEq/L at 100 mL/h | 7/17 |
| 7/16 | Cefuroxime 250 mg po Q12h | |
| 7/14 | Guaifenesin 100 mg/dextromethorphan 10 mg; use 2 tsp po Q4-6h prn cough | |
| 7/14 | Acetaminophen 650 mg po Q4-6hprn T > 101 | |
| 7/14 | Albuterol MDI prn SOB | |

# HOSPITAL PATIENT CASE 5

| | |
|---|---|
| **Patient Name:** Earnright, Richard | **Admission Date:** 8/5/13 |
| **Gender:** M    **Race:** Jamaican | **Weight:** 174 lb    **Height:** 5'10" |
| **Allergies:** NKDA | |

**Chief Complaint:** "I can't breathe, and I feel really tired"

**HPI:**

RE is a 65-yo Jamaican male with a significant history of repeated inpatient admissions for heart failure exacerbations. He presents to the ER with a 4-day history of increasing SOB and fatigue. He is presently using three pillows to sleep comfortably at night (increased from his normal of two pillows). He complains of cough, difficulty walking without getting short of breath, weakness, and swollen feet and ankles. He also admits to a 10-lb weight gain over the last month. RE is also quick to admit that he rarely remembers to get his prescriptions refilled when they run out and doesn't follow the diet that was suggested to him.

| **PMH:** | **PSH:** |
|---|---|
| Heart failure (diagnosed 2006) | Glaucoma laser surgery (right eye) × 3 |
| Glaucoma (right eye) | |
| Hypertension (since age 30) | |
| Hyperlipidemia (? duration) | |
| Hemorrhoids (since 2001) | |
| Diverticulitis (diagnosed 2001) | |

| **Family History:** | **Social History:** |
|---|---|
| Mother deceased age 50, heart attack | (+) history of tobacco (2 packs per day since age 18) |
| Father deceased age 78, Parkinson disease | (+) history of ETOH (since age 18; heavy alcohol use in the past, but only social drinking now per patient) (−) illicit drug use |

| **Home Medications:** | **ROS/PE:** | |
|---|---|---|
| Lipitor 10 mg po daily | General: | WDWN male with significant SOB |
| Enteric-coated aspirin 325 mg po daily | Vitals: | BP: 146/80, HR: 100 RR: 26, T 97 |
| Lasix 20 mg po daily | HEENT: | Blind in right eye |
| Vasotec 5 mg po daily | Neck: | (+) JVD |
| Pred Forte 1 gtt OD four times per day | CV: | (+) mild CP; heart regular rate and rhythm; (+) S3 gallop |
| Atropine 1 gtt OD bid | Lungs: | inspiratory rales bilaterally |
| Timolol XE 1 gtt OD daily | ABD: | (+) BS; nontender, mildly distended |
| Alphagan 1 gtt OD tid | GU: | (+) hemorrhoids; (−) occult blood |
| Truspot 1 gtt OD tid | EXT: | 2+ pitting edema to ankles bilaterally |
| | Neuro: | AAA × 3 |

## LABORATORY RESULTS

| Date: | 8/5 Admission | | 8/6 | | 8/7 | 8/8 |
|---|---|---|---|---|---|---|
| Time: | 1500 | 2100 | 0300 | 0600 | 0600 | 0600 |
| BP | 146/80 | | | 153/92 | 142/83 | 140/83 |
| HR | 100 | | | 99 | 98 | 96 |
| RR | 26 | | | 25 | 25 | 24 |
| $T_{max}$ | 97 | | | 98.1 | 97.9 | 98.2 |
| Na | 133 | | | 134 | 135 | 136 |
| K | 3.3 | | | 3.5 | 3.6 | 3.6 |
| Cl | 101 | | | 100 | 100 | 102 |
| $CO_2$ | 28 | | | 26 | 26 | 25 |
| BUN | 20 | | | 19 | 19 | 19 |
| SCr | 1.1 | | | 1.3 | 1.2 | 1.1 |
| Glucose | 98 | | | 100 | 101 | 99 |
| WBC | 8.7 | | | | | |
| Hgb | 15.2 | | | | | |
| Hct | 43.6 | | | | | |
| Platelets | 350 | | | | | |
| MCV | 87 | | | | | |
| MCHC | 33 | | | | | |
| RDW | 14.2 | | | | | |
| CK | 43 | 47 | 45 | | | |
| CKMB | – | – | – | | | |
| Troponin I | <0.3 | <0.3 | <0.3 | | | |
| Ca | | | 9.2 | | | |
| Mg | 1.8 | | | | | |
| $PO_4$ | 3.5 | | | | | |

## Hospital Medication Summary

| Start Date | Medication Dose/Route/Frequency | D/C Date |
|---|---|---|
| 8/5 | All eye drops as per home doses | |
| 8/5 | Atorvastatin 10 mg po daily | |
| 8/5 | Enteric-coated aspirin 325 mg po daily | |
| 8/5 | Enalapril 5 mg po daily | 8/6 |
| 8/5 | Furosemide 40 mg IV bid | 8/6 |
| 8/5 | Potassium chloride extended release 20 mEq po daily | |
| 8/6 | Furosemide 20 mg IV daily | 8/7 |
| 8/6 | Enalapril 10 mg po daily | |
| 8/7 | Furosemide 20 mg po daily | |
| 8/5 | NTG 0.4 mg tab SL Q5 minutes × 3 prn chest pain | |
| 8/5 | Morphine 2 mg/0.5 mL IV Q4h prn chest pain | 8/6 |
| 8/5 | Acetaminophen 650 mg po Q4-6h prn fever/pain/headache | |

## Hospital Patient Case 6

| | | | |
|---|---|---|---|
| **Patient Name:** Bowen, Francine | | **Admission Date:** 3/2/13 | |
| **Gender:** F | **Race:** African American | **Weight:** 96 lb | **Height:** 5'4" |
| **Allergies:** PCN | | | |

**Chief Complaint:** "My leg hurts, and it isn't getting better"

**HPI:**
FB is an 83-yo AAF who presents to the ER with complaints of a swollen and painful left lower extremity. She noticed that her leg seemed swollen about 1 week prior to arrival. For the past 3 days, however, the swelling has worsened and is painful. The leg is also extremely red and warm to touch.

| **PMH:** | **PSH:** |
|---|---|
| HTN × 10 years | TAH at age 56 |
| DM × 20 years | |

| Family History: | Social History: |
|---|---|
| Mother deceased at age 80, "ulcer" Father deceased at age 78, HTN/DM | (−) ETOH (+) tobacco (1 pack per week) (−) illicit drug use |

| Home Medications: | ROS/PE: | |
|---|---|---|
| Cardizem CD 240 mg po daily Lantus 15 units HS | General: | Thin AAF in NAD |
| | Vitals: | BP: 165/92 HR: 75 RR: 18, T: 100.6 |
| | HEENT: | (+) cataracts bilaterally |
| | Neck: | (−) JVD; (−) goiter |
| | CV: | RRR |
| | Lungs: | Clear to auscultation bilaterally |
| | ABD: | (+) BS |
| | GU: | occult blood (−) |
| | EXT: | significant peripheral neuropathy present bilaterally; LLE swollen to mid calf, warm to touch, diffuse redness, no obvious abrasions or cuts; poor nail and foot care |
| | Neuro: | AAA × 3 |

## LABORATORY RESULTS

| Date: | 3/2 Admission | | 3/3 | | 3/4 | 3/5 | 3/6 | 3/7 |
|---|---|---|---|---|---|---|---|---|
| Time: | 1800 | 0600 | 1200 | 2400 | 0600 | 0600 | 0600 | 0600 |
| BP | 165/92 | 157/89 | 139/90 | 160/90 | 156/87 | 143/82 | 140/82 | 141/79 |
| HR | 75 | 87 | 79 | 82 | 80 | 75 | 77 | 77 |
| RR | 18 | 20 | 20 | 20 | 19 | 19 | 19 | 20 |
| $T_{max}$ | 100.6 | 100.4 | 99.8 | 100.1 | 99.6 | 99.2 | 98.9 | 99.1 |
| Na | 136 | 136 | | | 134 | 135 | 135 | 135 |
| K | 4.4 | 4 | | | 3.9 | 4 | 4.1 | 4.1 |
| Cl | 98 | 100 | | | 100 | 101 | 99 | 100 |
| $CO_2$ | 26 | 28 | | | 28 | 27 | 27 | 28 |

| | | | | | | | | |
|---|---|---|---|---|---|---|---|---|
| BUN | 16 | 15 | | | 10 | 11 | 11 | 10 |
| SCr | 1.4 | 1.3 | | | 1.3 | 1.3 | 1.3 | 1.2 |
| Glucose | 163 | 122 | 201 | 110 | 145 | 172 | 106 | 133 |
| WBC | 12.2 | 12 | | | 11.2 | 10.9 | 9.8 | 9.2 |
| Hgb | 13.2 | 13 | | | 13.1 | 13.2 | 12.9 | 13 |
| Hct | 40.3 | 39.8 | | | 40.2 | 39 | 40.1 | 40.3 |
| Platelets | 272 | 270 | | | 275 | 300 | 289 | 288 |
| PMN | 87 | 86 | | | 86 | 82 | 73 | 74 |
| Lymphs | 9.7 | 8.5 | | | 8.2 | 8.1 | 7.6 | 7.5 |
| Bands | 2 | 3 | | | 2 | 2 | 3 | 2 |
| Albumin | 3.8 | | | | | | | |
| HgbA1C | | 9.2 | | | | | | |

## HOSPITAL MEDICATION SUMMARY

| Start Date | Medication Dose/Route/Frequency | D/C Date |
|---|---|---|
| 3/2 | Clindamycin 600 mg IV Q8h | 3/3 |
| 3/2 | Diltiazem CD 240 mg po daily | |
| 3/2 | Novolin R ACHS (see sliding scale protocol) | |
| 3/3 | Lisinopril 2.5 mg po daily | |
| 3/3 | Vancomycin 1 g IV Q12h | 3/3 |
| 3/4 | Vancomycin 750 mg IV Q24h | 3/5 |
| 3/4 | Potassium chloride extended release tablet 20 mEq po daily | 3/5 |
| 3/7 | Vancomycin 750 mg IV Q48h | |
| 3/2 | Acetaminophen 500 mg po Q4-6h prn fever/pain | |

CHAPTER

16

# Managed Care

*Sherry Clayton, Karen Martin, Kathryn Shalek*

**Objectives: Upon completion of the chapter and exercises, the student pharmacist will be able to**

1. Identify the goals and types of managed care organizations.
2. Illustrate managed care business management techniques.
3. Explain formulary management, drug utilization review, and disease state management.
4. Discuss outcomes research.
5. Identify current directions in managed care.

---

### Patient Encounter

Discussion (based on the Patient Encounter from Chap. 2, pages 18-19):

A 26-year-old African American Gold Medal Olympic bicyclist was struck by a car, flung 30 feet into the air, and fell into an embankment. He was training for his second Olympic trial and was well known in the community as being devoted to his sport. He was unconscious at the scene. After stabilization in the hospital, it was determined that his spinal cord was completely severed below T10. He sustained a serious head injury, but it was anticipated that he would probably be able to talk and communicate his wishes over time. However, a long rehabilitation period was anticipated for the head injury with uncertain degree of return to full preaccident mental abilities, and the paraplegia was permanent. During his recovery period, he needed surrogates (proxies) to make his decisions for him because of his temporary lack of decision-making capacity. The patient had several medical complications including pneumonia and urosepsis. After several weeks, several family members, including his wife, who was the main surrogate decision maker, voiced their concern that the patient,

*(continued on next page)*

---

given his athletic prowess, would "never want to be a cripple" and suggested that, because of the patient's poor quality of life, antibiotics be withheld and the patient be allowed to "die with dignity." Both the patient and his wife were avid athletes, and the subject of paraplegia had never been discussed. Because of his love of the sport and their life style of athleticism, she was sure he would not want to be a "cripple." You, as the pharmacist, are approached by the family to cease administration of antibiotics.

The goals of the managed care organizations are as follows:

> Prevent disease.
> Focus attention on wellness.
> Improve medication therapy.
> Base decisions on the entire population versus the individual.
> Cost containment.

> Are there programs a managed care organization could promote to prevent bicycle accidents for the members they serve?
> What would the programs entail and how would they be implemented?
> Would a program to prevent bicycle accidents fit into a larger accident prevention program?
> What would an accident prevention program include?

## INTRODUCTION

Managed care organizations (MCOs) can trace their beginnings back to prepaid health plans in the early 1900s. These early group prepaid practices were the model and precursors for our current health maintenance organizations (HMOs). The HMO Act of 1973 authorized federal funds to help develop HMOs and preempted state laws that prohibited prepaid plans. At the close of 1996, there were over 600 HMOs in the United States with 25% of the population as subscribers or members.[1] The National Committee for Quality Assurance (NCQA) (http://www.accesspharmacy.com/Content.aspx?searchStr= national+committee+on+quality+assurance&aid=6494862#6494867 {subscription required}), a nonprofit organization, formed in 1990 as well. The NCQA seal is a symbol that a program is accredited and has passed rigorous comprehensive review, is well organized, and has met quality standards.[2] NCQA measures health plan performance through a set of performance metrics, the Health Plan Employer Data and Information Set (HEDIS) (http://www.accesspharmacy.com/Content.aspx?searchS tr=health+plan+employer+data+and+information+set&aid=56791744#56791754 {subscription required}).[3]

---

**TABLE 16.1. GOALS OF MANAGED CARE ORGANIZATIONS[6]**

Prevent disease.

Focus attention on wellness.

Improve medication therapy.

Base decisions on the entire population versus the individual.

Control cost.

---

Much of the US population receives health insurance coverage through their place of employment. Costs of health insurance were escalating in the 1980s because of inflation, new technology, and an aging population, causing employers to look for strategies in cost containment. As a result, employers found they could achieve cost control by shifting from traditional indemnity insurance to more tightly managed plans during the 1990s.[4] Today, managed care is the most common delivery mechanism of health care.

Managed care is a system to deliver health care to contain costs and to improve the quality and the access to medical and pharmacy care (Table 16.1). Managed care pharmacy strives to deliver effective medications through innovative and comprehensive programs while improving overall health care for the member.[5]

Various types of MCOs exist. They include HMOs, preferred provider organizations (PPOs), point-of-service (POS) plans, exclusive provider organizations (EPOs), hybrid plans, consumer directed health plans (CDHP), and pharmacy benefit managers (PBMs). Managed care delivery may include one or a combination of these models (Table 16.2).

---

**TABLE 16.2. TYPES OF MANAGED CARE ORGANIZATIONS[6]**

Health Maintenance Organizations (HMO)

- Staff model
- Group model
- Network model

Independent Practice Association (IPA)

Preferred provider organization (PPO)

Point-of-service (POS)

Exclusive provider organization (EPO)

Consumer-directed health plan (CDHP)

Pharmacy benefit manager (PBM)

- In HMO plans (http://www.accesspharmacy.com/Content.aspx?searchStr=health+maintenance+organizations&aid=56180494#56180533 {subscription required}), members prepay a premium to receive comprehensive medical services provided by physicians or other medical providers under contract. Several subtypes are under the umbrella of HMOs. In the staff model, physicians are employees of the HMO and patients are able to obtain services only through these limited providers. The providers see members in the HMO's own facilities. Most of these staff models are no longer in existence. In the group model, the HMO contracts with a multi-specialty medical group that provides care to the member. The physicians are employees of the group practice. This medical group may work exclusively with the HMO or it may provide services to non-HMO patients as well. A network model HMO contracts with multiple physician groups to provide a broad range of services for their members. The independent practice association (IPA) model is the most common. In this model, a group of independent practicing physicians maintains their own offices, yet contracts their services to HMOs, other MCOs, and insurance companies, typically providing services to both HMO and non-HMO plan participants.
- PPO plans (http://www.accesspharmacy.com/Content.aspx?searchStr=preferred+provider+organizations&aid=56180494#56180531plans {subscription required}), another type of MCO, including a contracted network of physicians and hospitals from which the member may choose. These PPOs offer less control over providers than HMOs.
- POS plans are a hybrid of a PPO and an HMO. Members may go out of network, if they choose, for an increased deductible or co-payment. EPO plans are similar in structure to PPO plans, but limit the physicians and facilities that patients may use and limit or do not cover out of network services.
- A CDHP combines a high deductible health plan (HDHP) with a tax advantaged health reimbursement arrangement or a health savings account (HSA). A HSA is tax-exempt money set aside to pay for qualified medical expenses for the individual. Insurers typically supply consumers with web-based tools to allow them to compare quality and costs of different services to help them actively make the best health-care purchase.
- A PBM acts on behalf of the insurer, MCO, or government program to help maximize appropriate drug utilization and contain costs. A PBM provides a combination of clinical and business services.

Millions of people receive their health-care benefits through government programs. Many of these programs, administered collaboratively between the public and private sector, increasingly utilize managed care goals and tools to help maintain quality while controlling costs.

Medicaid, established in 1965 by the Social Security Act, provides general public assistance to the poor and disabled. While the federal government's Centers for Medicare and Medicaid Services (CMS) establish guidelines for these programs, the states determine their own eligibility and administrative procedures. Both federal and state dollars fund Medicaid.[7]

**TABLE 16.3. COMPONENTS OF MEDICARE[8]**

| | |
|---|---|
| Part A—Hospital Insurance (HI) | • Inpatient hospital services<br>• Some nursing home services<br>• Some home health -care costs<br>• Hospice |
| Part B—Supplemental Medical Insurance (SMI) | • Physician services<br>• Outpatient hospital services<br>• Home health services not covered under Part A<br>• Durable medical equipment<br>• Ambulance services |
| Part C—Medicare Advantage health plan options | Allows beneficiaries to enroll in private plans other than the traditional Medicare program<br>• Private fee for-service (PFFS)<br>• HMOs<br>• PPOs |
| Part D—Prescription drug coverage | Outpatient prescriptions<br>• Traditional Medicare with a freestanding prescription drug plan (PDP)<br>• Medicare Advantage Prescription Drug (MAPD) plan which integrates medical and prescription benefits |

The Social Security Act of 1965 also established Medicare (http://www.accesspharmacy.com/Content.aspx?searchStr=medicare&aid=56795503 {subscription required}) that pays a major proportion of medical costs for those aged 65 years and older.[8] Younger persons may also qualify for Medicare coverage if they have permanent disabilities or end-stage renal disease. Before 2003, the Medicare benefit consisted of three parts: Parts A, B and C (Table 16.3). The Medicare Modernization Act of 2003 (MMA) established Part D, a prescription drug benefit, which was fully implemented in 2006.

The Medicare Part D plan consists of an initial deductible, followed by a 25% coinsurance up to a certain amount of the drug spend (eg, $4000 for 2013).[8] A catastrophic threshold for drug spend is set at a higher amount (eg, $6400). The beneficiary is responsible for the total cost of any drugs in the coverage gap, also known as the donut hole. In the example given, the coverage gap occurs when the drug spend is $4000 to $6400. After the catastrophic threshold is met, the coinsurance drops to 5%. Expect these amounts to be adjusted in the future.

Purchase of supplemental insurance can help cover deductibles, coinsurance, and other services not covered under the various parts of Medicare. Some low-income recipients may also qualify for Medicaid (ie, dual eligible).

## BUSINESS SERVICES IN MANAGED CARE

The business services utilized by MCOs are integral to the prudent use of health-care resources. To achieve the goals of managed care there must be a balance of quality and cost. Although the strategies and tools mentioned in this section save cost, they also tie into quality components.

It is important to assess the financial risk that an MCO will incur by providing health benefits to a specific population. This process is called underwriting and helps determine the appropriate premium and co-pay amounts for each beneficiary. The medical loss ratio (MLR) indicates the profitability or loss for each contract and equals the total health-care expenditures divided by the total premium income (MLR Fig. 16.1). The industry considers a MLR of around 90% acceptable.[6]

A brief description of some basic MCO industry strategies is presented. An MCO sets up and administers various benefit designs that define eligibility, drug coverage, and co-pays. Some benefits may require annual deductibles or coinsurance to give members more incentives to choose cost-effective medications. Mandatory generic-use policies are becoming commonplace. Network development is an essential function provided by MCOs to ensure that their members are able to receive a broad range of services from physicians, hospitals, and ancillary providers, including retail, mail, and specialty pharmacies. Contractual arrangements spell out the standards and policies that the provider must follow, as well as the reimbursement rates. The MCO supports its clinical decisions and objectives by making the best possible financial arrangements with drug manufacturers to keep the drug benefit affordable. The MCO's ability to influence physician prescribing through their formulary enables them to receive rebates that are performance based. Of course, actual claims data processing is undertaken by the MCO as well.

One of the most useful tools that an MCO utilizes is reporting performance measures. These measures may include total and average prescription costs, utilization, administrative fees, rebates, generic dispensing rate, formulary compliance rate, number of member complaints, number of prior authorization approvals, customer service wait times, average turnaround on mail, network adequacy, and member satisfaction and retention. It is easy to see how closely some of these measures are tied to quality.

One of the most important performance measures for monitoring drug utilization is per member per month (PMPM Fig. 16.2). It is found by dividing the total claim cost for prescription drugs (minus the member co-payment) by the number of covered members. This is essentially the cost of the drug benefit. Ingredient costs, higher member co-payments, larger elderly populations, and higher generic and formulary utilization are significant contributors to the PMPM.[6]

**Figure 16.1.** Medical loss ratio (MLR).

$$MLR = \frac{\text{Total health-care expenditures}}{\text{Total premium income}}$$

**Figure 16.2.** Per member per month (PMPM).

$$\text{PMPM} = \frac{\text{Total claim cost for prescription drugs (minus member co-payment)}}{\text{Number of covered members}}$$

This calculation can also be done on a yearly basis and becomes per member per year (PMPY).[6]

## CLINICAL TOOLS IN MANAGED CARE

MCOs utilize many clinical tools to assist in the improvement of the quality of patient care while containing cost. Three tools, formulary management, drug utilization reviews (DURs), and disease state management (DSM), will be discussed here.

### Formulary Management

A formulary (http://www.accesspharmacy.com/Content.aspx?searchStr=formulary &aid=55674872#55674880 {subscription required}), as defined by American Society of Health-System Pharmacists (ASHP), is "...a continually updated list of medications and related information, representing the clinical judgment of physicians, pharmacists, and other experts in the diagnosis, prophylaxis, or treatment of disease and promotion of health." Formulary management is an ongoing process that allows for identification of the most medically appropriate and cost effective drug therapy. Frequently, an evidence-based process is used to select the medications that offer the best therapeutic outcomes while minimizing potential risks. Formulary management is not unique to managed care. Hospitals, acute care facilities, home care settings, and long-term-care facilities may have formularies as well.[9]

The Pharmacy and Therapeutics (P&T) Committee is responsible for deciding which drugs are included on a formulary as well as managing, updating, and administering it. This committee is comprised of physicians, pharmacists, and other professionals in the health-care field. The P&T Committee must meet regularly to keep the formulary current. They review medical and clinical literature, relevant patient experience and utilization of medications, current therapeutic guidelines, economic data, provider recommendations, and safety. The committee's first task is to look for medications that are clinically safe and effective. Once this has been ascertained, secondary measures such as cost, supplier services, and any unique attributes of the product may be taken into consideration for the formulary decision.

There are three main types of formularies (Table 16.4). An open formulary provides coverage for all medications, both formulary and non-formulary. Patients may incur additional out of pocket expenses for using non-formulary drugs. This additional expenditure encourages physicians to prescribe formulary agents. In a closed formulary system, only a limited number of drugs are available and non-formulary drugs are not covered by the plan. Exceptions are made for access to non-formulary

**TABLE 16.4. TYPES OF FORMULARIES**[10]

| | |
|---|---|
| Open formulary | Provides coverage for all medications regardless of whether or not they are listed on the formulary. Some products may not be covered (eg, over-the-counter agents or cosmetic products). |
| Closed formulary | A limited number of drugs are available and non-formulary drugs are not covered. |
| Partially/selectively closed formulary | Similar in structure to an open formulary; however, a few selected drugs are not covered. |

medications when medically appropriate or necessary. The structure of a partially or selectively closed formulary is similar to an open formulary; however, a few selected drugs are not covered. Formularies help the organization differentiate between superior products and those with marginal benefit for efficient use of resources.[10]

Many prescription plans use a tiered co-pay structure that encourages use of generic and preferred brand drugs. While three-tier formularies are currently the most common type, many larger MCOs and PBMs are experimenting with four or five tiered structures (Table 16.5).[10]

Medicare programs may offer a closed formulary, with non-formulary drugs available only through an exception or appeal process; however, CMS specifies certain criteria for a Medicare formulary. It must cover at least two drugs within each pharmacologic category and one drug within each key drug type based on US Pharmacopoeia (USP) definitions. In addition, all or substantially all of the drugs in six classes of clinical concern must be covered (antidepressants, antipsychotics, anticonvulsants, chemotherapeutics, immunosuppressants, and HIV/AIDS drugs).[8]

**TABLE 16.5. EXAMPLE OF FORMULARY CO-PAYMENT TIERS**[10]

| | Tier 1 | Tier 2 | Tier 3 | Tier 4 | Tier 5 |
|---|---|---|---|---|---|
| Type of drugs included | Generic | Preferred formulary brand | Non-preferred/ Non-formulary brand | Lifestyle or cosmetic | Self-injectables |
| Co-payment (defined amount paid by the member each time a service is rendered) | Lowest fixed amount (eg, $15) | Intermediate fixed amount (eg, $30) | Highest fixed amount (eg, $60) | Coinsurance (eg, a percentage of the total cost of product paid by the member) | Coinsurance (eg, a percentage of the total cost of product paid by the member) |

---

**TABLE 16.6.** SEVEN PRINCIPLES OF DUR[12]

1. The primary emphasis must be to enhance quality of care for patients by assuring appropriate drug therapy.

2. The criteria and standards must be clinically relevant.

3. The criteria and standards must be nonproprietary and must be developed and revised through an open professional consensus process.

4. The interventions must focus on improving therapeutic outcomes.

5. Confidentiality of the relationship between patients and practitioners must be protected.

6. Principles must apply to the full range of activities, including prospective, concurrent, and retrospective drug use evaluation.

7. Must be structured to achieve the principles of DUR.

---

## Drug Utilization Review

DUR is a vital tool used by MCOs to help promote the appropriate and effective use of medications that create positive patient outcomes (Table 16.6). DUR is an ongoing, systematic process that looks at data before, during, and after dispensing medication to the patient. DUR helps to control costs by decreasing the number of medications prescribed inappropriately or unnecessarily as well as by helping physicians conform to established guidelines.[11] Seven principles of DUR were accepted by the American Medical Association (AMA), the American Pharmaceutical Association (APhA), and the Pharmaceutical Research and Manufacturers of America (PhRMA).[12]

There are five, commonly agreed upon steps that comprise DUR delineated in Table 16.7.

DUR may be classified into three different categories based on the timing of the process: prospective, concurrent, and retrospective review (Table 16.8).

---

**TABLE 16.7.** FIVE STEPS OF DUR[11,13]

1. Identify optimal drug use. Optimal drug use should be determined based on objective and measurable diagnoses and drug-specific criteria.

2. Measure the actual use of medications. This is primarily obtained from prescription drug claims.

3. Compare optimal and actual medication use. This identifies discrepancies in patient's therapy or in a physician's prescribing patterns.

4. Take action to correct the identified discrepancies or problems.

5. Evaluate the effectiveness of the DUR process.

| TABLE 16.8. CATEGORIES OF DRUG UTILIZATION REVIEW (DURS)[11,13] | |
|---|---|
| Prospective DUR | Reviews performed before a medication is dispensed to a patient. |
| Concurrent DUR | Reviews performed at the time of dispensing or during the course of treatment. |
| Retrospective DUR | Reviews performed after the patient has received the medication. |

- Prospective reviews are done before a medication is dispensed to a patient. Guideline development and education are also forms of prospective DUR. Academic detailing and provision of physician report cards can encourage prescribers to change their patterns, strive for quality improvement, and save costs.
- Concurrent reviews are performed at the time of dispensing or during the course of treatment. These reviews are performed routinely when pharmacists verify medication dosages, directions, interactions, therapeutic duplications, contraindications, and drug allergies. Prior authorizations restrict access to certain medications until specific criteria are met. This restricted access assures that the medication is being used appropriately and is being taken by those individuals who may benefit most from its use.[14]
- Retrospective reviews are performed after the patients receive the medications and are designed to flag drug-related problems. Since this review is carried out after the dispensing process is complete, over and underutilization of drug therapy can be analyzed.

## Disease State Management

DSM is a method used to improve quality of life and reduce health-care costs associated with chronic and costly medical conditions. DSM is an integrated system that combines pharmaceutical care, practice guidelines, data management, and patient and provider interventions. The goal is to identify and treat chronic disease states in an attempt to slow the progression, prevent complications, minimize treatment variability, and ultimately improve patient care. DSM encourages active participation in health care through proper medication use, symptom monitoring, and changed behavior. Chronic conditions that are commonly a part of DSM include diabetes mellitus (DM), congestive heart failure (CHF), chronic obstructive pulmonary disease (COPD), coronary artery disease (CAD), asthma, and hypertension (HTN). In contrast, medication therapy management (MTM) programs optimize the therapeutic drug outcomes for all conditions the patient may have and not a single disease state.[15] CMS mandates that MTM be undertaken for Medicare beneficiaries with chronic diseases, on multiple medications, and who are likely to incur drug costs in excess of a standard specified amount per year.[8]

## OUTCOMES RESEARCH

Outcomes research (http://www.accesspharmacy.com/Content.aspx?searchStr=
outcomes+research&aid=55671826 {subscription required}) evaluates a medical
treatment in regards to clinical, economic, or humanistic results. Examples of outcome measurements are disease cure, hospital admission rates, outpatient visits, patient functional status, or ability to perform activities of daily living. One component
of outcomes research is pharmacoeconomic (PE) evaluation. Different cost analyses
describe PE evaluations as illustrated in Table 16.9. Outcomes research helps to determine how to improve care in a given population, with consideration of cost effectiveness and cost efficiency of health-care resources.[16]

Comparative effectiveness research (CER) determines the value of different
interventions or therapies using existing clinical trial data or new pragmatic trials
to prevent, diagnose, treat, or monitor health conditions. CER provides information
to determine best options in health care.[17]

**TABLE 16.9.  METHODS USED IN ECONOMIC EVALUATIONS[5]**

| Method of Economic Evaluation | Description |
| --- | --- |
| Cost-minimization analysis (CMA) http://www.accesspharmacy.com/Content .aspx?searchStr=cost-minimization+analysis &aid=56791957#56791965 (subscription required) | Compares costs of interventions that are considered therapeutically equivalent. |
| Cost-benefit analysis (CBA) http://www.accesspharmacy.com/Content .aspx?searchStr=cost-benefit+analysis& aid=56791957#56791966 (subscription required) | Determines the benefits of an intervention and converts the benefit to a dollar amount. |
| Cost-effectiveness analysis (CEA) http://www.accesspharmacy.com/Content .aspx?searchStr=cost-effectiveness+analysis& aid=56791957#56791967 (subscription required) | Determines if competing strategies have an advantage based on cost and clinical outcome. |
| Cost-utility analysis (CUA) http://www.accesspharmacy.com/Content .aspx?searchStr=cost-utility+analysis&aid= 56791957#56791968 (subscription required) | A form of CEA that assesses the patient's functional status or quality of life. |
| Cost of illness analysis (COI) http://www.accesspharmacy.com/Content .aspx?searchStr=cost+of+illness+evaluation &aid=7965069#7965079 (subscription required) | Measures the economic impact of a disease or condition on society. Also called a cost-consequence model. |

## CURRENT DIRECTIONS AND THE VALUE OF MANAGED CARE

Innovative use of technology (electronic prescribing), new ways of organizing pharmacy (specialty pharmacy), and patient care delivery (patient-centered medical homes, PCMH) and the implementation of the Affordable Care Act (ACA) are part of the changing landscape of managed care.

### Electronic Prescribing

Electronic prescribing (http://www.accesspharmacy.com/Content.aspx?searchStr= electronic+prescribing&aid=56791582#56791587 {subscription required}), or e-prescribing, is "the use of computing devices to enter, modify, review, and output or communicate drug prescriptions." It allows for the transfer of prescription information between the health plan, prescriber, and pharmacy.[18] Benefits of e-prescribing are numerous and its use is gaining momentum. The federal government has already recognized its importance, and has offered incentive plans for providers who use the technology "meaningfully" (eg, to improve safety, quality, and efficiency).[19] One of the most important advantages to e-prescribing is improved accuracy. It uses a standardized data entry format to generate a legible and "clean" prescription. It allows the prescriber to access the patient's medication profile and electronic medical record, as well as appropriate prescribing guidelines as the prescription is written. E-prescribing applications also address issues with formulary adherence, DUR, and quantity limits before the prescription is submitted to the pharmacy. Pharmacies benefit from more streamlined work flow and improved efficiency.[20]

While e-prescribing provides distinct advantages, there are some challenges as well. Some of these challenges include financial consideration, adapting national standardization, and integration with other office interfaces. There is also the need to monitor for new types of prescribing errors created by the system's inflexible ordering formats and fragmented screen displays.[20] These challenges are being addressed, and the use of e-prescribing will continue to increase as the benefits to patients, pharmacies, prescribers, and health plans are recognized.

### Specialty Pharmacy

http://www.accesspharmacy.com/Content.aspx?searchStr=specialty+pharmacy& aid=56798512 (subscription required)

Although there is no universally accepted definition of specialty pharmaceutical products, there are some attributes common among them. These characteristics include, targeting chronic disease states, high cost, special handling requirements, reimbursement complexities, increased clinical support, customized dosing, and complex delivery methods. To address these challenges, specialty distributers and pharmacies were created. Shifting specialty pharmaceutical products to these venues allows for more focused expertise not readily available through traditional retail and mail order pharmacies (Table 16.10).

| TABLE 16.10. FUNDAMENTAL SERVICES EMPLOYED TO MAXIMZE THE VALUE OF SPECIALTY PHARMACEUTICALS[21,22] | |
|---|---|
| Medication management | • Includes the use of prior authorization and step-therapy to encourage the use of preferred products, to promote the appropriate use of medications for FDA-approved indications, and to reduce the incidence of adverse events.<br>• Also involves the ongoing monitoring of disease progression, lab test results, and other pertinent clinical outcomes. |
| Patient management | • Refers to the education of patients, which is particularly important for those products that are self-administered. This service necessitates pharmacist involvement to promote patient adherence, adverse event monitoring, and coordination of changes in therapy. |
| Cost management | • Includes, but not limited to, bulk purchasing and variations in benefit design. Examples of variations in benefit design include placing co-payments on a higher tier and increasing the percentage of coinsurance paid by the patient. |
| Distribution | • Takes into consideration special handling to maintain the integrity of the product during delivery processes and addresses the need for non-drug supplies such as syringes, needles, and disposable containers. |

## Patient-Centered Medical Home

http://www.accesspharmacy.com/Content.aspx?searchStr=medical+home&aid=56180623#56180774 (subscription required)

Coordination of care for an individual patient through a team-based collaboration between health-care professionals is known as PCMH.[23] Key components of a PCMH are a personal physician, a focus on the whole person, access to quality care, and active decision-making on the part of the patient regarding their own health. Up-to-date information technology and free exchange of health information is crucial to the success of these types of programs. Managed care tools potentially affect all components of a PCMH.

## The Affordable Care Act (ACA)

The health reform law, known as the ACA, was signed into law in March 2010. It was structured around insurance reform (broader coverage, more benefits and protection, lower costs) and health system reform (improved quality and efficiency, focus on public health and prevention). The creation of insurance exchanges allows consumers

**TABLE 16.11. EXAMPLES OF STAKEHOLDER INVOLVEMENT IN MANAGED CARE[6]**

| Stakeholders | Sharing of Financial Risk/ Impact on Cost | Commitment to Excellence/ Impact on Quality |
|---|---|---|
| Health-care providers<br>• Physician<br>• Hospital<br>• Pharmacy | • Accept discounted reimbursement rates | • Take advantage of performance incentives (Pay for Performance, P4P)<br>  • Generic and formulary prescribing/ dispensing rates<br>  • HEDIS measures |
| Health plans<br>• Employer group<br>• Medicaid<br>• Medicare | • Incur lower premiums for using cost-saving benefit designs<br>  • Formulary limitations<br>  • Tiered co-pays<br>  • Prior authorization<br>  • Mail service dispensing | • Choose MCOs that meet national quality standards<br>• Promote appropriate DUR programs<br>• Promote DSM/MTM programs |
| Members | • Remit premium payments<br>• Incur fees to access care<br>  • Co-payment<br>  • Coinsurance<br>  • Deductible | • Undertake health and wellness education to make informed decisions |

and businesses to comparison-shop for the best plan to meet their needs. Most Americans will be required to obtain coverage or pay a penalty. Other provisions of the law specify a minimum set of benefits, allow children to stay on their parents' plan until age 26, and prevent denial of coverage based on pre-existing conditions. Some provisions of the law are already in effect, others will be phased in over time.[24]

## STAKEHOLDER INVOLVEMENT IS CRUCIAL TO THE SUCCESS OF MANAGED CARE

Managed care has become the primary health -care delivery method in the United States.[6] In order for the system to function efficiently; all stakeholders need to share in the financial risk (Table 16.11). In addition, they must be committed to the provision of excellent care. The balance between cost and quality is essential for the prudent use of limited health-care resources.

## ACADEMY OF MANAGED CARE PHARMACY

The Academy of Managed Care Pharmacy (AMCP) is a national professional society that was founded in 1988 by eight pharmacists. In 2012, the Academy has more than

6000 members nationwide. AMCP's mission is to empower its members to serve society by using sound medication management principles and strategies to improve health care for all. Its members share the common goal of ensuring positive health-care outcomes through quality, and accessible and affordable pharmaceutical care. The AMCP web site provides late-breaking industry news, internship opportunities, and information on managed-care residencies as well as links to a wide variety of published sources of information. They developed the AMCP Format for Formulary Submissions to standardize a set of essential information (dossier) needed by the MCO from pharmaceutical manufacturers when evaluating their product for both clinical and economic outcomes. AMCP publishes *The Journal of Managed Care Pharmacy*, a leading periodical in the field.[25] Pharmacists are encouraged to participate in the professional society that supports their practice.

## FOR MORE INFORMATION

### Web Sites

Academy of Managed Care Pharmacy *www.amcp.org*
American Pharmaceutical Association *www.pharmacist.com/*
American Society of Health-System Pharmacists *www.ashp.org*

## GLOSSARIES

Department of Health and Human Services Glossary
*https://www.healthcare.gov/glossary/*
Academy of Managed Care Pharmacy
*http://www.amcp.org/ManagedCareTerms/*

## ACKNOWLEDGMENT

The authors wish to acknowledge the contributions of Darlene M. Mednick, Tracy S. Hunter, and Cristina E. Bello to this chapter.

## APPLICATION EXERCISES

1. What are the goals of a managed care organization?
2. What types of managed care organizations are in the US market?
3. How is per member per month (PMPM) calculated and why is it important?
4. What is a formulary? What are the types of formularies? How is a formulary an effective tool for an organization?
5. What are the five steps of Drug Utilization Review (DUR)? What are the categories of DUR?
6. What is the goal of Disease State Management (DSM) and how is it achieved?

7. How does outcomes research evaluate a medical treatment and why is this important?
8. What are some of the examples of stakeholder involvement in managed care and why are they important?

## REFERENCES

1. Tufts Managed Care Institute: A Brief History of Managed Care. Available at http://www.thci.org/downloads/BriefHist.pdf. Accessed March, 2014.
2. About NCQA. National Committee for Quality Assurance. Washington, DC, 2012. Available at http://www.ncqa.org/tabid/675/Default.aspx. Accessed March, 2014.
3. HEDIS & Performance Measurement. National Committee for Quality Assurance. Washington, DC, 2012. Available at http://www.ncqa.org/HEDISQuality Measurement.aspx. Accessed March, 2014.
4. Kuttner R. The American health care system—employer sponsored health coverage. *N Engl J Med.* 1999;340:248–252.
5. Academy of Managed Care Pharmacy. Mapping your career in managed care pharmacy. Academy of Managed Care Pharmacy. Alexandria, VA; 2009. Available at http://www.amcp.org/InformationForSec.aspx?id=9033. Accessed March, 2014.
6. Navarro RP, Cahill JA. Role of managed care in the U.S. healthcare system. In: Navarro RP, ed. *Managed Care Pharmacy Practice.* 2nd ed. Sudbury, MA: Jones and Bartlett Publishers; 2009:1–16.
7. Owens MK. Medicaid pharmacy benefit management. In: Navarro RP, ed. *Managed Care Pharmacy Practice.* 2nd ed. Sudbury. MA: Jones and Bartlett Publishers; 2009:427–457.
8. Reissman D. Medicare pharmacy benefits. In: Navarro RP, ed. *Managed Care Pharmacy Practice.* 2nd ed. Sudbury. MA: Jones and Bartlett Publishers; 2009:459–475.
9. Tyler LS, Cole SW, May JR, et al. ASHP Guidelines on the Pharmacy and Therapeutics Committee and the Formulary System. *Am J Health-Syst Pharm.* 2008;65:1272–1283.
10. The Academy of Managed Care Pharmacy's Concepts in Managed Care Pharmacy: *Formulary Management.* Academy of Managed Care Pharmacy. Alexandria, VA; 2009. Available at http://www.amcp.org/Sec.aspx?id=5399. Accessed March, 2014.
11. The Academy of Managed Care Pharmacy's Concepts in Managed Care Pharmacy: *Drug Use Review.* Academy of Managed Care Pharmacy. Alexandria, VA; 2009. Available at http://www.amcp.org/Sec.aspx?id=5399. Accessed March, 2014.
12. Principles of drug-use review approved by APhA, AMA, and PMA. *Am J Hosp Pharm.* 1991;48:2062.
13. Thomas N, Larson LN, Bell NN. *Pharmacy Benefits Management.* Brookfield, WI: International Foundation of Employee Benefit Plans, Inc.; 1996.

14. The Academy of Managed Care Pharmacy's Concepts in Managed Care Pharmacy: *Prior Authorization*. Academy of Managed Care Pharmacy. Alexandria, VA; 2012. Available at http://www.amcp.org/Sec.aspx?id=5399. Accessed March, 2014.

15. The Academy of Managed Care Pharmacy's Concepts in Managed Care Pharmacy. *Disease Management*. Alexandria, VA; 2012. Available at http://www.amcp.org/Sec.aspx?id=5399. Accessed March, 2014.

16. The Academy of Managed Care Pharmacy's Concepts in Managed Care Pharmacy. *Outcomes Research*. Alexandria, VA; 2012. Available at http://www.amcp.org/Sec.aspx?id=5399. Accessed March, 2014.

17. Agency for Healthcare Research and Quality. What Is Comparative Effectiveness Research? Agency for Healthcare Research and Quality. Rockville, MD; 2012. Available at http://effectivehealthcare.ahrq.gov/index.cfm/what-is-comparative-effectiveness-research1/. Accessed March, 2014.

18. Navarro RP, Hailey R. Overview of prescription drug benefits in managed care. In: Navarro RP, ed. *Managed Care Pharmacy Practice*. 2nd ed. Sudbury. MA: Jones and Bartlett Publishers; 2009:17–46.

19. Fabius R, MacCracken L, Pritts J. Vocabulary of Healthcare Reform. January 2012. Truven Health Analytics. Available at http://img.en25.com/Web/TruvenHealth Analytics/TH%2011482_0712_VocabHealthReform_WP_web.pdf. Accessed March, 2014.

20. The Academy of Managed Care Pharmacy's Concepts in Managed Care Pharmacy. *Electronic Prescribing*. Alexandria, VA; 2012. Available at http://www.amcp.org/Sec.aspx?id=5399. Accessed March, 2014.

21. Johnson KA, Siegel JM. Specialty Pharmaceuticals. In: Navarro RP, ed. *Managed Care Pharmacy Practice*. 2nd ed. Sudbury. MA: Jones and Bartlett Publishers; 2009:151–180.

22. The Academy of Managed Care Pharmacy's Concepts in Managed Care Pharmacy. *Specialty Pharmaceuticals*. Alexandria, VA; 2012. Available at http://www.amcp.org/Sec.aspx?id=5399. Accessed March, 2014.

23. AMCP. The Patient-Centered Medical Home. Academy of Managed Care Pharmacy. Alexandria, VA; 2012. Available at: http://www.amcp.org/WorkArea/DownloadAsset.aspx?id=10704. Accessed March, 2014.

24. American Public Health Association (APHA). ACA Basics and Background. Available at: http://www.apha.org/advocacy/Health+Reform/ACAbasics/. Accessed March, 2014.

25. AMCP. History of AMCP. Academy of Managed Care Pharmacy. Alexandria, VA; 2012. Available at http://www.amcp.org/InformationForSec.aspx?id=8821. Accessed March, 2014.

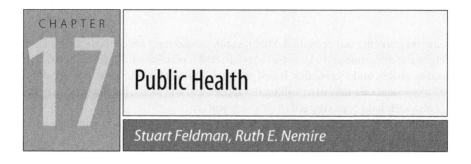

CHAPTER

17

# Public Health

*Stuart Feldman, Ruth E. Nemire*

**Objectives: Upon completion of the chapter and exercises, the student pharmacist will be able to**

1. Define public health.
2. Identify areas in public health where pharmacists are leading participants of the health-care team.
3. Identify partners for pharmacists in order to promote the health of their communities.
4. Describe collaborative pharmacy practice models that can be implemented to manage and prevent disease.
5. Identify public health content in your curriculum.

## INTRODUCTION

Pharmacists play an important role in the public's health but often think of their activities in the narrower framework of traditional pharmacy practice. This chapter provides an overview and background on public health specialty areas and organizations. While progressing through your school or college curriculum, take note of all of the areas of practice that now address promotion of wellness, and positive healthy behaviors. Think how the practice of pharmacy will continue to address public health issues. Take action now to become involved to improve the health of Americans, and others around the globe. An Internet search for a definition of public health results in a large number of returns. In general, a definition of public health includes such terms as protecting and improving the health of a community, disease prevention, health education, control of communicable diseases, application of sanitary measures, and monitoring of environmental hazards. The Association of Schools and Programs of Public Health's (ASPPH)[1] web site (http://www.whatispublichealth.org/what/index.html) provides a comprehensive definition. Overall, public health professionals are concerned with protecting the health of entire populations. These populations can be as small as a local neighborhood, or as big as an entire country. Public health professionals work to prevent problems from happening or reoccurring through implementing educational programs, developing policies, administering services, and conducting research, in contrast to clinical professionals, such as physicians and nurses, and pharmacists who focus primarily on treating individuals after they become sick or injured. Public health practitioners are concerned with limiting health disparities and a large part of public health practice is the fight for health-care equity, quality, and accessibility. Based on the definition of public health, it is clear that all pharmacists are now in a position to support, and add to, the role that public health pharmacists have been engaged in for many years.

The study of public health is highly varied and encompasses many academic disciplines and is comprised of five core areas:

1. *Biostatistics*
2. *Epidemiology*
3. *Environmental Health*
4. *Health Services Administration/Management*
5. *Social and Behavioral Science/Health Education*

In addition to the five core topics, other areas of public health where pharmacists make an impact include:

- *Maternal and Child Health*
- *Nutrition*
- *International/Global Health*
- *Public Health Laboratory Practice*
- *Public Health Policy*
- *Public Health Practice*

The following sections provide an introduction to each of the areas with respect to what topics are relevant, and the impact of public health professionals in that area.


## PUBLIC HEALTH SPECIALTY AREAS

### Biostatistics

Biostatistics is used to identify trends in disease outbreaks, or outcomes that may lead to life-saving measures. Statistical procedures are often used to create graphs and tables that allow for inferences to be made across populations and geographical areas to determine whether a disease has been introduced or become prevalent. Biostatistics is integral to determining trends in disease and prevention measure outcomes. Epidemiologists use biostatistics to report findings, and discuss evidence.[1]

### Epidemiology

Epidemiologists determine what causes a disease or spike in injuries across a population. These public health specialists ask question like what the risk is about, who is at risk, and how to prevent accidents and injuries. They study demographic and social trends that influence disease and injury. These public health professionals may evaluate new treatments for injury or prevention of disease outbreak. Epidemiologists first discussed the outbreak of the West Nile virus. The salmonella outbreaks during the years 2008 and 2009 are examples of times when epidemiologists are called to review outbreak of disease. Epidemiologists were responsible for the 1964 Surgeon General's report on smoking tobacco. Their insight and evidence stating the harmful effects of smoking changed history in the United States and elsewhere. Biostatistics is used to support the findings of the epidemiologist.[1]

## Environmental Health

Constructed and natural environments influence our health, and public health professionals ask how we reduce these risk factors? Environmental risk factors are associated with causing diseases such as asthma, cancer, and food poisoning. Chemistry, toxicology, and engineering specialists have combined their expertise to look for answers to questions concerning public health.

Environmental health is broad in scope and so it is often broken down into smaller areas of concern that can be addressed across or within organizations.[1]

These areas are:

- Air quality
- Food protection
- Radiation protection
- Solid waste management
- Hazardous waste management
- Water quality
- Noise control
- Environmental control of recreational areas
- Housing quality
- Vector control

## Health Services Administration/Management

Politics, business, and science are all combined to manage the human and fiscal resources for delivering public health services. The professionals in these roles may specialize in planning, organization, or policy formation in addition to budget and finance.[1]

## Social and Behavioral Science/Health Education

Behavioral science/health education focuses on creating programs to persuade people to make healthy choices in their daily lives. These educational endeavors may include development of community-wide education programs that promote lifestyle changes and research of complex health issues. Professionals in this area may review health services and promote more efficient use, and they may develop programs to encourage adoption of patient self-care programs. Areas of mental health, aging and prevention of disease, public health practice, and education are specialty areas found within the field of behavioral sciences.[1]

## Maternal and Child Health

These public health professionals deal with all areas of education, advocacy and research for women and children.[1]

## Nutrition

Those who specialize in nutritional research and education examine how populations are affected by their eating habits, nutrients, and available food. Much work is needed in terms of the study of obesity and the consequences, as it is a public health problem across the globe. The science of nutrition improves public health from the standpoint of promoting health and prevention of disease.[1]

## International/Global Health

The specialists in this area of public health are concerned with the differences in cultures and countries worldwide. Globalization links health outcomes more closely to one another than ever before in history. Travel has opened up new public health issues as people and food move across borders. Disease is spread more quickly than in the past due to ability of people to move across continents in aircraft, and on sea. The severe acute respiratory syndrome (SARS) epidemic is an example of how rapidly disease can spread, and the consequences of globalization on prevention of disease.[1]

## Public Health Laboratory Practice

Professionals who work in laboratories such as "bacteriologists, microbiologists, and biochemists test biological and environmental samples in order to diagnose, prevent, treat, and control infectious diseases in communities."[1] Safety of food and water is a concern to these individuals. These scientists also screen for the presence of disease within communities, and are asked to respond to emergencies such as bioterrorism.[1]

## Public Health Policy

Professionals in public health policy work to improve the public's health through legislative action at the local, state, and federal levels.[1]

## Public Health Practice

"Public health is an interdisciplinary field and professionals in many disciplines such as nursing, medicine, veterinary medicine, dentistry, and pharmacy routinely deal with public health issues. A degree in public health practice enables clinicians to apply public health principles to improve their practice."[1]

*Student Pharmacy Public Health Practice Exercise*
Using the table below to make entries, and the listed areas of public health defined above, write a reflection on how these areas may be applied to pharmacy. An example is given for environmental health.

| Public Health Area | Pharmacy Application |
|---|---|
| Environmental health<br>Air<br>Water<br>Interaction between environment and genetics | My practice is in an urban area and many of the older buildings have layers of lead paint on the walls. I can start a program in the pharmacy, in cooperation with the local health department or environmental community organization like WE ACT, to provide information on lead effects on children and adults, how to get tested, and contact information for the health department. |
| Biostatistics | |
| Epidemiology | |
| Behavioral science/ health education | |
| Maternal and child health | |
| Nutrition | |
| Public health policy | |

## PUBLIC HEALTH ORGANIZATIONS AND INSTITUTIONS

Public health organizations are an excellent source of information about the profession. Becoming involved in these organizations leads to development of networks which are important for you now and in the future. There will be opportunities for improving the health of the community in many of your introductory and advanced practice experience courses. The public health organizations are platforms for a pharmacist to advocate for a role in the public health arena for the profession. Membership in one of these organizations is an excellent way to stay current with local, state, and national or global activities. Active engagement in the organization provides a means for direct involvement in association activities and leadership.

### American Public Health Association

The American Public Health Association (APHA) web site (apha.org)[2] describes the organization as follows:

"The American Public Health Association is the oldest, largest, and most diverse organization of public health professionals in the world and has been working to improve public health since 1872. The Association aims to protect all Americans and their communities from preventable, serious health threats and strives to assure community-based health promotion and disease prevention activities and preventive health services are universally accessible in the United States. The American Public Health Association represents a broad array of health professionals and others who care about their own health and the health of their communities."[2]

APHA represents a collective voice for public health. There are two publications of the APHA, a peer-reviewed *American Journal of Public Health* and a newspaper *The Nation's Health*. The leadership communicates public health science and practice issues and topics to the members and others who read the journal and newspaper.[2]

Members of APHA include health officials, educators, environmentalists, policymakers, and other health providers who work in government offices, clinics, community organizations, and educational institutions. Members have multiple opportunities to be involved at both the national and local levels of the APHA.[2]

## Association of Schools and Programs of Public Health

ASPPH represents the Council on Education for Public Health (CEPH)-accredited schools and programs of public health.[3] This organization promotes faculty and administration in schools and programs to advance the education and research of public health.[3] The association web site (aspph.org) is an excellent source of information about public health and public health education.

## World Health Organization

The World Health Organization (WHO) is a component of the United Nations (UN) and is the directing and coordinating authority for health for the UN.[4] The WHO is responsible for providing leadership on global health matters, shaping the global health research agenda, setting norms and standards for health and disease prevention, articulating evidence-based policy options, providing technical support to countries, and monitoring and assessing health trends. The WHO web site (www.who.int/en/)[4] is a source of information on global health and an excellent resource for data and statistics on international health topics. More information on programs available from WHO are discussed in Chapter 18.

## Centers for Disease Control and Prevention

The mission of Centers for Disease Control and Prevention (CDC) is to collaborate to create the expertise, information, and tools that people and communities need to protect their health—through health promotion, prevention of disease, injury and disability, and preparedness for future health threats.[5] It was founded as the Communicable Disease Center on July 1, 1946, in Atlanta Georgia. The CDC is a part of the Department of Health and Human Services (HHS) of the United States government with headquarters in Atlanta, Georgia. The CDC has a global outreach and responsibility for coordinating with other global health promotion and disease prevention agencies.[6] The CDC promotes vaccination schedules for children and adults, provides information for travelers, and has educational materials available for use by health-care professionals for the public.

CDC seeks to accomplish its mission by working with partners throughout the nation and the world to:

- monitor health,
- detect and investigate health problems,
- conduct research to enhance prevention,
- develop and advocate sound public health policies,
- implement prevention strategies,
- promote healthy behaviors,
- foster safe and healthful environments,
- provide leadership and training.[5]

A review of the CDC web site (www.cdc.gov) will provide many opportunities for you to envision, as a student pharmacist and soon to be practitioner, how you can play an important role in protecting the public's health.

The CDC has a published program guide for pharmacists (http://www.cdc.gov/dhdsp/programs/nhdsp_program/docs/Pharmacist_Guide.pdf)[7]

## Food and Drug Administration

The Food and Drug Administration (FDA) is an agency within HHS and consists of nine centers. "The FDA is responsible for protecting the public health by assuring the safety, efficacy, and security of human and vetxterinary drugs, biological products, medical devices, our nation's food supply, cosmetics, and products that emit radiation. The FDA is also responsible for advancing the public health by helping to speed innovations that make medicines and foods more effective, safer, and more affordable; and helping the public get the accurate, science-based information they need to use medicines and foods to improve their health."[8]

A history of the FDA can be found on their web site, http://www.fda.gov/AboutFDA/WhatWeDo/History/default.htm.[9] I encourage you to read the history as it provides an excellent background into the agency responsible for regulating all prescription drugs in the United States. Important to add to your knowledge of public health is the FDA's role in food safety, nonprescription medications, radiation-emitting devices, animal and veterinary products, and so on. This information is available on the FDA web site.[8] The news items posted on the FDA site often relate to public health issues that pharmacists can promote, and provide education in their practices both as students and licensed pharmacists.

## HEALTHY PEOPLE 2020

Healthy People 2020 refers to a set of health objectives created over the last 40 years based on a 1979 Surgeon General's report for the United States population. Healthy People 2020 is built on initiatives pursued over the past three decades. Healthy People 2020 was developed through a broad consultation process, built on the best scientific knowledge, and designed to measure programs over time.[10] The document and ideals can be used by many different people, leaders of States, communities, and professional organizations to help create programs to improve health for a defined population. Healthy People 2020 reveals the assessment of major risks to health and wellness, changing public health priorities, and emerging issues related to our nation's health preparedness and prevention.[10]

Every 10 years, HHS leaders leverage scientific insights and lessons learned from the past decade, along with new knowledge to update the Healthy People document. The review of the last Healthy People 2010 is available in full at the CDC web site (http://www.cdc.gov/nchs/data/hpdata2010/hp2010_final_review.pdf). The data from the report indicates that 71% of the Healthy People goals for the population were improved or met during the period from 1997 to 2008. There was an overall reduction in deaths from coronary heart disease and stroke.[11]

The American College of Clinical Pharmacy (ACCP) produced and published a White Paper "Healthy People 2010: Challenges, Opportunities, and a Call to Action for America's Pharmacists" in 2004.[12] A committee of pharmacist professionals classified each of the 28 Healthy People 2010 primary focus areas into one of four categories according to the perceived role of pharmacists in meeting the specified objectives (Table 17.1). An analysis was conducted for each of 14 focus areas that the committee had placed into a category of 1 or 2 (ie, those for which

### TABLE 17.1.  HEALTHY PEOPLE 2010 FOCUS AREAS BY CATEGORY[12]

| Category | Perceived Role of Pharmacists in Meeting Objectives | Focus Areas |
|---|---|---|
| 1 | Pharmacists' role is well established. Leadership role is well documented in the literature and/or positive outcomes data are available. Pharmacists are active in these areas, receive adequate education or specialized training, and have adequate manpower. | Diabetes mellitus<br>Heart disease and stroke<br>Immunization and infectious diseases[a]<br>Medical product safety<br>Respiratory diseases |
| 2 | Pharmacists are active in these areas but have not yet established a leadership role. A leadership role is possible or may be emerging. Pharmacists are capable and reasonably well positioned to assume a leadership role. Currently, documentation of pharmacist's role is insufficient and/or outcomes data are limited. | Access to quality health services[a]<br>Arthritis, osteoporosis, and chronic back conditions<br>Cancer<br>Chronic kidney disease<br>Family planning<br>Health communication<br>Human immunodeficiency virus[a]<br>Tobacco use[a]<br>Mental health and mental disorders[a] |

**TABLE 17.1.** HEALTHY PEOPLE 2010 FOCUS AREAS BY CATEGORY[12] (*Continued*)

| Category | Perceived Role of Pharmacists in Meeting Objectives | Focus Areas |
|----------|------------------------------------------------------|-------------|
| 3 | Opportunities exist for pharmacists involvement but primarily in a supportive role. Future leadership role is possible, but only if additional efforts are made and if existing barriers (eg, inadequate training, insufficient manpower) are addressed. | Disability and secondary conditions<br>Educational and community-based programs<br>Maternal, infant, and child health[a]<br>Nutrition and overweight[a]<br>Physical activity and fitness[a]<br>Sexually transmitted diseases[a]<br>Substance abuse[a] |
| 4 | Little or no role exists for pharmacists in these areas, and opportunities for expansion are limited. | Environmental health[a]<br>Food safety<br>Injury and violence prevention[a]<br>Occupational safety and health<br>Oral health<br>Public health infrastructure<br>Vision and hearing |

[a]Focus areas with objectives designated as Leading Health Indicators. (With permission from ACCP. Copyright 2004 Pharmacotherapy Publications, Inc.)

a pharmacy role is already well established or for which pharmacists are capable and reasonably well positioned to assume a leadership role). A comprehensive literature review was completed to identify pharmacists' contributions toward each of the 28 focus areas.

The ACCP White Paper discussion underscores the fact that the Healthy People 2010 document did not address many areas where pharmacists have potential to play an important role. The authors reported that little or no role exists for pharmacists in these areas, and opportunities for expansion are limited (Category 4). These focus areas included:

Environmental health
Food safety
Injury and violence prevention
Occupational safety and health
Oral health
Public health infrastructure
Vision and hearing

Based on information and practices of pharmacists in some areas in 2013, some of the topics placed in Category 4, like environmental health, injury and violence prevention and recognition, oral health, and public health infrastructure, will need to be reexamined.

The committee placed opportunities for pharmacists' in Category 3 if pharmacists are involved, but primarily in a supportive role. Future leadership roles are possible, but only if additional efforts are made and if existing barriers to the success of programs (eg, inadequate training, insufficient manpower) are addressed. Included in this category are:

Disability and secondary conditions
Educational and community based programs
Maternal, infant, and child health
Nutrition and overweight
Physical activity and fitness
Sexually transmitted diseases
Substance abuse

Categories 3 and 4 are areas where pharmacists may impact the public's health.[12] These topics and areas of practice are now being included in college of pharmacy curricula and student pharmacists are becoming engaged in improving practice in these areas.

## Society for Public Health Education

The Society for Public Health Education (SOPHE) web site (www.sophe.org) describes the organization. "The mission of SOPHE is to provide global leadership to the profession of health education and health promotion and to promote the health of society."[13]

The organization promotes healthy behaviors, healthy environments, and advocates for federal budget prevention dollars, health literacy, tobacco education and health equity across all populations.

## PUBLIC HEALTH IN THE PHARMACY CURRICULUM

### Doctor of Pharmacy Programs

The Accreditation Council for Pharmacy Education (ACPE) includes public health as one of the major competencies necessary for students graduating from a school or college of pharmacy. The competency to "Promote health improvement, wellness, and disease prevention in cooperation with patients, communities, at-risk populations, and other members of an interprofessional team of health care providers"[14] must be recognized by all schools and colleges in the United States, and those American schools seeking accreditation outside of the boundaries of the United States. The Doctor of Pharmacy curricula in schools and colleges are inclusive of public health although the outcomes and competencies designed may not exactly match the wording of the ACPE.

The methods for introduction and practice of the theories and skills of public health vary across the country. Faculty members from schools and colleges are involved in public health in a variety of ways. Faculty members have practices that include prevention, pediatrics, nutrition, smoking cessation, policy, disaster medical teams, and epidemiology. Student pharmacists can be involved with public health practices during their experiential education courses, by doing research with a faculty member, and through service to any one of the many student pharmacist organizations.

## Master of Public Health

As you seek to be more involved in public health activities, it is appropriate to examine the educational background that will be helpful to you. The background offered by the Master of Public Health (MPH) degree provides coursework and practicums that will help develop skills in the public health arena. The content areas can be offered in stand-alone courses or in an integrated fashion. Key content includes many of the previously mentioned public health specialties. There are multiple programs offering online courses leading to degrees in public health.

## Epidemiology

Core functions of the discipline can be categorized into five areas:

1. Exploring the existence or occurrence of an exposure or a disease within a group or population.
2. Conducting disease surveillance and recognizing potential disease epidemics.
3. Describing if differences exist in the occurrence of exposure and/or disease in subgroups of the same population or different populations.
4. Identifying and then quantifying the effect of the causation of disease.
5. Testing interventions that may aid in disease identification or mitigation in a population.

An understanding of epidemiology is useful to pharmacists involved with any aspect of disease prevention or treatment. Knowledge and ability to interpret biostatistics allows a pharmacist to make learned judgment as to the quality of data for studies involving prevention and treatment of disease.

## Environmental Health

Understanding environmental health has grown in importance with the recent focus on emergency preparedness and response. Nationwide, many pharmacists are engaged in preparing and responding to a natural or terrorist-induced disaster. The principles of exposure, risk assessment, and toxicology are important to active engagement by pharmacists on the emergency preparedness team.

## Behavioral Health

A pharmacist's involvement in mental health is a major asset to public health. From the traditional role played in medication and adherence management to providing information on mental illness to patients and caregivers, pharmacists through their community involvement are equipped to play a significant role in community awareness of mental illness and the treatment involved. Advanced courses in psychology and sociology broaden the background beyond the traditional pharmacology and therapeutics experiences.

## Cultural Competence

Health-care professionals will practice in diverse communities and interact with patients and caregivers, whose life experiences may differ greatly from the provider. An understanding of the differences among cultures, religious groups, and individuals is critical to the delivery of appropriate and understood patient care. The National Center for Cultural Competence (NCCC)[15] web site descriptions of the critical factors in the provision of culturally competent health-care services include understanding of the:

- beliefs, values, traditions, and practices of a culture;
- culturally defined, health-related needs of individuals, families, and communities;
- culturally based belief systems of the etiology of illness and disease and those related to health and healing; and
- attitudes toward seeking help from health-care providers.[14]

## Disease Prevention and Health Promotion

This is one area where pharmacists are already and will continue to impact the public's health.

Chronic diseases—such as heart disease, cancer, and diabetes—are the leading causes of death and disability in the United States. Chronic diseases account for 70% of all deaths in the United States, which is 1.7 million each year. Heart disease, cancer and stroke account for more than 50% of all deaths each year.[16] Excessive alcohol consumption is the third leading preventable cause of death in the United States, behind diet and physical activity and tobacco.[17]

These chronic diseases also cause major limitations in daily living for almost 1 out of 10 Americans or about 25 million people. Arthritis is the most common cause of disability, with nearly 19 million Americans reporting activity limitations.[18]

Although chronic diseases are among the most common and costly health problems, they are also among the most preventable. Adopting healthy behaviors such as eating nutritious foods, being physically active, and avoiding tobacco use can prevent or control the devastating effects of these diseases."[19]

The CDC web site (http://www.cdc.gov/nccdphp/) provides data on the costs of chronic disease.[20] In 2005, 133 million people, almost half of all Americans lived with at least one chronic condition. The medical care costs of people with chronic diseases account for more than 75% of the nation's $2 trillion medical care costs.

*Student Pharmacist Practice Exercise*

As an exercise, list behaviors that have the potential to either increase or decrease health outcomes. List the steps you would take to reinforce healthy behaviors or alter nonhealthy activities. Describe how these interventions can be carried out in community pharmacies, in institutional practice, in clinics, or with community-based groups.

## CONCLUSION

The public health is everyone's business because it affects the workplace, health-care costs across the globe, and many chronic diseases that are preventable. As a student and future pharmacist the responsibility lies with you to become informed, involved, advocate for the role of the pharmacist as a public health professional and practitioner, and to be a public health professional. As a student pharmacist getting involved in providing education to improve health literacy, addressing public health issues such as osteoporosis, obesity, asthma, and diabetes, will enable you to learn about the treatment and prevention of diseases, practice your clinical skills, and become adept at advocacy. There are a variety of areas of public health, such as epidemiology, environmental health, safety, laboratory, maternal and child, and disaster preparedness, where you can specialize as a pharmacist.

## REFERENCES

1. The Association of Schools of Public Health. Available at http://www.whatis publichealth.org/about/index.html. Accessed March, 2014.
2. American Public Health Association. Available at http://apha.org/. Accessed March, 2014.
3. The Association of Schools of Public Health. Available at http://www.aspph.org. Accessed April 17, 2014.
4. World Health Organization. Available at http://www.who.int/en/. Accessed March, 2014.
5. Centers for Disease Control and Prevention. Available at http://www.cdc.gov/. Accessed March, 2014.
6. European Centre for Disease Prevention and Control. Available at http://ecdc .europa.eu/en/Pages/home.aspx. Accessed March, 2014.
7. Partnering with Pharmacists in the Prevention and Control of Chronic Diseases. Available at http://www.cdc.gov/dhdsp/programs/nhdsp_program/docs/ Pharmacist_Guide.pdf. Accessed March, 2014.
8. Food and Drug Administration. Available at http://www.fda.gov/. Accessed March, 2014.

9. FDA History. Food and Drug Administration. Available at http://www.fda.gov/AboutFDA/WhatWeDo/History/default.htm. Accessed March, 2014.

10. Healthy People. Available at http://www.healthypeople.gov/. Accessed March, 2014.

11. Healthy People 2010 Final Review. Available at http://www.cdc.gov/nchs/data/hpdata2010/hp2010_final_review.pdf. Accessed March, 2014.

12. Calis KA, Hutchison LC, Elliott ME, et al. Healthy People 2010: Challenges, Opportunities, and a Call to Action for America's Pharmacists. *Pharmacotherapy*. 2004;24(9):1241–1294.

13. Society for Public Health Education. Available at www.sophe.og. Accessed March, 2014.

14. ACPE https://www.acpe-accredit.org/pdf/S2007Guidelines2.0_ChangesIdentifiedInRed.pdf. Accessed March, 2014.

15. National Center for Cultural Competence. Available at http://nccc.georgetown.edu/. Accessed March, 2014.

16. Kung HC, Hoyert DL, Xu JQ, Murphy SL. Deaths: final data for 2005. National Vital Statistics Reports 2008;56(10). Available at http://www.cdc.gov/nchs/data/nvsr/nvsr56/nvsr56_10.pdf. Accessed March, 2014.

17. Mokdad AH, Marks JS, Stroup DF, Gerberding JL. Actual causes of death in the United States, 2000. *JAMA*. 2004;291(10):1238–1245.

18. Centers for Disease Control and Prevention. Prevalence of doctor-diagnosed arthritis and arthritis-attributable activity limitation—the United States, 2003–2005. MMWR 2006;55:1089–1092. Available at http://www.cdc.gov/mmwr/preview/mmwrhtml/mm5540a2.htm. Accessed March, 2014.

19. Wu SY, Green A. *Projection of Chronic Illness Prevalence and Cost Inflation*. Santa Monica, CA: RAND Health; 2000.

20. Chronic disease prevention and health promotion. Centers for Disease Control and Prevention. Available at http://www.cdc.gov/nccdphp/. Accessed March, 2014.

CHAPTER

18

# Taking it to the Streets: Reducing Health Disparities through Domestic and Global Outreach to the Underserved

*Kelly L. Scolaro, Lisa Inge Stewart, Hazel H. Seaba*

**Objectives: Upon completion of the chapter and exercises, the student pharmacist will be able to**

1. Explain two types of organizations that address health disparities.
2. Identify and describe the mission and scope of selected organizations that work to reduce health disparities and provide care to underserved populations.
3. Analyze the role of the pharmacist as an advocate for the profession and for underserved patients.
4. Categorize the key elements of developing and participating in an academic outreach project.
5. Identify the knowledge and skills necessary to participate in an interprofessional team whose goal is to develop services for an identified population.
6. Recognize the importance of reflection exercises in outreach projects.

## INTRODUCTION

There are times when taking the practice to the people can address health disparities more efficiently, than if pharmacists wait for the people to come to them. The world is small and motivated pharmacists can address not only local but also global health issues. This chapter is not about the practice of pharmacy in other countries nor is it a step-by-step guide to design an outreach or mission trip. This chapter is an overview of how to reduce health disparities in your own country or others, by understanding organizations that serve the underserved, by becoming an advocate for the profession of pharmacy and underserved patients, and by participating in outreach opportunities. You should take advantage as often as possible to participate in courses, outreach missions, or other global experiences that allow you to stretch your knowledge both medically and culturally.

## ORGANIZATIONS

Representatives from various organizations that address the needs of the underserved frequently contact pharmacists seeking partnerships for funding, supplies, or volunteer services. These organizations are a great way for student pharmacists to get involved in addressing health disparities. However, before getting involved in any organization, it is important to understand how the organization is defined, its mission, and its scope of service.

Organizations that typically address health disparities and serve the underserved usually fall into two categories: not-for-profit/nonprofit organizations (NPO) or charitable foundations.[1,2] The categories are mostly defined by how and where funds are directed (Table 18.1).

Included in this chapter is a short list of NPOs that support global health-care initiatives to reduce health disparities. Some of the most renowned organizations included in this chapter are government sponsored and provide disease-state statistics or provide funding for research to advance public health initiatives. The Centers for Disease Control and Prevention (CDC), and the World Health Organization (WHO) are examples of this kind of NPO (Table 18.2).[3-7]

Charitable foundations may be independent organizations, faith based initiatives, or part of a business, service, or professional organization. Some of the first outreach projects in history were initiated by various religious faiths. Faith based outreach projects are usually plentiful and can be easily found in almost every region where there is a School or College of Pharmacy. Some business and professional organizations build separate foundation accounts from various revenue streams and use the foundation accounts to support research projects aimed at reducing health disparities and to provide gifts that benefit the underserved. Examples of different foundations are listed in Table 18.3.[8-12]

## ADVOCACY FOR THE PROFESSION

As a student pharmacist, you bear a responsibility to advocate for the profession. This means that you work for the benefit of the profession to affect laws, practice, and public perception. One way of advocating for the profession is demonstrating how pharmacists can make a difference in caring for the underserved locally and globally (Table 18.4). You can make a difference by taking part in community leadership, and participation in pharmacy, public health, and other professional organizations' efforts to reduce health disparities (Table 18.5). The National Association of Chain Drug Stores (NACDS) has developed NACDS RxIMPACT a grassroots program to help pharmacists and student pharmacists understand issues and provide tools to help them advocate for the profession.[13] The American Pharmacists Association Academy of Student Pharmacists (APhA-ASP) provides unique opportunities for student pharmacists to get involved in advocacy efforts through patient care projects such as Operation Immunization and their partnership with the International

**TABLE 18.1. DEFINING ORGANIZATIONS[1,2]**

| Type | Definition | Country Specific | Regulated by Law | United States | Canada |
|---|---|---|---|---|---|
| Nonprofit Organization (NPO) Not-for-profit Some organizations are adopting the name "Civil Society Organization" rather than using the term profit. | Supports or engages in public or private activities solely for that purpose, without commercial or monetary profit. May be volunteer or charitable. Money earned is put back into organization for growth. Does not issue stock or pay dividends. | Yes | Legal requirements followed for establishment<br>• Purpose<br>• Economic activity<br>• Supervision and management provisions<br>• Representation<br>• Accountability and Auditing provisions<br>• Provisions for the amendment of the statutes or articles of incorporation<br>• Provisions for the dissolution of the entity<br>• Tax status of corporate and private donors<br>• Tax status of the foundation | 501(c)(3)-Tax code allows tax exemption status and donations. | |
| Charitable Foundation | Varies but usually established to provide a public benefit | Yes including regional | Yes<br>Legal requirements followed for establishment<br>• Purpose of the foundation<br>• Economic activity<br>• Supervision and management provisions<br>• Accountability and Auditing provisions<br>• Provisions for the amendment of the statutes or articles of incorporation<br>• Provisions for the dissolution of the entity<br>• Tax status of corporate and private donors<br>• Tax status of the foundation | Distinguishes between Public and Private, mostly with regard to tax law. 501(c)(3)-Tax code allows tax exemption status and donations. | May be public or private but is a charity. Regulated by the Canada Revenue Agency. |

**TABLE 18.2. GOVERNEMENT NONPROFIT ORGANIZATIONS[3-7]**

| Organization | Home Page URL | Comments |
|---|---|---|
| Centers for Disease Control and Prevention (CDC) | http://www.cdc.gov/ | The CDC is a component of the United States Department of Health and Human Services. There are multiple offices within the CDC responsible for improving environmental health factors, public health, and coordinating health information services. The Coordinating office for Global Health has a mission is to provide leadership and work to increase life expectancy, and increase the global preparedness to prevent and control naturally occurring and man-made threats to health. |
| European Centre for Disease Prevention and Control (ECDC) | http://ecdc.europa.eu | This organization was established in 2005 to improve infection control in Europe. The mission is to identify, assess, and communicate threats to humans from infectious disease. |
| Health Canada | http://www.hc-sc.gc.ca/index-eng.php | Agency responsible for implementation of disease prevention and wellness programs in Canada. Objectives of the organization are to:<br>• Prevent and reduce risks to individual health and the overall environment;<br>• Promote healthier lifestyles;<br>• Ensure high quality health services that are efficient and accessible;<br>• Integrate renewal of the health-care system with longer term plans in the areas of prevention, health promotion and protection;<br>• Reduce health inequalities in Canadian society; and<br>• Provide health information to help Canadians make informed decisions. |
| Pan-American Health Organization | http://www.paho.org/hq | PAHO is an international public health agency that focuses on improving health and living standards in the Americas (North, South, and Central). PAHO is part of the United Nations system. |
| World Health Organization (WHO) | http://www.who.int/en/ | WHO is the directing and coordinating authority for health within the United Nations system. The WHO provides leadership on global health, shapes health research agendas, sets standards, sets agenda for evidence-based policy options, provides technical support to countries and monitors health trends. The agenda of the WHO health organization is to promote partnerships, foster health security, strengthen health systems and improve performance. |

**TABLE 18.3.** CHARITABLE FOUNDATIONS[8-12]

| Organization | Home Page URL | Comments |
|---|---|---|
| **Bill and Melinda Gates Foundation** | http://www .gatesfoundation .org | There are two simple values that lie at the core of the foundation's work:<br>The core values of the foundation's work:<br>• All lives—no matter where they are being lived—have equal value.<br>• To whom much is given, much is expected |
| **Clinton Foundation** | http://www .clintonfoundation .org/ | The mission of the foundation is to strengthen the capacity of people in the United States and throughout the world to meet the challenges of global interdependence.<br>Programs developed and supported by the Foundation include:<br>• Health Security<br>• Economic Empowerment<br>• Leadership Development and Citizen Service<br>• Racial, Ethnic, and Religious Reconciliation |
| **Global Health Council** | http://www .globalhealth .org/ | The Council works to ensure that all who strive for improvement and equity in global health have the information and resources they need to succeed. Key Issues of the Council include<br>• Women's Health<br>• Child Health<br>• HIV/AIDS<br>• Infectious Disease<br>The organization offers membership to NGO organizations, health professionals and students, Corporate, and University organizations |
| **Management Sciences for Health (MSH)** | http://www.msh .org/ | The mission of MSH is to save lives and improve the health of the world's poorest and most vulnerable people by closing the gap between knowledge and action in public health.<br>• Programs that support leaders in developing countries create stronger management systems improving health services for the greatest impact. |

*(continued)*

**TABLE 18.3.** CHARITABLE FOUNDATIONS[8-12] (*Continued*)

| Organization | Home Page URL | Comments |
|---|---|---|
| **Rotary International Foundation** | http://www .rotary.org | The mission is to enable Rotarians to advance world understanding, goodwill, and peace through the improvement of health, the support of education, and the alleviation of poverty.<br>• Funding of the Health Hunger and Humanity grant has supported 280 projects in 75 countries since 1978 at a cost of 74 million dollars |

**TABLE 18.4.** ADVOCATING FOR THE PROFESSION

Define the appropriate role and scope of practice for the pharmacist in the delivery of patient care and practice.

Assist other health-care professionals in rendering high quality care and measuring the effectiveness of that care.

Work to convey the value of the practice of pharmacy and the appropriate role of pharmacists to other professionals, policymakers, and the public.

Advocate for appropriate payment for medication therapy management.

Participate in development and dissemination of practice knowledge by participation in local, national and global organizations.

Pharmaceutical Students' Federation (IPSF).[14,15] IPSF offers student exchange and WHO internship opportunities. The APhA-ASP's web site also offers a wealth of information and links to issues important for pharmacists and the profession. Being an advocate for the profession is an imperative responsibility of being a professional.

## ADVOCACY FOR THE UNDERSERVED PATIENT

Student pharmacists' advocacy for underserved patients evolves and matures through experience. Advocacy for underserved patients can be as simple as calling a physician to develop the most economical and appropriate treatment plan or educating a patient on generic alternatives. Table 18.6 provides other examples of advocacy. By working with local health departments, offering medication-assistance group sessions, volunteering at a free clinic, or developing or participating in a medical mission, you are advocating for the patient who has limited access to care and medications. In the broader sense, advocating for specific patient groups is equally important. For example, underserved children are a particular concern in both developed and less developed countries. Becoming involved in groups

**TABLE 18.5.  PROFESSIONAL ORGANIZATIONS**[14–20]

| Organization | Home Page URL | Comments |
|---|---|---|
| American Pharmacists Association (APhA) | www.pharmacist.com | Oldest national organization of pharmacists in the United States. APhA provides a forum for discussion, consensus building, and policy setting for the profession of pharmacy. |
| International Pharmaceutical Association (FIP) | https://www.fip.org | Sets global pharmacy standards through professional and scientific guidelines, policy statements and declarations, as well as through its collaboration with other international organizations, including the World Health Organization (WHO) and other United Nations agencies. |
| International Pharmaceutical Students' Federation (IPSF) | http://www.ipsf.org/ | IPSF is the leading international advocacy organization of pharmacy students promoting improved public health through provision of information, education, networking, and a range of publication and professional activities. |
| | | Students may join as individual members. The American Pharmacists Association is a full Member. |
| World Health Professions Alliance (WHPA) | http://www.whpa.org/ | The World Health Professions Alliance is a unique alliance of dentists, nurses, pharmacists, and physicians to address global health issues striving to help deliver cost-effective quality health care worldwide. |
| | | The organization represents the members of the FIP, World Medical Association, International Council of Nurses and the World Dental Federation and has developed consensus statements, and annual conferences on topics of concern. |
| National Association of Free and Charitable Clinics | http://nafcclinics.org/ | To locate free clinics or inquire about volunteering. |
| | | A nonprofit 501c(3) organization whose mission is solely focused on the issues and needs of the more than 1,200 Free and Charitable Clinics in the United States. The NAFC is an effective advocate for the issues and concerns of Free and Charitable Clinics, their volunteer workforce of doctors, dentists, nurses, therapists, pharmacists, nurse practitioners, technicians and other health-care professionals, and the patients served by Free and Charitable Clinics in communities throughout the nation. |

*(continued)*

**TABLE 18.5.** PROFESSIONAL ORGANIZATIONS[14-20] (*Continued*)

| Organization | Home Page URL | Comments |
|---|---|---|
| **Volunteers in Medicine** | http:// volunteersinmedicine .org/ | Volunteers in Medicine (VIM) is the only national nonprofit dedicated to building a network of sustainable free primary health-care clinics for the uninsured in local communities within multiple cities in the United States. |
| **International Volunteer Program Association (IVPA)** | http://www .volunteerinternational .org | IVPA is an association of nongovernmental organizations involved in international volunteer work and internship exchanges. IVPA is an association of volunteer sending organizations, not a volunteer program. |
|  |  | Membership with IVPA is a distinguished mark of excellence, in that organizations are expected to uphold the Principles and Practices as guidelines for good programming as well as meet stringent membership criteria. |

**TABLE 18.6.** ADVOCATING FOR PATIENTS

Coverage for and access to medications and treatment services by a pharmacist.

Coverage for and access to immunizations and vaccine services by a pharmacist.

Support efforts to ensure culturally competent care to diverse populations.

Work to protect the privacy of patients' medical records in clinical settings, informational databases and other venues.

Disseminate clinically relevant findings from basic and clinical research to pharmacists, other health-care professionals, and the public.

Develop materials to improve health literacy and individual patient education.

Recognize the need of populations both local and globally who are unable to meet their needs for medication and treatment; work to reduce disparities.

Participate in organizations whose mission is to strengthen public health infrastructure, create emergency preparedness, and respond for disaster management.

like the Pediatric Pharmacy Advocacy Group can help children in need.[21] In the end, it is about making sure there is proper access to pharmacists who can provide individuals with medication therapy management, access to medication at a cost that is affordable, and team support for health care and improved public health.

## TAKING THE PRACTICE TO THE STREETS, HILLSIDES, AND MOUNTAIN TOP VILLAGES

### Academic Opportunities

There may be opportunities at your school or college to enroll in a course or earn academic credit for local or global outreach work. These types of opportunities will enhance your knowledge and skills about the practice of pharmacy in areas where populations have limited or no access to medical care. If an opportunity does not already exist, student pharmacists may want to inquire about creating one. Several web sites, such as The American Association of Colleges of Pharmacy Global Pharmacy Education Special Interest Group and the Forum on Education Abroad (paid membership required to access publications), contain many helpful documents that may assist in the creation, implementation, and assessment of academic experiences involving global outreach work.[22,23]

There are several key elements of academic outreach opportunities (Table 18.7).[24-26] Clear goals and objectives must be part of any work that is accomplished for academic credit. Course goals and objectives, that successfully meld caring for the underserved with educating and sensitizing students to their role as a global citizen, may attract funding sources. Partnerships between the school/college, NPO or other third-party organization, and the targeted community are needed.

| TABLE 18.7. ESSENTIAL COMPONENTS TO INTERNATIONAL COURSE DEVELOPMENT[24-26] | |
| --- | --- |
| **Ethics and Integrity** | • Choice of Partner<br>• Sustainability of Partnership<br>• Respect for Ethos |
| **Mission, Policies, and Procedures** | • Institution has mission and commitment to domestic and international service<br>• Formal affiliation agreement or memorandum of understanding<br>• Assessment of need by local residents<br>• Authorization to operate in Country (visa, Ministry of Health)<br>• IRB approval (Host and Local) |
| **Academic Framework** | • Academic credit desired or needed<br>• Academic goals and coursework in addition to service<br>• Pre-site or in-country time for orientation<br>• Supervision by health-care professional<br>• Assessment<br>• Opportunity for scholarship |
| | *(continued)* |

TABLE 18.7.  ESSENTIAL COMPONENTS TO INTERNATIONAL COURSE
            DEVELOPMENT[24-26] (*Continued*)

| | |
|---|---|
| **Organizational and Program Resources** | • Participants: education and skill sets<br>• Student selection process<br>• Fundraising for organizational /program resources<br>• Cost to participants<br>• Travel documents (passports, visas)<br>• Language requirements |
| **Health, Safety, and Security** | • Country political stability and security<br>• Weather conditions (hurricane-monsoon-rainy season, winter)<br>• Insurance<br>• Risk management<br>• Vaccine and travel medication (prophylactic and acute care)<br>• Emergency procedures |
| **Medical Mission or Site** | • Pharmacy patient care health/wellness, public health goals<br>• Administrative structure<br>• Population to be served<br>• Local transportation responsibilities<br>• Management of drug supply<br>• Reference materials<br>• Assessment of patient outcomes |

A signed memorandum of understanding, a document that outlines roles of the partners, is necessary to define responsibilities and shared and individual risks. Funding sources for the outreach project need to be identified and may include local fundraising by students and faculty or requesting funds from one of the organizations identified earlier in the chapter. Identifying and targeting the needs of the community is another key element. Needs should be identified by the community members and can be done by working directly with the community or indirectly through a third-party organization. After the needs are identified, faculty and student pharmacists should determine, with leaders from the community, how to meet the need. Faculty and students can then work together to align the academic needs of the proposed experience with the needs of the community. Needs may range from manpower to build a sewer, targeted disease state treatment, or prophylaxes of helminth infections or vaccines to comprehensive health-care activities. The academic experience must also have defined policies and procedures to ensure patients are treated ethically.[26] Students should be educated about ethical dilemmas (Chap. 2) they may face during the experience and how to appropriately respond. They should also be aware of disciplinary procedures in case of an ethics breach.

## PREPARATION FOR OUTREACH TRIPS

Whether an outreach trip is planned for a local or an international community, there is much preparation that needs to occur. It is important to understand that the health of those patients that you will interact with is dependent upon a number of factors present in their individual families, the communities where they live and their country's health policies. It is essential that you spend time studying the cultural, social, economic and political conditions of your patients' environment. The World Health Professions Alliance has created a handbook that may be helpful when preparing for trips.[27]

Initially determine the type and prevalence of medical conditions found in the geographic area or cultural environment where you will be offering your services.[24] Interventions may include pharmaceutical treatment of identified conditions, health education for non-pharmacological treatment, or even prevention via medications or vaccines. If pharmacological interventions will be made, your team will need to select and obtain the essential medications necessary to treat indigenous medical conditions and work with local health officials to ensure follow-up care.[28,29] The WHO identifies an "essential medication" as a medication which satisfies the priority health-care needs of the population while also taking into account effectiveness, affordability, and sustainability within the current health-care system.[30]

While carrying out preparation for potential medical interventions, it is also necessary to think about the team's safety in terms of disease prevention and physical hazards. It is advisable to consult at least one web site that addresses international travel such as the CDC or WHO to identify vaccinations and other prophylactic agents needed before, during, and after travel.[31] Information pertaining to physical safety concerns can be found at the US Department of State international travel information web site[32] or may be available through your university's international student office. Reviewing passport expiration dates, medical coverage and emergency medical insurance is necessary as well before leaving the country.

## GETTING THERE

Travel of any type with a group can be intimidating at best and international group travel presents new challenges for leaders and participating student health-care professionals. When identifying methods of group travel, the team leaders should identify methods of safe transportation within the country (ie, to and from the identified clinic or outreach site). Not only will transportation for the team, along with all of their personal belongings, need to be arranged, but extra space will also be necessary for packing the items necessary to accomplish the planned intervention. Regulations pertaining to the transportation of medications into the target country must be identified. Compliance will avoid having these items seized by local customs officials. While the option to purchase medications at your final destination may be attractive, concerns about cost and quality need to be determined.[28,29,33] Team leaders also need to identify housing for the team. Housing options may include hotels, hostels, community buildings, community members' homes, or hammocks under the open sky.

## Practicing in Underserved Areas

Once partnership, preparation, and safety issues are addressed, and a team is prepared to embark on an outreach trip, or work week in an underserved area, the excitement and anticipation are high. The limits of student pharmacists' activities are defined by their state internship license.[34] Despite predefined roles, these kinds of activities require that participants be adaptable, flexible, and ready to step into other roles that come along during the trip. Although they seem to be mundane tasks, making sure supply boxes are all accounted for and people are all where they should be will fill mornings and evenings in preparation for the next day's work. As a student health-care professional, you will be addressing the needs of the community and your team. However, your own health and safety needs must be kept in mind. Getting enough sleep, dressing appropriately for the climate, keeping water and nutritional snacks (ie, protein bars) on hand for days when meals times may vary, will make it easier to learn and function as a team member.

## Reflection

Reflection is often a forgotten element of outreach work. Whether you engage in an outreach project for academic credit or not, reflection is necessary. Reflection improves learning, offers a means of providing feedback to faculty members and future students, and is a part of becoming a master practitioner.[35] Ideally, reflection should be done during all stages of an outreach project and not just relegated to the end of a project or trip. Reflection activities can be an individual or a group effort. Reflection can be in the form of assigned questions from a faculty member or a personal journal that you write in for 5 to 10 minutes every day. Reflection topics may include preparation activities, day-to-day work activities, personal views of the population served, group interactions with the underserved population, and team's overall interaction and effectiveness. One basic format for reflection is a three-part structure; what, so what, and now what.[36] "What" is an accurate, objective description of the event or interaction. "So what" is a subjective account of your feelings and reactions. "Now what" links your pharmacy knowledge to the experience you have just had and prepares you for future activities and experiences. A SOAP format for reflection and further discussion of reflection in community service appears in Chapter 3. Reflection increases our ability to understand ourselves in the context of our work and develops critical thinking skills—a hallmark of seasoned, master professionals.

## CONCLUSION

While you are in school, there will likely be opportunities to participate in outreach programs locally or internationally that will affect the lives of those who do not have access to health care or other basic resources for living. These opportunities may or may not help fulfill an academic credit need. Regardless of academic credit, the opportunity will enable you to stretch your skills and gain knowledge of populations, disease states, or cultures not previously in your vocabulary. Many organizations are available to help you get involved and you will need to understand the differences in their structure, function, and funding. As a student pharmacist, strive to become involved in organizations enabling you to become an advocate for the profession and the individual patient in ways that make you comfortable. Advocacy is a professional responsibility and can manifest itself locally or globally through your actions.

Participating in development and implementation of a local or global outreach project can be personally, as well as professionally, rewarding. To achieve this rewarding experience you must keep in mind the prerequisites for a successful mission, such as focusing on the needs of the partner, establishing a strong academic framework, creating a sound organizational agenda, and protecting the health and safety of team members throughout (Table 18.7). Finally, use reflection to integrate your experiences into your professional fabric. Reflect on what you learned, how you learned it, and what you will do with the knowledge you gained.

*You must be the change you wish to see in the world.*

*Mahatma Gandhi*

## APPLICATION EXERCISES

1. What is the difference between a nonprofit organization and a charitable foundation?
2. Describe two major global health initiatives of the Bill and Melinda Gates Foundation.
3. Using the Internet, find reliable organizations that provide safety, travel, and health information for students participating in an international course. What are the travel and safety recommendations for travel to Tanzania?
4. What issues and questions should be addressed in journal entries that will lead to learning from global experiences?
5. Create an outline with headings and subheadings for a written report or oral presentation that presents and analyzes the outcomes of a global mission trip.

## REFERENCES

1. United States Department of the Treasury: Internal Revenue Service. Available at http://www.irs.gov/charities/content/0,,id=96986,00.html. Accessed March, 2014.

2. Canada Revenue Agency: Charities and Giving. Available at http://www.cra-arc.gc.ca/chrts-gvng/menu-eng.html. Accessed March, 2014.

3. Centers for Disease Control and Prevention. Available at http://www.cdc.gov/. Accessed March, 2014.

4. World Health Organization. Available at http://www.who.int/en/. Accessed March, 2014.

5. European Centre for Disease Prevention and Control. Available at http://www.ecdc.europa.eu/en/Pages/home.aspx. Accessed March, 2014.

6. Health Canada. Available at http://www.hc-sc.gc.ca/index-eng.php. Accessed March, 2014.

7. Pan-American Health Organization. Available at http://www.paho.org/hq. Accessed March, 2014.

8. Bill and Melinda Gates Foundation. Available at http://www.gatesfoundation.org. Accessed March, 2014.

9. Clinton Foundation. Available at http://www.clintonfoundation.org/. Accessed March, 2014.

10. Rotary International. Available at http://www.rotary.org. Accessed March, 2014.

11. Global Health Council. Available at http://www.globalhealth.org/. Accessed March, 2014.

12. Management Sciences For Health. Available at http://www.msh.org/about-us/index.cfm. Accessed March, 2014.

13. National Association of Chain Drug Stores RxIMPACT. Available at http://capwiz.com/nacds/home/index. Accessed March, 2014.

14. American Pharmacists Association Academy of Student Pharmacists. Available at http://www.pharmacist.com. Accessed March, 2014.

15. International Pharmaceutical Student's Federation (IPSF). Available at http://www.ipsf.org. Accessed March, 2014.

16. International Pharmaceutical Association. Available at https://www.fip.org. Accessed March, 2014.

17. World Health Professions Alliance. Available at http://www.whpa.org. Accessed March, 2014.

18. National Association of Free and Charitable Clinics. Available at http://nafcclinics.org/. Accessed March, 2014.

19. Volunteers in Medicine. Available at http://volunteersinmedicine.org/. Accessed March, 2014.

20. International Volunteer Program Association. Available at http://www.volunteerinternational.org. Accessed March, 2014.

21. Pediatric Pharmacy Advocacy Group (PPAG). Available at http://www.ppag.org/. Accessed March, 2014.

22. American Association of Colleges of Pharmacy Global Pharmacy Education Special Projects and Information. Available at http://www.aacp.org/governance/SIGS/global/Pages/GlobalPharmacyEducationSpecialProjectsandInformation.aspx. Accessed March, 2014.

23. Forum on Education Abroad. Available at http://www.forumea.org/index.cfm. Accessed March, 2014.

24. Ward C.T., Nemire R.E., Daniel K.P. The development and assessment of a medical mission elective course. *Am J Pharm Educ* 2005; 69(3) Article 50.

25. Standards of good practice for education abroad. The Forum on Education Abroad. 4th ed. 2011.

26. Code of ethics abroad. The Forum on Education Abroad. 2nd ed. 2011.

27. A Publication from the World Health Professions Alliance: A core competency framework for international health consultants. 2007. Available at http://www.whpa.org/pub2007_IHC.pdf. Accessed March, 2014.

28. Brown DA, Ferrill MJ. Planning a pharmacy-led medical mission trip part 1: focus on medication acquisition. *Ann Pharmacother.* 2012;46:751–9.

29. Hogerzeil HV. The concept of essential medicines: lessons for rich countries. *BMJ.* 2004;329:1169–1172.

30. World Health Organization. WHO policy perspectives on medicines- the selection of essential medications. 2002. Geneva, Switzerland.

31. World Health Organization: International Travel and Health. Available at http://www.who.int/ith/en/. Accessed March, 2014.

32. United States Department of State: International Travel Information. Available at http://travel.state.gov/travel/cis_pa_tw/cis_pa_tw_1168.html. Accessed March, 2014.

33. World Health Organization. Effective medicines regulation: ensuring safety, efficacy and quality. *Policies and Perspectives on Medicine,* 2003. Available at http://whqlibdoc.who.int/hq/2003/WHO_EDM_2003.2.pdf. Accessed March, 2014.

34. Herman RA. Global health outreach: pharmacist handbook for short term mission projects. Christian Pharmacists Fellowship International. Bristol, TN. March 2001. Available at www.cpfi.org. Accessed March, 2014.

35. Moon JA. A handbook of reflective and experiential learning: theory and practice. RoutledgeFalmer. 2004.

36. Hampton M. Reflective writing: a basic introduction. University of Portsmouth Department for Curriculum Quality Enhancement. August 2010. Available at http://www.servicelearning.umn.edu/info/reflection.html. Accessed March, 2014.

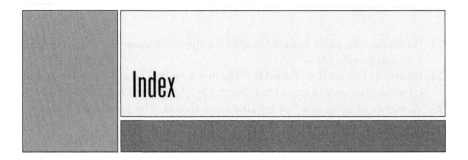

# Index

Note: Page numbers followed by *f* indicate figures; page numbers followed by *t* indicate tables.